NEW RESEARCH ON PHARMACOGENETICS

NEW RESEARCH ON PHARMACOGENETICS

LINDA P. BARNES
EDITOR

Nova Biomedical Books
New York

For permission to use material from this book please contact us:
Telephone 631-231-7269; Fax 631-231-8175
Web Site: http://www.novapublishers.com

Library of Congress Cataloging-in-Publication Data

Available upon request

ISBN 13: 978-1-60021-056-3
ISBN 10: 1-60021-056-2

Published by Nova Science Publishers, Inc. ✦ New York

Contents

Preface		**vii**
Chapter I	**The Transformation of Pharmacogenetics into Pharmacogenomics Reinforces Personalized Medicine Towards Pharmacotyping for Improved Patient Care** *Ioannis S. Vizirianakis*	**1**
Chapter II	**Development, Analysis and Use of Pharmacogenomic Time Series for Pharmacokinetic/Pharmacodynamic Modeling of Multi-Tissue Polygenic Responses to Corticosteroids** *Richard R. Almon, Debra C. DuBois, Jin Y. Jin, Zhenling Yao, Anasuya Hazra, Mahesh Samtani, Grayson Snyder, William Piel and William J. Jusko*	**39**
Chapter III	**Clinical Applications of Pharmacogenetics: Genetic Polymorphisms and Neuroleptic Malignant Syndrome** *Chiaki Kawanishi*	**83**
Chapter IV	**Genetic Detection of Antimicrobial Resistance Determinants in Gram-Positive Cocci** *Toshinobu Horii*	**103**
Chapter V	**A Special Bibliography**	**123**
Index		**585**

Preface

The terms pharmacogenomics and pharmacogenetics tend to be used interchangeably, and a precise, consensus definition of either remains elusive. Pharmacogenetics is generally regarded as the study of genetic variation that gives rise to differing response to drugs, while pharmacogenomics is the broader application of genomic technologies to new drug discovery and further characterization of older drugs. Pharmacogenetics considers one or at most a few genes of interest, while pharmacogenomics considers the entire genome. Much of current clinical interest is at the level of pharmacogenetics, involving variation in genes involved in drug metabolism with a particular emphasis on improving drug safety. This new book presents leading-edge research in this dynamic field.

Chapter I - Pharmacogenetics has been transformed into pharmacogenomics through the use of genomic technologies in clinical practice, whereas research in this area is now focusing on the identification of new genomic drug targets and exploitation of genetic variations contributing to inter-individual variability of drug response. Interestingly, pharmacogenomics deals with the genomic aspects implicated in both pharmacodynamic and pharmacokinetic drug effects in the body. Such direction obviously leads pharmacology into a merger with molecular biology and biotechnology, in order genome-wide analytical techniques to be used in pharmacological research to assess at the molecular level genes, RNA transcripts, proteins, and/or metabolic pathways, (i.e. genome, transcriptone, proteome, metabolome) involved in drug actions. Furthermore, pharmacogenomics attempts to establish specific gene and protein expression profiles for different tissues and organs associated with disease pathophysiology and drug response variability in individuals. As a matter of fact, pharmacogenomics data are now considered useful and valuable information for new-targeted drug development and improved patient care, thus ensuring personalized medicine to be achieved in clinical practice. Although this experimental design in pharmaceutical research and drug delivery represent painstaking and time-consumable processes, the recent development of new sophisticated high-throughput tools for extracting, analyzing and mining genomic data gives new hopes for pharmacogenomics to be finally applied in healthcare. This chapter comprehensively discusses the progress that is being made towards this direction and presents the achievements already happened that might eventually lead pharmacotyping to be established in routine patient care in the years to come.

Chapter II - Many drugs either directly or indirectly alter the expression of genes. Such changes in gene expression can be the consequences of cascades of molecular events in time often involving many tissues. The molecular cascades in complex biological systems usually result in polygenic phenomena related to either the efficacious or adverse effects of the drug. Mechanism-based pharmacokinetic/pharmacodynamic (PK/PD) modeling provides a tool for formulating testable quantitative hypotheses relevant to such aspects of drug treatment as dosing and dosing regimen. In order to develop such models for polygenic phenomena it is necessary that a large amount of data be acquired within the context of a single experimental paradigm so that realistic temporal relationships between events can be evaluated. Gene arrays when used in a time series construct provide a powerful tool for generating the magnitude of organized temporal data necessary for constructing PK/PD models of complex polygenic phenomena. Such models can then serve as a transcriptional scaffold onto which translational and post-translational events can be placed. The intent is to construct a realistic motion picture of the phenomena that can be used to devise regimens of drugs or combinations of drugs that maximize efficacy while minimizing adverse effects. Obtaining data from gene arrays that can be used to develop PK/PD models is dependant on the appropriate resolution of several considerations. The first is the construct of the time series. The second is data mining to identify the percentage of the genes whose expression is affected by the drug. The third is cluster analysis in order to group genes with similar temporal signatures. The fourth is text mining to place these genes in functionally relevant clusters. The last is placing the vast amount of data into a relational organization that allows for reasonable navigation amongst the different levels of information. The nature and some limited approaches to resolution of these problems is addressed using the synthetic glucocorticoid, methylprednisolone, with a rich time series following a bolus dose of drug and analysis of multiple tissues from the same animals.

Chapter III - Psychiatrists and pharmacologists have recently investigated the factors underlying differences between patients in efficacy and adverse effects of neuroleptic drugs. Prediction and prevention of likely adverse drug reactions are a vitally important goal for medication safety. At present, however, treatment still must be stopped or changed occasionally in response to severe drug reactions. Among these adverse reactions, neuroleptic malignant syndrome is a potentially lethal complication of neuroleptic administration that is characterized by hyperthermia, extrapyramidal signs, altered consciousness, and multiple manifestations of autonomic dysfunction. Mortality was estimated to exceed 70% when the syndrome initially was recognized. In addition to acquired risk factors, genetic predisposition toward neuroleptic malignant syndrome has been suggested by clinical observations. Genetic association studies have sought to identify polymorphisms influencing susceptibility to neuroleptic malignant syndrome, especially with respect to the dopamine D2 receptor, serotonin receptor, and cytochrome P450 2D6. Certain case reports, and data suggesting associations between NMS and genetic polymorphisms/haplotypes of the dopamine D2 gene have paved the way toward understanding the pathophysiology of the syndrome. Neuroleptic malignant syndrome might have a include heterogeneous nature, with common characteristic symptoms but multiple causative mechanisms. More large controlled genetic studies of neuroleptic malignant syndrome and related conditions are needed. Genetic data should be analyzed together with detailed clinical information. Such a productive pharmacogenetic studies should permit reconsideration of the entity of neuroleptic malignant syndrome.

Chapter IV - Antimicrobial resistance is a clinical problem in treating bacterial infections. Antimicrobial-resistant Gram-positive cocci include methicillin-resistant *Staphylococcus aureus* (MRSA), methicillin-resistant coagulase-negative staphylococci (MRCNS), penicillin-resistant *Streptococcus pneumoniae* (PRSP), and vancomycin-resistant enterococci (VRE). MRSA and VRE also are recognized as important nosocomial pathogens. Spread of antimicrobial resistance determinants by gene transfer can cause emergence of antimicrobial-resistant Gram-positive cocci (horizontal spread).

MRSA produces penicillin-binding protein (PBP)2' (PBP2a) encoded by the *mecA* gene, which confers resistance to all -lactams. MRCNS, similarly resistant, also produce PBP2'. MRSA can show concurrent resistance to fluoroquinolones and/or aminoglycosides. Fluoroquinolone resistance is determined mainly by mutations within the *gyrAB* and *grlAB* genes respectively encoding subunits of DNA gyrase and those of DNA topoisomerase IV, or by increased expression of the *norA* gene encoding a drug efflux protein, NorA. Fluoroquinolone resistance is associated with mutations in specific regions of the *gyrAB* and *grlAB* genes termed quinolone resistance-determining regions (QRDRs). Aminoglycoside resistance is conferred by aminoglycoside-modifying enzymes (AMEs) encoded by the *aac(6')-aph(2")*, *ant(4')-I*, and *aph(3')-III* genes.

Among *S. pneumoniae*, prevalence of isolates resistant to β-lactams such as penicillins and cephems, macrolides, and fluoroquinolones has increased worldwide. *S. pneumoniae* resistant to β-lactams emerged through recombination events between the PBP genes of *S. pneumoniae* and those of closely related species. PRSP has multiple alterations in PBPs, which are associated with a mosaic of PBP gene alleles. Resistance of *S. pneumoniae* to macrolides involves target site modification by a 23S rRNA-methylating enzyme encoded by the *ermB* gene and an efflux pump formed by membrane-associated proteins encoded by the *mefA* gene.

Enterococcus faecalis and *Enterococcus faecium* resistant to glycopeptides such as vancomycin and teicoplanin are referred to as VRE, which attain glycopeptide resistance in association with acquisition of *van* gene clusters located in a conjugative element. Genotypes include *vanA*, *vanB*, and *vanD*. VRE synthesize peptidoglycan precursors with pentapeptide side chains terminating in D-Ala-D-Lac, to which glycopeptides bind more poorly than that to D-Ala-D-Ala. Synthesis of D-Ala- D-Lac depsipeptide is catalyzed by VanA, VanB, and VanD ligases respectively encoded by the *vanA*, *vanB*, and *vanD* genes. Antimicrobial therapy for VRE infections is difficult since VRE can develop concurrent resistance to penicillins and aminoglycosides.

We can reliably detect these antibiotic resistance determinants by advanced genetic techniques based mainly on polymerase chain reactions (PCR), DNA-DNA hybridization, and nucleotide sequencing. Antimicrobial resistance determinants detected by PCR with or without DNA-DNA hybridization include the *mecA* gene in MRSA and MRCNS, the PBP genes and the *mefA* and *ermB* genes in *S. pneumoniae*, the *van* genes in VRE, and the AME genes in *S. aureus* and enterococci. Fluoroquinolone resistance of *S. aureus* and *S. pneumoniae* commonly is determined by nucleotide sequencing in the regions (QRDRs) coding for DNA gyrase and topoisomerase IV. Genetic methods, including new methods such as real-time PCR and DNA microarray systems, should guide antimicrobial therapy against infections caused by Gram-positive cocci by early prediction of antimicrobial susceptibility patterns of the isolate. Moreover, information regarding these genotypic traits will contribute identification of nosocomial infections caused by antimicrobial-resistant Gram-positive cocci.

In: New Research on Pharmacogenetics
Editors: Linda P. Barnes, pp. 1-38

ISBN: 1-60021-056-2

Chapter I

The Transformation of Pharmacogenetics into Pharmacogenomics Reinforces Personalized Medicine Towards Pharmacotyping for Improved Patient Care

Ioannis S. Vizirianakis*

Laboratory of Pharmacology, Department of Pharmaceutical Sciences, Aristotle University of Thessaloniki, GR-54124 Thessaloniki, Greece

Abstract

Pharmacogenetics has been transformed into pharmacogenomics through the use of genomic technologies in clinical practice, whereas research in this area is now focusing on the identification of new genomic drug targets and exploitation of genetic variations contributing to inter-individual variability of drug response. Interestingly, pharmacogenomics deals with the genomic aspects implicated in both pharmacodynamic and pharmacokinetic drug effects in the body. Such direction obviously leads pharmacology into a merger with molecular biology and biotechnology, in order genome-wide analytical techniques to be used in pharmacological research to assess at the molecular level genes, RNA transcripts, proteins, and/or metabolic pathways, (i.e. genome, transcriptone, proteome, metabolome) involved in drug actions. Furthermore, pharmacogenomics attempts to establish specific gene and protein expression profiles for different tissues and organs associated with disease pathophysiology and drug response variability in individuals. As a matter of fact, pharmacogenomics data are now considered useful and valuable information for new-targeted drug development and

* Address correspondence to this author at the Laboratory of Pharmacology, Department of Pharmaceutical Sciences, Aristotle University of Thessaloniki, GR-54124 Thessaloniki, Greece; Tel., +30-2310-997658; Fax, +30-2310-997645; Email: ivizir@pharm.auth.gr

improved patient care, thus ensuring personalized medicine to be achieved in clinical practice. Although this experimental design in pharmaceutical research and drug delivery represent painstaking and time-consumable processes, the recent development of new sophisticated high-throughput tools for extracting, analyzing and mining genomic data gives new hopes for pharmacogenomics to be finally applied in healthcare. This chapter comprehensively discusses the progress that is being made towards this direction and presents the achievements already happened that might eventually lead pharmacotyping to be established in routine patient care in the years to come.

Keywords: Genotyping, Haplotyping, Personalized medicine, Pharmacogenetics, Pharmacogenomics, Pharmacotyping, Pharmacotherapy, Drug efficacy, Drug safety.

1. Introduction

The concept of maximum efficacy and safety upon drug delivery is of major concern in clinical practice since the establishment of pharmacology as a basic medical and pharmaceutical discipline. For instance, this approach in pharmacotherapy has been partly achieved several years now and at least for some administered drugs, through the application of therapeutic drug monitoring in clinical pharmacology and the development of pharmacogenetics [1, 2]. Nowadays however, this situation is further expanded towards covering all the field of pharmaceutical care, thus making the long-term aim of pharmacotherapy to ensure drug efficacy and safety to come, more or less, closer into reality. This happens due to the rapid development of genomic technologies and their use in pharmacotherapy and healthcare. For example, it is now well accepted that in terms of drug toxicity many adverse drug reactions (ADRs) arise because of inter-individual genetic differences in drug metabolism, transport, ion channels, receptors, and other drug targets [2, 3]. The completion of the whole-genome sequencing projects for several organisms and the evolution of genomic technologies offered new tools for extracting drug-related information through the emergence of pharmacogenomics in recent years [4-7]. Pharmacogenomics aims to prevent most, if not all, ADRs by giving the ability to any healthcare provider to test each patient before a drug was ever administered to this individual, a practice that lead to individualized therapy or tailored drug treatment. As a matter of fact, if this happen, the ideal situation for anticipating and minimizing toxicity related to drug delivery in routine patient care will come to reality [3]. Collectively, this approach in pharmacotherapy belongs to the broader concept of personalized medicine that is a major challenge happening in healthcare nowadays. Major goals of personalized medicine are considered the anticipation and minimization of the individual risk of disease onset and progression as well as individualized drug therapy for improved patient care [8].

The genomic era is now a reality, since high-quality and comprehensive sequences of the human genome as well as other organisms are available recently and the efforts for extracting genetic information of practical value in health and pharmaceutical care is still a fascinating expectation for the public [9]. The unprecedented level of information that is now offered at the molecular level for several cellular functions and biochemical pathways generate new hopes for better and more effective therapeutic intervention in order to cure complex and multifactorial illnesses, like cancer, cardiovascular disorders and neurodegenerative diseases. In addition, these advances and challenges in pharmaceutical research have added new knowledge in both drug's pharmacology and delivery systems' technology in such a way that are transforming several issues of routine clinical practice and causing positive changes in the healthcare system and pharmacotherapy outcome [10, 11].

These scientific efforts have had a huge impact on our understanding of disease pathophysiology and of drug actions at the molecular level, thus changing pharmacology and therapeutics into a more biology- and biotechnology-oriented direction. Moreover, the capability to predict drug-drug interactions and the emergence of ADRs in clinical practice are considered as fundamental aspects in modern pharmacology and therapeutics. The elucidation of specific genetic factors predisposing to individual drug-drug interactions, ADRs, or drug disposition also gives new dimensions to drug delivery [12-15]. As a matter of fact, the application of genotyping data in clinical pharmacology can move drug prescription towards pharmacotyping, a process that might be an interesting step for improving patient care, at it has been reported recently [3].

Overall, by using the principles of pharmacogenomics, personalized medicine and pharmacotyping in clinical practice and monitoring their impact on current drug development and delivery will obviously allow genomic data to be co-evaluated with clinical data to improve healthcare and to be finally accepted by the public and the society in general. In this respect, the clinical use of genomic data for routine drug prescription, the training of future healthcare professionals and the integration of molecular medicine into clinical trials for new drug development have to be clearly addressed and defined in this new environment. Also, the need for extensive discussions about the ethical, societal and economic impacts arising from the application and the use of genomic data into patient care is now, more than ever, a necessity. In any case however, it is expected that major influences from the use of genomic technologies will happen in disease diagnosis and drug delivery in the years to come. The tools will be provided by functional genomics enabling the extraction of genomic information applicable to clinical practice from sequencing data generated from the completion of several whole-genome projects [9]. This area already represents an expanding body of information on genes and proteins implicated in drug response heterogeneity, whereas several databases have been created that contain a considerable amount of genomic data of clinical relevance (Box 1).

Box 1. Databases with functional genomics data related to genetic disorders, gene polymorphisms and drug response variability

1) David Nelson's Cytochrome P450 Homepage <http://drnelson.utmem.edu/CytochromeP450.html>
2) Human Cytochrome P450 Nomenclature Website <http://www.imm.ki.se/CYPalleles>
3) The SNP Consortium-High-density maps of SNPs in the human genome <http://snp.cshl.org>
4) Entrez SNP <http://www.ncbi.nlm.nih.gov/entrez/query.fcgi?db=snp>
5) Pharmacological Targets Database (PTbase) <http://research.bmn.com/ptbase>
6) The "Online Mendelian Inheritance in Man" (OMIM) database (catalog of human genes and genetic disorders) <http://www.ncbi.nlm.nih.gov/entrez/query.fcgi?db=OMIM>
7) The International HapMap Research Project with haplotyping data of the human genome <http://www.hapmap.org/>
8) The official database of the International Union of Pharmacology (IUPHAR) on Receptor Nomenclature and Drug Classification <http://www.iuphar-db.org/iuphar-rd/index.html>
9) The Pharmacogenetics and Pharmacogenomics Knowledge Base (PharmGKB) (It is an integrated resource database that contains genomic data, molecular, cellular as well as clinical phenotype data related to drug response) <http://www.pharmgkb.org/>
10) The Endogenous GPCR List (A. Schonbrunn and D. L. Steffen) <http://www.tumor-gene.org/GPCR/gpcr.html>
11) GPCRDB: An Information System for G Protein-Coupled Receptors (GPCRs) (Version 8) <http://www.gpcr.org/>
12) NucleaRDB: An Information System for Nuclear Receptors (Version 4) <http://receptors.ucsf.edu/NR/>
13) The Wnt Gene Homepage (Wnt proteins form a family of highly conserved secreted signaling molecules that regulate cell-to-cell interactions during embryogenesis. Wnt genes and Wnt signaling are also implicated in cancer) <http://www.stanford.edu/~rnusse/wntwindow.html>
14) Genomic glossaries and Taxonomies - Evolving Terminology for Emerging Technologies (Mary Chitty, Cambridge Healthtech Institute) <http://www.genomicglossaries.com/>

2. Pharmacogenetics Research: The Transition from One-Gene to Whole-Genome Studies in Recent Years

The response of an organism to drugs had being challenging scientists through the years and it must be considered as one aspect of the overall responses that living species exert to different environmental impacts and stressors within an ever-changing environment. In this respect, our knowledge to drug actions in the body goes in parallel with the scientific advances focusing to elucidate mechanisms and processes that contribute to the existence of life. Thus, if we consider the scientific achievements that mainly influenced the drug discovery and development era during the 20th century, then it will be clearly defined that besides the fundamental influences coming from the advances in chemistry, physiology and pharmacology, specific contributions occurred at different times from other health-related disciplines as these were being expanded through the years [16]. Such examples are microbiology at the 30s and 40s, biochemistry at the 50s and 60s and molecular biology with recombinant DNA (rDNA) technology from the mid of 70s and onwards. In parallel, and during this period, pharmacology has been developed into a basic and fundamental discipline in health-related sciences by gathering, creating and analyzing drug-related information, thus expanding and enriching our knowledge of how the different drug classes exert their effects in the body. In this regard, the development of pharmacology led to the emergence of new disciplines by impinging on the molecular mechanisms implicated in pharmacokinetics and pharmacodynamics effects of drugs, including undesirable drug responses like drug inefficiency, ADRs and toxicity. As a matter of fact, the term pharmacogenetics had been coined about 45 years ago in 1959 by Friedrich Vogel to describe the inherited pattern of differential drug response seen in certain individuals [17] (for terminology in pharmacogenetics, pharmacogenomics and other drug-related areas see the web site: http://www.genomicglossaries.com/). However, at that time no one could predict the tremendous progress achieved thus far especially within the last couple decades with drug-related knowledge to reach extraordinary levels nowadays and give some fascinating results connecting specific drug action with individual gene variants. Actually, the evolution of molecular genetics and genomic technologies has transformed pharmacogenetics especially during the last decade of the 20th century. Of equal relevance however, is the fact that this transformation in the drug-related era has opened up new directions towards the application of personalized medicine in clinical practice. This is a long-term desirable target in pharmacotherapy and drug delivery in clinical practice that might reach to reality nowadays (see the following sections of this paper).

Pharmacogenetics deals with inherited variations of drug effects in the body. At the beginning, however, the most common examples of inter-individual drug responses relevant to pharmacogenetic research were that related to inherited enzyme deficiencies implicated in the occurrence of specific diseases. From that point of view, probably the first example of pharmacogenetic disorder described ever was that referred by the ancient Greek mathematician Pythagoras (580-500 BC) who noted that certain, but not all, individuals develop hemolytic anemia in response to the ingestion of uncooked fava beans, an effect now known to be associated with glucose-6-phosphate dehydrogenase (G6PD) deficiency (the flavism disorder) [18]. Actually, the example of G6PD can also be considered as the first pharmacogenetic trait that applied in 1956 in routine pharmaceutical care by screening patients for erythrocyte G6PD deficiency prior to initiating primaquine delivery for the therapy of malaria [19, 20]. However, the involvement of a genetic component into biochemical processes linked to enzyme deficiencies resulting to drug response variability was first supported by Gorrod and Oxon in 1902. These ideas were further refined by Arno

Motulsky in 1957 who suggested the implication of genetic factors in certain toxic drugs reactions observed in individual patients. Such historic aspects of pharmacogenetic research have been recently presented in several review articles and they present the scientific efforts that created the solid ground in which the modern genomic drug-related disciplines were emerged [18, 19, 21]. By following up chronologically these scientific breakthroughs, it is obvious that these efforts became successful by merging experimental data from different disciplines, e.g. chemistry, biochemistry, physiology, biology, and pharmacology that enable the improvement of new drug discovery and development era as well as pharmaceutical care in clinical practice. These trends in pharmacogenetics research apply even to the recent years where the genomic and other technologies, like combinatorial chemistry, high throughput screening, bioinformatics and nanotechnology, are changing and enriching the scientific basis of all biology-oriented disciplines included drug-related ones.

As it has already been discussed, the approach of analyzing at the molecular level differences seen in drug response obviously depends on the existed knowledge and techniques in biology and chemistry that give the background in order the major pharmacogenetic discoveries to emerge through the years. The rapid progress, however, achieved in molecular biology since 1975 generated some fascinating results related to specific cellular processes implicated in drug effects in the body. Furthermore, this information created new sophisticated technologies applicable to different scientific areas including the new drug discovery and development era, as well as the health and pharmaceutical care sectors in general. As a matter of fact, new disciplines emerged to cover such advances in a way to further expand this information by taking advantage of both applied and basic knowledge through the unprecedented flood of genetic information entering the health sciences. In this respect, pharmacogenomics emerged as the new discipline that bridges molecular biology with pharmacology [4]. Pharmacogenomics is a major development that is taking place in pharmaceutical sciences today with the progressive transition from genetics to genomics and the attempt to analyze the whole genome of an organism and correlate genotyping with specific drug actions [6]. In other words, pharmacogenomics seems to be the next step in pharmacogenetics that, as it has already been mentioned, historically has been referred to drug response in relation to individual genetic variation amongst patients. The recent technological advances through the combined use of DNA microarray (DNA chip) technology and automated DNA sequencing now permits the detection of specific single-nucleotide variants, the so-called single nucleotide polymorphisms (SNPs), in several genes involved in drug response [22]. Since, the genome from two unrelated person share of over 99.9% identity in their DNA sequences consisting of more than 3 billion base pairs, the rest 0.1% gives the variability seen in humans and in some degree accounts for the observed inter-individual drug response and disease susceptibility. Moreover, recent data support the notion that groups of SNPs and other variants (DNA deletions of insertions) in a considerably longer sequence of nucleotides are inherited together in a stretch of DNA (haplotypes), thus making the efforts to correlate genotypes with specific phenotypic variations in disease diagnosis and drug action more easily attainable by researchers and applicable into clinical practice [23]. These advances are likely improving pharmacodynamics by differentiation of the conventional clinical diagnosis and drug selection into separate molecular subtype groups within patients suffering the same disease, a result that can eventually improve patient care.

3. Inter-Individual Variability in Drug Response: The Understanding of the Genetic Basis Implicated in this Pharmacological Phenomenon

It has long been recognized by healthcare providers and patients that individuals often respond differently to the same drug, both in terms of efficacy and toxicity [24]. This heterogeneity in drug response is of important relevance in pharmacotherapy, since it often results in drug inefficiency or toxicity, e.g. the emergence of severe ADRs that can ultimately lead to the removal of the drug from the market. This situation is also crucial in drug discovery era, since it causes the discontinuation of several drug candidates at early stages during the drug development process. Collectively, it has been estimated that for approved drug delivery therapies the percentage of all patients that effectively respond to pharmacotherapy significantly varies. In particular, it is proposed that 20-40% of patients with depression respond inefficiently to pharmacotherapy (poor/non-responders), 40-75% with asthma, 50-75% with diabetes, 70-100% with cancer (referring to breast, lung and brain), 20-70% with duodenal ulcer, 30-75% with hyperlipidemia, 10-70% with hypertension, 30-60% with migraine, 20-50% with osteo/rheumatoid arthritis and 25-75% with schizophrenia [25]. Of equal importance are the results for the incidence and the severity of ADRs in clinical practice. In a meta-analysis from 39 prospective studies from U.S. hospitals it has been proposed that 6.7% of hospitalized patients developed ADRs during pharmacotherapy and 0.32% showed fatal ADRs, the latter causing about 100,000 deaths per year in U.S.A. [26]. This notion is further strengthened by the report released from the Institute of Medicine in December 1999 showing that nearly 98.000 deaths in U.S.A. annually were attributed to medication errors including ADRs [27]. In addition, about 10-17% of patient hospitalizations are directly related to the emergence of ADRs, an effect that poses patient pharmaceutical care and safety as a fundamental issue in each healthcare system [28]. The importance of the incidence of ADRs in hospitalized patients was further confirmed in a European study, conducted in a Department of Internal Medicine in a Norwegian hospital. In particular, in a two-year period of study and from 732 deaths reported amongst the 13,993 in-patients, 133 of those were directly attributed to ADRs observed during pharmacotherapy [29]. This result gives almost 10 deaths per 1000 hospitalized patients, a number that obviously stresses towards the need of improving drug efficacy and minimizing toxicity in the healthcare system.

Of major concern is thus, for the reasons outlined above, the understanding of the molecular mechanisms underlined drug response variability. The causes for this inter-individual heterogeneity in clinical pharmacology and incidence of ADRs include several potential risk factors that contribute differently to this phenomenon and are related to the disease pathophysiology and severity, possible drug or nutrient interactions, concomitant illnesses, specific organ function, age, or even lifestyle [2] (Fig. 1). Genetic factors influencing both pharmacokinetics and pharmacodynamics drug response also contribute to inter-individual variability, whereas their importance has been greatly appreciated by the emergence of pharmacogenomics and personalized medicine [23].

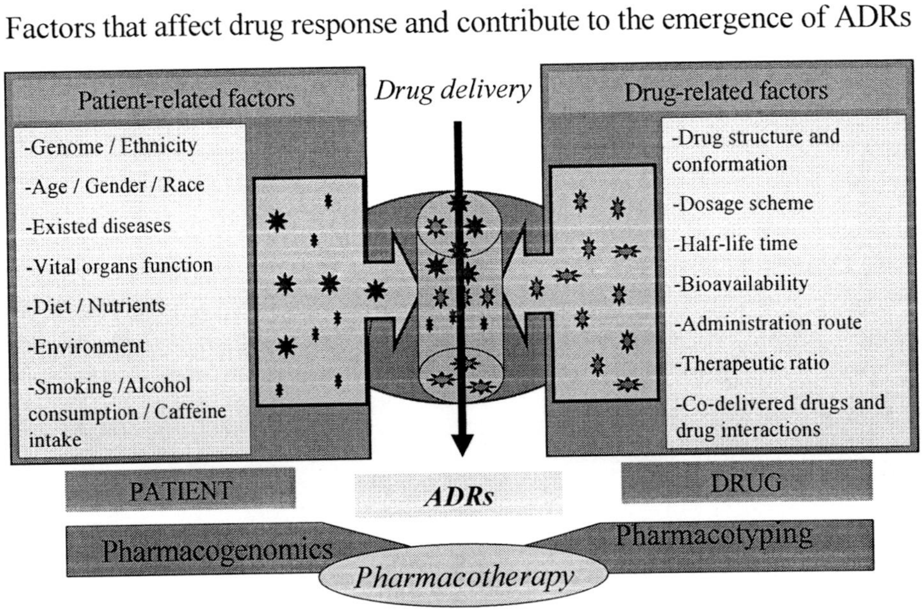

Figure 1. Diagrammatic presentation of patient and drug related factors that influence drug response and contribute to the emergence of ADRs in patient care. Several factors related either to patient status and physiology, or to drug properties and delivery modulate pharmacotherapy outcome in patient care. The recent advances made through the development of genomic technologies, it is expected to change drug delivery in a way of improving patient care, an effect that ultimately can establish pharmacotyping as a new dimension in pharmacotherapy

The underlined genetic nature of some toxic reactions to drugs or xenobiotics and the notion that, at least in part, the variability in drug response may be inherited have long been recognized in pharmacology during the past several years [3, 10, 18]. However, in recent years the correlation of genetic variations with altered drug efficacy and toxicity in certain individuals indicates that personalized medicine in drug therapy can be applied to some if not all people. Exploitation of genomic information related to genes that encode either drug metabolizing enzymes, drug receptors, or drug transporters is now well accepted in modern therapeutics [30]. It is also now known that specific genetic variations, for example, clearly account for monogenic (one gene involved) disorders, like cystic fibrosis, Huntington's disease and Duchenne's muscular dystrophy [31]. Moreover, as it will be presented in the following sections, individual genetic variations of genes encoding cytochrome P450 (CYP) enzymes, (e.g. CYP1A2, CYP2D6, CYP3A4), drug receptors (G-protein coupled receptors; GPCRs), ion channels (e.g. HERG), and drug transporters (e.g. P-glycoprotein; P-gp) play a crucial role in defining and ensuring drug efficacy and safety for individual patients in clinical practice [32-34] (Table 1).

Table 1. Examples of clinically relevant genetic polymorphisms associated with altered drug response and/or ADRs

Polymorphic gene	Drug	Effect	Reference
CYP2C9	Warfarin Phenytoin Tolbutamide, glipizide	Bleeding risk Toxicity Hypoglycemia	[2, 15]
CYP2C19	Proton pump inhibitors (e.g. Omeprazole)	Altered drug response	[150]
CYP2D6	Fluoxetine Codeine	Toxicity Toxicity	[2, 15]
Dihydropyrimidine dehydrogenase	5-Fluorouracil	Toxicity	[32, 87]
MDR1 (or *ABCB1*)	Antiepileptic drugs	Drug resistance	[32, 74]
TPMT	6-Mercaptopurine, 6-thioguanine, Azathioprine	Toxicity	[15, 71, 88]
β_2-Adrenergic receptors ($\beta_2 AR$)	β_2-agonists (e.g. albuterol)	Altered drug response	[70, 82]
5-Lipoxygenase (*ALOX5*)	Zileuton, Montelukast	Altered drug response	[151]
Angiotensin-converting enzyme (*ACE*)	β-blockers (e.g. propranolol)	Altered drug response	[53, 54, 56]
Apolipoprotein E4 (*APOE4*)	Tacrine	Altered drug response	[24]
α-Adducin	Diuretics (thiazides)	Altered drug response	[56]
Angiotensin II type I-receptor (*AT-1*)	Losartan	Altered drug response	[53]
UDP-glucuronosyltransferase 1A1 (*UGT1A1*)	Irinotecan	Toxicity	[32, 73]
Human leukocyte antigen (*HLA*)	Abacavir	Hypersensitivity	[105, 106]
Glutathione-S-transferases (*GSTs*), XPD and XRCC1 (genes of the DNA excision-repair system)	Platinum chemotherapeutic agents	Altered drug response	[85, 87]
Glutathione-S-transferases (*GSTs*)	D-penicillamine	Altered efficacy	[152]
N-acetyltransferases (*NATs*)	Sulfonamides Isoniazid, procainamide, hydralazine	Hypersensitivity Toxicity	[13, 72]
Serotonin *5-HT2A, 2C* receptors	Clozapin	Altered efficacy	[153]
KCNH2 (HERG potassium channel)	Quinidine Cisapride	Long-QT syndrom Torsade de pointes	[154]
KCNQ1 (KvLQT1 potassium channel)	Terfenadine, Disopyramide	Long-QT syndrome	[155]

4. The Emergence of Pharmacogenomics in the 90's and the Advances in New Drug Discovery and Development Technologies

During the last couple decades of the past century, healthcare professionals were confronted with an expanding body of information as well as an impressive number of technological advances related to drug development, therapy and clinical practice. The advent of recombinant DNA (rDNA) technology has provided several new methods, revealed novel molecular targets and created DNA-based diagnostics for screening and developing new biotechnology-based drugs as well as improving drug response and patient care. Furthermore, new innovative therapeutics are reaching the market, or are under development, including potential new classes of drugs, like antisense oligonucleotides, ribozymes and aptamers (synthetic nucleic ligands) [35-38]. Furthermore, new-sophisticated drug delivery systems are evolved through the use of micro- and nano-particles prepared with blends of biodegradable and polycationic polymers to formulate drugs and to enhance drug bioavailability in the body [39-42].

Overall, the impact of biotechnology on pharmaceutical research *via* the development of pharmaceutical biotechnology opened up new dimensions into our ability to develop new therapeutics and led to the genesis of new exciting research areas of work in many disciplines and technologies [5, 10, 43, 45]. In particular, further to the advent of pharmacogenomics, other advances related to pharmacology and pharmaceutical research are: a) The DNA microarray (DNA chip) technology that permits the expression analysis of thousands of genes in order to identify those variants correlated with human disease pathogenesis as well as drug response [46]; b) The availability of bioinformatic tools to analyze the load of genomic data and identify novel molecular drug targets with unique structural domains and specific functional motifs including genes and proteins implicated in drug actions [47]; c) The application of new genetic approaches for gene and protein therapy protocols and development of fascinating site-specific drug delivery systems [40, 41]; d) The use of combinatorial chemistry that allows the synthesis of large libraries of low molecular weight compounds for high-throughput screening (HTS) in order to discover pharmacodynamic active agents [48]; and e) Finally, last but not least, the application of proteomics, functional and structural genomics, expression genetics, and genome mapping for the analysis and functional characterization of all potential genes and proteins serving as drug receptors, or other biological functions [49]. Furthermore, by the completion of several whole-genome sequencing projects including that of HGP, new applications for mapping and analyzing SNPs throughout the genome for their functional and therapeutic relevance and the use of new sophisticated inducible gene expression systems have been recently evolved [22, 46, 50]. Such achievements already generated several databases to include functional genomics data that can further be used for pharmacogenomics studies (Box 1). This procedure obviously facilitate the identification of new drug targets, whose number is estimated to increase from about 500 nowadays to more than 3000 in the near future [10, 16]. Therefore, major attempts in pharmaceutical research are now focusing on finding and exploiting potential genomic targets for drug development. The tools used for new drug structure design and their pharmaceutical production have also positively influenced by the elucidation of specific molecular mechanisms and pathways implicating gene polymorphisms that determine why patients respond differently to drugs, or why some drugs show adverse effects or interactions in specific group of patients. However, with all these advances covering the whole era of pharmaceutical research and development the need for better ways to retrieve and analyze the mass of data generated is now, more than ever, a fundamental issue in drug discovery area [51, 52]. As a matter of fact, the development and application of new bioinformatics tools to approach these issues of data mining would also greatly influence the integration of genomic information into clinical practice and help the information-based medicine to be applied in routine patient care.

5. The Concept of Personalized Medicine Applied in Pharmacotherapy and Therapeutics

The aims of personalized medicine are focusing on minimizing the risk of disease onset and anticipating disease progression for individual patients, as well as trying to apply individualized drug therapy in clinical practice [8]. Regarding the first task, the isolation and functional characterization of specific genes and their variants (alleles) by the application of genomic technologies have empowered the ability to further exploit the role of various genomic factors contributing to pathogenesis of complex and polygenic diseases e.g. cardiovascular disorders, Alzheimer's disease (AD) and asthma. Alternatively and more interestingly, specific variants of these genes have been found either to predispose for, or to contribute, or even to increase the susceptibility of individual persons for the disease development and progression. There have been several attempts in the past few years to establish specific polymorphic gene variants at pharmacodynamic loci predisposing to cardiovascular diseases or affect drug response such as angiotensin-converting enzyme (ACE), angiotensin II type-1 receptor (AT-1), apolipoprotein E (APOE), α-adducin, and adrenergic receptors that could alternatively be used to improve pharmacotherapy of heart disorders [53-56]. For example, the identification of several genes whose function is associated with diseases like hypertrophic or dilated cardiomyopathy, human long-QT syndrome and essential hypertension give new insights on the molecular basis of the heart disease progression and may help in orienting the proper drug therapies in a given population [57-59]. Among them are included genes encoded for β-myosin heavy chain, cardiac troponins and α-tropomyosin in hypertrophic cardiomyopathy, dystrophin, tafazzin and actin in dilated cardiomyopathy, cardiac sodium channel (SCN5A) and potassium channel (HERG) in long-QT syndrome as well as ACE, α-adductin, angiotensinogen and β_2-adrenergic receptor (β_2AR) in essential hypertension.

The structural and functional genomics analysis of AD has recently identified several genetic loci that potentially contribute into disease pathophysiology in cooperation with both environmental and epigenetic factors [60]. In particular, genetic predisposition to AD development is demonstrated either for genes whose variants exhibit a mendelian inheritance pattern e.g. the amyloid precursor protein (APP), and the presenilin-1 (PS1) and -2 (PS2), or for those considered to be potential susceptibility genes contributing to AD predisposition, e.g. APOE, ACE, interleukin-1α (IL1α), nitric oxide syntase-3 (NOS3), low density lipoprotein-related protein 1 (LRP1) and α-2-macroglobulin (A2M). Furthermore, recent results have shown that specific genotypes and haplotypes may cause different drug response rates in individual AD patients receiving cholinesterase inhibitors and/or non-cholinergic agents used for the treatment of AD. [24, 60] Although this progress in AD genomics suggests that pharmacogenomics could be a suitable platform applied for the molecular diagnosis, identification of new drug targets, improvement of drug therapy and also analysis of complex and polygenic disorders, however much work is still needed in order these efforts to be finally achieved in clinical practice. Of equal importance and obviously confirmatory to this hypothesis are some successful experimental efforts related to pharmacogenomics and molecular diagnosis of other complex diseases like cancer and asthma (Table 1) [61-65]. However, of crucial contribution must be considered the use of both genetic- and clinical-related knowledge on the way towards applying genomic information for therapeutic intervention. Although this direction needs rather a multidisciplinary approach in order to be finally achieved, however, a recently published study has clearly shown that it is an affordable task. In particular, the maintenance warfarin dose was estimated through an algorithm generated by evaluating at the same time several clinical, pharmacogenetic and demographic factors that were obtained before the warfarin initiation therapy be applied to patients [66]. Overall, similar approaches it is expected to be finally used in clinical practice giving hope in the years to come that the association of unique genetic markers with specific drug delivery even for the therapy of complex diseases is a realistic approach and can be achieved in routine healthcare.

A question, however, that arises from genomic studies is related to the time and the manner by which the application of pharmacogenomics principles will be generally established in clinical practice for therapeutic intervention. This question is crucial but the answer is not simple. So, in order to address such dilemmas, several examples of applied pharmacogenomics research will be outlined below. The first one is related with the CYP enzymes involved in drug metabolism. With the completion of HGP there were characterized 57 putative functional genes encoding different CYP enzymes and 58 pseudogenes [67, 68] (see also the website: http://drnelson.utmem.edu/CytochromeP450.html). In addition, a different number of CYP enzyme genes has also been identified in the genome of various organisms ranging from 323 in rice and 249 in arabidopsis thaliana (or thale cress as it is commonly known) to 102 in mouse and 54 in dog [18, 68]. Furthermore, the existed complexity at the genomic level in the field of drug metabolism is additionally complicated by considering the high number of polymorphic variants discovered for these genes and especially those belonging into families 1-3. In particular, the major human CYP enzymes involved in drug metabolism include CYP1A2, CYP2A6, CYP2B6, CYP2C8, CYP2C9, CYP2C19, CYP2D6, CYP2E1, CYP3A4 and CYP3A5 that exhibit several polymorphic sites with clinical significance (see the website: http://www.imm.ki.se/cypalleles). Interestingly, polymorphic enzymes that mainly account for ~40% of CYP-mediated drug metabolism are those of CYP2C9, CYP2C19 and CYP2D6 and, for this reason, are considered very important in pharmacotherapy by making problematic the application of a general drug dosing scheme for the drugs whose disposition is determined by these enzymes [18]. Indeed, several experimental studies of applied pharmacogenomics research have already been published that correlate specific CYP gene variants with altered drug efficacy and safety and clearly shade light on the elucidation of the molecular mechanisms involved in inter-individual drug response seen amongst patients suffering the same disease.

Interestingly and in addition to CYP gene variants already characterized, specific genetic polymorphisms were also analyzed in genes encoding P-gp, GPCRs, thiopurine methyltransferase (TPMT), ACE, arylamine N-acetyltransferases (NATs) and/or UDP-glucuronosyltransferases (UGTs) in just to mention a few, which have also been shown to correlate with the modulation of drug response and incidence of ADRs in humans [32-34, 54, 69-73], (Table 1). To better clarify the manner by which such gene variants contribute to the pharmacotherapy outcome some experimental data will be discussed. P-gp is an ATP-dependent efflux pump belonging to the superfamily of ABC transporters, which include 48 already identified members in human. The role of P-gp in limiting intestinal, brain and placental transport, as well as in biliary and urinary excretion of its substrates is now well recognized. Thus, variations in its gene (*MDR1* or *ABCB1*) existed in several individuals may influence drug disposition and alter drug response [32, 69]. In this respect, specific mutations are detected in several regions of *MDR1* including domains of the transmembrane part (5, 6, 11, and 12 domains), or the intracellular and extracellular loops, or even the ATP binding sites. Although these genetic variations can affect the function of P-gp as transporter by altering its binding with drugs and other xenobiotics, however the clinical relevance of all the characterized genotypes of *MDR1* in certain individuals and ethnic populations has not been extensively studied [32]. Confirmatory to this situation, is one specific polymorphism detected on *MDR1* and designated as ABCB1-C3435T which has been characterized recently and it was shown to be well associated with the variability of drug response seen during antiepileptic pharmacotherapy [74]. On the other hand, and of equal clinical importance is the fact that the accumulated knowledge thus far regarding P-gp cellular function in certain organs clearly shows that most of P-gp drug-substrates are also metabolized by CYP3A4, and these two systems are co-localized in tissues with a major role in drug disposition like small intestine and liver [69, 75, 76]. This evidence must also be clinically evaluated in close relation to the recent data indicating that some nutrients or phytopharmaceutical preparations, (e.g. St John's Wort; Hypericum Perforatum), can modify P-gp and CYP3A4 expression and function and thus they might interfere and influence phenotype-genotype correlation studies upon their concomitant delivery with the drugs being studied [32, 77]. This proposal, however, can alternatively be applied to pharmacotherapy to predict drug-drug or drug-nutrient interactions ensuring drug response and improving patient outcome, whereas it can also be integrated into clinical pharmacology teaching courses to implement rational drug prescription in clinical practice [28, 78-80]. At the same time, further functional characterization of specific P-gp gene variants and elucidation of the molecular mechanisms underlined their involvement in inter-individual drug variability are expected to give new insights towards the selective modulation of P-gp function in blood-brain barrier for optimizing therapeutic intervention and improving patient pharmaceutical care [81].

It is well recognized nowadays that there is a significant inter-individual variability in the therapeutic responses of drugs binding to GPCRs, like adrenergic receptors in the general population [70]. For example, thirteen SNPs were identified in the promoter and the coding region of β_2AR gene and found to be organized into twelve haplotypes. Some of these haplotypes have shown significant divergence in different ethnic populations and this fact is associated with the bronchodilator response to β_2-agonists in patients with asthma [82]. Since asthma is considered a polygenic disease, several other gene variants have also been shown to contribute to pharmacotherapy outcome in asthmatics in addition to *β_2AR* polymorphisms. The genes whose several alleles are implicated in altered anti-asthmatic drug response include those of 5-lipoxygenase (*ALOX5*) for zileuton, muscarinic receptor-2 (M_2) and 3 (M_3) for muscarinic antagonists (e.g. ipratropium bromide), glucocorticoid receptor for glucocordicoids (e.g. prednisolone, beclomethasone) and phosphodiesterase-4A (*PDE4A*) and 4D (*PDE4D*) for theophylline delivery [83]. Collectively, it is now known the complex genetic nature underlined the drug response in patients with asthma. In this respect, the example of β_2AR gene polymorphisms will be further discussed in close relation to several structural and functional elements of the receptor itself that have been recently defined. In particular, the elucidation of several aspects related to the molecular mechanisms of β_2AR signaling has added new information of pharmacological importance about structure and function relationships, as well as coupling of this receptor to its multiple effectors [84]. Like all GPCRs, β_2AR has 7 transmembrane-spanning domains, an extracellular amino-terminus with 3 intra-connecting extracellular loops, and an intracellular carboxy-terminus with 3 intracellular loops. Structural and functional analysis has been identified several amino-acids as absolutely necessary for β-agonist binding [84]. This knowledge implement recent pharmacogenomics data from genomic studies estimating that as much as 60% of inter-individual variability in anti-asthmatic drug response observed with β_2-agonist delivery might involve genetic factors modulating pharmacotherapy outcome. However, more systematic efforts must be undertaken in order to fully elucidate the underlined mechanisms for improving asthma patient care in clinical practice [70]. By impinging on these molecular mechanisms it would be possible to identify and uncover novel structural and functional aspects of the β_2AR signaling pathway of clinical importance. Of particular interest in this direction are considered recent data showing that key role for high-affinity and full-agonist activation of the receptor is mediated through interactions of agonist molecules with the amino-acids Asp113, Ser204, Ser207 and Asn293. In parallel, several attempts have been focused towards understanding the pharmacological phenomenon related to drug-receptor binding known as "inverse agonism", an event known to occur in GPCRs. Such efforts have been recently reinforced by the accumulation of new data implicating several aspects of GPCRs binding with their effectors that allow better evaluation of the β_2-agonist inter-individual response to improve their efficacy and safety [85, 86].

Another example of personalized medicine applies to cancer pharmacotherapy. Recent progress in cancer pharmacogenomics suggests that it is possible to improve chemotherapy outcome for specific anticancer drugs, like 5-fluorouracil (5-FU), irinotecan and platinum agents [87]. In particular, specific polymorphisms in the genes encoding the enzymes dihydropyrimidine dehydrogenase and thymidylate synthase have been shown to influence the efficacy and toxicity of 5-FU in certain individuals, although their applicability into clinical practice by selecting patients who are likely to tolerate and respond to 5- FU therapy still remains very complicated [32]. Furthermore, it has been proposed that polymorphisms in the promoter region of the gene encoded UDP-glucuronosyltransferase 1A1 (*UGT1A1*) may be clinically useful for predicting severe toxicity to irinotecan for certain individuals, thus improving its efficacy and safety outcomes [32, 73]. Also, in the case of platinum chemotherapeutic agents (cisplatin, carboplatin, oxaliplatin) several polymorphic genes have been implicated in their efficiency and toxicity. These genes are the *XPD* and *XRCC1* that encode proteins involved in the cellular DNA excision repair system and that of glutathione-S-transferases (GSTs). Although these results can be considered as positive indicators for the improvement of cancer patient care, additional work must be done in order the general applicability and acceptance of genetic information related to platinum agents response to be established in clinical practice.

Furthermore, additional data in the area of cancer pharmacotherapy exist that are of pharmacogenomic interest. One of the most studied examples of applied pharmacogenomics that clearly shows how the translation of genomic information is being transferred to guide patient therapeutics is related to TPMT gene polymorphisms. Interestingly, specific TPMT gene variants have been isolated and clinically validated in studies showing that their presence is associated with high risk of toxicity in individuals taking thiopurine drugs (6-mercaptopurine, 6-thioguanine, azathioprine) [71, 88, 89]. At present, eight TPMT alleles have been identified, including three variant alleles designated as TPMT*2 (with G238C mutation), TPMT*3A (with G460A and A719G mutations) and TPMT*3C (with A719G mutation) that account for about 80-95% of intermediate or low TPMT enzymatic activity, and for this reason, they are analyzed during genotyping and haplotyping population studies [71]. The pharmacogenomic data regarding the TPMT deficiency correlated well with drug toxicity and were so clear and convincing that helped the Clinical Pharmacology Subcommittee of FDA to organize in October 2002 a public hearing for implementing the prescription of thiopurine-related drugs with pharmacogenomic data in order to minimize patients' risk for developing toxic drug effects (90). However, at a critical review in the subsequent meeting of the FDA's Oncology Drug Advisory Committee held in July 2003, pediatricians did not agree to recommend in advance TPMT gene testing before the initiation of 6-mercaptopurine delivery to children suffering from acute lymphoblastic leukemia (ALL) [91]. The proposal for the need of a genetic test was based on the pharmacogenomic data suggesting that the calculation of drug dosage scheme could be achieved though the use of the identified TPMT genotypes in each child. The difficulty for applying a genetic test in clinical practice was further demonstrated by the discussions following the attempts to apply TPMT pharmacogenomic data in routine drug prescription. Such discussions have been extended even to the need and usefulness of the genetic testing as compared with the traditional biochemical tests e.g. the use of a red-cell assay for the detection of TPMT enzyme deficiency [8]. The expression of such thoughts against usefulness of pharmacogenomics in improving patient care clearly shows the different perspectives that several investigators or clinicians share on this type of research and poses the difficulties that these new concepts of drug delivery will meet before their general acceptance in routine clinical practice. To ascertain for applied pharmacogenomics a final succeed, more systematic work is undoubtedly needed in order the translation of genomic data into clinical formalities to lead into the wide use of genetic testing with high quality and validity outcomes, thus ensuring specific dosage recommendations of individual drugs in routine pharmaceutical care [32, 92].

6. The Application of Genotypic-Haplotypic and Gene Expression Data to Pharmacotherapy and Pharmaceutical Research

As it has already been discussed, genomic technologies provide valuable techniques for uncovering the molecular mechanisms leading to pathogenesis and phenotype of specific human diseases. In this frame of genetic research, new genes, proteins and genetic variations can be detected in individuals, since the new technology allows the screening thousands of genes simultaneously. Genotyping and haplotyping analysis of individuals can identify specific gene variations and correlate them with drug effects, an approach that can obviously lead to individualized drug therapy (Fig. 2). Furthermore, the conventional concept applied in drug therapy, (considering patients suffering of the same disease as homogenous population and using similar drug therapy of all patients), is changing in the genomic era. Under the new technologies and personalized medicine, each one of the patients is being handled as an individual, a practice that applies differentiation in pharmacotherapy.

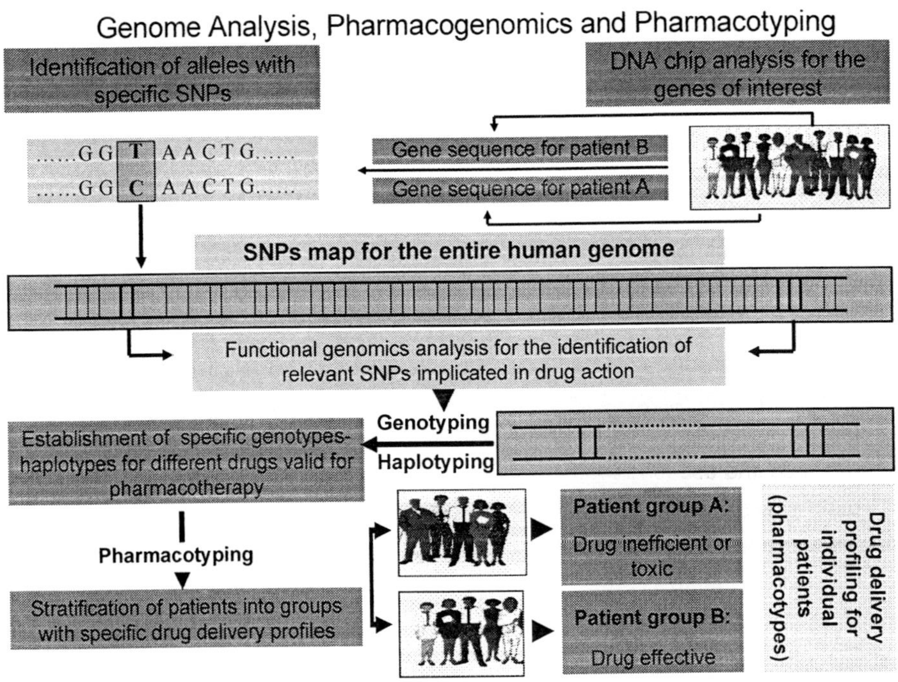

Figure 2. Diagrammatic presentation of the different steps applied in pharmacogenomics that ultimately lead to pharmacotyping. The establishment of specific haplotypes of genes implicated in drug actions, (carrying not only SNPs, as shown in this diagram, but even deletion or insertion variations), by functional genomics and their subsequent use in clinical practice could eventually result in the generation of specific pharmacotyping profiles for individual patients to improve patient care. In order this process to be finally successful at the end, considerable progress in functional genomics area must be done in the future, in parallel with the more thorough understanding of the mechanisms underlined gene molecular networks that are involved in vital cellular processes like proliferation, differentiation and apoptosis (see text for details)

Questions regarding genomic analysis and the application of genotyping-haplotyping data in healthcare are of major concern for various aspects in clinical pharmacology and therapeutics. Some thoughts are discussed below. Although the prospects for basic research in pharmacogenomics and the generation of considerable amounts of data look very promising, their incorporation into clinical practice is quite challenging [93]. Furthermore, detailed analysis of the molecular actions of drugs has clearly shown that medicines exert their effects *via* specific "molecular networks" involving several genes and proteins [12, 15, 94]. The genetic basis underlined the response of an organism to delivered drugs is also determined by the interaction of genes with drugs, as it is illustrated in Fig. 3. This interplay between genes and drugs also implies that their interaction can modulate the pharmacotherapy outcome through either genetic variation, or drug-regulated gene expression that consequently leads to phenotypic variation, e.g. differential pharmacological response. This must also be considered on the light of recent evidence indicating that gene expression can also be affected by environmental factors, like epigenetics phenomena including DNA methylation, histone acetylation and RNA interference (RNAi) mechanisms, which it is now well known that represent crucial processes for establishing a specific gene expression pattern in the cell [95-97] (Fig. 3). The latter is a result that might also contribute into more inter-individual variability of drug response. Overall, both environmental and genomic factors finally contribute to drug response variability and cause drug inefficiency or toxicity to the organism (Fig. 4). In addition, the fundamental role of epigenetic events and the molecular alterations that might cause them and/or underlie altered gene expression in health and disease has been clearly shown especially for cancer. Such an experimental approach gives the chance for the exploitation of epigenetic mechanisms as potential anticancer therapeutics [95-99]. Especially, small interfering RNAs (siRNA) which are the effector molecules of the RNAi pathway discovered in 1998, represent one of the most recent additions to the wide repertoire of nucleic acid molecules used to silence gene expression in a specific manner and whose application as tools for large-scale genotypic-phenotypic screens to study complex biological phenomena as well as the development of new potential therapeutics has already given new insights of an unprecedented importance in terms of clinical relevance and use [97, 98].

Before however, these new challenges to become available in routine clinical practice the underlined complexity of pharmacotherapy outcome in clinical practice has to be primarily resolved by applying genomic tools to analyze gene expression patterns in different health or disease states enabling then pharmacogenomics to establish specific genetic variation profiles for individual drug response. This fact highlights even more the existing complexity in modern pharmacology, and makes the possibility of applying personalized medicine into clinical practice difficult, although an achievable task. The application of genotyping-haplotyping data to improve patient care it is depicted in Fig. 2 by considering the example of SNPs analysis for the stratification of patients suffering the same disease into different genomic groups for better pharmacotherapy outcome. Furthermore, the efforts towards correlating genotyping-haplotyping data with drug response are closely related with the efforts aiming to identify new genomic drug targets for pharmaceutical research [16, 100]. But in order these tasks to proceed, new technological advances permitting faster and less expensive application of whole genome sequencing and genome-wide analysis must happen within the next few years. If this achieved, a major enforcement to personalized medicine application for everyday health and pharmaceutical care would be given.

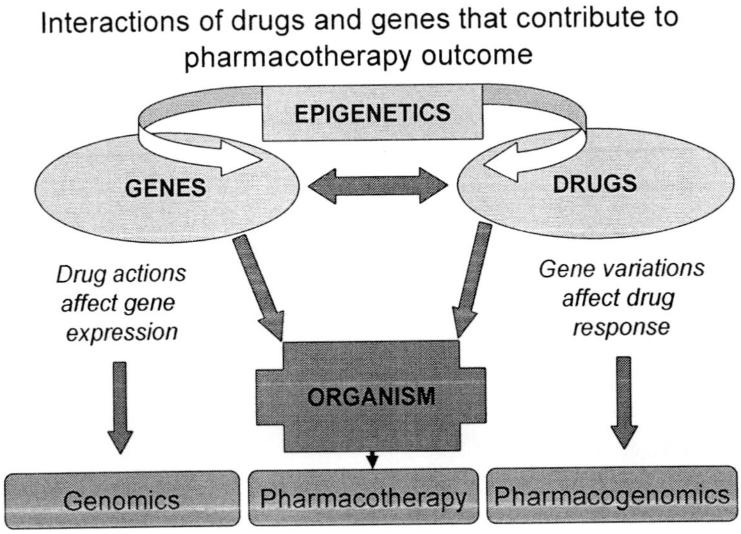

Figure 3. The role of epigenetic regulation in the interplay of genes with drugs to modulate pharmacotherapy outcome. Inter-individual variability of drug response can be affected by specific gene variations that modulate drug effects and in close relation to the ability of drugs to also change gene expression. However the latter, it is known to be regulated by epigenetic phenomena, like DNA methylation, histone acetylation and RNA interference (RNAi), thus contributing into the observed inter-individual variability of drug response. As a matter of fact, the complexity underlined the pharmacotherapy outcome in clinical practice can be resolved by functional genomics through the analysis of gene expression in health or disease states, and pharmacogenomics through the correlation of genetic variation with drug response

Another issue concerning the application of genotyping-haplotyping data in pharmacotherapy is related to the need of minimizing the incidence of ADRs. To achieve full benefits from the application of pharmacogenomics, the prediction of possible drug-drug and drug-nutrient interactions, or even emergence of ADRs must also be attained [101-103]. ADRs remain a major clinical problem, since they contribute either to drug withdrawal from the market, or to patient hospitalizations, thus increasing the time for in-patients and the healthcare cost, or even cause a significant number of deaths per year. However during the previous years, evidence exists to show that the application of pharmacogenomic concepts might have beneficial effects towards reducing ADRs in clinical practice [2, 90, 102]. Such an example is related to the use of antiretroviral agent abacavir in which about 5% of HIV patients experience a potentially severe hypersensitivity reaction [104].

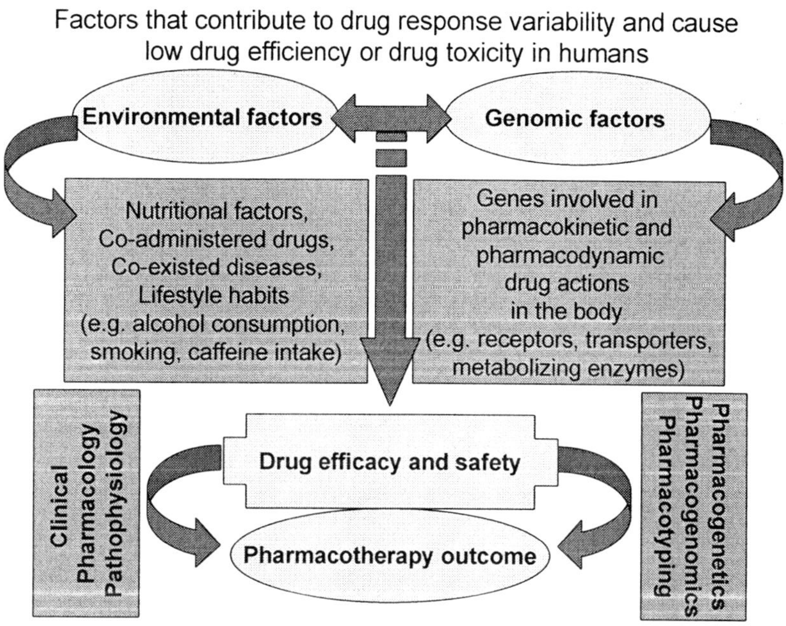

Figure 4. Environmental and genomic factors influence drug efficiency and toxicity in patient care. Several environmental and genomic factors modulate the drug efficiency and toxicity and affect pharmacotherapy outcome. Such a connection clearly shows the existed complexity that finally determines the drug response in the body. Also, several health and drug related specialties including pharmacogenomics and pharmacotyping, contribute towards resolving this complexity at the molecular level and to use the information obtained into clinical practice and healthcare

Recently published pharmacogenomic data have convincingly shown that a specific polymorphism in human leukocyte antigen (HLA) region is highly associated with the incidence of the abacavir-related hypersensitivity reaction [105, 106]. This result can lead to additional pharmacogenomic studies concerning the possible associations of major histocompatibility complex genotypes with idiosyncratic and allergic reactions to other antiretroviral drugs thus improving their efficacy and safety [107]. This direction could also finally lead to the establishment of a genetic test for personalized medicine of HIV-1 nucleoside reverse-transcriptase inhibitors, although considerable criticism has also been raised over how such research should be incorporated in pharmacotherapy [104].

7. Pharmacotyping and the Drug Prescription Process in the Post-Genomic Era: How Realistic Is this to Be Achieved in the Near Future?

For the most of the 20th century, many healthcare providers thought genetics as an esoteric academic specialty with no substantial projections or even scientific branches coming into the clinic; that notion is nowadays at least dangerously outdated. More interestingly, inspiring thoughts urging the need for all healthcare providers to understand the concepts of genetic variability, its interactions with the environment and implication for patient care are now becoming a routine part in many medical and pharmaceutical disciplines [31]. Especially as it has already been mentioned, pharmacogenomics brought new ideas regarding drug delivery and healthcare in clinical practice by connecting genomics with pharmacology and therapeutics [4]. Following this, the concept of personalized medicine was introduced in such a rigorous way into healthcare practice that it was rapidly created high expectations in the public for its immediate clinical application, especially after the completion of the HGP. But, in order these expectations to be converted into reality and the feasible clinical applicability of genomic technologies to be generally applied into routine clinical practice, major scientific and technological efforts it is needed to come together from different scientific areas. This direction obviously means that the progress in this area must follow the same successful and traditional ways of human knowledge that gave in the past the scientific breakthroughs already changed the basis for many specialties, but with the tools and approaches now available enabling the more detailed, integrated and sometimes sophisticated analysis at the molecular, or even at the supra-molecular, level of crucial cellular functions like proliferation, differentiation, and apoptosis. However, in such an approach well-documented and insightful opinions and thoughts that primarily express a somehow discoursing view of the future as well as the ability of pharmacogenomics principles to be successfully delivered into clinical practice, or even more interestingly, discuss the constraints that exist on the way of bringing personalized medicine into a reality, clearly help in setting up priorities and focusing on targets that ultimately facilitate and accelerate future developments and achievements in this era.

Another aspect related to pharmacogenomics and personalized medicine is the way by which the unprecedented load of the genomic information available at the molecular level it has to be easily and rapidly transformed into a type-form readily applicable in the healthcare sector and used by the medical practitioner or other specialties. Indeed, the fast growing accumulation of genomic data concerning drug action is a real challenge needed to be clarified in terms of the development of suitable tools capable of analyzing such information in a manner to be readily compatible for clinical use. This is of great importance in current drug delivery and biomedicine. In such a case, the validation of the genomic data mining processes will totally be based on the development of computerized systems and data integration systems in order these then to support the clinical transformation of the gathered genotyping and haplotyping profiling data from individual patients before making such information applicable into the routine patient care. Moving towards personalized medicine also means the existence of tools and molecular diagnostics capable of assessing genome-related clinical information in laboratory medicine to make the extracted information easily applicable by the physician. This is a very difficult task, since before the transfer of techniques from genomic-related research laboratories to those used for the routine analysis of clinical samples in diagnostic laboratories, these techniques must be firstly assessed for their ethical, social and cost-benefit consequences [108]. As a consequence, the gradual integration of technologies transferring genomic information into clinic needs the development of carefully selected and evaluated specific genetic markers for the diagnosis of disease and prediction of drug response, as well as the use and application of genome-wide linkage analysis capable for genotyping, gene array, proteomics, transcriptomics and metabolomics profiling [109, 110]. These developments of laboratory medicine should also highlight the way that must be undertaken in order to assure the level of quality and validity needed in genetic and molecular diagnostics tests [111]. If this being confirmed in practice, then the individualized drug delivery profiling based on patient's clinical, genomic and bioinformatics data will be achieved in pharmacotherapy, e.g. to what is referred as pharmacotyping [3] (Fig. 5).

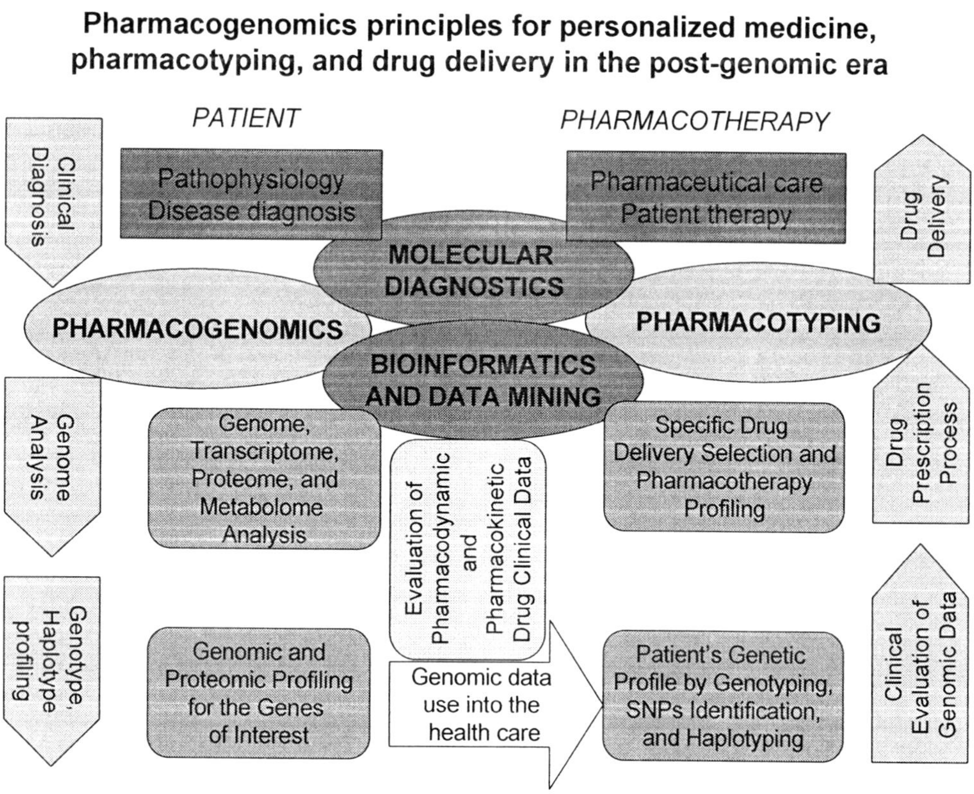

Figure 5. Personalized medicine and pharmacotyping are major directions of drug delivery in the post-genomic era. The advances achieved by pharmacogenomics, bioinformatics and molecular diagnostics greatly influence healthcare towards the establishment of pharmacotyping in drug delivery. Furthermore as it is shown above, patient clinical diagnosis is facilitated by the application of genomic technologies through the validation of specific genotyping- haplotyping profiles relevant for clinical use that ultimately can improve pharmacotherapy outcome. Of major interest however, should be considered the compatibility forms with which the clinical and genomic drug-related data enter the information-mining platforms to create individual pharmacotyping profiles in routine clinical practice (see text for details)

Furthermore, the advent of specialized techniques coming from the advances of functional genomics will greatly influence the application of genomic information in laboratory and clinical practice. This also means that unified platforms must be developed in order to permit compatibility in handling different data gathered from unrelated sources like those of drug databases, clinical trials, DNA sequencing and functional genomic analysis in a way to ultimately support the clinical application of pharmacogenomics, personalized medicine and pharmacotyping in routine clinical practice [3].

But what is the reality now and how far away do we really are from seeing pharmacogenomics, personalized medicine and pharmacotyping to be applied in routine clinical practice? This is a question that all the clinicians want to know the answer. However, on the other hand, for the scientists working in pharmacogenomics and pharmaceutical research era this question seems to be more a challenge than a substantial one in terms of scientific interest. Of course, the answer is negative for the foreseeable near future although some scientists predict the applicability of such approaches in the healthcare system in 1-2 decades by now. Whatever this will be happened, specific scientific and technological breakthroughs regarding the clinical use of gemonic data must be firstly achieved in order then these advances to push methodology forward in making success for improved patient care. These individual scientific steps represent painstaking and time-consumable processes that will also need more thorough understanding of the mechanisms implicated in disease pathophysiology and drug response as well as basic biological processes that affect cell functions like cellular proliferation, differentiation, apoptosis, communication, motility and renewal. The latter related to crucial cellular functions, would greatly enhance the exploitation of specific macromolecules underlined the pharmacokinetics and pharmacodynamics effects of the drugs in the body, including specific molecular interactions, their multifunctional properties, their tertiary structure formation and the signaling pathways being involved. These properties are considered very crucial for better structural design and development of molecules as potential drug candidates. Efforts to this direction applied during the previous years already led researchers to uncover some interesting molecular mechanisms involved in such vital cellular functions like apoptosis, differentiation and proliferation, thus permitting nowadays the development of new drugs in the areas, among others, of oncology, cardiovascular disorders and degenerative diseases [53, 112-114]. The better knowledge for the molecular mechanisms underlying drug response is achieved, the bigger benefits in pharmaceutical care in terms of drug efficacy and safety will be expected. The example of cancer pharmacogenomics will be further discussed in terms of applicability of pharmacotyping and the concerns raised and are related to the complexity of cellular functions as outline above.

8. Cancer Pharmacogenomics and Pharmacotyping: The Road Towards Elucidating Cellular Complexity

Of special interest related to the application of pharmacotyping in cancer pharmacogenomics are issues concerning the development of drug resistance, since this phenomenon affects the pharmacotherapy outcome and of course the healthcare cost. The underlined mechanisms leading to the emergence of cancer drug resistance are also negatively influencing the general application of personalized medicine, pharmacogenomics and pharmacotyping and restrict specific drug efficiency designed and entered the clinical practice. Over the past several years, several novel exploitable targets for cancer drug development have been revealed that recently resulted into the development of some innovative drugs already applied to clinical practice. Such targets include enzymes like tyrosine kinases involved in signal transduction pathways, genes regulating apoptosis and differentiation of malignant cells, cell-lineage transcriptional factors, angiogenesis factors and unique proteins driving the cell cycle machinery [115-119]. For example, the development of Gleevec/Glivec (imatinib mesylate) as an effective agent inducing apoptosis for the treatment of patients suffering chronic myelogenous leukemia (CML) represents such a bright example of molecularly targeted anticancer therapeutics [120]. Gleevec is a selective inhibitor of Bcr-Abl fusion tyrosine kinase specifically being present in CML patients that result from a reciprocal translocation between chromosomes 9 and 22. This translocation causes the genetic fusion of *bcr* with exon-1 of *c-abl* resulting in a defect known as Philadelphia chromosome. Although the use of Gleevec give very impressive and promising results for the therapy of CML as well as for other tumors by inhibiting also the kinase c-kit, however, the development of drug resistance causes a real restriction point into its clinical use for all CML patients [121]. This is partially attributed to the occurrence of specific mutations in the gene encoding the Bcr-Abl fusion tyrosine kinase, a result that poses the drug resistance development of major concern in modern cancer pharmacotherapy.

The problems confronted in clinical practice from the development of drug resistance in the case of Gleevec, clearly support the notion for the exploitation of alternative and more sophisticated ways in order to better cure cancer patients. Also, it stresses the need for better understanding of the molecular mechanisms of vital cellular processes before pharmacotyping can be generally applied. In this respect, and in order to avoid such undesirable effects, the development and use of drugs that can induce simultaneously differentiation and apoptosis of leukemia cells it has also been suggested [119]. Both processes result in restricted cell growth and thus represent a desirable target for the development of new cancer therapeutics. Indeed, the recent advances in molecular biology of cancer opened up new directions for studying and analyzing complex processes to be turned out to exploitable targets for novel treatments in clinical practice. For example, the process of cell renewal in leukemia versus that of cell differentiation and/or apoptosis appears to be linked somehow to each other, thus giving hope both differentiation and apoptosis can be simultaneously activated in order to serve as potential platforms for developing combined therapeutic approaches [119, 122, 123]. In addition, the use of model cellular systems for more detailed analysis of the function of genes and the elucidation of their specific interactions in normal and disease state represent a useful experimental design of clinical significance, as it has been recently shown for murine erythroleukemia (MEL) cells [119, 123]. All this knowledge it is expected also to help towards elucidating the complexity underlined drug response at the molecular level. Interestingly to this direction, but for breast cancer therapy, a great progress has been recently occurred by revealing the structural interactions of the drug Herceptin and its receptor HER2. Herceptin is a humanized monoclonal antibody (known as trastuzumab) which approved by the FDA in 1998 for breast cancer treatment and represents the first genomic-research-based targeted anti-cancer therapeutic entered the clinical practice [118]. Its effects are achieved through the binding in the HER2 receptor, (also known as Neu, or ErbB2), a member of the epidermal growth factor receptor (EGFR; also known as ErbB) family of tyrosine kinases and its prescription is based on the expression level of HER2 in the patient's tumor tissue (individualized therapy) [124]. The recent elucidation of the crystal structure of the entire extracellular regions of HER2 complexed with the Herceptin antigen-binding fragment (Fas), gives new information on the drug-receptor structural interactions and this knowledge may lead in better drug design and development of new therapeutics of this type [125]. Furthermore, such studies envisage the better understanding of cancer biology at the molecular level and permit specific pharmacogenomics studies to help establishing pharmacotyping in cancer therapy. In particular, such an interesting step related to human breast cancer progression is considered to be the recently published data on the gene expression profiles of the pre-malignant, pre-invasive, and invasive stages of this type of tumor [126]. Through this approach of genomic analysis the better understanding of disease pathogenesis is expected and the identification of specific genomic targets for better drug development could be achieved. Moreover, by analyzing gene expression profiles in cancer pharmacotherapy treatments it would be possible to characterize molecular gene networks that in turn might have some clinical relevance for improving patient care. This happened in the case of ALL where 124 genes were identified to discriminate between different treatments of chemotherapeutic agents (methotrexate and mercaptopurine), a result that can be reversely applied afterwards, in order individualize therapy to be based on the expression level of such genes. This direction implies the application of genomic analysis of the identified genes for each ALL patient before initiating therapy with the referred drugs [127]. This procedure that utilizes the transcriptional profiling analysis has been recently proposed as one way for applying pharmacogenomics in cancer pharmacotherapy [128]. In any case however, by enriching our knowledge in the molecular biology of cancer will ensure better pharmacological interventions to be achieved in the near future.

To resume the data already discussed, some further thoughts of practical value related to several aspects of the potential application of pharmacotyping will be presented. As it has been already mentioned, genetic variations detected in genes encoding proteins implicated in drug action could affect their function and thus might result in altered drug response (e.g. decreased metabolism, inadequate intracellular transport, impaired function on target site, etc). As a matter of fact, the detection of SNPs or other variations and establishment of specific haplotypes for several genes could explain why one patient responds well in drug therapy, while another does not, or even why some people experience serious ADRs (Fig. 2). Overall, if our understanding to these idiosyncratic pharmacological effects is finally achieved, then drug prescription would be greatly influenced. In fact, this will be a major transition in pharmacotherapy since pharmacotyping will be finally achieved, meaning that the physician could be based on patient's genotyping-haplotyping analysis data for initiating and maintaining drug dosage therapeutic scheme for individual patients [3]. But at which extent the pharmacotherapy outcome can be improved by pharmacotyping? One consequence coming from the establishment of pharmacotyping could be the better drug selection and dosage profiling in personalized medicine (Fig. 5). Since, the future prescription process is expected to be done by the physician in a fully computerized environment with the aid of genomic and bioinformatic information concerning patient status, pharmacotyping could better ensure drug efficacy and safety. Such a case also means a transition from a drug-selection process mainly based on the physician's own experience, into a more, highly integrated, information and computer-aided pharmacotherapy, thus making drug delivery digitized, more efficient and safer. It is evident however that the genetic information derived from pharmacogenomics studies must be incorporated into clinical practice in such a way to assess simultaneously, besides drug efficiency, the risk of ADRs attributed to specific drug specimens. Furthermore, the identification of functional SNPs and establishment of specific haplotypes for genes implicated in drug response, or ADRs, could also be used as a marker for drug prediction effects in a given individual, or even for a specific group of patients. In this way, a standard framework for information-based medicine must firstly be developed, in order this later to support an infrastructure for personalized medicine to achieve pharmacotyping in routine pharmaceutical care. The likelihood of the ultimate success in this endeavor is difficult to be predicted. However, the recent advances in *in silico* molecular modeling used during the drug development process to predict the absorption, distribution, metabolism and excretion (ADME) data of potential drug candidates, it clearly indicates that also the prediction of drug effects in the body is a realistic expectation and may be achieved in the years to come [129-131].

9. Pharmaceutical and Medical Education for Future Healthcare Providers

All the advances already described regarding the genomic and other technologies and their application in clinical practice have changed drug-related disciplines into a more biology- and biotechnology-based direction. It is obvious that the future of healthcare providers and their competitiveness in the job market will clearly depend, at least in part, on their ability to integrate into their practice new molecular diagnostic biomarkers as well as molecular and bioinformatic technologies applied to analyze, extract, evaluate and finally validate genomic information of clinical relevance. For example, the advantage for pharmacologists to apply the principles of personalized medicine seems to go in parallel with the application of pharmacogenomics and pharmacotyping aspects in routine clinical practice. More interestingly, all these achievements and challenges in pharmaceutical research that have already discussed in previous sections have added new knowledge in pharmacology and now stress for the need of appropriate adjustments of education and curricula in medical and pharmacy faculties [132-134]. These recent reports analyze the new roles that healthcare providers have to play in the changing environment of drug therapy and clinical practice and the need for their better education in pharmacogenomics and personalized medicine. It is evident that better training in pharmacology of future medical and pharmacy students will be achieved by the development of new curricula based on the integration of new drug-related genomic and bioinformatic technologies into the teaching process. However, healthcare educators already face up difficulties in teaching pharmacogenomics and personalized medicine as well as in trying to give future practitioners the knowledge to keep them update with recent advances on several drug-related areas. The classical background bridge of physiology with pharmacology needed in order students to understand drug-related actions and effects in the body has now expanded to include the knowledge coming from biochemistry, molecular biology, genetics and finally genomics. This knowledge is considered now crucial for more thorough understanding of several aspects of drug delivery in clinical practice in order to improve the skills of future practitioners for better selection, dosage and co-administration of drugs for individual patients. Undoubtedly, this need for better training in pharmacogenomics for both educators and healthcare providers will be in increasing demands in the years to come, since developments are achieving by genomic technologies in all drug-related areas are rapidly introduced and applied into healthcare and clinical practice [3, 132]. This is a very difficult task however, since in the case of pharmacology it means the development and introduction of new interactive computer-assisted learning methods related to genes and genomes into the teaching process which would have to be organized into an already tight timetable for completing both theory and practice [132, 136-138]. Finally, another challenging issue in the design of new curricula will be to instruct the students to keep pace with the new scientific knowledge rapidly influencing drug-related aspects even after their graduation. Such profound changes in pharmacotherapy are expected to eventually enter the clinical practice, thus affecting modern medicine and pharmacy [132, 133, 139]. Finally, the positive consequences in clinical practice will be greatly enhanced by imperatively incorporating the fundamental principles of pharmacogenomics, personalized medicine and pharmacotyping into the core curricula of pharmacy and medicine. And for sure, this will be beneficial both for health and pharmaceutical care, as well as for the society and the public in general.

10. Ethical, Societal and Economic Aspects Related to Pharmacogenomics Research and Its Application to Clinical Practice

The continuing scientific developments in the era of pharmacogenomics research and their unprecedented potentiality to empower the improvement of healthcare by ensuring drug efficacy and safety will eventually make routine genotyping and haplotyping analysis a standard procedure in clinical practice. However, before the widespread clinical use of pharmacogenomics principles in routine clinical practice and pharmacotyping in drug prescription process, several ethical, societal and economical aspects have firstly to be addressed [140, 141]. Issues related to legislation and regulatory mechanisms for conducting genome-based clinical research are of major concern in the society, especially the healthcare and regulatory authorities all over the world. These aspects include the concepts of informed consent, privacy and anonymity of persons subjected to pharmacogenomics analysis. In addition, problems of intellectual property rights applied to the genetic material collected and used for genotyping-haplotyping analysis in order to lead into new drug development, pharmacotyping and improvement of patient care will be raised in the years to come [142]. Furthermore, it is noteworthy that these societal and ethical issues of pharmacogenomics research also share ecomomic projections with major impact to the whole health and pharmaceutical care sectors and they must be clearly addressed accordingly. In this respect and besides its clinical consequences, genomic information nowadays may be used to pharmacoeconomic studies in a way to predict and evaluate healthcare cost, a result that for all healthcare payers is of major concern. This must be done, however, with caution, unbiased and by taking into consideration primarily the ethical and societal issues related to pharmacogenomics research. An example of this application type of pharmacogenomics is considered to be the ε4 allele of APOE gene located on chromosome 19 that has been shown to modulate tacrine pharmacotherapy outcome (Table 1). Also, ε4 allele is a potential susceptibility marker for heart disease, stroke and AD [24, 60]. In addition to this profound pharmacogenomics interest, ε4 allele has been recently evaluated in terms of pharmacoeconomics analysis on the possibility to be used as a measure for healthcare cost [143]. Although such studies are still few, undoubtedly it is expected that they will be in increasing numbers in the near future.

It is evident that the application of pharmacotyping in the drug prescription process requires the medical practitioner must have to look into patient's genetic privacy based on previous pharmacogenomics studies confirming the validity of what specific genotypes-haplotypes are compatible with what drug. However, pharmacogenomics data show that genetic variations and traits implicated in altered drug response are usually different amongst populations from various part of the world [1, 18]. So, an obvious question then rises. How do a pharmacogenomics-based molecular diagnostic test can be clinically tested and validated in order to be applied for all populations around the world, by taking apart the patient's ethnic origin? Furthermore, the same question seems to apply in the case of the drug development process and the criticism raised regarding the use of pharmacogenomics criteria for the stratification of patients recruited in clinical trials in order to gain better benefits from the response of the drug being tested [140]. In addition, the development of DNA-based molecular diagnostics by no mean must dismiss the utilization of classical biochemical tests such as measurement of enzymatic activity, but they have to work in parallel. As molecular diagnosis is getting simpler, cheaper and readily automated, then the application of pharmacogenomics will become more easily integrated in clinical practice. Undoubtedly, as the field of pharmacogenomics and personalized medicine continues to expand towards the development of relevant clinical research data, more issues will be raised for the society that they will need to be addressed. However, until pharmacogenomics research to be generally accepted in patient care, its beneficial clinical impact together with the ethical and societal aspects raised must be taken into consideration by all scientists being involved and the clinicians must work towards its clinical use to be compatible with the good clinical practice guidelines. Furthermore, issues related either to quality or validation of the genetic tests that could be applied in therapeutics must be clearly addressed, before the usage of genomic information in routine patient care.

11. Perspectives and Future Directions

Phenotypic variation within a species arises from differences in the genetic makeup between individuals, whereas the tendency of genes to mutate is the key to evolution and the existence of biodiversity in living organisms. Nowadays, the progress in biomolecular and genomic technologies achieved thus far facilitate the analysis and exploitation of genetic variations for therapeutic intervention. This fact has also paved the way for pharmacogenomic strategies to be developed and applied in clinical practice for improved patient care. However, after the completion of the HGP, scientists confront major challenges by trying to translate genomic results into relevant transformative clinical data to achieve major impacts in health and pharmaceutical care. But consequently, in order these directions in medical genetics, pharmacogenomics and personalized medicine to be fully beneficial for the public in routine patient care, several issues must firstly be addressed, concerning either the education and training of next generation health care professionals, or the development of suitable methods that would permit the smooth integration of genomic information in clinical practice, or even the awareness of the public in ethical and societal aspects concerning this type of scientific work [144, 145].

Pharmacogenomics research especially that related to polygenic and multifactorial diseases in order to become a reality in the near future, it must first address the existed biological complexity derived from the interplay and contribution of multiple environmental and genetic risk factors implicating several genes and signal transduction pathways. However, by using genomic information to create tools for perturbing gene function it will be possible to undertake systematic genome-wide functional screens to examine the contribution of every gene to a biological process. This basic experimental approach of functional genomics is reaching to reality through the generation of the first genome-wide functional screens for two model organisms *Caenorhabditis elegance* and *Drosophila melanogaster* [146]. These high-throughput techniques offer unique approaches for functional genomics and they promise the rapid elucidation of the function of each gene characterized by the whole-genome sequencing projects. In addition, this genomic information can be further exploited to drug-related genes like CYPs. Regarding the CYP polymorphisms and their clinical application for improved pharmacotherapy outcome, it will be greatly enhanced by the elucidation of enzyme crystal structures and subsequently the generation of more accurate pharmacophore models for the exploitation of binding properties of metabolized drugs. Such achievements happened recently with the enzyme CYP2C9 whose crystal structure was elucidated with bound warfarin (a drug substrate for CYP2C9) and the proposal of a new pharmacophore model for enzyme CYP2D6 [147, 148]. Therefore, by haplotyping analysis of specific genes, whose function in disease pathophysiology and consequently their pharmacological importance has been established, may lead to a further advancement in drug delivery by improving patient outcome in pharmaceutical care. As a matter of fact, the clinical integration of genomic data will be greatly advanced by careful design and experimentation of pharmacogenomic studies, ensuring genetic test quality, evaluating and validating the data in routine patient care, and finally positively affecting the rate by which genotyping data are transformed into personalized medicine, thus achieving pharmacotyping concepts as a future dimension of drug delivery [156].

Another future advancement that obviously depends upon the application of genomic technologies in clinical practice through the advent of personalized medicine will be the development and use in clinical practice of highly selective, in terms of their pharmacological response, multi-target drugs in order to avoid undesirable drug-related effects like the development of drug resistance and toxicity. Such strategy has been already applied for the development of more specific and effective drugs used to combat cancer [149]. Multi-target drugs represent a special group including either individual chemical molecules or macromolecules (developed as drugs) and are designed in such a way to modulate simultaneously several receptor-like motifs, e.g. those located either onto the same protcin and give multifunctional capacities to that entity, or on different proteins that, however, are implicated in, or constitute a downstream network pathway involved in different cellular functions. To move forward in designing selective and effective multi-target drugs, the need for extracting basic knowledge related to multifunctional properties of specific macromolecules contributing to cells economy, as well as the inter- and intra-convergence routes of individual signaling pathways that modulate the better orchestration of cell structure and function will be in stressing demands in the years to come. To this respect, by learning how to mimic cellular economy in the use of molecules and their functional flexibility, the drug discovery era will certainly gain new insights towards getting by on challenges of multi-target drug development for improved patient care.

References

[1] Ingelman-Saundberg, M., Oscarson, M. and McLellan, R.A. (1999). Polymorphic human cytochrome P450 enzymes: an opportunity for individualized drug treatment. *Tends Pharmacol. Sci.*, 20, 342-349.

[2] Meyer, U. A. (2000). Pharmacogenetics and adverse drug reactions. *Lancet*, 356: 1667-1671.

[3] Vizirianakis, I. S. (2004). Challenges in current drug delivery from the potential application of pharmacogenomics and personalized medicine in clinical practice. *Cur. Drug Deliv.* 1: 73-80.

[4] Housman, D. and Ledley, F. D. (1998). Why pharmacogenomics? Why now? *Nature Biotechnol.,* 16: 2-3.

[5] Evans, W. E., and Relling, M. V. (1999). Pharmacogenomics: Translating functional genomics into rational therapeutics. *Science*, 286: 487-491.

[6] McLeod, H. L. and Evans, W. E. (2001). Pharmacogenomics: Unlocking the human genome for better drug therapy. *Annu. Rev. Pharmacol. Toxicol.*, 41: 101-121.

[7] Roses, A. D. (2000). Pharmacogenetics and the practice of medicine. *Nature*, 405: 857-865.

[8] Nebert, D. W., Nebert, L. J. and Vesell, E. S. (2003). Pharmacogenomics and "individualized drug therapy": High expectations and disappointing achievements. *Am. J. Pharmacogenomics* 3: 361-370.

[9] Collins, F. S., Green, E. D., Guttmacher, A. E., Guyer, M. S. (2003). A vision for the future of genomics research. *Nature*, 422: 835-847.

[10] Emilien, G., Ponchon, M., Caldas, C., Isacson, O. and Maloteaux, J. M. (2000). Impact of genomics on drug discovery and clinical medicine. *Q. J. Med.* 93: 391-423.

[11] Norton, R. M. (2001). Clinical pharmacogenomics: applications in Pharmaceutical RandD. *Drug Discov. Today*, 6: 180-185.

[12] Müller, M. (2003). Pharmacogenomics and drug response. *Int. J. Clin. Pharmacol. Ther.*, 41: 231-240.

[13] Pirmohamed, M. and Park, B. K. (2001). Genetic susceptibility to adverse drug reactions. *Trends Pharmacol. Sci.*, 22: 298-305.

[14] Ginsburg, G. S. and McCarthy, J. J. (2001). Personalized medicine: revolutionizing drug discovery and patient care. *Trends Biotechnol.*, 19: 491-496.

[15] Evans, W. E. and McLeod, H. L. (2003). Pharmacogenomics--drug disposition, drug targets, and side effects. *N. Engl. J. Med.*, 348: 538-549.

[16] Drews, J. (2000). Drug discovery: A historical perspective. *Science* 287: 1960-1964.

[17] Vogel, F. (1959). Moderne probleme der humangenetik. *Ergeb. Inn. Med. Kinderheilk*, 12: 52-125.

[18] Ingelman-Sundberg, M. (2004). Pharmacogenetics of cytochrome P450 and its applications in drug therapy: the past, present and future. *Trends Pharmacol. Sci.*, 25: 193-200.

[19] Müller, M. (2003). Pharmacogenomics and the complexity of drug response. *Int. J. Clin. Pharmacol. Ther.*, 41: 231-240.

[20] Carson, P. E., Flanagan, C. L., Ickes, C. E. and Alving, A. S. (1956). Enzymatic deficiency in primaquine-sensitive erythrocytes. *Science,* 124: 484-485.

[21] Rusnak, J. M., Kisabeth, R. M., Herbert, D. P., McNeil, D. M. (2001). Pharmacogenomics: a clinician's primer on emerging technologies for improved patient care. *Mayo Clin. Proc.*, 76: 299-309.

[22] McCarthy, J. J. and Hilfiker, R. (2000). The use of single-nucleotide polymorphism in pharmacogenomics. *Nature Biotechnol.*, 18: 505-508.

[23] Weinshilboum, R. (2003). Inheritance and drug response. *N. Engl. J. Med*, 348: 529-537.

[24] Manasco, P. K., Rieser, P., Renegar, G. and Mosteller, M. (2002). Pharmacogenetics and the genetic basis of ADRs. In *Pharmacovigilance*, Mann R. D. and Andrews, E. B. (eds.), John Wiley and Sons, Ltd, West Sussex, pp. 516-553.

[25] Silber, B. M. (2003). Pharmacogenomics, biomarkers, and the promise of personalized medicine. In *Pharmacogenomics*, Kalow, W., Meyer, U. A., and Tyndale, R. F. (eds.), pp. 11-31, Marcel Dekker, Inc., New York.

[26] Lazarou, J., Pomeranz, B. H. and Corey, P. N. (1998). Incidence of adverse drug reactions in hospitalized patients: a meta-analysis of prospective studies. *JAMA* 279: 1200-1205.

[27] Kohn, L. T., Corrigan, J. M. and Donaldson, M. S. (eds.) (2000). To Err is human: Building a safer health system. Committee on Quality of Health Care in America, Institute of Medicine, The National Academy Press, Washington, DC.

[28] Flockhart, D. A. and Tanus-Santos, J. E. (2002). Implications of cytochrome P450 interactions when prescribing medication for hypertension. *Arch. Intern. Med.*, 162: 405-412.

[29] Ebbesen, J., Buajordet, I., Erikssen, J., Brors, O. Hilberg, T., Svaar, H. and Sandvik, L. (2001). Drug-Related Deaths in a Department of Internal Medicine. *Arch. Intern. Med.* 161: 2317-2323.

[30] Jazwinska, E. C. (2001). Exploiting human genetic variation in drug discovery and development. *Drug Discov. Today*, 6: 198-205.

[31] Guttmacher, A. E., and Collins, F. S. (2002). Genomic medicine – A primer. *N. Engl. J. Med.* 347: 1512-1520.

[32] Schwab, M., Eichelbaum, M. and Fromm, M. F. (2003). Genetic polymorphisms of the human MDR1 drug transporter. *Annu. Rev. Pharmacol. Toxicol.*, 43: 285-307.

[33] Sadee, W., Hoeg, E., Lukas, J. and Wang, D. (2001). Genetic variations in human G protein-coupled receptors: implications for drug therapy. *AAPS PharmSci.*, 3(3):E22 (available at: http://www.pharmsci.org).

[34] Desta, Z., Zhao, X., Shin, J-G. and Flockhart, D. A. (2002). Clinical significance of the cytochrome P450 2C19 genetic polymorphism. *Clin. Pharmacokinet.*, 41: 913-958.

[35] Burgstaller, P., Jenne, A. and Blind, M. (2002). Aptamers and aptazymes: accelerating small molecule drug discovery. *Curr. Opin. Drug Discov. Devel.*, 5: 690-700.

[36] Read, M. L. Farrow, P. J. and Seymour, L. W. (2003). Emerging developments in RNA therapeutics. *Expert Opin. Ther. Targets*, 7: 299-303.

[37] James, W. (2001). Nucleic acid and polypeptide aptamers: a powerful approach to ligand discovery. *Curr. Opin. Pharmacol.*, 1: 540-546.

[38] Sullenger, B. A. and Gilboa, B. A. (2002). Emerging clinical applications of RNA. *Nature*, 418: 252-258.

[39] Pillai, O. and Panchagnula, R. (2001). Polymers in drug delivery. *Curr. Opin. Chem. Biol.*, 5: 447-451.

[40] Chien, Y. W. and Lin, S. (2002). Optimisation of treatment by applying programmable rate-controlled drug delivery technology. *Clin. Pharmacokinet.*, 41: 1267-1299.

[41] Braeckmans, K., De Smedt, S. C., Leblans, M., Pauwels, R. and Demeester, J. (2002). Encoding microcarriers: present and future technologies. *Nat. Rev. Drug Discov.*, 1: 447-456.

[42] Torchilin, V. P. and Lukyanov, A. N. (2003). Peptide and protein drug delivery to and into tumors: challenges and solutions. *Drug Discov. Today*, 8: 259-266.

[43] Debouck, C. and Goodfellow, P.N. (1999). DNA microarrays in drug discovery and development. *Nature Genetics* 21(Suppl.), 48-50.

[44] Sander, C. (2000). Genomic medicine and the future of health care. *Science*, 287: 1977-1978.

[45] Schmitz, G., Aslanidis, C. and Lackner, K. J. (2001). Pharmacogenomics: implications for laboratory medicine. *Clin. Chim. Acta*, 308: 43-53.

[46] Hardiman, G. (2004). Microarray platforms-comparisons and contrasts. *Pharmacogenomics*, 5: 487-502.

[47] Searls, D. B. (2000). Using bioinformatics in gene and drug discovery. *Drug Discov. Today*, 5: 135-143.

[48] Myers, P. L. (1997). Will combinatorial chemistry deliver real medicines? *Curr. Opin. Biotechnol.*, 8: 701-707.

[49] Lee, K. H. (2001). Proteomics: a technology-driven and technology-limited discovery science. *Trends Biotechnol.*, 19: 217-222.

[50] Fussenegger, M. 2001. The impact of mammalian gene regulation concepts on functional genomic research, metabolic engineering, and advanced gene therapies. *Biotechnol. Prog.*, 17: 1-51.

[51] Landro, J. A., Taylor, I. C. A., Stirtan, W. G., Osterman, D. G., Kristie, J., Hunnicutt, E. J., Rae, P. M. M. and Sweetnam, P. M. (2000). HTS in the new millenium: The role of pharmacology and flexibility. *J. Pharmacol. Toxicol. Methods*, 44: 273-289.

[52] Searls, D. B. (2000). Using bioinformatics in gene and drug discovery. *Drug Discov. Today,* 5: 135-143.

[53] Cadman, P. E. and O'Connor, D. T. (2003). Pharmacogenomics of hypertension. *Cur. Opin. Nephrol. Hypertens.*, 12: 61-70.

[54] Rudnicki, M. and Mayer, G. (2003). Pharmacogenomics of angiotensin converting enzyme inhibitors in renal disease--pathophysiological considerations. *Pharmacogenomics,* 4: 153-162.

[55] Humma, L. M. and Terra, S. G. (2002). Pharmacogenetics and cardiovascular disease: impact on drug response and applications to disease management. *Am. J. Health-Syst. Pharm.*, 59: 1241-1252.

[56] Anderson, J. L., Carlquist, J. F., Horne, B. D. and Muhlestein, J. B. (2003) Cardiovascular pharmacogenomics: current status, future prospects. *J. Cardiovasc. Pharmacol. Ther.*, 8: 71-83.

[57] Ferrari, P. (1998). Pharmacogenomics: a new approach to individual therapy of hypertension? *Cur. Opin. Nephrol. Hypertens.*, 7: 217-222.

[58] Ferrari, P. and Bianchi, G. (2000). The genomics of cardiovascular disorders. *Drugs*, 59: 1025-1042.

[59] Nakagawa, K. and Ishizaki, T. 2000. Therapeutic relevance of pharmacogenetic factors in cardiovascular medicine. *Pharmacol. Therapeut.* 86, 1-28.

[60] Cacabelos, R. (2004). The application of functional genomics to Alzheimer's disease. *Pharmacogenomics*, 4: 597-621.

[61] Ulrich, C. M., Robien, K. and Mcleod, H. L. (2003). Cancer pharmacogenetics: Polymorphisms, pathways and beyond. *Nat. Rev. Cancer*, 3: 912-920.

[62] Loktionov, A. (2004). Common gene polymorphisms, cancer progression and prognosis. *Cancer Lett.*, 208:1-33.

[63] Stearns, V., Davidson, N. E. and Flockhart, D. A. (2004). Pharmacogenetics in the treatment of breast cancer. *Pharmacogenomics J.*, 4: 143-153.

[64] Palmer, L. J., Silverman, E. S., Weiss, S. T. and Drazen, J. M. (2002). Pharmacogenetics of asthma. *Am. J. Respir. Crit. Care Med.*, 165: 861-866.

[65] Peisong, G., Mao, X-Q, Enomoto, T., Feng, Z., Gloria-Bottini, F., Bottini, E., Shirakawa, T., Sun, D. and Hopkin, J. M. (2004). An asthma-associated genetic variant of STAT6 predicts low burden of ascaris worm infestation. *Genes Immunity*, 5: 58-62.

[66] Gage, B. F., Eby, C., Milligan, P. E., Banet, G. A., Duncan, J. R. and McLeod, H. L. (2004). Use of pharmacogenetics and clinical factors to predict the maintenance dose of warfarin. *Thromb. Haemost.*, 91: 87-94.

[67] Wrighton, S. A., Schuetz, E. G., Thummel, K. E., Shen, D. D., Korzekwa, K. R. and Watkins, P. B. (2000). The human CYP3A subfamily: practical considerations. *Drug Metab. Rev.*, 32: 339-361.

[68] Nelson, D. R., Zeldin, D. C., Hoffman, S. M., Maltais, L. J., Wain, H. M. and Nebert, D. W. (2004). Comparison of cytochrome P450 (CYP) genes from the mouse and human genomes, including nomenclature recommendations for genes, pseudogenes and alternative-splice variants. *Pharmacogenetics* 14: 1-18.

[69] Sakaeda, T., Nakamura, T. and Okumura, K. (2003). Pharmacogenetics of MDR1 and its impact on the pharmacokinetics and pharmacodynamics of drugs. *Pharmacogenomics*, 4: 397-410.

[70] Small, K. M., Tanguay, D. A., Nandabalan, K., Zhan, P., Stephens, J. C. and Liggett, S. B. (2003). Gene and protein domain-specific patterns of genetic variability within the G-protein coupled receptor superfamily. *Am. J. Pharmacogenomics*, 3: 65-71.

[71] McLeod, H. L. and Siva, C. (2002). The thiopurine S-methyltransferase gene locus -- implications for clinical pharmacogenomics. *Pharmacogenomics,* 3: 89-98.

[72] Meisel, P. (2002). Arylamine N-acetyltransferases and drug response. *Pharmacogenomics*, 3: 349-366.

[73] Guillemette, C. (2003) Pharmacogenomics of human UDP-glucuronosyltransferase enzymes. *Pharmacogenomics J.*, 3: 136-158.

[74] Siddiqui, A., Kerb, R., Weale, M. E., Brinkmann, U., Smith, A., Goldstein, D. B., Wood, N. W. and Sisodiya, S. M. (2003). Association of multidrug resistance in epilepsy with a polymorphism in the drug-transporter gene ABCB1. *N. Engl. J. Med.*, 348: 1442-1448.

[75] Doherty, M. M. and Charman, W. N. (2002). The mucosa of the small intestine: how clinically relevant as an organ of drug metabolism? *Clin. Pharmacokinet.*, 41: 235-253.

[76] Lin, J. H. and Yamazaki, M. (2003). Role of P-glycoprotein in pharmacokinetics: clinical implications. *Clin. Pharmacokinet.*, 42: 59-98.

[77] Ioannides, C. (1999). Effect of diet and nutrition on the expression of cytochromes P450. *Xenobiotica*, 29: 109-154.

[78] Flockhart, D. A,; Yasuda, S. U., Pezzullo, J. C., Knollmann, B. C. (2002). Teaching rational prescribing: a new clinical pharmacology curriculum for medical schools. *Naunyn-Schmiedeberg's Arch. Pharmacol.*, 366: 33-43.

[79] Bailey, D. G., Dresser, G. K. and Bend, J. R. (2003). Bergamottin, lime juice, and red wine as inhibitors of cytochrome P450 3A4 activity: comparison with grapefruit juice. *Clin. Pharmacol. Ther.*, 73: 529-537.

[80] Lin, J. H. (2003). Drug-drug interaction mediated by inhibition and induction of P-glycoprotein. *Adv. Drug Deliv. Rev.*, 55: 53-81.

[81] Bredel, M. and Zentner, J. (2002). Brain-tumour drug resistance: the bare essentials *Lancet Oncol.*, 3: 397-406.

[82] Drysdale, C. M., McGraw, D. W., Stack, C. B., Stephens, J. C., Judson, R. S., Nandabalan, K., Arnold, K., Ruano, G. and Liggett, S. B. (2000). Complex promoter and coding region beta 2-adrenergic receptor haplotypes alter receptor expression and predict in vivo responsiveness. *Proc. Natl. Acad. Sci. U. S. A.,* 97: 10483-10488.

[83] Hall, I. P. (2002). Pharmacogenetics, pharmacogenomics and airway disease. *Respir. Res.*, 3: 10.

[84] Liggett, S. B. (2002). Update on current concepts of the molecular basis of beta2-adrenergic receptor signaling. *J. Allergy Clin. Immunol.*, 110: S223-S227.

[85] Strange, P. G. (2002). Mechanisms of inverse agonism at G-protein-coupled receptors. *Trends Pharmacol. Sci.*, 23: 89-95.

[86] Kenakin, T. (2002). Efficacy at G-protein-coupled receptors. *Nature Rev. Drug Discov.*, 1: 103-110.

[87] Watters, J. W. and McLeod, H. L. (2003). Cancer pharmacogenomics: current and future applications. *Biochim. Biophys. Acta*, 1603: 99-111.

[88] Coulthard, S. A. and Hall, A. G. (2001). Recent advances in the pharmacogenomics of thiopurine methyltransferase. *Pharmacogenomics J.*, 1: 254-261.

[89] Krynetski, E. Y. and Evans, W. E. (2000). Genetic polymorphism of thiopurine S-methyltransferase: molecular mechanisms and clinical importance. *Pharmacology*, 61: 136-146.

[90] O'Kane D. J., Weinshilboum, R. M. and Moyer, T. P. (2003). Pharmacogenomics and reducing the frequency of adverse drug events. *Pharmacogenomics*, 4: 1-4.

[91] Marshall, E. (2003). Preventing toxicity with a gene test. *Science,* 302: 588-590.

[92] Coulthard, S. A., Hogarth, L. A., Little, M., Matheson, E. C., Redfern, C. P., Minto, L. and Hall, A.G. (2002). The effect of thiopurine methyltransferase expression on sensitivity to thiopurine drugs. *Mol. Pharmacol.*, 62: 102-109.

[93] Goldstein, D. B. (2003). Pharmacogenetics in the laboratory and the clinic. *N. Engl. J. Med.*, 348: 553-556.

[94] Ginsburg, G. S. and McCarthy, J. J. (2001). Personalized medicine: revolutionizing drug discovery and patient care. *Trends Biotechnol.*, 19: 491-496.

[95] Robertson, K. D. and Wolffe, A. P. (2000). DNA methylation in health and disease. *Nature Rev. Genet.*, 1: 11-19.

[96] Johnstone, R. W. (2002). Histone-deacetylase inhibitors: Novel drugs for the treatment of cancer. *Nature Rev. Drug Discov.*, 1: 287-299.

[97] Mittal, V. (2004). Improving the efficiency of RNA interference in mammals. *Nature Rev. Genet.*, 5: 355-365.

[98] Dorsett, Y. and Tuschl, T. (2004). siRNAs: Applications in functional genomics and potential as therapeutics. *Nature Rev. Drug Discov.*, 3: 318-329.

[99] Baylin, S. B. and Jones, P. A. (2002). The fundamental role of epigenetic events in cancer. *Nature Rev. Genet.*, 3: 415-428.102.

[100] Halapi, E. and Hakonarson, H. (2002). Advances in the development of genetic markers for the diagnosis of disease and drug response. *Expert Rev. Mol. Diagn.* 2: 411-421.

[101] Liddle, C. and Robertson, G. R. (2003). Predicting inductive drug-drug interactions. *Pharmacogenomics,* 4: 141-152.

[102] Phillips, K. A., Veenstra, D. L., Oren, E., Lee, J. K., and Sadee, W. (2001). Potential role of pharmacogenomics in reducing adverse drug reactions: a systematic review. *JAMA*, 286: 2270-2279.

[103] Güzey, C. and Spigset, O. (2002). Genotyping of drug targets: a method to predict adverse drug reactions? *Drug Safety*, 25: 553-560.

[104] Lindpaintner, K. (2002). The importance of being modest--reflections on the pharmacogenetics of abacavir. *Pharmacogenomics*, 3: 835-838.

[105] Mallal, S., Nolan, D., Witt, C., Masel, G., Martin, A. M., Moore, C., Sayer, D., Castley, A., Mamotte, C., Maxwell, D., James, I. and Christiansen, F. T. (2002). Association between presence of HLA-B*5701, HLA-DR7, and HLA-DQ3 and hypersensitivity to HIV-1 reverse-transcriptase inhibitor abacavir. *Lancet*, 359: 727-732.

[106] Hetherington, S., Hughes, A. R., Mosteller, M., Shortino, D., Baker, K. L., Spreen, W., Lai, E., Davies, K., Handley, A., Dow, D. J., Fling, M. E., Stocum, M., Bowman, C., Thurmond, L. M. and Roses, A. D. (2002). Genetic variations in HLA-B region and hypersensitivity reactions to abacavir. *Lancet*, 359: 1121-1122.

[107] Telenti, A., Aubert, V. and Spertini, F. (2002). Individualising HIV treatment-pharmacogenetics and immunogenetics. *Lancet,* 359: 722-723.

[108] Hall, A. G., Coulthard, S. A. and Irving, J. A. (2003). Molecular diagnostics: a healthcare perspective. *Expert Rev. Mol. Diagn.*, 3: 13-16.

[109] Halapi, E. and Hakonarson, H. (2002). Advances in the development of genetic markers for the diagnosis of disease and drug response. *Expert Rev. Mol. Diagn.*, 2: 411-421.

[110] Johnson, J. A. and Evans, W. E. (2002). Molecular diagnostics as a predictive tool: genetics of drug efficacy and toxicity. *Trends Mol. Med.*, 8: 300-305.

[111] Dequeker, E., Ramsden, S., Grody, W. W., Stenzel, T. T. and Barton, D. E. (2001). Quality control in molecular genetic testing. *Nature Rev. Genet.*, 2: 717-723.

[112] Evans, W. E. and Johnson, J. A. (2001). Pharmacogenomics: the inherited basis for interindividual differences in drug response. *Annu. Rev. Genomics Hum. Genet.*, 2: 9-39.

[113] Johnson, J. A. and Terra, S. G. (2002). Beta-adrenergic receptor polymorphisms: cardiovascular disease associations and pharmacogenetics. *Pharm Res.*, 19: 1779-1787.

[114] Traxler, P. (2003). Tyrosine kinases as targets in cancer therapy - successes and failures. *Expert Opin. Ther. Targets*, 7: 215-34.

[115] Tenen, D. G. (2003). Disruption of differentiation in human cancer: AML shows the way. *Nature Rev. Cancer*, 3: 89-101.

[116] Graf, T. (2002). Differentiation plasticity of hematopoietic cells. *Blood*, 99: 3089-3101.

[117] Hockenbery, D. M., Giedt, C. D., O'Neill, J. W., Manion, M. K. and Banker, D. E. (2002). Mitochondria and apoptosis: New therapeutic targets. *Adv. Cancer Res.*, 85: 203-242.

[118] Fischer, O. M., Streit, S., Hart, S. and Ullrich, A. (2003). Beyond Herceptin and Gleevec. *Cur. Opin. Chem. Biol.*, 7: 490-495.

[119] Tsiftsoglou, A. S., Pappas, I. S. and Vizirianakis, I. S. (2003). Mechanisms involved in the induced differentiation of leukemia cells. *Pharmacol Ther.*, 100: 257-290.

[120] Capdeville, R., Buchdunger, E., Zimmermann, J., and Matter, A. (2002). Clivec (STI-571, imatinib), a rationally developed, targeted anticancer drug. *Nature Rev. Drug Discov.,* 1: 493-502.

[121] Cowan-Jacob, S. W., Guez, V., Fendrich, G., Griffin, J. D, Fabbro, D., Furet, P., Liebetanz, J., Mestan, J. and Manley, P. W. (2004). Imatinib (STI571) resistance in chronic myelogenous leukemia: molecular basis of the underlying mechanisms and potential strategies for treatment. *Mini Rev. Med. Chem.*, 4: 285-299.

[122] Domen, J. (2001). The role of apoptosis in regulating hematopoietic stem cell numbers. *Apoptosis*, 6: 239-252.

[123] Tsiftsoglou, A. S., Pappas, I. S., and Vizirianakis, I. S. (2003). The developmental program of murine erythroleukemia cells. *Oncol. Res.*, 13: 339-346.

[124] Lindpaintner, K. (2002). The impact of pharmacogenetics and pharmacogenomics on drug discovery. *Nature Rev. Drug Discov.*, 1: 463-469.

[125] Cho, H-S., Mason, K., Ramyar, K. X., Stanley, A. M., Gabelli, S. B., Denney, D. W. Jr and Leahy, D. J. (2003). Structure of the extracellular region of HER2 alone and in complex with the Herceptin Fab. *Nature*, 421: 756-760.

[126] Ma, X. J, Salunga, R., Tuggle, J. T., Gaudet, J., Enright, E., McQuary, P., Payette, T., Pistone, M., Stecker, K., Zhang, B. M., Zhou, Y. X., Varnholt, H., Smith, B., Gadd, M., Chatfield, E., Kessler, J., Baer, T. M., Erlander, M. G. and Sgroi, D. C. (2003). Gene expression profiles of human breast cancer progression. *Proc. Natl. Acad. Sci. U. S. A.*, 100: 5974-5979.

[127] Cheok, M. H., Yang, W., Pui, C. H., Downing, J. R., Cheng, C., Naeve, C. W., Relling, M. V. and Evans, W. E. (2003). Treatment-specific changes in gene expression discriminate in vivo drug response in human leukemia cells. *Nature Genet.*, 34: 85-90.

[128] Slonim, D. K. (2001). Transcriptional profiling in cancer: the path to clinical pharmacogenomics. *Pharmacogenomics*, 2: 123-136.

[129] Attar, M. and Lee, V. H. (2003). Pharmacogenomic considerations in drug delivery. *Pharmacogenomics*, 4: 443-461.

[130] Van de Waterbeemd, H. and Gifford, E. (2003). ADMET in silico modeling: towards prediction paradise? *Nature Rev. Drug Discov.*, 2: 192-204.

[131] Weigl, B. H., Bardell, R. L. and Cabrera, C. R. (2003). Lab-on-a-chip for drug development. *Adv. Drug Deliv. Rev.*, 55: 349-377.

[132] Vizirianakis, I. S. (2002). Pharmaceutical education in the wake of genomic technologies for drug development and personalized medicine. *Eur. J. Pharm. Sci.*, 15: 243-250.

[133] Gurwitz, D., Weizman, A. and Rehavi, M. (2003). Education: Teaching pharmacogenomics to prepare future physicians and researchers for personalized medicine. *Trends Pharmacol. Sci.*, 24: 122-125.

[134] Brock, T. P., Valgus, J. M., Smith, S. R., and Summers, K. M. (2003). Pharmacogenomics: implications and considerations for pharmacists. *Pharmacogenomics*, 4: 321-330.

[135] Wieczorek, S. J. and Tsongalis, G. J. (2001). Pharmacogenomics: will it change the field of medicine? *Clin. Chim. Acta*, 308: 1-8.

[136] Hughes, I., Hollingsworth, M., Jones, S. J. and Markham, T. (1997). Knowledge and skills needs of pharmacology graduates in first employment: how do pharmacology courses measure up? *Trends Pharmacol. Sci.*, 18: 111-116.

[137] Landro, J. A., Taylor, I. C., Stirtan, W. G., Osterman, D. G., Kristie, J., Hunnicutt, E. J., Rae, P. M. and Sweetnam, P. M. (2000). HTS in the new millennium: the role of pharmacology and flexibility. *J. Pharmacol. Toxicol. Methods,* 44: 273-289.

[138] Rodriguez, R., Vidrio, H., Lopez-Martinez, E., Contreras, E. and Valenzuela, F. (1997). Changing the countenance of pharmacology courses in medical schools. Changing the countenance of pharmacology courses in medical schools. *Trends Pharmacol. Sci.*, 18: 314-318.

[139] Ross, J. S. and Ginsburg, G. S. (2002). Integrating diagnostics and therapeutics: revolutionizing drug discovery and patient care. *Drug Discov. Today*, 7: 859-864.

[140] Issa, A. M. (2002). Ethical perspectives on pharmacogenomic profiling in the drug development process. *Nat. Rev. Drug Disc.,* 1: 300-308.

[141] Kalow, W. and Motulsky, A. G. (2001). General conclusions and future directions. In *Pharmacogenomics* (eds.) Kalow, W., Meyer, U. A. and Tyndale, R. F., pp. 389-395, Marcel Dekker Inc., New York.

[142] Issa, A. M. (2000). Ethical considerations in clinical pharmacogenomics research. *Trends Pharmacol. Sci.*, 21: 247-250.

[143] Taylor, D. H. Jr. (2003). Caution in the use of the apolipoprotein E ε4 allele as a predictor of healthcare cost. *Expert Rev. Pharmacoeconomics Outcomes Res.*, 3: 569-573.

[144] Varmus, H. (2002). Getting ready for gene-based medicine. *N. Engl. J. Med.*, 347: 1526-1527.

[145] Weber, W. W., Caldwell, M. D. and Kurth, J. H. (2003). Edging toward personalized medicine. *Cur. Pharmacogenomics*, 1: 193-202.

[146] Carpenter, A. E. and Sabatini, D. M. (2004). Systematic genome-wide screens of gene function. *Nature Rev. Genet.*, 5: 11-22.

[147] Williams, P. A., Cosme, J., Ward, A., Angove, H. C., Matak-Vinkovic, D. and Jhoti, H. (2003). Crystal structure of human cytochrome P450 2C9 with bound warfarin. *Nature,* 424: 464-468.

[148] Guengerich, F. P., Miller, G. P., Hanna, I. H., Martin, M. V., Leger, S., Black, C., Chauret, N., Silva, J. M., Trimble, L. A., Yergey, J. A. and Nicoll-Griffith, D. A. (2002). Diversity in the oxidation of substrates by cytochrome P450 2D6: lack of an obligatory role of aspartate 301-substrate electrostatic bonding. *Biochemistry*, 41: 11025-11034.

[149] Vorshavsky, A. (1998). Codominant interference, antieffectors, and multitarget drugs. *Proc. Natl. Acad. Sci. U.S.A.*, 95: 2094-2099.

[150] Furuta, T., Shirai, N., Sugimoto, M., Ohashi, K. and Ishizaki, T. (2004). Pharmacogenomics of proton pump inhibitors. *Pharmacogenomics*, 5: 181-202.

[151] Drazen, J. M., Yandava, C. N., Dube, L., Szczerback, N., Hippensteel, R., Pillari, A., Israel, E., Schork, N., Silverman, E. S., Katz, D. A. and Drajesk, J. (1999). Pharmacogenetic association between ALOX5 promoter genotype and the response to anti-asthma treatment. *Nature Genet.*, 22: 168-170.

[152] Layton, M. A., Jones, P. W., Alldersea, J. E., Strange, R. C., Fryer, A. A., Dawes, P. T. and Mattey, D. L. (1999). The therapeutic response to D-penicillamine in rheumatoid

arthritis: influence of glutathione S-transferase polymorphisms. *Rheumatology*, 38: 43-47.

[153] Arranz, M. J., Munro, J., Birkett, J., Bolonna, A., Mancama, D., Sodhi, M., Lesch, K. P., Meyer, J. F., Sham, P., Collier, D. A., Murray, R. M. and Kerwin, R. W. (2000). Pharmacogenetic prediction of clozapine response. *Lancet,* 355: 1615-1616.

[154] Anantharam, A., Markowitz, S. M. and Abbott, G. W. (2003). Pharmacogenetic considerations in diseases of cardiac ion channels. *J. Pharmacol. Exp. Ther.*, 307: 831-838.

[155] Tsai, Y. J. and Hoyme, H. E. (2002). Pharmacogenomics: the future of drug therapy. *Clin. Genet.*, 62: 257-264.

[156] Vizirianakis, I. S. (2005). Improving pharmacotherapy outcomes by pharmacogenomics: from expectation to reality? *Pharmacogenomics*, 6: 701-711.

In: New Research on Pharmacogenetics
Editors: Linda P. Barnes, pp. 39-81
ISBN: 1-60021-056-2

Chapter II

Development, Analysis and Use of Pharmacogenomic Time Series for Pharmacokinetic/Pharmacodynamic Modeling of Multi-Tissue Polygenic Responses to Corticosteroids

Richard R. Almon, Debra C. DuBois, Jin Y. Jin, Zhenling Yao, Anasuya Hazra, Mahesh Samtani, Grayson Snyder, William Piel and William J. Jusko

Department of Biological Sciences (RRA, DCD, GS, WP) and Department of Pharmaceutical Sciences (RRA, DCD, JYJ, ZY, AH, MS, WJJ), State University of New York at Buffalo, Buffalo NY

Abstract

Many drugs either directly or indirectly alter the expression of genes. Such changes in gene expression can be the consequences of cascades of molecular events in time often involving many tissues. The molecular cascades in complex biological systems usually result in polygenic phenomena related to either the efficacious or adverse effects of the drug. Mechanism-based pharmacokinetic/pharmacodynamic (PK/PD) modeling provides a tool for formulating testable quantitative hypotheses relevant to such aspects of drug treatment as dosing and dosing regimen. In order to develop such models for polygenic phenomena it is necessary that a large amount of data be acquired within the context of a single experimental paradigm so that realistic temporal relationships between events can be evaluated. Gene arrays when used in a time series construct provide a powerful tool for generating the magnitude of organized temporal data necessary for constructing PK/PD models of complex polygenic phenomena. Such models can then serve as a transcriptional scaffold onto which translational and post-translational events can be placed. The intent is to construct a realistic motion picture of the phenomena that can be used to devise regimens of drugs or combinations of drugs that maximize efficacy while minimizing adverse effects. Obtaining data from gene arrays that can be used to develop

PK/PD models is dependant on the appropriate resolution of several considerations. The first is the construct of the time series. The second is data mining to identify the percentage of the genes whose expression is affected by the drug. The third is cluster analysis in order to group genes with similar temporal signatures. The fourth is text mining to place these genes in functionally relevant clusters. The last is placing the vast amount of data into a relational organization that allows for reasonable navigation amongst the different levels of information. The nature and some limited approaches to resolution of these problems is addressed using the synthetic glucocorticoid, methylprednisolone, with a rich time series following a bolus dose of drug and analysis of multiple tissues from the same animals.

Introduction

Corticosteroids have potent anti-inflammatory, anti-proliferative and immunosuppressive effects that define their pharmacological use as immunosuppressant and anti-inflammatory agents [1-3]. These synthetic glucocorticoids are used therapeutically for a variety of conditions including transplantation (bone marrow, liver, and kidney), asthma, nephrotic syndrome, Crohn's disease, lupus, multiple sclerosis, dermatomyositis, arthritis, inflammatory bowel disease, leukemia and non-Hodgkin's lymphoma. Beneficial effects deriving from inhibition of the immune system are accompanied by adverse effects that include hyperglycemia, dyslipidemia, muscle wasting, hypertension, nephropathy, fatty liver, and an increased risk of atherosclerosis [4-8]. Both beneficial and adverse effects derive from the pharmacological exaggeration of the physiological effects of glucocorticoids.

Physiologically, the hypothalamic/pituitary/adrenal (HPA) axis and its primary effector hormones, the glucocorticoids, impact virtually every tissue. Normally circulating glucocorticoids vary in a circadian pattern with a peak during the active wake period and a trough during the inactive sleep period [9-11]. However, stress can increase glucocorticoids in circulation during both the peak and trough periods. Three tissues that are highly important to systemic influences of glucocorticoids are the liver, kidney, and skeletal muscle. Together these three tissues play major roles in energy substrate availability, distribution, and utilization. They also have major impacts on blood volume, content, and distribution. Understanding glucocorticoid effects on these three tissues provides the basis for appreciating many of the adverse effects resulting from the pharmacological use of corticosteroids.

Physiological Effects of Glucocorticoids: Liver, Kidney, Skeletal Muscle

The liver provides the most fundamental protection for the brain in that it stores glucose in the form of glycogen and releases it to maintain adequate amounts in circulation. Glucose is the fundamental energy substrate for the brain and unlike many tissues the brain does not store glycogen. The brain is dependant on the constant delivery of glucose by the circulation. If glucose concentration in circulation is inadequate, then the brain rapidly dysfunctions. The liver is the only organ that stores and releases glucose to maintain adequate circulating levels. However, maintenance of systemic glucose concentrations is not solely dependant on liver glycogen stores. The liver is also one of only two tissues that are capable of synthesizing glucose from non-carbohydrate sources. Gluconeogenesis is essentially the reverse of glycolysis in which glucose is synthesized from pyruvate starting with a variety of substrates, but predominantly from amino acid carbon and glycerol derived from fats. Gluconeogenesis requires the expression of three specific enzymes to circumvent the irreversible steps in glycolysis. The first enzyme is phosphoenolpyruvate carboxykinase (PEPCK) the rate-limiting enzyme, which circumvents the irreversible step in the conversion of oxaloacetate to phosphoenolpyruvate. The oxaloacetate is formed from pyruvate by the enzyme pyruvate carboxylase, which is not unique to gluconeogenesis. The second, enzyme is fructose-1,6-bisphosphatase (F1,6BPase) which converts fructose-1,6-bisphosphate to fructose-6-phosphate. The last enzyme is glucose-6-phosphatase (G6Pase), which converts glucose-6-phosphate to glucose. The transcription of all three of these enzymes in liver is greatly enhanced by glucocorticoids [12-16].

A major substrate for gluconeogenesis is amino acid carbon. The use of amino acid carbon for gluconeogenesis requires both removal and disposal of ammonia. Removal of ammonia is accomplished by amino acid transaminases. These enzymes remove the ammonia from the amino acid, transferring it to α-ketoglutarate to form glutamate. Removal of ammonia from alanine, the second most abundant amino acid in circulation, yields pyruvate, which can be used directly for gluconeogenesis. Removal of ammonia from glutamine, the most abundant amino acid in circulation, yields glutamate. Glutamate is a major carrier of nitrogen for the formation of urea, which occurs through an additional transaminase reaction, regenerating α-ketogluterate in the process. Urea serves as the non-toxic carrier of ammonia. Urea formation involves alterations in the expression of both cytoplasmic and mitochondrial proteins. It is well documented that glucocorticoids alter the expression of many genes involved in urea formation [12, 17-19]. Changes in the expression of many proteins such as the transaminases by glucocorticoids is direct while others such as carbamyl phosphate synthetase and arginase are indirect by way of glucocorticoid enhancement of the expression of other transcription factors such as CCAAT/enhancer binding protein beta (C/EBPβ) [19].

Just as the liver is central to the control of systemic carbohydrate storage and distribution it is also pivotal to the control, storage and distribution of fats. Fats represent the largest source of stored energy in the body. Fat is either of dietary origin or is synthesized from excess carbohydrate. Of particular importance is the role of cholesterol in the distribution of fats. The liver is the only tissue that can dispose of large amounts of cholesterol through its production of bile. In conjunction with the production of bile acids, the liver also has the capacity to produce very substantial amounts of cholesterol. Apolipoproteins synthesized in the liver are used to assemble and distribute lipoproteins containing triglycerides and cholesterol esters to other tissues in the form of VLDL, which is degraded to form LDL. Cholesterol can then be recovered by the liver through LDL receptors. The liver also receives cholesterol from other tissues in the form of HDL by way of HDL receptors. The control of this process is under complex hormonal and dietary control. In general glucocorticoids promote the distribution of fats and reduce the uptake of cholesterol by the liver. The transcriptional influence of glucocorticoids is both direct through a glucocorticoid regulatory element (GRE) and indirect by way of their influence on the expression of other transcription factors such as sterol regulatory element-binding proteins (SREBP-1) [20, 21].

In addition to apolipoproteins from which lipoproteins are constructed the liver also produces a variety of serum proteins. These proteins range from albumin and carrier proteins for steroids and vitamin D to proteins involved in certain specific systemic processes. For example, the liver produces a variety of proteins that either promote immune/inflammatory responses such as elements of the compliment cascade, or inhibit aspects of the response such as macroglobins. The liver also produces proteins such as fibrinogen that are involved in blood clotting. The expressions of many of these proteins are also influenced by glucocorticoids [22-26].

The major function of the kidney is to balance blood volume with the small molecule quality of the blood. Regulation of kidney function is a multifaceted balancing of small molecules and ion concentrations with blood volume and blood pressure. The kidney is also the only tissue other than the liver that expresses the enzymes necessary for gluconeogenesis. However, gluconeogenesis in the kidney is relevant not only to the production of glucose from amino acid carbon but also to systemic acid-base balance. Ammonia (NH_3) removed from the carbon skeletons of amino acids is uncharged and freely diffuses across the tubule membrane. In conditions of acidosis, hydrogen ions are pumped across the tubule membrane and form ammonium ions (NH_4^+), which because of their charge are trapped and removed from the blood. Glucocorticoids are capable of binding to both the glucocorticoid and the mineralocorticoid receptors in the kidney [27, 28]. Physiologically, the mineralocorticoid receptor is protected from endogenous glucorticoid binding by the enzyme 11 beta-hydroxysteroid dehydrogenase (11β-HSD), which converts cortisol and corticosterone to hormonally inactive cortisone and 11-dehydrocorticosterone. However, in conditions in which 11β-HSD is deficient or natural glucocorticoids are excessive, cortisol (humans) or corticosterone (rodents) have potent mineralocorticoid effects resulting in sodium retention and increased blood volume [29, 30].

Skeletal muscle represents about 40 percent of the protein mass of most mammals. The apparent functions of the musculature, movement and posture, are subservient to its metabolic function as the primary source of amino acid carbon for gluconeogenesis in the liver and kidney. Under the influence of glucocorticoids skeletal muscle is shifted into a net degradative state yielding excess free amino acids [31-34]. The net degradation is duc to both increased degradation of and a reduced synthesis of proteins. Glucocorticoids enhance the expression of proteins of the ubiquitin proteosome degradative system [35-38] while at the same time they reduce the anabolic influences of insulin, insulin like growth factor-1 (IGF-I), and growth hormone [39-43]. Contractile proteins, which represent 70 to 80 percent of total muscle protein, are disproportionately lost and are thus the major systemic contributor of amino acid carbon. Glucocorticoids also enhance the expression of the enzyme glutamine synthetase, which converts glutamate to glutamine [44-47]. Glutamine serves as the major systemic carrier of ammonia to the liver and kidney for disposal. The removal of amino acid carbon from the musculature is not equally distributed amongst all muscles. The more active tonic postural muscle fibers contribute less than the less active phasic muscle fibers involved in movement. The musculature is also responsible for about 70-80% of the insulin-directed glucose disposal [48]. Finally control of the distribution of blood to the musculature is important in the regulation of blood pressure.

Corticosteroid Pharmacology: Liver, Kidney and Skeletal Muscle

Corticosteroids are a major class of the immunosuppressive/anti-inflammatory drugs. Of the three tissues sensitive to steroid regulated gluconeogenesis, only the liver also directly contributes significantly to the immunosuppressive/anti-inflammatory effects of corticosteroids. However, all three tissues contribute collectively to the adverse effects of these drugs. In addition, corticosteroids have significant adverse effects on these tissues individually.

A major adverse effect of corticosteroids is steroid diabetes [4, 5, 7, 43]. Excessive corticosteroid directed wasting of the musculature provides amino acid carbon for excessive gluconeogenesis in the liver and kidney. Uptake of the large amount of glucose produced by the liver and kidney into the musculature is greatly decreased due to a glucocorticoid-induced decrease in insulin sensitivity (insulin resistance). The newly synthesized glucose is therefore maintained in circulation. Insulin resistance in the musculature is caused by the change in the expression of many genes. Decreases in the expression of proteins such as insulin receptor substrate-1 along with increases in the expression of genes such as protein-tyrosine phosphatase type 1B inhibit the insulin-signaling cascade [49-53]. Other changes in gene expression impair the ability of skeletal muscle to carry out glycolysis. For example, there is an increased expression of the enzyme pyruvate dehydrogenase kinase isoenzyme 4, which inactivates the mitochondrial pyruvate dehydrogenase complex necessary for the disposal of pyruvate [54, 55]. Some changes are direct while others are the result of changes in the expression of transcription factors such as the reduced expression of SREBP-1c [21, 56].

Corticosteroid treatment causes an elevation in plasma levels of triglycerides and cholesterol [57, 58]. Corticosteroids enhance the already large capacity of the liver to synthesize cholesterol. The rate-limiting enzyme in the synthesis of cholesterol is 3-hydroxy-3-methylglutaryl-CoA reductase. Hepatic cholesterol pools are a major factor regulating the expression of this enzyme [59, 60]. Data are available demonstrating the ability of corticosteroids to reduce the number of liver LDL receptors thus reducing the ability of the liver to take up LDL cholesterol [61, 62]. This suggests the possibility that the reduced uptake of cholesterol from plasma depletes liver cholesterol pools sufficiently to indirectly enhance the expression of 3-hydroxy-3-methylglutaryl-CoA reductase causing the liver to produce more cholesterol, which is necessary for bile acid synthesis. Another gene that has been implicated in corticosteroid dysregulation of systemic cholesterol metabolism is SREBP-1c, which is up-regulated by insulin and down-regulated by corticosteroids [20].

Corticosteroids also cause hypertension [4, 5, 63, 64]. In part, this may be due to atherosclerosis resulting from the chronic elevation of LDL cholesterol. However, another contributing factor may be the interaction of the corticosteroid with the mineralocorticoid receptor. Although the non-fluorinated corticosteroids can be inactivated by 11β-HSD, pharmacological doses may exceed the capacity of this enzyme in the kidney thus permitting such corticosteroids to enhance salt and water retention. Corticosteroids also reduce blood flow to the musculature, which would further contribute to hypertension.

Associated with these systemic adverse effects, corticosteroids have other detrimental effects on all three tissues. They cause increased deposition of fat in the liver, muscle wasting, and kidney hypertrophy and nephropathy [4, 5]. The effects on the kidney in part can be attributed to direct effects of the corticosteroids but in part may be due to diabetes and hypertension. The major difficulty in parsing causal molecular relationships for the complex systemic effects caused by corticosteroids is the diverse origins of the available data. A large proportion of the data is derived from cell culture studies in which corticosteroids are applied for a period of time and changes in the expression of particular genes are noted. Although useful, these studies do not consider the fact that other factors in the environmental milieu such as other hormones and substrates often modulate the cellular response to corticosteroids. Even when these factors are added, they are not presented in the temporal sequence extant *in vivo*. Similarly, the available *in vivo* data is derived from many different animals subjected to a wide variety of dosing regimens.

Time Series Data: Defining Causal Molecular Cascades

Complex systemic phenomena such as diabetes, arteriosclerosis, and hypertension do not develop as the result of a single dose of drug. However, each dose of a drug initiates molecular events in time that if perpetuated by repeated dosing results in the development of the complex adverse systemic phenomena. For many years we have used a time series design to evaluate cascades of molecular events in time initiated by the corticosteroid, methylprednisolone (MPL) [44, 45, 65-68]. These studies were initiated with adrenalectomized rats where the expression of the corticosteroid responsive gene has a stable baseline, diverges from that baseline, and returns to the initial value. The standard experiment is designed with multiple controls and at least three animals at each of 16 time points over a seventy-two hour period. The distribution of time points is not equal over the time series as experience indicates that many events occur during the early time period following dosing but some changes in gene expression require up to seventy-two hours for complete recovery of baseline. This approach has been applied extensively to evaluating the temporal response of the enzyme tyrosine aminotransferase (TAT) in liver and glutamine synthetase (GS) in skeletal muscle. Measurements include MPL kinetics, the glucocorticoid receptor (GR), GR mRNA, TAT mRNA and activity (liver), and GS mRNA and activity (skeletal muscle).

Pharmacokinetic/Pharmacodynamic Models: Constructing Quantitative Hypotheses for Molecular Cascades

Figure 1 shows the kinetics of methylprednisolone following a single bolus dose to a population of adult male ADX rats. Plasma MPL concentrations vs. time were described by a biexponential equation:

$$C_{MPL}=C_1 \cdot e^{-\lambda_1 \cdot t}+C_2 \cdot e^{-\lambda_2 \cdot t} \quad (1)$$

where C_1 and C_2 are intercept coefficients, λ_1 and λ_2 are slopes. Parameters were estimated by least-squares fitting using the ADAPT II program by the maximum likelihood method.

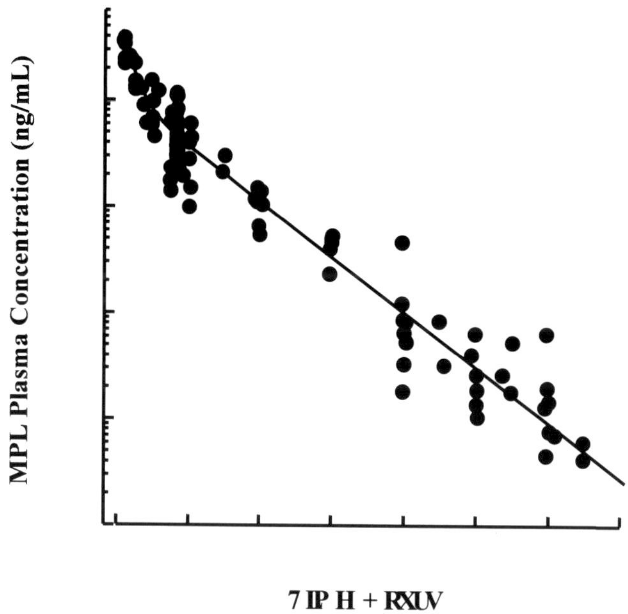

Figure 1. Plasma concentrations of methylprednisolone versus time after 50 mg/kg iv bolus dose of methylprednisolone in rats. Symbols represent actual data points, and the solid line represents fitting of those points to a biexponential function

Figure 2 provides a schematic of the events involved in the gene mediated effects of corticosteroids at the cellular level. The drug enters the cell by diffusion where it interacts with the glucocorticoid receptor (GR) forming drug receptor complex (DR) causing its release from a protein complex and activation. The activated DR enters the nucleus (DRN) where it dimerizes and interacts with GREs in the DNA. The consequences of this interaction can be either a decrease or an increase in production of a specific mRNA. If enhanced expression, then the mRNA must leave the nucleus and be used to synthesize the protein. If reduced expression, then there will be a period of time based on the degradation rate of the message before the reduced expression is reflected as reduced protein. If the gene products influenced are transcription factors, then the change in protein can itself become the controlling factor changing the expression of other genes.

Mechanism-based PK/PD modeling is a systematic approach for characterizing these types of turnover responses. Such modeling can be used to explain how drugs might induce their effects not only by direct interactions with receptors, but also by the ability of this interaction to affect the fate of endogenous compounds and the subsequent effects that are mediated by those substances. The four basic models of Dayneka and colleagues [69] formalize PK/PD modeling of responses generated by indirect mechanisms of action.

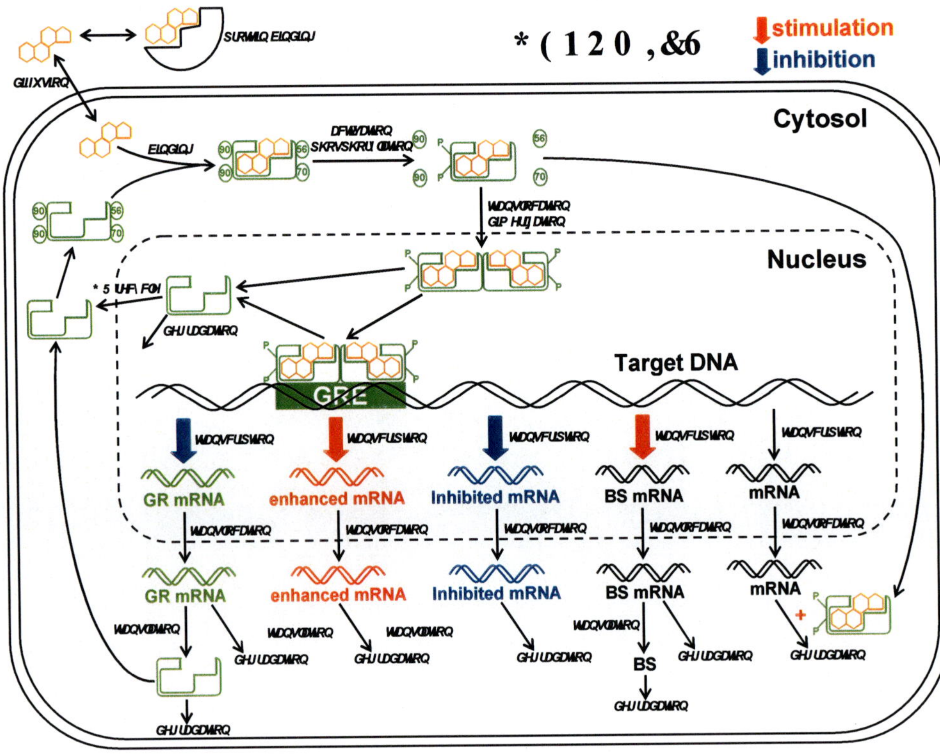

Figure 2. Schematic for corticosteroid receptor/gene mediated effects

The basic premise of such modeling is that a measured response (R) to a drug may be produced by indirect mechanisms; for example, factors controlling the input or production of the response variable (k_{in}) may be either inhibited or stimulated, or the determinants of loss of the response variable (k_{out}) may be inhibited or stimulated. The rate of change of the response over time with no drug present can be described by:

$$\frac{dR}{dt} = k_{in} - k_{out} \cdot R \qquad R(0) = R_0 \tag{2}$$

where k_{in} represents the zero-order constant for production of the response and k_{out} defines the first-order rate constant for loss of the response. It is assumed that k_{in} and k_{out} fully account for production and loss of the response. The response variable R may be a directly measured entity or an observed response, which is immediately proportional to the concentration of R. In Fig. 3, Models I and II represent inhibitory processes that operate according to the classical inhibitory function, I(t)

$$I(t) = 1 - \frac{I_{\max} \cdot C_P}{C_P + IC_{50}} \tag{3}$$

where C_P represents the plasma concentration of the drug as a function of time and IC_{50} is the drug concentration which produces 50% of maximum inhibition achieved. Accordingly, the rate of change of drug response in Model I can be described by

$$\frac{dR}{dt} = k_{in} \cdot I(t) - k_{out} \cdot R \tag{4}$$

Model II describes drug response that results from inhibition of the factors controlling the dissipation of response variable according to

$$\frac{dR}{dt} = k_{in} - k_{out} \cdot I(t) \cdot R \tag{5}$$

Note that in Models I and II, $I_{max} = 1$ for maximum inhibition is implied by the assumption that inhibition can completely negate the functioning of the affected factors, i.e., when $C_P >> IC_{50}$, I(t) approaches zero. In addition, note that I(t) approaches unity when $C_P << IC_{50}$.

In Figure 3, Model III and Model IV represent processes that stimulate the factors controlling drug response and operate according to the stimulation function, S(t)

$$S(t) = 1 + \frac{S_{max} \cdot C_P}{SC_{50} + C_P} \tag{6}$$

where S_{max} represents the maximum effect attributed to the drug and SC_{50} represents drug concentration producing 50% of the maximum stimulation achieved at the effect site. When $C_P >> SC_{50}$, the net effect approaches the maximal value of S_{max} plus the baseline constant. On the other hand, when $C_P << SC_{50}$, the net effect approaches the baseline effect, i.e., $S(t) \approx 1$.

Model III represents drug response that accrues from stimulation of the factors that control the production of the response variable according to

$$\frac{dR}{dt} = k_{in} \cdot S(t) - k_{out} \cdot R \tag{7}$$

When drug response is attributed to factors controlling the dissipation of the response variable, Model IV describes the rate of drug response by

$$\frac{dR}{dt} = k_{in} - k_{out} \cdot S(t) \cdot R \tag{8}$$

As stationarity is assumed for all models, the response variable (R) begins at a predetermined baseline value (R_0), changes with time following drug administration, and eventually returns to R_0. Thus

$$k_{in} = k_{out} \cdot R_0 \tag{9}$$

which reduces the number of operative parameters in these models. Equations (3) and (6) entail an assumption that drug effects correlate directly to plasma drug concentrations; thus, C_P can be generated using classical pharmacokinetic models describing drug input and disposition rates.

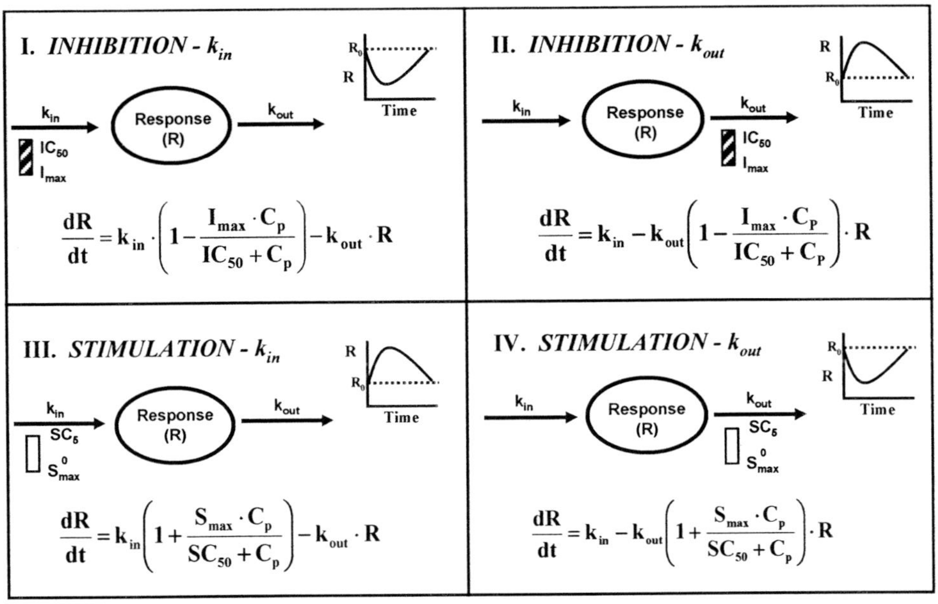

Figure 3. Four basic mechanism-based indirect effect models for drug action

In these models, R represents the measured response variable while the site of action represents a separate locus where the mechanism of action controls either stimulation or inhibition of the designated controlling process (k_{in} or k_{out}).

Indirect Pharmacokinetic/Pharmacodynamic Models: Application to Gene Expression

Our laboratories have been involved extensively in modeling corticosteroid pharmacodynamics using both TAT in the liver and GS in the skeletal muscle as PD markers. Modeling the genomic effects of CS has been an evolving process. Since 1986, a series of mechanism-based PK/PD models have been proposed to describe the gene-mediated effects of steroids in terms of receptor down-regulation and enzyme induction in rats [44, 45, 65-68, 70, 71]. These models evolved over time with the addition of mRNA measurements and more extensive studies in terms of dosages used and duration of tissue sampling. Several basic pharmacodynamic elements were integrated in these models including receptor binding, signal transductions, and tolerance development due to receptor down-regulation. The most recent "fifth-generation model" is shown in Figure 4 using TAT as the PD marker. The results of the application of this model are shown in Figure 5 as follows: (a) pharmacokinetics, (c) GR mRNA repression, (d) receptor dynamics, (e) TAT mRNA induction, and (f) its enzyme induction in liver upon acute dosing of MPL in ADX rats (4, 6). Also shown (Figure 5b) is the simulated profile of drug-receptor complexes in the nucleus (DR(N)), which acts as the major driving force for genomic effects of corticosteroids.

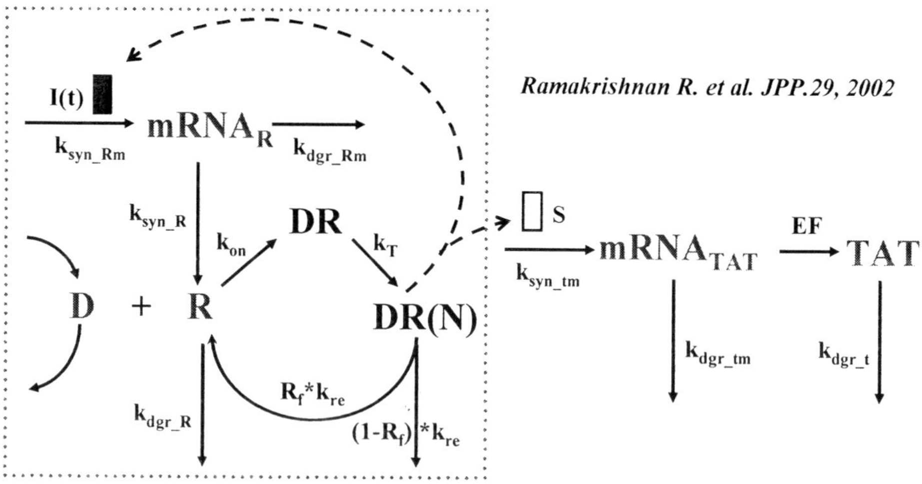

Figure 4. Fifth-generation model for corticosteroid regulated gene-mediated effects in liver

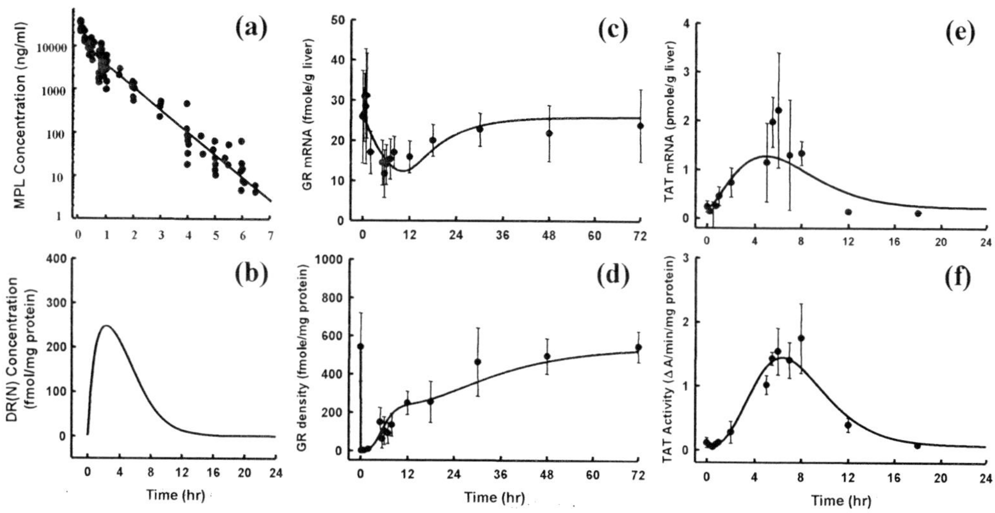

Figure 5. Plots of plasma MPL concentrations (top left), nuclear bound drug-receptor (bottom left), GR mRNA (top middle), GR activity (bottom middle), TAT mRNA (top right) and TAT activity (bottom right) in rat liver as a function of time after a 50 mg/kg iv dose of MPL

Gene Arrays: High Throughput Data Collection for PK/PD Modeling

Data used to develop the models such as described in the previous section were obtained from a rich time series following a single bolus dose of drug and the measurement of one gene at a time. However, phenomena such as steroid diabetes involve many genes in different tissues. Gene arrays provide a method of measuring the expression of mRNA for thousands of genes simultaneously using a single uniform platform. Applied within the context of a rich time series, the results can be used to construct pictures of the transcriptional events in time that cause phenomena such as steroid diabetes. This "motion picture" of transcriptional events can then be used as a scaffold for translational and post-translational events as they become available. Just as protein measurements were used to construct models prior to the availability of mRNA measurement, the wealth of mRNA data available from gene arrays can be used to develop models reflecting previous findings and in anticipation of further protein data.

We have generated time series gene array data for rat liver, skeletal muscle, and kidney following *in vivo* dosing with corticosteroids, and analysis of that data is ongoing. For these experiments liver, skeletal muscle (gastrocnemius), and kidney samples were obtained from a previously performed animal study in our laboratory, which was designed for construction of PK/PD models [44, 66]. Briefly, male adrenalectomized (ADX) Wistar rats (Rattus rattus) weighing 225–250 g were obtained from Harlan Sprague-Dawley (Indianapolis, IN). Animals were allowed free access to rat chow (Agway, RMH 1000) and 0.9% NaCl drinking water. They were housed in a room with a 12 h light/12 h dark cycle, a constant temperature of 22° C and were allowed to acclimatize to this environment for at least 1 week. One day prior to the study, all rats were subjected to right external jugular vein cannulation under light ether anesthesia. Four animals were designated as controls (i.e., zero time samples) and were cannulated but received vehicle only. All remaining animals received a single 50 mg/kg dose of methylprednisolone sodium succinate (Pharmacia-Upjohn Company, Kalamazoo, Mich.) via the cannula over 30 s. Rats (3) were sacrificed by exsanguinations under anesthesia at 0.25, 0.5, 0.75, 1, 2, 4, 5, 5.5, 6, 7, 8, 12, 18, 30, 48, 72 hr after dosing. The sampling time points were selected based on earlier studies describing GR dynamics and enzyme induction in liver and skeletal muscle. Four cannulated vehicle treated rats were sacrificed as controls (data represented as time zero). Tissue samples were rapidly excised, flash frozen in liquid nitrogen, and stored at -80°C. Frozen tissues were ground into powder using a liquid nitrogen chilled mortar and pestle.

Isolated RNA from each individual tissue from each individual animal was used to prepare target according to manufacturer's protocols. The biotinylated cRNAs from liver and muscle were hybridized to individual Affymetrix GeneChips® Rat Genome U34A (Affymetrix, Inc., Santa Clara, CA), which contained 8799 probe sets. The kidney samples were hybridized to individual Rat Genome 230A chips, which contain 15923 probe sets. The Affymetrix arrays used have the advantage of having multiple measurements per gene (11 probe pairs or more per transcript). However, this same redundancy leads to many different interpretations of probe sets to determine a signal for each gene (probe set algorithms), and controversy regarding the sensitivity and specificity of resulting signals, as well as appropriate normalization methods [72]. We have used the Affymetrix Microarray Suite 5.0 (MAS5.0) algorithm, which places a relatively high penalty for mismatch hybridization, favoring specificity over sensitivity [73]. This entire data set has been submitted to the NCBI Gene Expression Omnibus database (GSE490) and is also available online at http://microarray.cnmcresearch.org/pgadatatable.asp) [74].

The approach to data mining was developed based on our use of gene arrays as a technique for high throughput data collection within the context of a rigidly controlled time series paradigm. The Affymetrix oligonucleotide microarrays use sequence information and photolithograpy-directed combinatorial chemical synthesis to develop probe sets for the genes of interest. Each probe set consists of a series of short oligonucleotide sequences and an identical partner sequence, except for a single base mismatch in the center. The mismatch sequence provided a unique background for each sequence in the series. MAS5.0 (Affymetrix, Inc., Santa Clara, CA) was used for initial data acquisition and basic analysis. In this first step, a "call" of *Present* (P), *Absent* (A), or *Marginal* (M) was determined for each probe set on each chip based on the comparison of the matched and mismatched pairs for the gene sequence. The results were normalized for each chip using a distribution of all genes around the 50th percentile. The results from the first step were entered into the program GeneSpring 6.2 ® (Silicon Genetics, Redwood City, CA). This robust software provides a number of tools for visualization and analysis of time series data. One such tool for both hierarchical clustering and visualization is the gene tree approach described by Eisen [75] as modified by the GeneSpring software. This algorithm can be used to construct a dendrogram of genes with similar patterns. A negative aspect of this tool, and most time series data mining tools, is the assumption that the points in the time series are equally spaced. However, to design our 72 hr time series in this manner would have ignored the richness of biological information during the early period following dosing of the drug. Notwithstanding this drawback, gene trees provide an excellent method of visualizing the progression of the data analysis. In order for this and other tools to be used it was also necessary to transform the data so that the values for all probe sets were within the same range. To accomplish this, values for each individual probe set on each chip were expressed as a ratio of the mean of the four control values for that gene, which we refer to as "normalized intensity". Thus the average of each probe set has a value of 1 at zero time and either increases, decreases, or remains unchanged relative to controls over the time series.

Figure 6 (top left) shows the gene tree derived from the GeneSpring program for the entire skeletal muscle dataset (8799 probe sets at 17 time points). This tree was constructed using Pearson correlation. The x-axis presents the 17 time points studied in rank order from left to right. Vehicle controls are nominally referred to as time zero. As pointed out above, each time point is equally spaced and therefore does not represent the true temporal relationship between points. The y-axis presents the mean of the normalized value at each time point for each of the individual probe sets, represented by color and clustered by similarity. In this view, the color yellow represents a value of "1", progression towards red represents values that exceed "1", and progression towards blue represents values that decline towards zero. The intensity of the color reflects the intensity of the original signal. To the immediate left of the gene tree is a schematic tree of the relationship of all probe sets to each other based on expression pattern similarity (represented in green). On the left side of the gene tree but spatially separated is what is referred to as a "marquee view" in the GeneSpring software.

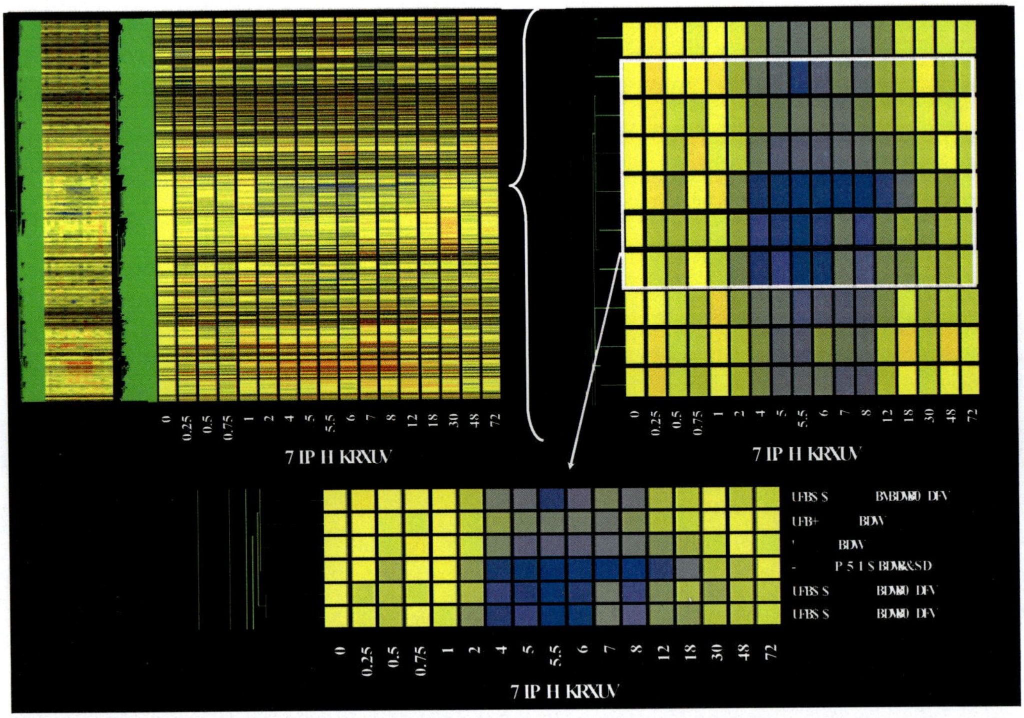

Figure 6. Gene tree representation of entire dataset of mRNA expression in skeletal muscle as a function of time following MPL treatment. The gene tree represents the averaged normalized values of each of 8799 probe sets at 17 different time points following MPL treatment, grouped by pattern similarities. The y-axis represents individual probe sets, with color representing relative intensities (yellow represents no change from control, progression towards red indicates increased expression, and progression towards blue represents decreased expression versus control values). The x axis ranks the samples in sequence of time following MPL treatment. The top left panel represents the entire dataset, while the top right and bottom panels present successive zoom in views of the areas highlighted

This marquee view can be used to navigate the view of the main gene tree. Although the gene tree representation of the entire dataset is of limited value for examining individual gene patterns of regulation, it does illustrate two points. First, within the entire dataset are a vast number of genes represented by black (no expression in skeletal muscle regardless of treatment) or by the color yellow across the entire timeframe studied. This latter group of genes exhibits no temporal regulation by the drug (i.e. their expression does not deviate from control values following drug dosing) and represents probe sets that we wish to filter from the data set. This gene tree does reflect segregation of similarly regulated genes and demonstrates that similar patterns of regulation do exist. For example, groups of intense red or blue represent clusters of genes with similar up- or down-regulation respectively. Figure 6 (top right) provides a zoom in view of one such clustering of down-regulated probe sets. The location of this group of probe sets on the entire gene tree is indicated by the white bracket. Figure 6 (bottom) shows an even closer zoom in on five probe sets in this grouping with similar patterns. In this case three probe sets for the gene myristoylated alanine rich protein kinase C substrate (AA955167, AA899253, AA925762) segregate close to each other, which demonstrates the optimal functioning of gene tree clustering. The location of these probe sets in the top right panel is indicated by the white rectangle. Figure 7 provides gene trees for the entire liver and kidney data sets. It should be recalled that the kidney data set was developed using the newer R230A rat chip with 15,923 probe sets while the muscle and liver datasets were developed using the older U34A chips that only contain 8799 probe sets.

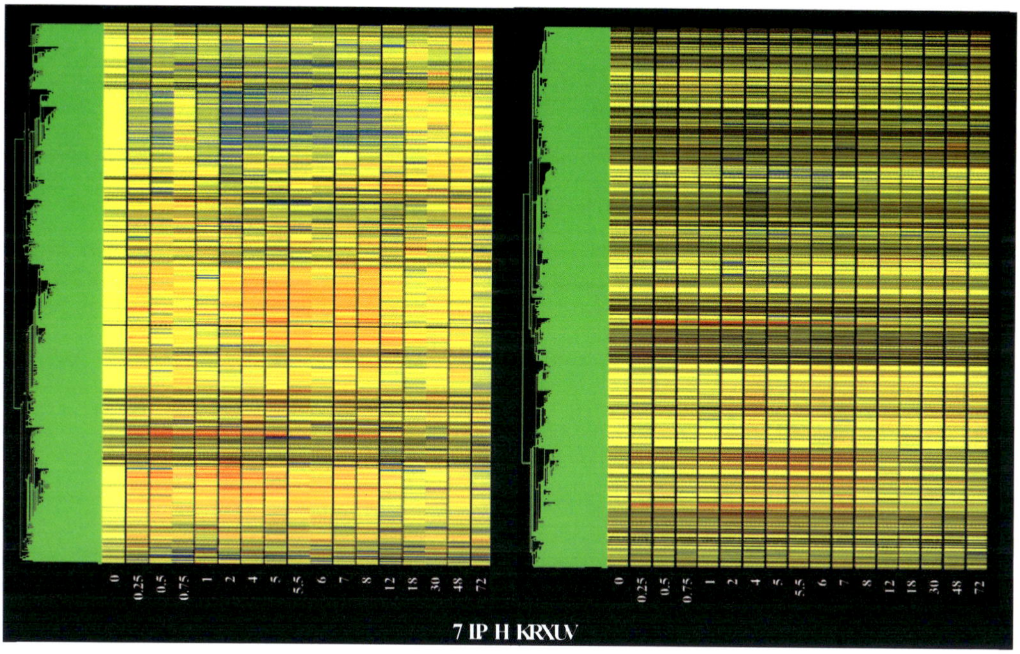

Figure 7. Gene tree representation of filtered datasets of mRNA expression showing corticosteroid-regulated probe sets in liver (left) and kidney (right) as a function of time following MPL treatment

Data Mining: Identifying Regulated Probe Sets

Mining such time series datasets presents uniquely different problems from those encountered when microarrays are used to distinguish one group from another (eg. cancerous versus non-cancerous tissues). For those applications one attempts to define a pattern or fingerprint that distinguishes with very high probability one group from another [76-81]. In many cases it is the pattern of gene expression rather than the relationship between the genes that is the important focus. In the present application of microarrays the problem is sorting through the vast amount of data to identify probe sets with temporal patterns of change in expression that indicate that the gene is regulated in response to the drug. In this case the causal relationship between the genes whose expression is changing in response to the drug is of paramount importance. For example the drug may change the expression of a particular transcription factor, which in turn alters the expression of downstream genes. For this reason the most important aspect of the mining approach is to avoid discarding valuable data. This is of particular importance because each identified gene becomes the subject of extensive literature searches (text mining) in order that it can be placed into a temporal context of all other transcriptionally altered genes. The purpose of the endeavor is to use PK/PD modeling to develop a "motion picture" of the polygenic response to the drug.

For data mining, we used a series of "filtering" steps in an attempt to identify genes and eliminate probe sets that either are not expressed in skeletal muscle or are not responsive to MPL treatment. The first level of filtering was designed to eliminate probe sets not expressed in the tissue regardless of drug treatment (represented by very low intensity on the gene tree), and utilized the Affymetrix "call" feature. For this first filter, we eliminated all probe sets that did not receive a call of "P" on at least 4 chips. Although this is a very non-stringent filter, it did eliminate almost half of the probe sets from each of the three data sets. The second level of filtering was designed to eliminate probe sets that could not meet the basic criteria of a regulated probe. Specifically this filter was designed to eliminate probe sets whose average did not deviate from baseline by a certain value for a reasonable number of time points. After exploring a variety of filtering values and number of conditions using gene trees in the manner describe previously, we developed two filters that were designed to eliminate probe sets that were neither down- nor up-regulated. The first filter eliminated probe sets that could not meet a minimal criterion for down-regulation. Starting with the 4P filtered list we eliminated all probe sets that did not have average values below 0.65 in at least 4 conditions (time points). The next filter was designed to eliminate probe sets that could not meet a minimal criterion for up-regulation. Starting with the 4P filtered list, we eliminated all probe sets that did not have average values above 1.5 in at least 4 conditions (time points). There were a small number of probe sets in both the liver and skeletal muscle data sets that were not eliminated by either filter indicating both up- and down-regulation. These probe sets (which were present on both lists) suggest biphasic regulation, a phenomenon we have previously described [82]. The last filter we applied addressed the quality of the data. For this "quality control" filter we eliminated probe sets that did not meet two conditions. The first condition focused on the control chips. As indicated above our initial operation was to divide the value of each individual probe set on each chip by the mean of the values for that probe set on the four control chips. Therefore, the quality of the control data for each particular probe set is of paramount importance in defining regulation by the drug. The second condition focused on the remaining 16 time points. Using the standard deviation of the mean, this filter excluded all probe sets whose coefficient of variation (CV) for the control chips exceeded 50% and whose CV for more than 8 of the remaining 16 time points exceeded 50%. As an example, Figure 8 shows a gene tree constructed using Pearson correlation of the 653 probe sets from the skeletal muscle data set that were not eliminated by the series of filters. These filters eliminated 8146 probe sets from the skeletal muscle data set, 7299 probe sets from the liver data set and 14955 probe sets from the kidney data set. The remaining probe sets then became the focus of temporal clustering.

Clustering: Identifying Groups of Probe Sets with Similar Temporal Signatures

Most of the clustering algorithms currently in use are based on either Euclidian space (Self Organizing Maps (SOM)) or correlation (gene trees, K-means, and QT clustering). The problem with these algorithms is that they treat all time domains as equal elements. In our time series, time domains range from 0.25 hr in the beginning to 24 hr at the end of the 72 hr time period. In our opinion none of these clustering algorithms adequately deal with time series data. This opinion is based on the fact that all algorithms yield different results. This can be illustrated using the 653 probe sets identified in the muscle data set. Figure 8 shows the gene tree constructed using Pearson correlation. This provides a visualization tool for comparing clustering algorithms. If other clustering tools agree with the gene tree method then they should yield results with all probe sets in each cluster sitting next to each other on the tree. To the degree that this is not true then the algorithms disagree.

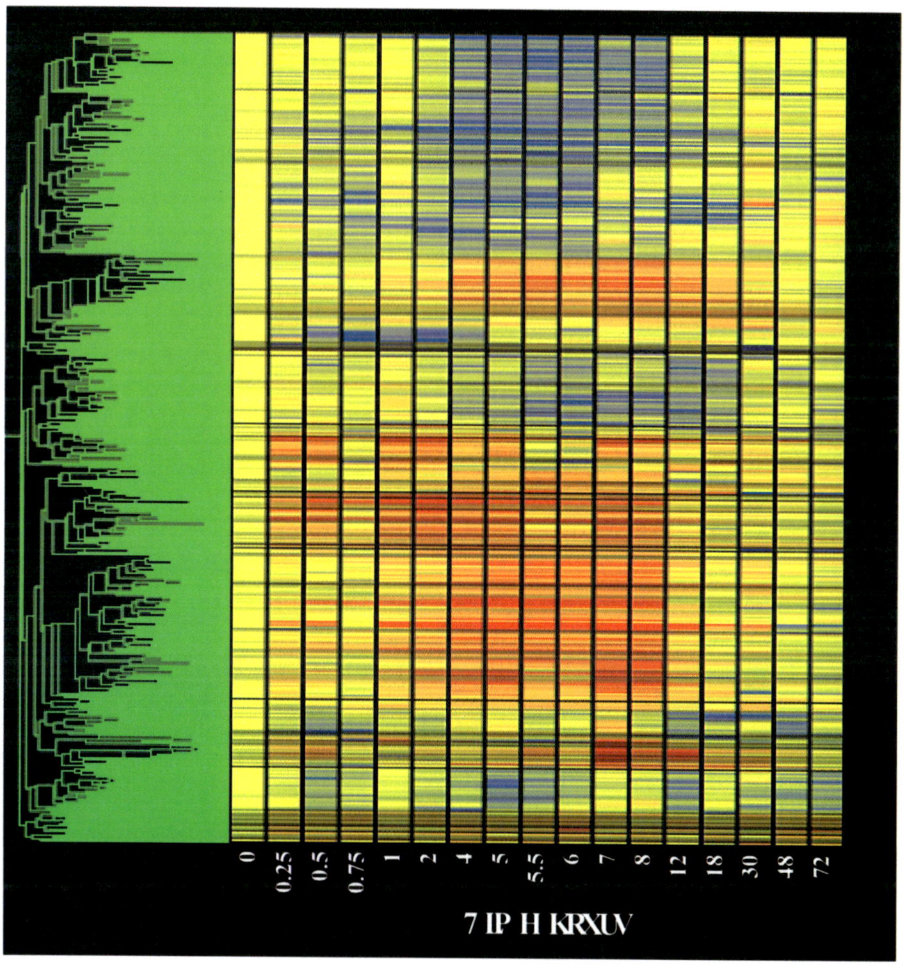

Figure 8. Gene trees of the 653 probe sets remaining in the skeletal muscle dataset after completion of all filtering steps described in the text

Figure 9 shows the results of a 3X2 SOM of the 653 probe sets mined from the skeletal muscle data set. The SOM algorithm uses Euclidian distance and requires that one arbitrarily decide how many clusters are extant in the data set. We chose six simply for purposes of illustration. This figure, which presents the six clusters in a gene tree format, demonstrates that SOM and the gene tree methodologies do not agree on the grouping of genes into temporal clusters. Figure 10 shows the same set of probe sets clustered using the correlation based K-means algorithm. Like SOM, this algorithm requires that an *a priori* judgment be made concerning the number of clusters extant in the data set. We chose six to be consistent with the SOM and Pearson correlation to be consistent with the gene tree. Again the groupings of the genes are different for all three methods. The last method we applied is QT clustering. This method is also based on correlation. However, this method does not require an *a priori* judgment on number of clusters but does require that one designate a minimum correlation coefficient and a minimum size of a grouping that will be accepted as a cluster. This method also allows for a remainder of probe sets that do not meet the designated constraints. Initially, we chose a Pearson correlation of 0.9 to be consistent with the gene tree and K-means analysis and a minimum cluster size of 10.

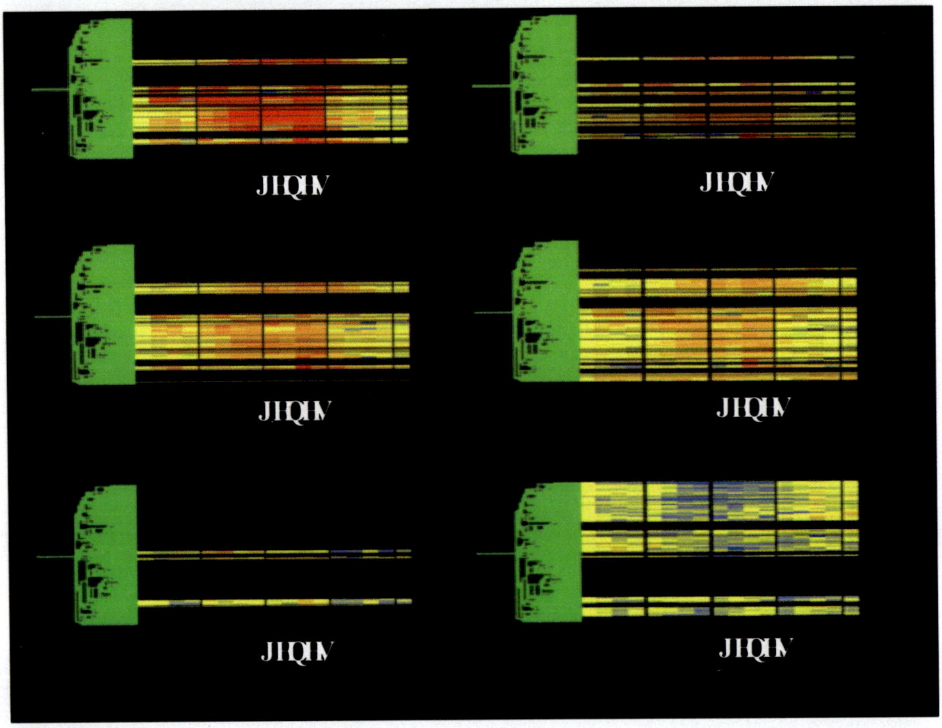

Figure 9. Gene trees of the six clusters obtained after applying Self Organizing Map clustering to the filtered skeletal muscle dataset

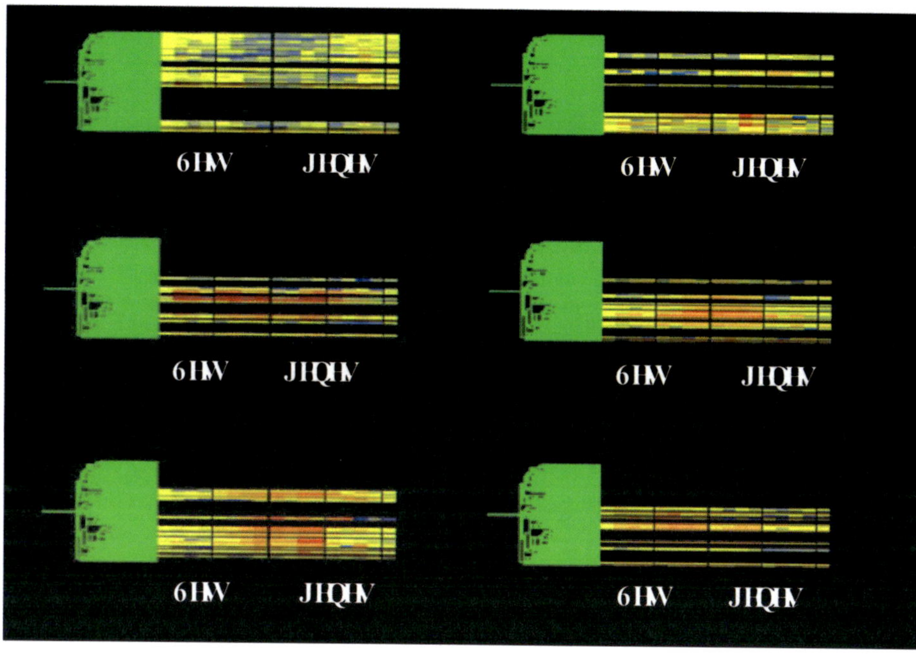

Figure 10. Gene trees of the six clusters obtained after applying K-means clustering to the filtered skeletal muscle dataset

Figure 11 shows that these constraints yielded only three small clusters and a remainder of 614 probe sets. Even in the case of the three small clusters, the probe sets are not all contiguous on the original gene tree. We reanalyzed the dataset maintaining the minimum cluster size at 10 but reducing the minimum Pearson correlation to 0.6. Figure 12 shows that this analysis yields 16 clusters with a remainder of 279 probe sets. The largest cluster contains 109 probe sets while three small clusters contain the designated minimum of 10 probe sets. The fundamental problem is that it is often posited that probe sets that cluster together reflect genes with common mechanisms of regulation. However, if different clustering algorithms yield significantly different results then this proposition is fallacious unless some cogent argument is put forth that one method is superior to the others. With respect to time series data, a major problem is that none of these algorithms actually treats time as proportional time. All time intervals are considered as equal elements for correlation or objects in Euclidian space. This distinction can be seen in Figures 13 and 14. Figure 13 is a linear plot of the largest QT cluster containing 109 probe sets. At the top is the centroid (average of all probe sets) of the cluster and at the bottom is a plot of all 109 probe sets together. The red color indicates this is an up-regulated cluster with a peak at about 6 hours. All probe sets appear to have approximately the same signature, with the primary difference being in the magnitude of the up-regulation. Similarly Figure 14 shows the second largest QT cluster, which contains 47 probe sets. At the top is the centroid of the cluster that shows a nadir at about six hours. The blue color indicates that this is a down-regulated cluster with a nadir at about 6 hours. Although it appears that the variation in magnitude is less than in the up-regulated cluster, it should be recalled that down-regulation has a much more limited range (1 – 0).

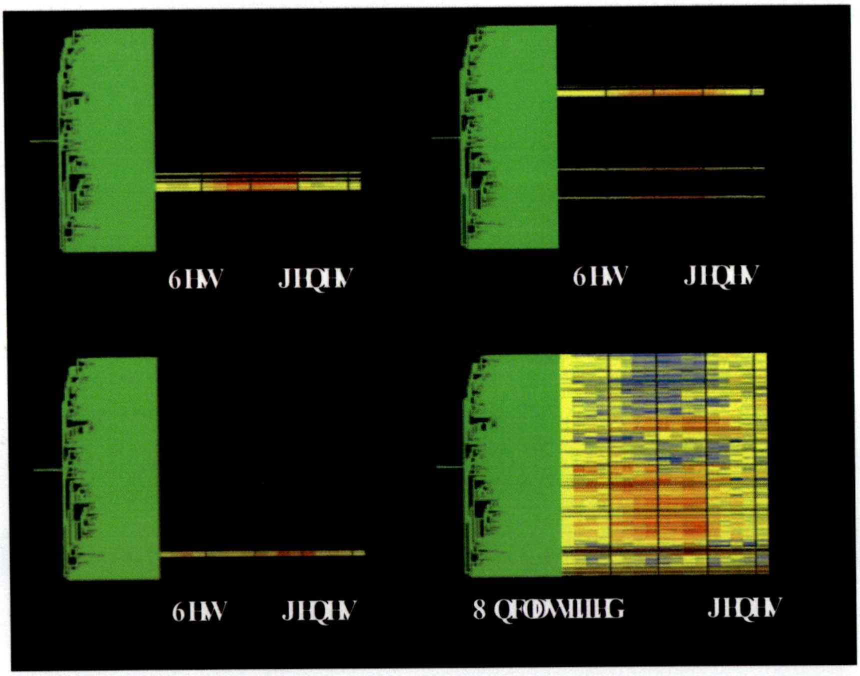

Figure 11. Gene trees of the four groups obtained after applying QT clustering with a correlation of 0.9 to the filtered skeletal muscle dataset

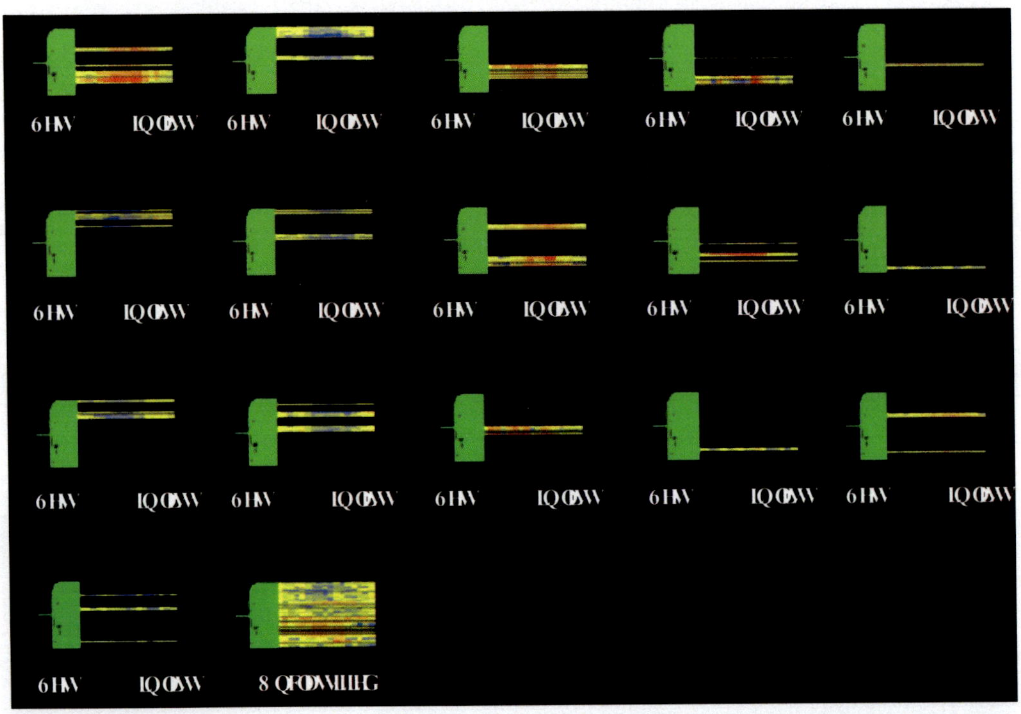

Figure 12. Gene trees of the seventeen groups obtained after applying QT clustering with a correlation of 0.6 to the filtered skeletal muscle dataset

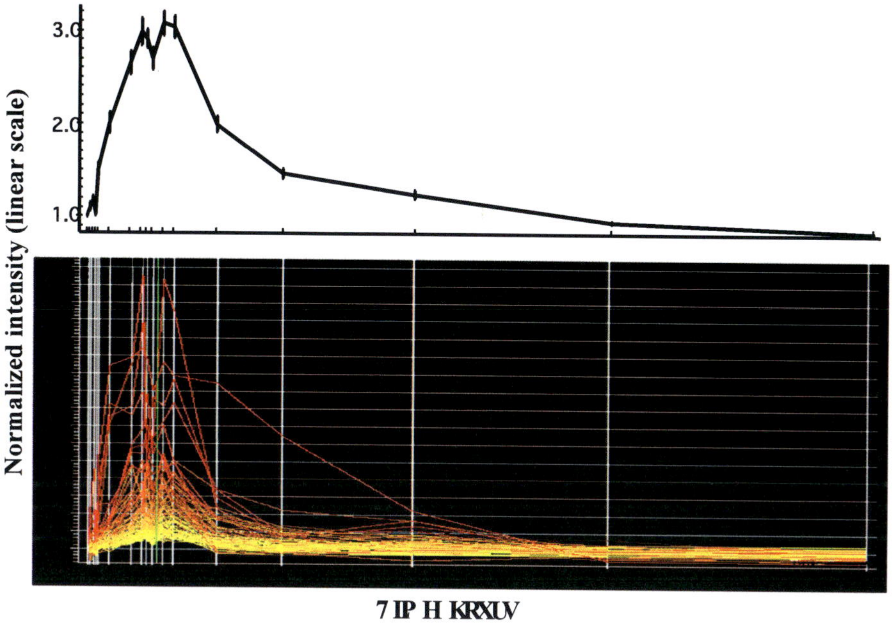

Figure 13. Linear plot of QT cluster containing 109 up-regulated probe sets (Figure 12, Set 1). The x-axis represents time after MPL administration, and the y-axis represents mean normalized probe intensities obtained from Affymetrix array analysis as described in the text. The bottom panel presents individual plots for each of the109 probe sets, while the top panel presents the centroid (average of all probe sets at each time point)

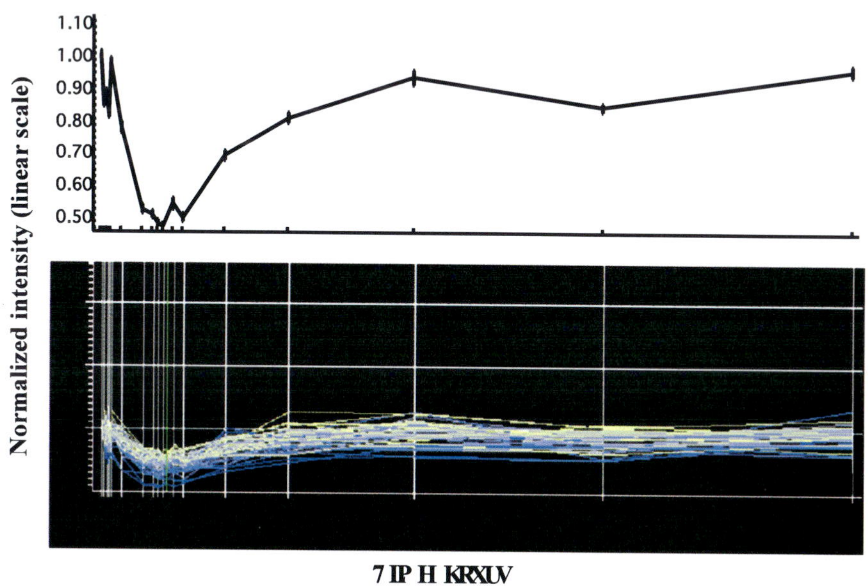

Figure 14. Linear plot of QT cluster containing 47 down-regulated probe sets (Figure 12, Set 2). The x-axis represents time after MPL administration, and the y-axis represents mean normalized probe intensities obtained from Affymetrix array analysis as described in the text. The bottom panel presents individual plots for each of the 47 probe sets, while the top panel presents the centroid (average of all probe sets at each time point)

The cluster shown in Figure 13 contains 4 probe sets for the enzyme glutamine synthetase. The locations of these four probe sets among the 109 probe sets in this cluster is highlighted in white on the blow up of the original tree presented in Figure 15. Although the top two GS probe sets are very close and the bottom two are contiguous, all four are not together. Figure 16 shows a linear plot of all four GS probe sets. Although not identical, all four GS probe sets have remarkably similar temporal signatures. We have previously measured, using quantitative Northern hybridization, GS in these same muscle samples and modeled the change in the expression of that message [44, 45]. Figure 17 shows the results of the original modeling of GS from data developed using quantitative Northern hybridization along with the fitting of these four probe sets to that same model. The inset table shows the fitting parameters for each set of data. The data generated with the gene arrays is quite similar to that obtained by the method of quantitative hybridization we developed more than ten years ago.

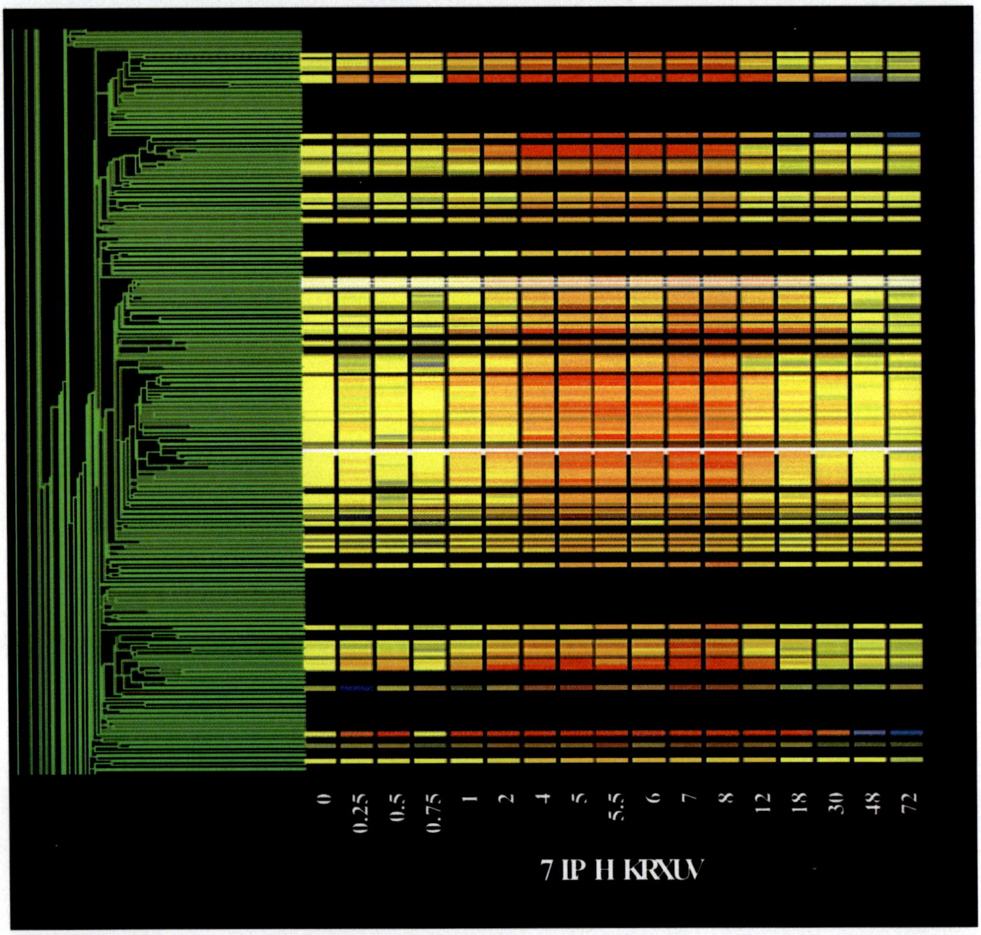

Figure 15. Gene tree showing the locations of 4 probe sets for glutamine synthetase (GS) following QT clustering of the filtered skeletal muscle dataset, applying a correlation of 0.6. The 4 probe sets for GS are highlighted in white

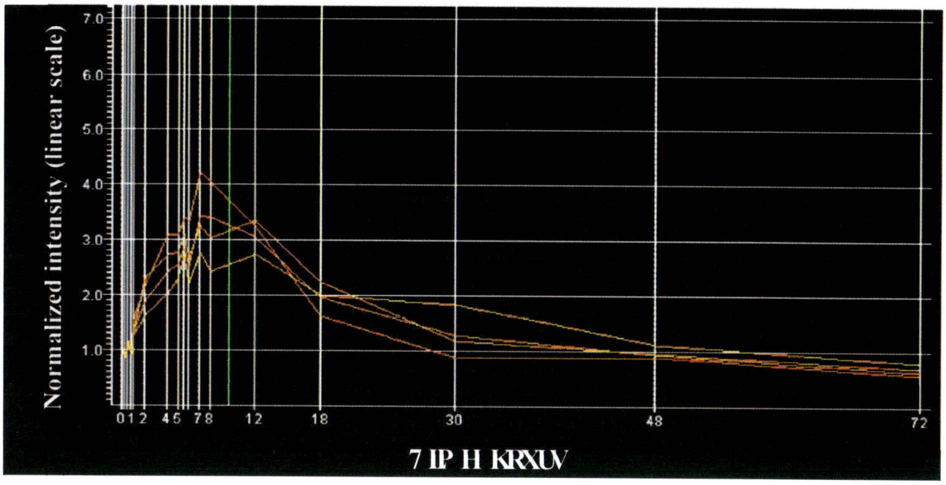

Figure 16. Linear plots of the 4 probe sets for glutamine synthetase (GS) from the skeletal muscle dataset. The x-axis represents time after MPL administration, and the y-axis represents mean normalized probe intensities obtained from Affymetrix array analysis as described in the text

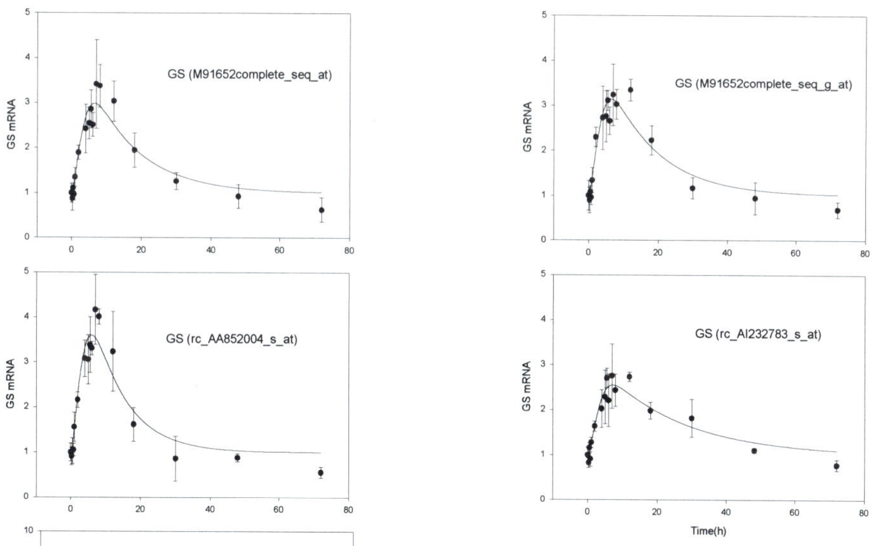

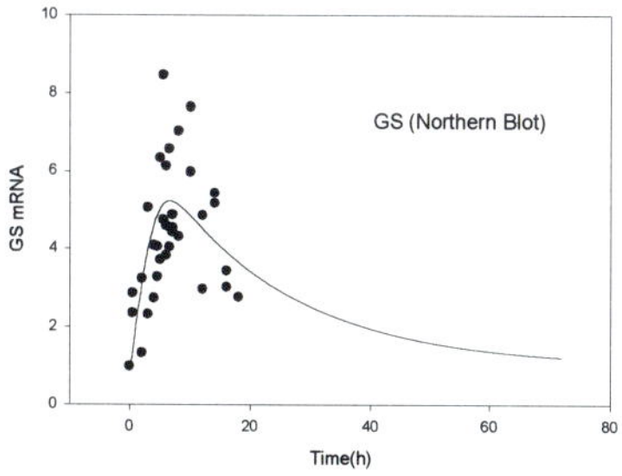

Accession Number	kout (1/h) Estimate	kout (1/h) CV%	S (1/(fmol/l/mg protein)) Estimate	S (1/(fmol/l/mg protein)) CV%
M91652complete_seq_at	**0.073**	20	**0.263**	15
M91652complete_seq_g_at	**0.071**	19	**0.288**	14
rc_AA852004_s_at	**0.104**	20	**0.267**	14
rc_AI232783_s_at	**0.043**	20	**0.307**	16
GS (Northern Blot)	**0.047**	42	**0.783**	33

Figure 17. Application of fifth-generation mechanism-based indirect effect model for corticosteroid-regulated gene mediated effects to the gene array data for the 4 individual glutamine synthetase probe sets, as well as similar data obtained by Northern hybridization. The x-axis represents time following MPL administration, and the y-axis represents GS mRNA expression. Symbols represent actual data points, while the solid line presents fitting of the data to the model

PK/PD Modeling of Gene Array Data

Previously, we reported an initial analysis of the liver data set described here [82]. Based on our fifth-generation model of steroid PK/PD, mechanistic models were developed to describe the time-pattern for 197 probes sets representing 143 responsive genes. As shown in Figure 18, the drug kinetics and receptor dynamics were modeled as before with the differential equations as follows:

$$\frac{dmRNA_R}{dt} = k_{s\_Rm} \cdot \left(1 - \frac{DR(N)}{IC_{50\_Rm} + DR(N)}\right) - k_{d\_Rm} \cdot mRNA_R \tag{10}$$

$$\frac{dR}{dt} = k_{s\_R} \cdot mRNA_R + R_f \cdot k_{re} \cdot DR(N) - k_{on} \cdot D \cdot R - k_{d\_R} \cdot R \tag{11}$$

$$\frac{dDR}{dt} = k_{on} \cdot D \cdot R - k_T \cdot DR \tag{12}$$

$$\frac{dDR(N)}{dt} = k_T \cdot DR - k_{re} \cdot DR(N) \tag{13}$$

where symbols represent the receptor mRNA ($mRNA_R$), the free cytosolic GR density (R), cytosolic drug-receptor complex (DR) and drug-receptor complex in nucleus (DR(N)). The rate constants in the equations include: zero-order rate of GR mRNA synthesis (k_{s_Rm}); the first-order rates of GR mRNA degradation (k_{d_Rm}), receptor synthesis (k_{s_R}) and degradation (k_{d_R}), translocation of the drug-receptor complex into the nucleus (k_T), and the overall turnover of DR(N) to cytosol (k_{re}); as well as the second-order rate constant of drug-receptor association (k_{on}). In addition, IC_{50_Rm} is the concentration of DR(N) at which the synthesis rate of receptor mRNA drops to 50% of its baseline value, and R_f is the fraction of free receptor being recycled. At time 0, the system yields the baseline equations as $k_{d\_Rm} = \frac{k_{s\_Rm}}{mRNA_R^0}$ and $k_{s\_R} = \left(\frac{R^0}{mRNA_R^0}\right) \cdot k_{d\_R}$, where $mRNA_R^0$ and R^0 are the baseline values of receptor mRNA and free cytosolic GR density.

Based on various mechanisms of corticosteroid action, six mathematical models were proposed to describe the typical gene expression patterns after acute MPL treatment in rat liver. In all of these models except *Model C*, target mRNA was assumed to be synthesized at zero-order rate k_{s_m}, and degraded at first-order rate k_{d_m} without drug administration:

$$\frac{dmRNA}{dt} = k_{s\_m} - k_{d\_m} \cdot mRNA \tag{14}$$

The message level was assumed to be at steady-state at time zero (control animals), yielding the baseline equation as $k_{s\_m} = k_{d\_m} \cdot mRNA^0$, where $mRNA^0$ was fixed as 1 for most of the genes.

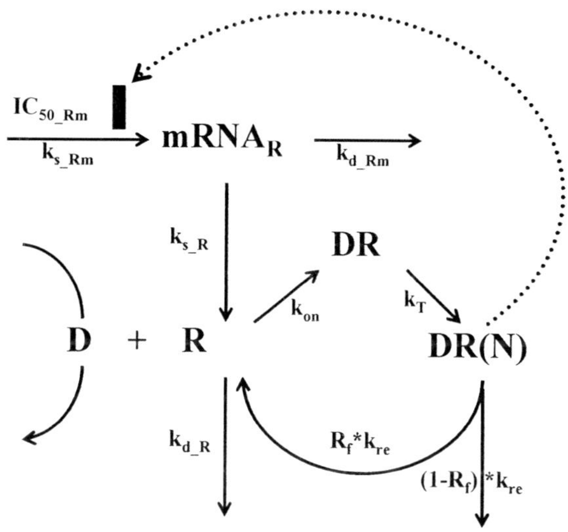

Figure 18. Schematic of model for MPL drug kinetics and corticosteroid receptor dynamics, which is common to the six models (presented in Figures 19-24) developed for pharmacogenomic effects of corticosteroids

Model A. Binding of the activated steroid-receptor complex (DR(N)) to the GRE in target DNA leads to direct enhanced expression of several genes, which were described as follows:

$$\frac{dmRNA}{dt} = k_{s\_m} \cdot (1 + S \cdot DR(N)) - k_{d\_m} \cdot mRNA \tag{15}$$

where the enhancement of transcription rate k_{s_m} is dependent on DR(N) concentration with a linear efficiency constant (S). This model described 32 probes representing 27 genes. Figure 19 presents the partial model structure and fitting of a representative gene.

Model B. Binding of DR(N) to the negative GRE leads to gene repression, which was described as follows:

$$\frac{dmRNA}{dt} = k_{s\_m} \cdot \left(1 - \frac{DR(N)}{IC_{50} + DR(N)}\right) - k_{d\_m} \cdot mRNA \tag{16}$$

where the inhibition of transcription rate k_{s_m} is dependent on DR(N) concentration, and IC_{50} represents the concentration of DR(N) at which mRNA synthesis rate drops to 50% of its baseline value. This model described 64 probes representing 42 genes. Figure 20 presents the partial model structure and fitting of a representative gene.

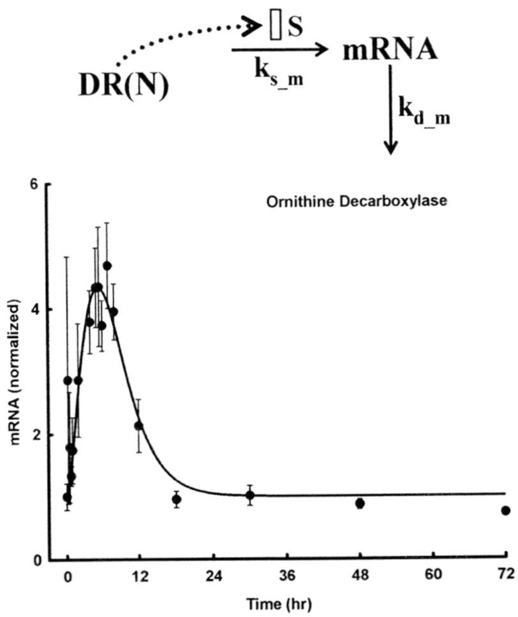

Figure 19. Model (top) for direct corticosteroid stimulation of mRNA by DR(N). This model was applied to 32 probe sets from the liver dataset; a representative example (ornithine decarboxylase) is presented (bottom). The x-axis represents time after MPL administration, and the y-axis represents mean normalized probe intensities obtained from Affymetrix array analysis as described in the text. Symbols represent actual data points, while the solid line presents fitting of the data to the model

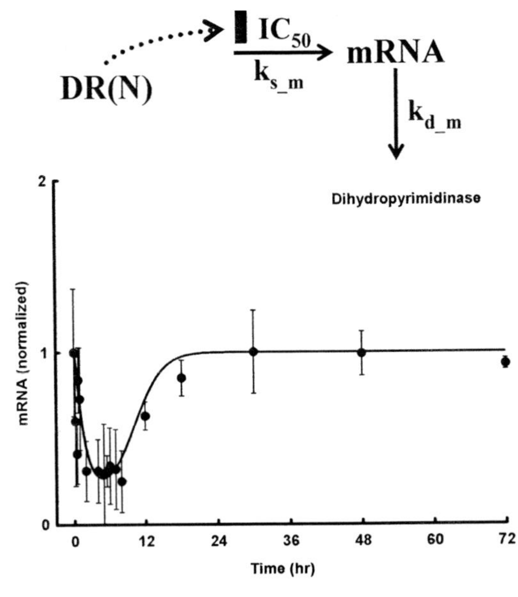

Figure 20. Model (top) for direct corticosteroid repression of mRNA by DR(N). This model was applied to 64 probe sets from the liver dataset; a representative example (dihydropyrimidinase) is presented (bottom). The x-axis represents time after MPL administration, and the y-axis represents mean normalized probe intensities obtained from Affymetrix array analysis as described in the text. Symbols represent actual data points, while the solid line presents fitting of the data to the model

Model C. The CS may also affect gene expression without binding to GRE. Steroid-receptor complex can directly or indirectly affect mRNA stability in cytosol. Furthermore, DR(N) may affect transcription of functional biosignals/transcription factors, such as C/EBP, therefore causing secondary alterations of genes controlled by these factors. Messages with induced degradation plus secondarily induced production were described as follows:

$$\frac{dmRNA_{BS}}{dt} = k_{s\_BSm} \cdot (1 + S_{BSm} \cdot DR(N)) - k_{d\_BSm} \cdot mRNA_{BS} \tag{17}$$

$$\frac{dBS_r}{dt} = k_{s\_BS} \cdot mRNA_{BS} - k_{d\_BS} \cdot BS_r \tag{18}$$

$$\frac{dmRNA}{dt} = k_{s\_m} \cdot (1 + S_{m\_s} \cdot BS_r) - k_{d\_m} \cdot (1 + S_{m\_d} \cdot DR) \cdot mRNA \tag{19}$$

where symbols represent the message ($mRNA_{BS}$) and protein (BS_r) level of the intermediate regulator BS. The extra rate constants in the equations include: zero-order rate of BS mRNA synthesis (k_{s_BSm}); the first-order rates of BS mRNA degradation (k_{d_BSm}), translation to BS protein (k_{s_BS}) and protein degradation (k_{d_BS}). The stimulation of BS transcription process k_{s_BSm} is dependent on DR(N) concentration with a linear efficiency constant (S_{BSm}). The stimulation of mRNA synthesis k_{s_m} is dependent on the relative changes of regulator BS with a linear efficiency constant (S_{m_s}). This stimulation is present even at baseline conditions. The mRNA degradation k_{d_m} in cytosol is regulated by DR concentration with a linear stimulation factor (S_{m_d}). At time zero, equations 18-20 yield the baseline equations as

$$k_{s\_BSm} = k_{d\_BSm} \cdot mRNA^0_{BS} \; k_{s\_BS} = \left(\frac{BS^0_r}{mRNA^0_{BS}} \right) \cdot k_{d\_BS} \text{ and}$$

$$k_{s\_m} = \frac{k_{d\_m} \cdot mRNA^0}{1 + S_{m\_s} \cdot BS^0_r} \tag{20}$$

where $mRNA_{BS}{}^0$ and $BS_r{}^0$ were fixed as 1. This model described 21 probes representing 18 genes. Figure 21 presents the partial model structure and fitting of a representative gene.

Model D. Genes with repressed transcription plus secondarily induced production were described as follows:

$$\frac{dBS_a}{dt} = k_1 \cdot (DR(N) - BS_a) \tag{21}$$

$$\frac{dmRNA}{dt} = k_{s\_m} \cdot \left(1 - \frac{DR(N)}{IC_{50\_s} + DR(N)} + S_s \cdot BS_a \right) - k_{d\_m} \cdot mRNA \tag{22}$$

where the intermediate regulator BS is described in a simplified fashion using a linear transduction model [83]. In this model, BS_a represents the absolute change of regulator level from the control. And this change is produced by DR(N) via first-order rate (k_1). Drug (DR(N)) and the regulator (BS_a) both act on mRNA synthesis independently. The IC_{50_s} represents the concentration of DR(N) which inhibits synthesis rate by 50% and S_s represents the efficiency of BS stimulation on transcription. The initial condition BS_a^0 was fixed as 0. This model described 48 probes representing 33 genes. Figure 22 presents the partial model structure and fitting of a representative gene.

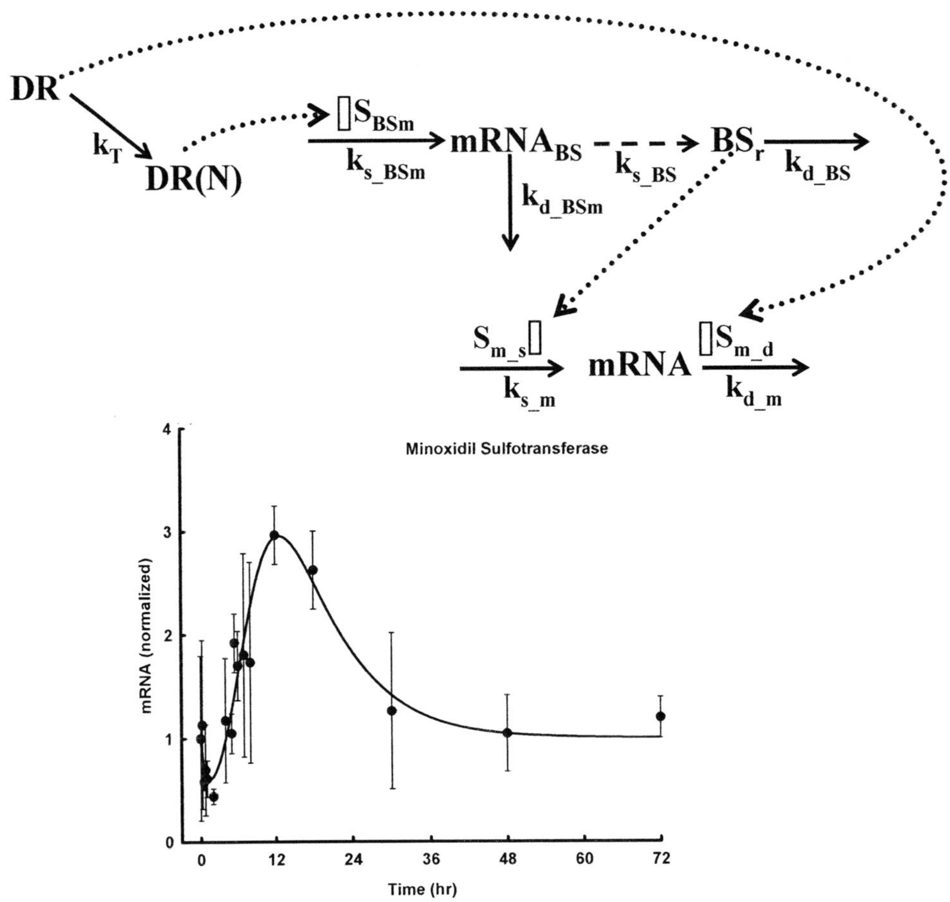

Figure 21. Model (top) for corticosteroid stimulation of mRNA by DR(N) effects on mRNA stability and induction of an intermediate regulator (BS). This model was applied to 21 probe sets from the liver dataset; a representative example (minoxidil sulfotransferase) is presented (bottom). The x-axis represents time after MPL administration, and the y-axis represents mean normalized probe intensities obtained from Affymetrix array analysis as described in the text. Symbols represent actual data points, while the solid line presents fitting of the data to the model.

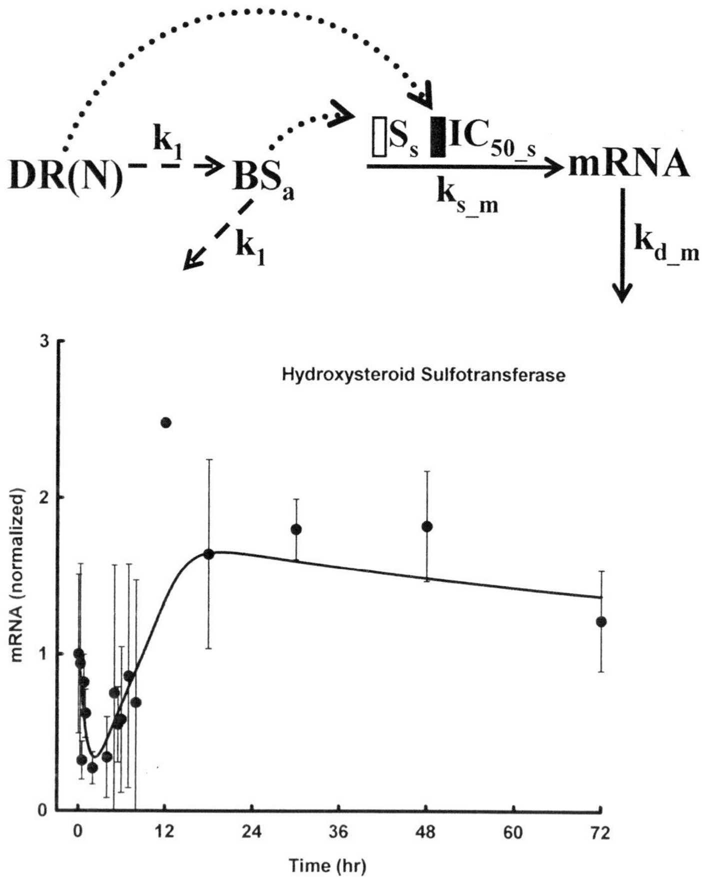

Figure 22. Model (top) for direct corticosteroid repression of mRNA by DR(N) followed by a secondary induced expression through induction of an intermediate regulator (BS). This model was applied to 48 probe sets from the liver dataset; a representative example (hydroxysteroid sulfotransferase) is presented (bottom). The x-axis represents time after MPL administration, and the y-axis represents mean normalized probe intensities obtained from Affymetrix array analysis as described in the text. Symbols represent actual data points, while the solid line presents fitting of the data to the model.

Model E. Genes with repressed transcription and secondarily repressed degradation were described as follows:

$$\frac{dBS_a}{dt} = k_1 \cdot \left(DR(N) - BS_a\right) \tag{23}$$

$$\frac{dmRNA}{dt} = k_{s\_m} \cdot \left(1 - \frac{DR(N)}{IC_{50\_s} + DR(N)}\right) - k_{d\_m} \cdot \left(1 - \frac{BS_a}{IC_{50\_d} + BS_a}\right) \cdot mRNA \tag{24}$$

where BS_a is characterized as in *Model D.* The IC_{50_s} represents the concentration of DR(N) which inhibits mRNA synthesis by 50%, and IC_{50_d} represents the changes of BS_a at which mRNA degradation rate drops to 50% of its baseline value. This model described 22 probes representing 20 genes. Figure 23 presents the partial model structure and fitting of a representative gene.

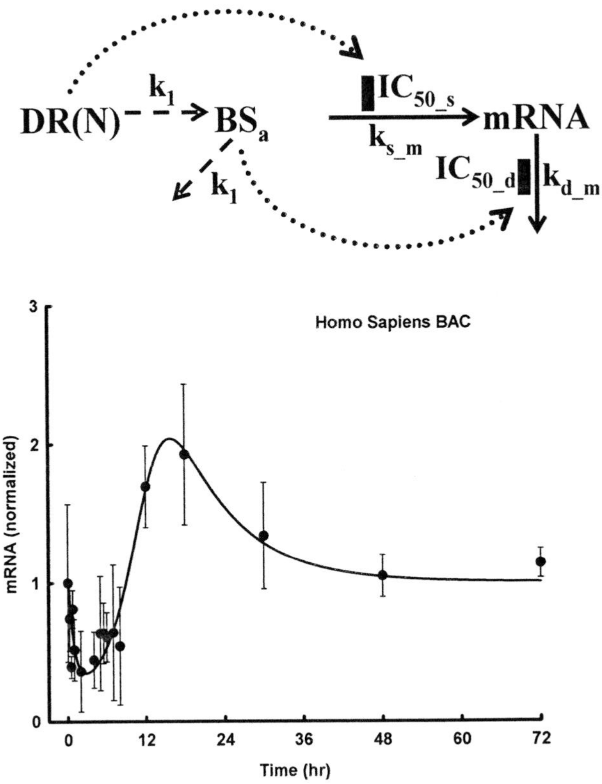

Figure 23. Model (top) for direct corticosteroid repression of mRNA by DR(N) followed by a secondary reduced degradation of that mRNA through induction of an intermediate regulator (BS). This model was applied to 22 probe sets from the liver dataset; a representative example (human BAC) is presented (bottom). The x-axis represents time after MPL administration, and the y-axis represents mean normalized probe intensities obtained from Affymetrix array analysis as described in the text. Symbols represent actual data points, while the solid line presents fitting of the data to the model.

Model F. Since whole liver was used in our study, it is likely that gene expression detected in our current gene array study also came from blood lymphocytes in the sample. As an immunosuppressant, CS is well-known to regulate immune-related genes in lymphatic cells. Recent data suggest the possibility of rapid membrane-initiated genomic effects via specific steroid membrane receptors, and the intracellular signaling in lymphocytes [84]. As CS also cause an acute effect on lymphocyte trafficking, it is possible that lymphocyte efflux from the liver bloodstream could also contribute to the changes of immune-related message levels. Immune-related genes with induced production were described as follows:

$$\frac{dCell_B}{dt} = k_{in\_C} \cdot \left(1 - \frac{D}{IC_{50\_C} + D}\right) - k_{out\_C} \cdot Cell_B \tag{26}$$

$$\frac{dmRNA_C}{dt} = k_{s\_m} \cdot (1 + S \cdot DR) - k_{d\_m} \cdot mRNA_C \tag{27}$$

$$mRNA = mRNA_C \cdot Cell_B \tag{28}$$

As reflected in Equation 26, lymphocytes from the lymphatic tissues enter into blood at a zero-order rate k_{in_C}, and return to the tissues at a first-order rate constant k_{out_C}. The CS instantaneously inhibit the movement of lymphocytes from tissues to blood, and IC_{50_C} represents the drug concentration which inhibits k_{in_C} by 50%. The immediately enhanced message level in single lymphocyte ($mRNA_C$) is described as induced production (k_{s_m}) by CS upon binding to its receptor via a linear efficiency constant (S). The total message level in liver sample (mRNA) is represented by the combination of mRNA in a single lymphocyte and total lymphocyte counts from blood source in the sample (multiplication). This model described 10 probes representing 5 genes. Figure 24 presents the partial model structure and fitting of a representative gene.

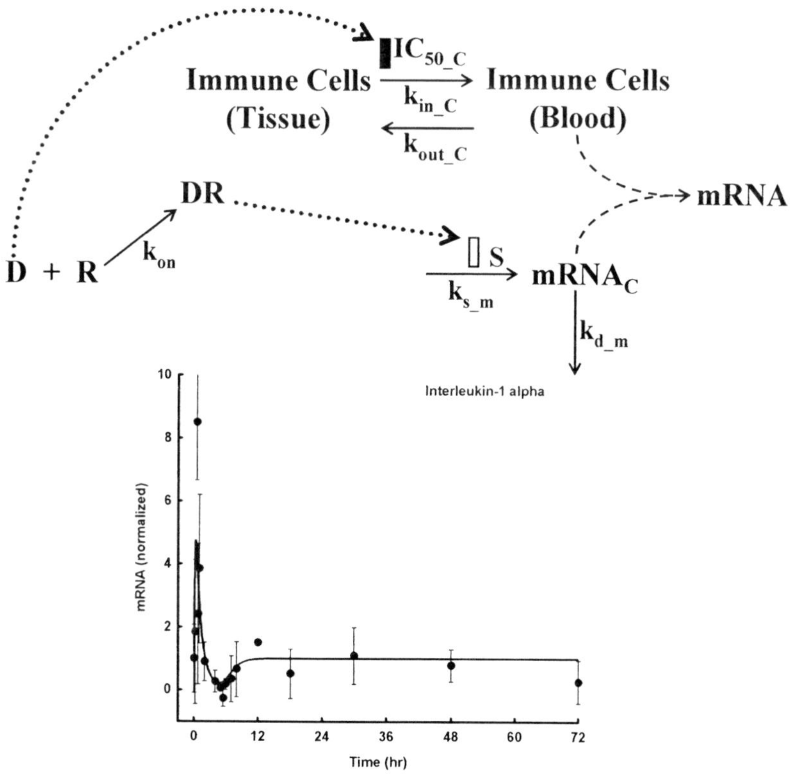

Figure 24. Model (top) for corticosteroid induction of mRNA via effects on lymphocyte trafficking. This model was applied to 10 probe sets from the liver dataset; a representative example (interleukin-1 alpha) is presented (bottom). The x-axis represents time after MPL administration, and the y-axis represents mean normalized probe intensities obtained from Affymetrix array analysis as described in the text. Symbols represent actual data points, while the solid line presents fitting of the data to the model

Text Mining

Assembling such models into a cohesive whole to address broader systemic phenomena such as insulin resistance requires that the temporal pattern of the change in the expression of one gene be put into the context of many others. Because of the wealth of information in the literature in most cases we can confirm that the expression of a specific gene in a particular tissue is influenced by corticosteroids in a particular way. However, mining the biomedical literature for relevant information presents some rather substantial problems. These problems stem from both the structure of the literature and limitations of the search engines available. One major problem is one of nomenclature. Literature searches start with a word-based query. However, a single gene product can have multiple names. Table 1 illustrates this point for a single enzyme, carbamoyl phosphate synthase that became of interest to us following the initial mining of the liver data set. This single enzyme can be found under 15 different names and two EC numbers. Keyword assignment to papers is in general non-standard and thus obscures rather than adds to the search process. When it comes to controlling molecules such as transcription factors entire separate non-overlapping literatures can exist because the factor was discovered and named more than once. An excellent illustration of this point are the the leucine zipper transcription factors, CCAAT/enhancer binding protein β and δ (C/EBPβ and C/EBPδ) which were also discovered and named Nuclear Factor Interleukin 6 (NFIL6) and Nuclear Factor Interleukin 6β (NFIL6β). Interestingly, even with the recognition discovered through sequence comparison many papers only use one name as a keyword. A second major problem relates to the nature of available search engines. The two major search engines available are PubMed and MEDLINE. Both have limited Boolean capabilities that can be used to in part address the nomenclature problem

Table 1. Nomenclature Problems

Carbamoyl phosphate synthase EC NUMBER 6.3.5.5	
RECOMMENDED NAME:	Carbamoyl-phosphate synthase (glutamine-hydrolysing)
SYSTEMATIC NAME:	Carbon-dioxide:L-glutamine amido-ligase (ADP forming, carbamate-phosphorylating)
SYNONYMS:	Carbamoyl phosphate synthase (glutamine)
	Carbamoyl phosphate synthetase (glutamine-hydrolyzing)
	Carbamoyl-phosphate synthetase (glutamine-hydrolysing)
	Carbamoylphosphate synthase
	Carbamoylphosphate synthetase
	Carbamoylphosphate synthetase II
	Carbamyl phosphate synthetase (glutamine)
	Carbamyl phosphate synthetase II
	CPS, CPSase, CPSase-A, CPSase-P
	EC 2.7.2.9 (formerly)
	Glutamine-dependent carbamyl phosphate synthetase
	Synthase, carbamoylphosphate (glutamine)
	Synthetase, carbamoylphosphate (glutamine-hydrolyzing)

For example, there are approximately 250,000 reports on glucocorticoids in the literature. To find all of them it is necessary to do independent searches on glucocorticoids, corticosteroids, cortisol, corticosterone, dexamethasone, prednisolone, betamethasone, and triamcinolone and combine the results with a Boolean "or". Interestingly methylprednisolone, the drug we used, will be included with prednisolone. The Boolean "and" can also be used to find papers that deal with more than one gene. Similarly the "neighboring" feature in PubMed is useful in finding papers that are relevant to more than one gene. Although there are text mining tools being developed, for the most part readily available tools relegate the process to a one-gene-at-a-time endeavor. The most important factor in this approach is what is now referred to as "domain knowledge". Such domain knowledge generally resides with very experienced people. Even when large groups of relevant citations are collected the final problem is to organize the information into a structure that can be navigated by individuals without extensive domain knowledge.

Data Management

Time series pharmacogenomic experiments with corticosteroids can generate large amounts of data. In our case, the three tissue types of interest are sampled at 16 time points plus four control animals, with each time point requiring three animals. Therefore, each experiment consumes up to 52 chips, which in the case of RU34A produces a total of about 0.5 million data points per scan, and in the case of R230A, about 1 million data points per scan. The result is a fairly substantial volume of data, especially considering that we seek to associate patterns in these data with copious quantities of auxiliary features, annotations, and attributes. For this reason we are custom developing a database application called CortBASE in order to store, handle, and manipulate these data.

The principal functions of CortBASE are (1) to store and organize the results of our experiments and to interface with other analysis software, such as GeneSpring; (2) to relate time series profiles with auxiliary features, annotations, and attributes so as to discover patterns that might suggest interesting biological connections; (3) to serve as a vehicle for building custom functions, filters, calculations, and graphical reporting instruments that are not found on commercial, off-the-shelf gene chip analysis software. CortBASE is currently implemented in a relational database management system and application development environment called 4th Dimension® (http://4d.com), which provides a rich graphical user environment that is friendly for biologists to interact with.

The Data Model

The observation points, in the form of signal magnitude and Affymetrix calls (as estimated by MAS5.0®), are stored in a *Data Points* table (Figure 25). This table is in a many-to-one relation with a *Chips* table (which stores information on the animal, tissue type, sacrifice time, and experimental treatment), and in a many-to-one relation with a *Probe Sets* table. The *Probe Sets* table is a focus point for all information that is known about Affymetrix probes, such as the Genbank Accession Number of the target sequence, the DNA sequence of the target, the location of the target in the rat genome, the UniGene ClusterID (which identifies clusters of sequences with identical 3' UTRs [85]), the RGD ID (the principle ID numbers used by the Rat Genome Database, http://rgd.mcw.edu/), LocusLink LocusIDs (a database of curated sequences and descriptive information about genes, [86]), and in cases of enzymes, the IUPAC-IUBMB EC numbers (http://www.chem.qmul.ac.uk/iubmb/enzyme/).

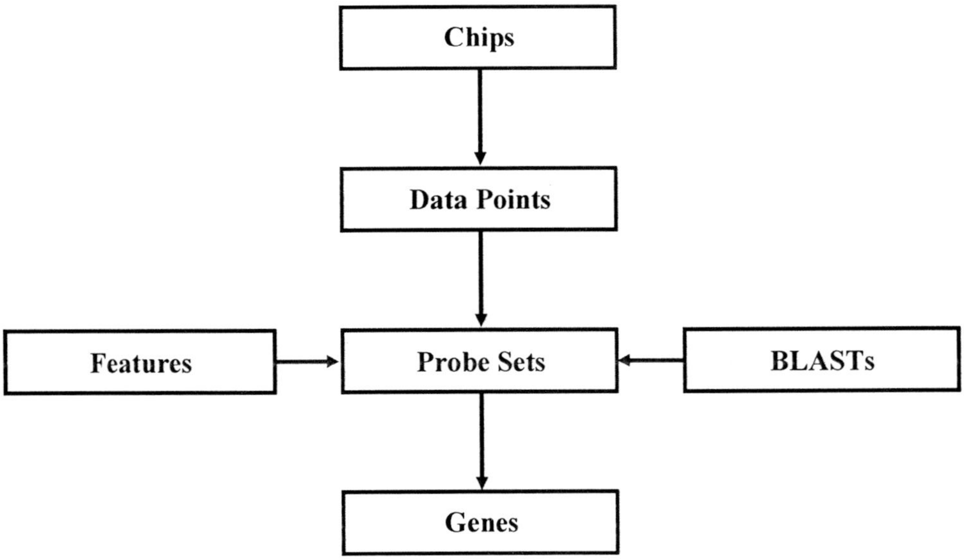

Figure 25. Data model showing the principal relationships among the major tables in CortBASE

Additional features related to probe sets are collectively stored in the *Features* table in a many-to-one relationship with the *Probe Set* table. This table stores the name of a feature type and an identifier for a specific feature along with a broader description of it. These features could include anything, but CortBASE has an uploading function specifically designed to import CVS-formatted annotation files that are periodically updated by Affymetrix. From these files, CortBASE imports the following features:

- *Blocks Protein Families* — multiply aligned segments corresponding to highly conserved regions of proteins [87].
- *Ensembl* — database of annotated metazoan genomes (http://www.ensembl.org).
- *Gene Ontology™ (GO)* — produces a species-independent controlled vocabulary for biological processes, cellular components, and molecular functions (http://www.geneontology.org/).
- *GenMAPP* — visualizes gene expression data on maps representing biological pathways and groupings of genes (http://www.genmapp.org).
- *InterPro* — a database of protein families, domains, and functional sites (http://www.ebi.ac.uk/interpro).
- *Pfam* — a database of multiple sequence alignments and hidden Markov models covering common protein domains and families

(http://www.sanger.ac.uk/Software/Pfam).
- *SCOP* — Structural Classification of Proteins (http://scop.mrc-lmb.cam.ac.uk/scop).
- *Swiss-Prot Knowledgebase* — an annotated protein sequence database (http://www.ebi.ac.uk/swissprot).

CortBASE also parses the results of BLAST searches buts stores the HSP hits in a separate table, *BLASTs*. Through a series of iterative joins, the *Features* table and the *BLASTs* table serve as edges linking probe set vertices into an interconnected Small-World network, possibly allowing for some novel forms of graph-based data mining [88, 89].

CortBASE also has a *Genes* table with the purpose of uniting data from probe sets that ostensibly target the same gene by way of a one-to-many relationship with the *Probe Set* table. Tools for synonymizing multiple probe sets under the same gene name, or assigning probe sets to different gene names, are linked to tools for exploring probe set relationships by way of shared features.

Cataloging Sets of Records

For any given table, CortBASE can store a set of flagged records, along with a searchable description of how the set was created and why. Any two sets of records for the same table can generate a third using standard set theory operations (i.e., *union*, *intersection*, and *complement*), and any set of records can be projected to another related table through a series of joins. Sets can be exported to GeneSpring or imported from GeneSpring by way of ASCII lists of probes. In this way, as sets of probes are identified as biologically meaningful, or as sets are identified as belonging to a certain expression profile model, these can be stored or operated on in conjunction with other sets.

Custom Filtering and Charting

As the need arises, we are adding filtering and charting tools that are specific to the needs of time series expression data. For example, we have a filter that selects for probe sets with time series profiles that are biologically meaningful, such as those with consecutively elevated or depressed levels of expression over a given number of time intervals. In addition, we have custom charting tools for making visual comparisons of expression profiles.

Steroid Diabetes, Transcriptional Dissection of a Polygenic Multi-Tissue Phenomena

Chronic corticosteroid treatment causes steroid diabetes, which is classified as a form of type 2 diabetes. Following a single bolus dose in our experimental paradigm there is both a transient hyperglycemia and a transient hyperinsulinemia. The origins of these systemic effects can be observed as transcriptional changes in liver, skeletal muscle, and kidney. In skeletal muscle there are elevations in proteolytic enzymes and a reduction in both the insulin signaling cascaade and IGF-I. The net effect of these changes would be a net degradation of protein, yielding amino acid carbon. There is also an enhanced expression of the enzyme glutamine synthetase that produces glutamine for the export of amino acid carbon from the muscle. There is also an enhanced expression of myostatin, which presages muscle atrophy. In the liver and kidney there is the enhanced expression of both amino acid transaminases as well as gluconeogenic enzymes. In the liver there is also an enhanced expression of enzymes of the urea cycle necessary for the disposal of the ammonia. Some of these changes occur quickly and are the result of the direct interaction of the activated receptor complex with a GRE. Others are delayed and are the consequence of enhanced expression of transcription factors such as C/EBPβ. The result is increased synthesis and release of sugar form the liver and kidney. Normally, skeletal muscle is responsible for about 80% of the insulin-directed glucose disposal. In the skeletal muscle there are many changes in gene expression that cause insulin resistance. Amongst these changes in gene expression are several transcription factors. These include decreases in the expression of SREBP-1c and RXRγ and increases in C/EBPβ, C/EBPδ, and PPARδ. Either directly or indirectly, the result is a reduced ability of muscle to import and use glucose and an increase in the use of lipids for energy production. The decreased capacity of muscle to import sugar is reflected in decreases in the expression of IRS-I and the enhanced expression of two phosphatases that dephosphorylate and inactivate the insulin kinase cascade. The reduced ability of muscle to use glucose is reflected by changes such as the enhanced expression of PDK4 and the reduced expression of mitochondrial glycerol-3-phosphate dehydrogenase 2 (mGDPH). There are even changes in the expression of genes that would reduce blood flow to the muscle. These changes include the enhanced expression of angiotensin converting enzyme (ACE) and endothelin-1. Together, these and other changes in gene expression in liver, skeletal muscle, and kidney not detailed here but in the dataset provide broad polygenic, multi-tissue picture of steroid diabetes. The challenge is to use the temporal signatures of these changes to construct PK/PD models of these changes that cause hyperglycemia and hyperinsulinemia.

Summary and Conclusions

Pathologies such as diabetes, hypertension, dyslipidemia, and arteriosclerosis caused by chronic corticosteroid treatment are complex phenomena involving altered expression of multiple genes in a number of different tissues. Of particular importance to the development of corticosteroid-induced adverse effects are the liver, kidney, and skeletal muscle. The majority of corticosteroid effects on these three tissues are caused by induced changes in gene expression. These changes in gene expression can be direct or indirect. A single dose of drug does not result in the same adverse effects seen with chronic dosing. However a single dose will transiently cause the same changes in gene expression that if perpetuated by multiple dosing will result in those pathological changes. A single bolus dose of corticosteroids in conjunction with an extended time series involving the sacrifice of multiple animals at each time point can provide a method for measuring a sequence of molecular events in time. Indirect effect mechanism based PK/PD modeling provides a tool for developing models and testable hypotheses concerning these sequences of molecular events in time. However, complex biological processes such as insulin resistance, dyslipidemia, and hypertension involve both multiple tissues and multiple genes in these tissues. In essence, such complex biological processes involve multiple parallel cascades of molecular events that converge and diverge in time. Gene arrays when used within a rigidly structured time series and measurements on multiple tissues from the same group of animals can provide the volume of organized data necessary for applying PK/PD modeling to such complex biological phenomena. This endeavor requires the development of new tools and approaches for data clustering, text mining, and data management and organization.

Acknowledgements

This work was supported by Grants GM 24211 and 1 P20 GM67650 from the National Institute of General Medical Sciences, NIH. This dataset was developed under the auspices of a grant from the NHLBI/NIH Programs in Genomic Applications U01 HL66614.

References

[1] J. Baxter. Advances in glucocorticoid therapy. *Adv. Intern. Med.* 317--349: (2000).

[2] J. M. Goust, H. Stevenson, R. Galbraith, and G. Virella. Immunosuppression and immunomodulation. *Immunology Series* 58: 465-80 (1993).

[3] B. Schimmer, and K. Parker. Adrenocorticotrophic hormones; adrenocortical steroids and their synthetic analogs; inhibitors of synthesis and actions of adrenocortical hormones. In: *Goodman and Gilman's the Pharmacological Basis of Therapeutics*, edited by J. Hardman, L. Limbird, B. Molinoff, R. Ruddon and A. Goodman-Gilman. New York: McGraw Hill, 1996, p. 1459-1486.

[4] M. Bialis, and P. Routledge. Adverse effects of corticosteroids. *Adverse Drug Reactions and Toxicological Reviews* 17: 227-235 (1998).

[5] A. Frauman. An overview of the adverse reactions to adrenal corticosteroids. *Adverse Drug Reactions and Toxicological Reviews* 15: 203-206 (1996).

[6] L. Locsey, L. Asztalos, Z. Kincses, F. Gyorfi, and C. Berczi. Dyslipidaemia and hyperlipidaemia following renal transplantation. *International Urology and Nephrology* 28: 419-30 (1996).

[7] R. M. Reynolds, and B. R. Walker. Human insulin resistance: the role of glucocorticoids. *Diabetes, Obesity and Metabolism.* 5: 5-12 (2003).

[8] J. A. Wald, and R. S. Farr. Abnormal liver-function tests associated with long-term systemic corticosteroid use in subjects with asthma. *Journal of Allergy and Clinical Immunology* 88: 277-8 (1991).

[9] S. House, S. Ruch, W. Koscienski, C. Rocholl, and R. Moldow. Effects of the circadian rhythm of corticosteroids on leukocyte-endothelium interactions in the AM and PM. *Life Sciences* 60: 2023-2034 (1997).

[10] A. Guyton. The Adrenocortical Hormones. In: *Medical Physiology*. Philadelphia: WB Saunders, 1986, p. 909-922.

[11] A. Chakraborty, W. Krzyzanski, and W. Jusko. Mathematical modeling of circadian cortisol concentrations using indirect response models: comparison of several methods. *J. Pharmacokinet. Biopharm.* 27: 559-575 (1999).

[12] R. Almon, and D. DuBois. Tyrosine Transaminase. In: *Wiley Encyclopedia of Molecular Medicine* John Wiley and Sons, 2002, p. 3297-3300.

[13] A. Eisenstein. Effects of adrenal cortical hormones on carbohydrate, protein, and fat metabolism. *American Journal of Clinical Nutrition* 26: 113-120 (1973).

[14] J. Gunn, R. Hanson, O. Meyuhas, L. Reshef, and F. Ballard. Glucocorticoids and the regulation of phosphoenolpyruvate carboxykinase (guanosine triphosphate) in the rat. *Biochem. J.* 150: 195-203 (1975).

[15] R. Hanson, and L. Reshef. Regulation of phosphoenolpyruvate carboxykinase (GTP) gene expression. *Ann. Rev. Biochem.* 66: 581-611 (1997).

[16] M. McMahon, J. Gerich, and R. Rizza. Effects of glucocorticoids on carbohydrate metabolism. *Diabetes-Metabolism Reviews* 4: 17-30 (1988).

[17] R. C. Andrews, and B. R. Walker. Glucocorticoids and insulin resistance: old hormones, new targets. *Clinical Science* 96: 513-23 (1999).

[18] M. Garlatti, M. Aggerbeck, J. Bouguet, and R. Barouki. Contribution of a nuclear factor 1 binding site to the glucocorticoid regulation of the cytosolic aspartate aminotransferase gene promoter. *Journal of Biological Chemistry.* 271: 32629-34 (1996).

[19] M. Takiguchi, and M. Mori. Transcriptional regulation of genes for ornithine cycle enzymes. *Biochem. J.* 312: 649-659 (1985).

[20] J. Horton, J. Goldstein, and M. Brow. SREBPs: activators of the complete program of cholesterol and fatty acid synthesis in liver. *J. Clin. Invest.* 109: 1125-1131 (2002).

[21] H. Shimano. Sterol regulatory element-binding protein family as global regulators of lipid synthetic genes in energy metabolism. *Vitamins and Hormones.* 65: 167-94 (2002).

[22] C. D. Klaassen. Induction of metallothionein by adrenocortical steroids. *Toxicology* 20: 275-9 (1981).

[23] D. M. Fowlkes, N. T. Mullis, C. M. Comeau, and G. R. Crabtree. Potential basis for regulation of the coordinately expressed fibrinogen genes: homology in the 5' flanking regions. *Proceedings of the National Academy of Sciences of the United States of America* 81: 2313-6 (1984).

[24] K. Kasutani, N. Itoh, M. Kanekiyo, N. Muto, and K. Tanaka. Requirement for cooperative interaction of interleukin-6 responsive element type 2 and glucocorticoid responsive element in the synergistic activation of mouse metallothionein-I gene by interleukin-6 and glucocorticoid. *Toxicology and Applied Pharmacology* 151: 143-51 (1998).

[25] G. S. Marks, J. K. Stephens, P. Fischer, and R. Morgan. Hormonal effects on the regulation of hepatic heme biosynthesis. *Mol. Cell. Biochem.* 25: 111-123 (1979).

[26] B. H. Pannen, and J. L. Robotham. The acute-phase response. *New Horizons* 3: 183-97 (1995).

[27] C. Edwards, P. Stewart, D. Burt, L. Brett, M. McIntyre, W. Sutanto, E. deKloet, and C. Monder. Localization of 11B-hydroxysteroid dehydrogenase-tissue specific promotor of the mineralocorticoid receptor. *Lancet* 986-989 (1988).

[28] J. Funder, P. Pearce, R. Smith, and A. Smith. Mineralocorticoid action: target tissue specificity is enzyme, not receptor, mediated. *Science.* 242: 583-585 (1988).

[29] T. Mune, F. Rogerson, J. Nikkila, A. Agarwal, and P. White. Human hypertension caused by mutations in the kidney isozyme of 11B-hydroxysteroid dehydrogenase. *Nature Genetics* 10: 394-399 (1995).

[30] P. Stewart, J. Corrie, C. Schackleton, and C. Edwards. Syndrome of apparent mineralocorticoid excess: a defect in the cortisol-cortisone shuttle. *J. Clin. Invest* 82: 340-349 (1988).

[31] R. R. Almon, and D. C. Dubois. Fiber-type discrimination in disuse and glucocorticoid-induced atrophy. *Medicine and Science in Sports and Exercise.* 22: 304-11 (1990).

[32] I. Kettelhut, S. Wing, and A. Goldberg. Endocrine regulation of protein breakdown in skeletal muscle. *Diabetes Metabol. Rev.* 4: 751-772 (1988).

[33] S. C. Ferrando AA, Sheffield-Moore M, Wolfe RR. Inactivity amplifies the catabolic response of skeleatl muscle to cortisol. *J. Clin. Endocrinol. Metab.* 84: 3515-3521 (1999).

[34] P. Sugden, and S. Fuller. Regulation of protein turnover in skeletal and cardiac muscle. *Biochem. J.* 273: 21-37 (1991).

[35] D. Auclair, Garrel, D.R., Chaouki Zerouala, A., Ferland, L.H. Activation of the ubiquitin pathway in rat skeletal muscle by catabolic doses of glucocorticoids. *Am. J. Physiol.* 272: C1007-C1016 (1997).

[36] S. V. Lecker SH, Mitch WE, Goldberg AL. Muscle protein breakdown and the critical role of the ubiquitin-proteasome pathway in normal and disease states. *J. Nutr.* 129: 227S-237S (1999).

[37] M. W. Du J, Wang X, Price SR. Glucocorticoids induce proteasome C3 subunit expression in L6 muscle cells by opposing the supression of its transcription by NFKB. *J. Biol. Chem.* 275: 19661-19666 (2000).

[38] S. C. Bodine, E. Latres, S. Baumhueter, V. K. Lai, L. Nunez, B. A. Clarke, W. T. Poueymirou, F. J. Panaro, E. Na, K. Dharmarajan, Z. Q. Pan, D. M. Valenzuela, T. M. DeChiara, T. N. Stitt, G. D. Yancopoulos, and D. J. Glass. Identification of ubiquitin ligases required for skeletal muscle atrophy. *Science.* 294: 1704-8 (2001).

[39] R. R. Almon, D. C. DuBois, E. H. Brandenburg, W. Shi, S. Zhang, R. M. Straubinger, and W. J. Jusko. Pharmacodynamics and pharmacogenomics of diverse receptor-mediated effects of methylprednisolone in rats using microarray analysis. *Journal of Pharmacokinetics and Pharmacodynamics.* 29: 103-29 (2002).

[40] C. Jux, K. Leiber, U. Hugel, W. Blum, C. Ohlsson, G. Klaus, and O. Mehls. Dexamethasone impairs growth hormone (GH)-stimulated growth by suppression of local insulin-like growth factor (IGF)-I production and expression of GH- and IGF-I-receptor in cultured rat chondrocytes. *Endocrinology* 139: 3296-305 (1998).

[41] J. M. Luo, and L. J. Murphy. Dexamethasone inhibits growth hormone induction of insulin-like growth factor-I (IGF-I) messenger ribonucleic acid (mRNA) in

hypophysectomized rats and reduces IGF-I mRNA abundance in the intact rat. *Endocrinology* 125: 165-71 (1989).

[42] T. Ohyama, Sato, M., Niimi, M., Hizuka, N., Takahara, J. Effects of short- and long-term dexamethasone treatment on growth and growth hormone (GH)-releasing hormone (GRH)-GH insulin-like growth factor-I axis in conscious rats. *Endocr. J.* 44: 827-835 (1997).

[43] V. G. Selyatitskaya, O. I. Kuz'minova, and S. V. Odintsov. Development of insulin resistance in experimental animals during long-term glucocorticoid treatment. *Bulletin of Experimental Biology and Medicine.* 133: 339-41 (2002).

[44] Y. N. Sun, L. I. McKay, D. C. DuBois, W. J. Jusko, and R. R. Almon. Pharmacokinetic/Pharmacodynamic models for corticosteroid receptor down-regulation and glutamine synthetase induction in rat skeletal muscle by a Receptor/Gene-mediated mechanism. *Journal of Pharmacology and Experimental Therapeutics.* 288: 720-8 (1999).

[45] L. I. McKay, D. C. DuBois, Y. N. Sun, R. R. Almon, and W. J. Jusko. Corticosteroid effects in skeletal muscle: gene induction/receptor autoregulation. *Muscle and Nerve.* 20: 1318-20 (1997).

[46] S. Max, J. Mill, K. Mearow, M. Konagaya, Y. Konagaya, J. Thomas, C. Banner, and L. Vitkovic. Dexamethasone regulates glutamine synthetase expression in rat skeletal muscles. *Am. J. Physiol.* 255: E397-E402 (1988).

[47] S. Abcouwer, B. Bode, and W. Souba. Glucocorticoids regulate rat glutamine synthetase expression in a tissue-specific manner. *J. Surgical Res.* 59: 59-65 (1995).

[48] H. A. Koistinen, and J. R. Zierath. Regulation of glucose transport in human skeletal muscle. *Annals of Medicine.* 34: 410-8 (2002).

[49] A. Shirakami, T. Toyonaga, K. Tsuruzoe, T. Shirotani, K. Matsumoto, K. Yoshizato, J. Kawashima, Y. Hirashima, N. Miyamura, C. R. Kahn, and E. Araki. Heterozygous knockout of the IRS-1 gene in mice enhances obesity-linked insulin resistance: a possible model for the development of type 2 diabetes. *Journal of Endocrinology.* 174: 309-19 (2002).

[50] G. Sesti. Insulin receptor substrate polymorphisms and type 2 diabetes mellitus. *Pharmacogenomics.* 1: 343-57 (2000).

[51] B. A. Zinker, C. M. Rondinone, J. M. Trevillyan, R. J. Gum, J. E. Clampit, J. F. Waring, N. Xie, D. Wilcox, P. Jacobson, L. Frost, P. E. Kroeger, R. M. Reilly, S. Koterski, T. J. Opgenorth, R. G. Ulrich, S. Crosby, M. Butler, S. F. Murray, R. A. McKay, S. Bhanot, B. P. Monia, and M. R. Jirousek. PTP1B antisense oligonucleotide lowers PTP1B protein, normalizes blood glucose, and improves insulin sensitivity in diabetic mice. *Proceedings of the National Academy of Sciences of the United States of America.* 99: 11357-62 (2002).

[52] B. J. Goldstein. Protein-tyrosine phosphatase 1B (PTP1B): a novel therapeutic target for type 2 diabetes mellitus, obesity and related states of insulin resistance. *Current Drug Targets - Immune Endocrine and Metabolic Disorders.* 1: 265-75 (2001).

[53] R. Di Paola, L. Frittitta, G. Miscio, M. Bozzali, R. Baratta, M. Centra, D. Spampinato, M. G. Santagati, T. Ercolino, C. Cisternino, T. Soccio, S. Mastroianno, V. Tassi, P. Almgren, A. Pizzuti, R. Vigneri, and V. Trischitta. A variation in 3' UTR of hPTP1B

increases specific gene expression and associates with insulin resistance.[erratum appears in Am J Hum Genet 2002 May;70(5):1388]. *American Journal of Human Genetics.* 70: 806-12 (2002).

[54] M. C. Sugden, and M. J. Holness. Therapeutic potential of the mammalian pyruvate dehydrogenase kinases in the prevention of hyperglycaemia. *Current Drug Targets - Immune Endocrine and Metabolic Disorders.* 2: 151-65 (2002).

[55] M. C. Sugden, K. A. Orfali, and M. J. Holness. The pyruvate dehydrogenase complex: nutrient control and the pathogenesis of insulin resistance. *Journal of Nutrition.* 125: 1746S-1752S (1995).

[56] I. Guillet-Deniau, V. Mieulet, S. Le Lay, Y. Achouri, D. Carre, J. Girard, F. Foufelle, and P. Ferre. Sterol regulatory element binding protein-1c expression and action in rat muscles: insulin-like effects on the control of glycolytic and lipogenic enzymes and UCP3 gene expression. *Diabetes.* 51: 1722-8 (2002).

[57] B. Staels, A. v. Tol, L. Chen, G. Verhoeven, and J. Auwerx. Variable effects of different corticosteroids on plasma lipids, apolipoproteins, and hepatic apolipoprotein mRNA levels in rats. *Artheriosclerosis and Thrombosis* 11: 760-769 (1991).

[58] R. Blum. Computer-assisted design of studies using routine clinical data. Analyzing the association of prednisone and cholesterol. *Annals Internal Med.* 104: 858-868 (1986).

[59] S. Balasubramaniam, A. Szanto, and P. Roach. Circadian rhythm in hepatic low-density-lipoprotein (LDL) receptor expression and plasma LDl levels. *Biochem. J.* 298: 39-43 (1994).

[60] J. Goldstein, and M. Brown. The cholesterol quartet. *Science.* 292: 1310-1312 (2001).

[61] O. A. Rayyes, A. Wallmark, and C. Floren. Additive inhibitory effect of hydrocortisone and cyclosporine on low-density lipoprotein receptor activity in cultured HepG2 cells. *Hepatology* 26: 967-971 (1997).

[62] A. Salter, S. Fisher, and D. Brindley. Binding of low-density lipoprotein to monolayer cultures of rat hepatocytes is increased ny insulin and decreased by dexamethasone. *FEBS Letters* 220: 159-162 (1987).

[63] B. Kennedy, H. Elayan, and M. G. Ziegler. Glucocorticoid hypertension and nonadrenal phenylethanolamine N-methyltransferase. *Hypertension.* 21: 415-9 (1993).

[64] H. Schacke, W. D. Docke, and K. Asadullah. Mechanisms involved in the side effects of glucocorticoids. *Pharmacology and Therapeutics.* 96: 23-43 (2002).

[65] A. Nichols, F. Boudinot, and W. Jusko. Second generation model for prednisolone pharmacodynamics in the rat. *J. Pharmacokinet. Biopharm.* 17: 209-227 (1989).

[66] Y. N. Sun, D. C. DuBois, R. R. Almon, and W. J. Jusko. Fourth-generation model for corticosteroid pharmacodynamics: a model for methylprednisolone effects on receptor/gene-mediated glucocorticoid receptor down-regulation and tyrosine aminotransferase induction in rat liver. *Journal of Pharmacokinetics and Biopharmaceutics.* 26: 289-317 (1998).

[67] Y. N. Sun, D. C. DuBois, R. R. Almon, N. A. Pyszczynski, and W. J. Jusko. Dose-dependence and repeated-dose studies for receptor/gene-mediated pharmacodynamics of methylprednisolone on glucocorticoid receptor down-regulation and tyrosine aminotransferase induction in rat liver. *Journal of Pharmacokinetics and Biopharmaceutics.* 26: 619-48 (1998).

[68] Z. Xu, Y. Sun, D. DuBois, R. Almon, and W. Jusko. Third-generation model for corticosteroid pharmacodynamics: roles of glucocorticoid receptor mRNA and tyrosine aminotransferase mRNA in rat liver. *J. Pharmacokinet. Biopharm.* 23: 163-181 (1995).

[69] N. Dayneka, V. Garg, and W. Jusko. Comparison of four basic models of indirect pharmacodynamic responses. *J. Pharmacokinet. Biopharm.* 21: 457-478 (1993).

[70] R. Ramakrishnan, D. C. DuBois, R. R. Almon, N. A. Pyszczynski, and W. J. Jusko. Fifth-generation model for corticosteroid pharmacodynamics: application to steady-state receptor down-regulation and enzyme induction patterns during seven-day continuous infusion of methylprednisolone in rats. *Journal of Pharmacokinetics and Pharmacodynamics.* 29: 1-24 (2002).

[71] R. Ramakrishnan, D. C. DuBois, R. R. Almon, N. A. Pyszczynski, and W. J. Jusko. Pharmacodynamics and pharmacogenomics of methylprednisolone during 7-day infusions in rats. *Journal of Pharmacology and Experimental Therapeutics.* 300: 245-56 (2002).

[72] T. A. B. P. W. Group. Expression profiling--best practices for data generation and interpretation in clinical trials. *Nature Reviews Genetics* 5: 229-237 (2004).

[73] J. Seo, M. Bakay, Y. Chen, S. Himler, B. Shneiderman, and E. Hoffman. Optimizing signal/noise ratios in expression profiling: project-specific algorithm selection and detection p value weighting in affymetrix microarrays. *Bioinformatics* Epublished ahead of print: (2004).

[74] R. R. Almon, J. Chen, G. Snyder, D.C DuBois, W.J. Jusko, and E.P. Hoffman. In vivo multi-tissue corticosteroid microarray time series available online at Public Expression Profile Resource (PEPR). *Pharmacogenomics* 4: 791-799 (2003).

[75] M. B. Eisen, P. T. Spellman, P. O. Brown, and D. Botstein. Cluster analysis and display of genome-wide expression patterns. *Proceedings of the National Academy of Sciences of the United States of America.* 95: 14863-8 (1998).

[76] G. Cojocaru, N. Friedman, M. Krupsky, P. Yaron, D. Simansky, A. Yellin, G. Rechavi, Y. Barash, A. Ben-Dor, Z. Yakhini, and N. Kaminski. Transcriptional profiling of non-small cell lung cancer using oligonucleotide microarrays. *Chest.* 121: 44S (2002).

[77] N. Friedman, and N. Kaminski. Statistical methods for analyzing gene expression data for cancer research. *Ernst Schering Research Foundation Workshop.* 109-31 (2002).

[78] N. Kaminski. Microarray analysis of idiopathic pulmonary fibrosis. *American Journal of Respiratory Cell and Molecular Biology.* 29: S32-6 (2003).

[79] C. Lock, G. Hermans, R. Pedotti, A. Brendolan, E. Schadt, H. Garren, A. Langer-Gould, S. Strober, B. Cannella, J. Allard, P. Klonowski, A. Austin, N. Lad, N. Kaminski, S. J. Galli, J. R. Oksenberg, C. S. Raine, R. Heller, and L. Steinman. Gene-microarray analysis of multiple sclerosis lesions yields new targets validated in autoimmune encephalomyelitis.[see comment]. *Nature Medicine.* 8: 500-8 (2002).

[80] K. T. Morgan, H. Ni, H. R. Brown, L. Yoon, C. W. Qualls, Jr., L. M. Crosby, R. Reynolds, B. Gaskill, S. P. Anderson, T. B. Kepler, T. Brainard, N. Liv, M. Easton, C. Merrill, D. Creech, D. Sprenger, G. Conner, P. R. Johnson, T. Fox, M. Sartor, E. Richard, S. Kuruvilla, W. Casey, and G. Benavides. Application of cDNA microarray technology to in vitro toxicology and the selection of genes for a real-time RT-PCR-

based screen for oxidative stress in Hep-G2 cells. *Toxicologic Pathology*. 30: 435-51 (2002).

[81] D. R. Rhodes, T. R. Barrette, M. A. Rubin, D. Ghosh, and A. M. Chinnaiyan. Meta-analysis of microarrays: interstudy validation of gene expression profiles reveals pathway dysregulation in prostate cancer. *Cancer Research*. 62: 4427-33 (2002).

[82] J. Y. Jin, R. R. Almon, D. C. DuBois, and W. J. Jusko. Modeling of corticosteroid pharmacogenomics in rat liver using gene microarrays. *Journal of Pharmacology and Experimental Therapeutics*. 307: 93-109 (2003).

[83] Y. Sun, and W. Jusko. Transit compartments versus gamma distribution function to model signal transduction processes in pharmacodynamics. *J. Pharm. Sci.* 87: 732-737 (1998).

[84] E. Falkenstein, H.-C. Tillmann, M. Christ, M. Feuring, and M. Wehling. Multiple actions of steroid hormones - a focus on rapid, nongenomic effects. *Pharm. Reviews* 52: 513-555 (2000).

[85] D. Wheeler, D. Church, and S. Federhenet. Database resources of the National Center for Biotechnology. *Nucl. Acids Res.* 31: 28-33 (2003).

[86] K. Pruitt, T. Tatusov, and D. Maglott. RefSeq and LocusLink: NCBI gene-centered resources. *Nucl. Acids Res.* 31: 34-37 (2003).

[87] J. Henikoff, E. Greene, S. Pietrokovski, and S. Henikoff. Increased coverage of protein families with the Blocks Database servers. *Nucl. Acids Res.* 28: 228-230 (2000).

[88] G. del Rio, T. F. Bartley, H. del-Rio, R. Rao, K. L. Jin, D. A. Greenberg, M. Eshoo, and E. Bredesen. Mining DNA microarray data using a novel approach based on graph theory. *FEBS Letters* 509: 230-234 (2001).

[89] A. Rzhetsky, and S. M. Gomez. Birth of scale-free molecular networks and the number of distinct DNA and protein domains per genome. *Bioinformatics* 17: 988-996 (2001).

In: New Research on Pharmacogenetics
Editors: Linda P. Barnes, pp. 83-102
ISBN: 1-60021-056-2

Chapter III

Clinical Applications of Pharmacogenetics: Genetic Polymorphisms and Neuroleptic Malignant Syndrome

Chiaki Kawanishi*
Department of Psychiatry, Yokohama City University School of Medicine

Abstract

Psychiatrists and pharmacologists have recently investigated the factors underlying differences between patients in efficacy and adverse effects of neuroleptic drugs. Prediction and prevention of likely adverse drug reactions are a vitally important goal for medication safety. At present, however, treatment still must be stopped or changed occasionally in response to severe drug reactions. Among these adverse reactions, neuroleptic malignant syndrome is a potentially lethal complication of neuroleptic administration that is characterized by hyperthermia, extrapyramidal signs, altered consciousness, and multiple manifestations of autonomic dysfunction. Mortality was estimated to exceed 70% when the syndrome initially was recognized. In addition to acquired risk factors, genetic predisposition toward neuroleptic malignant syndrome has been suggested by clinical observations. Genetic association studies have sought to identify polymorphisms influencing susceptibility to neuroleptic malignant syndrome, especially with respect to the dopamine D2 receptor, serotonin receptor, and cytochrome P450 2D6. Certain case reports, and data suggesting associations between NMS and genetic polymorphisms/haplotypes of the dopamine D2 gene have paved the way toward understanding the pathophysiology of the syndrome. Neuroleptic malignant syndrome might have a include heterogeneous nature, with common characteristic symptoms but multiple causative mechanisms. More large controlled genetic studies of neuroleptic

* Chiaki Kawanishi, M.D., Ph.D. Assistant Professor, Department of Psychiatry Yokohama City University School of Medicine, 3-9 Fukuura, Kanazawa-ku, Yokohama 236-0004, Japan. Phone: 81-45-787-2667. Fax: 81-45-783-2540. E-mail address: chiaki@yokohama-cu.ac.jp

malignant syndrome and related conditions are needed. Genetic data should be analyzed together with detailed clinical information. Such a productive pharmacogenetic studies should permit reconsideration of the entity of neuroleptic malignant syndrome.

Introduction

Pharmacotherapy has played a central role in treatment for mental disorders since chlorpromazine entered psychiatric practice use in the mid-1950s. Over the following 5 decades, many different classes of neuroleptics have been produced and used. Although neuroleptics have brought patients considerable benefits, psychiatrists nonetheless need to exercise caution with medications. For example, adverse reactions to neuroleptics commonly occur, often unpredictably and unpreventably; some of these events are potentially lethal or refractory. Table 1 lists of neuroleptic adverse reactions associated with neurotransmitter systems in the central nervous system (CNS). Some of these, including tardive dyskinesia, tardive dystonia, and neuroleptic malignant syndrome, have been incompletely understood in terms of mechanisms, and lack of definitive therapies. A new generation of antipsychotic drugs termed atypical neuroleptics, such as clozapine, olanzapine, quetiapine, risperidone, and perospirone, have been found to carry less risk of adverse effects including extrapyramidal symptoms and prolactin elevation [1]. However, complete prevention of adverse reactions is impossible. Effects such as body weight gain and hyperglycemia have emerged as potential problems in administration of some atypical neuroleptics [2, 3], and clozapine is associated with risk of life-threatening agranulocytosis [4].

Table 1. Potential neurologic symptoms of adverse reactions associated with neurotransmitter systems

1	Sedation
2	Dizziness
3	Depressive state
4	Postural tremor
5	Akathisia
6	Restless leg syndrome
7	Tardive dyskinesia
8	Orofacial dyskinesia
9	Rabbit syndrome
10	Tics
11	Acute dystonic movement
12	Tardive dystonia
13	Myoclonus
14	Convulsion
15	Neuroleptic malignant syndrome

In a meta-analysis, Lazarou et al. [5] reported frequency of adverse effects, irrespective of type of drug, in patients hospitalized from 1966 to 1996 in the United States; serious adverse reactions occurred in 6.7% of patients, and fatal adverse reactions in 0.32%. These data excluded cases of errors in drug administration, noncompliance, overdose, drug abuse, therapeutic failure, and questionable adverse reaction. Interindividual differences in responses to drugs in terms of both efficacy and adverse reactions are an important problem in pharmacotherapy; understanding the reasons for these diffrerences should lead to more rational and safe therapy. Age, pregnancy, diseases, lifestyle and habits, diet, and genetic predisposition are known to affect pharmacokinetics. Among these, genetic factors have been known to be a major contributor to interindividual differences in responses. Recent progress in pharmacogenetics has linked genetic polymorphisms of drug-metabolizing enzymes, drug transporters, and possibly drug-targeting molecules to interindividual variations in drug responses [6-9]. In terms of psychotropic drugs, interindividual responses involving efficacy, treatment resistance, and vulnerability to adverse reactions have been investigated from a pharmacogenetic point of view. This chapter surveys pharmacogenetic studies of neuroleptic malignant syndrome, one of the most severe adverse reactions to psychotropic drugs, including problems remaining to be solved and prospects for future advances. This consideration of neuroleptic malignant syndrome will begin with a summary of its clinical picture.

Neuroleptic Malignant Syndrome

Neuroleptic malignant syndrome (NMS), a severe and potentially lethal adverse reaction to neuroleptic administration, is characterized by hyperthermia, extrapyramidal signs, altered consciousness, and autonomic dysfunction including fluctuation of blood pressure, arrhythmia, dyspnea, diaphoresis, and incontinence [10]. A case report of "fatal hyperpyrexia" following administration of chlorpromazine might be the first description of NMS as a clinical entity [11]. Delay et al. [12, 13] further delineated this condition as "neuroleptic malignant syndrome", describing groups of symptoms. Mortality in NMS was estimated to exceed 70% when the syndrome first came to be recognized. While increased awareness of prodromal symptoms and prompt therapy has improved the prognosis, nevertheless mortality still is estimated to be in excess of 10% [14].

With increased recognition of NMS in the 1980s, hundreds of individual cases reports and a variety of clinical investigations have been reported. Several diagnostic criteria have been proposed [15]. Although no consensus criteria has been adopted, the criteria of Pope et al. [16], which cover a broad spectrum of features of the syndrome, are useful for both early detection of the NMS occurrence and as a definition for use in research (Table 2). Several prospective studies have reported NMS occurrence rates ranging from 0.07% to 2.2% of patients receiving neuroleptics [17]. The variability may reflect differences in institutional settings and diagnostic criteria. According to a survey in Japan, 89% of NMS episodes occurred in patients between 20 to 59 years old [18]. Gender probably has no significant influence on incidence. Ethnic differences have not been well examined, but regional practice preferences and changes over time are thought to be involved in some of these [10].

Considering that the occurrence data above were obtained from psychiatric units, NMS has proven less rare overall than initially thought. Recent NMS cases reported from clinical settings outside of neurologic and psychiatric units underscore the possibility of NMS anywhere that any neuroleptic drug is administered [19-21]. NMS may occur at any ages in parallel with the prevalence of psychotropic drug administration. Moreover, incomplete forms of NMS are likely to have been overlooked in all practice settings.

Table 2. Diagnostic criteria propsed by Pope et al. [16]

Hyperthermia:	Oral temperature of at least 37.5 in absence of other aetiology
Severe extrapyramidal effects characterized by two or more of the following:	1) lead pipe rigidity, 2) cogwheel rigidity 3) sialorrhoea 4) oclogyric crisis 5) retrocollis 6) opisthotonos 7) trismus 8) dysphagia 9) choreiform movements 10) dyskinetic movements 11) festnating gate flexor-extensor posturing
Autonomic dysfunction characterized bytwo or more of the following:	1) hypertension (at least 20 mmHg diastolic above the baseline) 2) tachycardia (at least 30 beats above baseline) 3) tachypnoea (at least 25/min) 4) diaphoresis 5) incontinence
For retrospective diagnosis:	Diagnosis of probable NMS is permissible if the remaining two of three items are met plus one of the following: clouded consciousnss; delirium; mutism; stupor or coma; leukocytosis (WBC greater than 15,000/mm^3); serum CK level greater than 300 U/ml)

In general, responses to drug treatment vary between individuals, and psychiatrists still note difficulty in predicting and preventing adverse reactions to neuroleptics. Even after minimizing acquired risk factors (described later), complete elimination of NMS is impossible. Even the new generation of atypical neuroleptics, which show less prominence of adverse reactions, nonetheless can cause NMS [22, 23].

Treatment of NMS

Pathogenetic and pathophysiologic mechanisms of NMS are not fully understood, and treatment of NMS remains empiric. Discontinuation and washout of the causative neuroleptic is the initial measure taken, accompanied by supportive care including physical cooling and cardiovascular support with continuous monitoring.

While no medication has been established as optimal treatment for NMS, certain agents such as bromocriptine, a dopamine receptor agonist, and dantrolene or diazepam both muscle relaxants, often are used based on clinical evidence [10]. Bromocriptine, given to reverse dopamine receptor antagonism caused by neuroleptics, has been reported to shorten the course of NMS and reduce mortality [24]. Muscle relaxants improve the abonormal muscle tonus in NMS. Intravenous administration of diazepam is safe and effective not only as a muscle relaxant but also for managing mental distress occurring as a reaction to NMS symptoms, and further for blunting residual psychotic symptoms [25-27]. A case report speculated a possibly direct effect of dantrolene on NMS showing improvement of electroencephalography [28]. One should consider whether a therapeutic agent treats NMS directly or moderates its symptoms, but in practice whether or not either dantrolene or diazepam has direct effects on NMS is undetermined. Combined use of a muscle relaxant and a postsynaptic dopamine agonist nonetheless may be most effective. Caroff et al. [29] suggested that electroconvulsive therapy (ECT) is effective in treating NMS as well the active psychiatric symptoms that had been observed in patients prior to NMS onset. Modern methods of modified nonconvulsive ECT might be a safe treatment of NMS, especially for NMS patients with prolonged NMS symptoms or severe psychotic symptoms [30].

A fuller understanding of the pathogenesis of NMS is important for both prevention of occurrence and establishment of a rational treatment.

Environmental Factors in Susceptibility to NMS

Certain predisposing conditions such as dehydration, malnutrition, and exhaustion are risk factors for development of NMS [31-35]. Psychomotor agitation, high or rapidly increasing neuroleptic doses, and frequent use of intramuscular injections are other risk factors that tend to be interrelated [31, 33]. Organic brain diseases and infectious diseases have been suggested to be risk factors, although this has not been fully assessed by a large-scale study [32-35]. Patients with organic brain diseases typically are naive to neuroleptics and other psychotropic drugs, which aggravates problems in risk prediction. Infections, on the other hand, could be a trigger if they significantly worsened the physical condition of the patient. In a somewhat similar situation, a patient whom we recently reported developed NMS following neuroleptic treatment after bone marrow transplantation for acute myeloid leukemia. Pretransplantation irradiation, chemotherapy, and graft-versus-host disease (GVHD) had resulted in both physical and mental stress [21]. Tanaka et al. reported NMS complicating treatment of delirium following surgery for soft palate cancer [19]. Such patients could be considered at high risk.

Minimizing risk factors and increasing awareness of NMS could decrease its incidence to some extent, and detection of prodromal symptoms could permit action to decrease morbidity. However, prediction and prevention are still difficult because no biologic marker is available for identifying individuals who are at increased risk for NMS.

Constitutional Factors Susceptibility to NMS

Even among patients with environmental risk factors, most do not develop NMS, while NMS often recurs despite absence or correction of acquired risk factors. Some patients appear to be intrinsically vulnerable to NMS, and genetic factors are thought to be involved. Further, a patient who has experienced NMS remains at increased risk [32, 37-40]. As NMS occurrence is relatively rare, multiple occurrences in a family also suggests a genetic predisposition. Deuschl et al. [41] reported NMS in twin brothers. Otani et al. [42] described occurrence of NMS in a woman and her two daughters. Manor et al. [43] reported NMS in siblings with type II gangliosidosis, an inherited metabolic disease. Increasing numbers of molecular genetic studies are being carried out, mainly representing mutation analyses and case-control genetic association studies. The results are described later in the chapter, after a consideration of some aspects of pathogenesis and pathophysiology of NMS.

The Mechanism of NMS

Mechanisms underlying NMS still are a matter of controversy. The only point of consensus is that the dopaminergic system in the brain is pivotal in the onset of NMS. The clinical potency of a given neuroleptics, especially against the positive symptoms of schizophrenia such as hallucinations and delusions is closely related to its dopamine receptor binding affinity [44]. All neuroleptics causing NMS act as antagonists at CNS dopamine receptors, especially the dopamine D2 receptor (DRD2), and sudden withdrawal of dopamine agonists occasionally causes events indistinguishable from NMS in patients with Parkinson's disease who have no neuroleptic exposure [10]. Other central neurotransmission pathways such as the serotonergic and cholinergic systems have been considered as contributors to NMS, either independently or probably together with the dopaminergic system [45, 46].

Monoamine turnover in the central nervous system can be estimated indirectly by measuring cerebrospinal fluid concentrations of the respective metabolites. Nishijima et al. [47] demonstrated low concentrations of both homovanillic acid (HVA; a metabolite of dopamine) and 5-hydroxyindoleacetic acid (5-HIAA; a metabolite of serotonin) in cerebrospinal fluid in the active phase of NMS and also after recovery. This observation does not necessarily conflict with the dopamine blockade theory. Importantly, single-photon emission computed tomography demonstrated intense occupancy of DRD2 in a patient with NMS [48].

In general, neuropathologic assessment has been central to investigation of pathogenesis and pathophysiology of CNS diseases and dysfunction. However, since neuropathologic studies of NMS have been few, sites of brain damage causing dysfunction in NMS have not been established. Under such conditions, agreement between two clinical neuropathologic studies is noteworthy. Iwabuchi et al. [49] and Lee et al. [50] both observed destruction of efferent pathways in the cerebellum at autopsy in individuals showing residual neurologic symptoms. Figure 1 schematically presents neuropathologic findings in NMS patients [49].

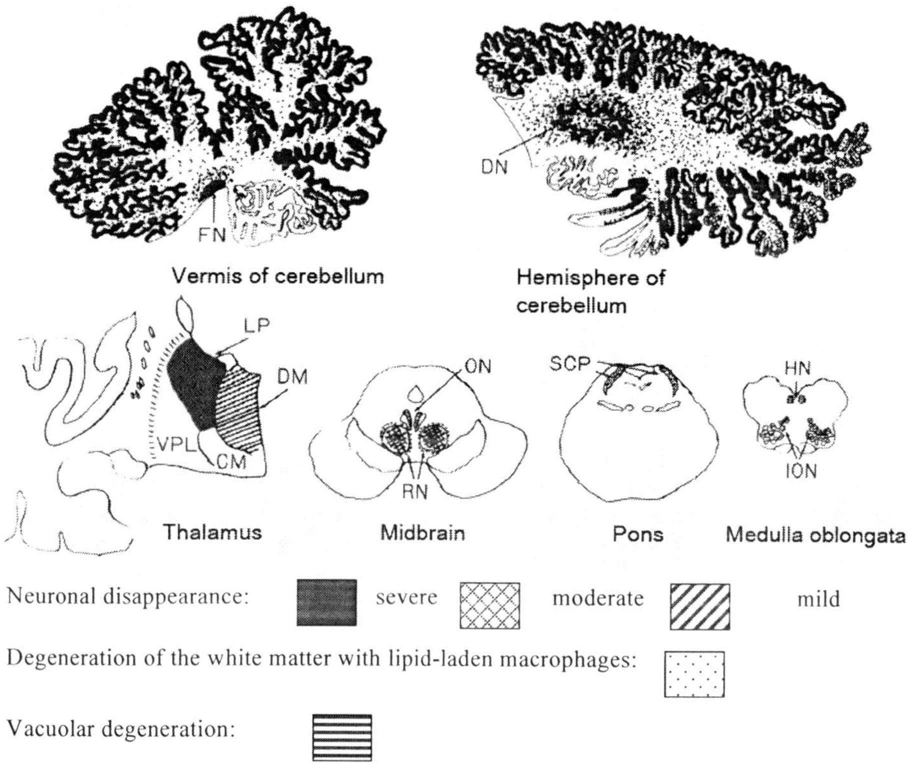

Figure 1. Schematic presentation of the neuropathological findings observe in two patients with NMS. The patients had shown a residual psychiatric symptom such as decreased spontaneity, and irreversible neuromuscler symptoms such as choreoathetoid movement and general muscle atrophy. They died from pneumonia [49]. CM: centromedian nucleus, DM: dorsomedial nucleus, DN: dentate nucleus, HN: hypoglossal nucleus, ION: inferior olivary nucleus, LP: lateral posterior nucleus, ON: oculomotor nucleus, RN: red nucleus, SCP: superior cerebellar peduncle, VPL: ventral posterior nucleus
Reproduced with permission

An alternative to central theories involves a preexisting muscle abnormality in NMS. This possibility has been suggested mainly by similarities in clinical manifestations between NMS and malignant hyperthermia, a life-threatening adverse reaction to inhalation anesthetics or succinylcholine. Malignant hyperthermia is inherited in autosomal dominant fashion and involves accelerated metabolism in skeletal muscle [51]. This disorder is characterized by hyperpyrexia, muscle rigidity, rhabdomyolysis, respiratory acidosis, and tachycardia. However, functional impairment of muscle is not central to NMS. Abnormal skeletal muscle contracture, which is observed in vitro in the halothane-caffeine test used in patients suspected to be predisposed to malignant hyperthermia, is not consistently observed in NMS patients [52]. Malignant hyperthermia is caused by mutations either in the ryanodine receptor gene or in other unidentified genes [51, 53]. Miyatake et al. [54] screened for several mutations of the ryanodine receptor gene, which had been shown to cause malignant hyperthermia, in 10 NMS patients, without finding any mutation. Further, successive occurrence of these two conditions in one patient has reported only once [55], so clinical similarities and the possibility of a common pathogenesis may have been exaggerated. Yet, generalized adverse drug reactions with hyperthermia might follow converging but presently unknown pathways [56-58], so malignant hyperthermia and NMS may share pathophysiologic if not etiologic features.

No single hypothesis proposed so far fully explains all aspects of NMS occurrence and symptomatology; instead, competing and complementary concepts have been hypothesized and disputed [59]. Table 3 lists various proposed mechanisms in NMS. The author has suggested that aberrant CNS neurotransmission followed by impaired drug metabolism could trigger occurrence of NMS, which may be a possibly heterogeneous condition involving different etiologies and early pathophysiologic mechanisms. Subsequently patients' courses may come to appear similar as subsequent events follow a common pathway.

Table 3. Proposed elements contributing to occurrence and pathophysiology of NMS

- Antagonism of the CNS dopaminergic nervous system
- Imbalance between CNS dopaminergic and serotonergic nervous systems
- Imbalance between CNS cholinergic and dopaminergic nervous systems
- Sympathoadrenal hyperreactivity
- Impairment of drug metabolism
- Preexisting muscle impairment, or the hypothesis that NMS and malignant hyperthermia are identical

Pharmacogenetic Approach to NMS

Before the 1990s, little attention had been paid to genetic aspects of adverse reactions to psychopharmacotherapy except for tardive dyskinesia, where familial occurrence had been investigated [60-62]. Accumulated reports of familial occurrence and advances in pharmacogenetics paved the way to a molecular genetic approach toward adverse reactions of neuroleptics. To date several adverse reactions to neuroleptics, such as extrapyramidal side effects [63, 64], clozapine-induced agranulocytosis [65], and body weight gain [66, 67] have been studied genetically. As a result, genetic polymorphisms of cytochrome P450 2D6, a drug metabolizing enzyme, have been associated with vulnerability to extrapyramidal side effects [63]. Tardive dyskinesia, perhaps the most troubling extrapyramidal side effect, showed possible associations with certain HLA types and with genetic polymorphisms involving dopamine D2/D3 receptors, serotonin 2A/2C receptors, manganese superoxide dismutase, and opioid receptors, as well as cytochrome P450 2D6 gene polymorphisms [68]. Recently, the pharamacogenetics of efficacy of psychotropic drugs and treatment resistance has become another focus of investigation. In mood disorders, genetic polymorphisms of the serotonin transporter have been linked to clinical response to antidepressants of the selective serotonin reuptake inhibitor group [69]. Genetic polymorphisms of serotonin 2A receptors have been linked to response to clozapine [70]. Some treatment resistance in mood disorders may depend on activity of cytochrome P450 2D6, which is affected by genetic polymorphisms [71]. Various case-control association studies have been carried out to investigate susceptibility to NMS. These pharmacogenetic studies have been designed from either a pharmacokinetic pharmacogenetic or a pharmacodynamic point of view.

NMS and Drug Metabolism

Cytochrome P450 2D6 (CYP2D6), an isozyme of the cytochrome P450 superfamily, is a major hepatic oxidative enzyme that metabolizes many drugs, including neuroleptics such as haloperidol, risperidone, aripiperazole, perphenazine, thioridazine, and zuclopenthixol, as well as most antidepressants [72]. CYP2D6 is highly polymorphic, and metabolism involving CYP2D6 shows marked interindividual variation. More than 70 polymorphic alleles have been identified in the CYP2D6 gene, which is localized on chromosome 22 (website, http://www.imm.ki.se/CYPalleles/CYP2D6.htm), and genotype-phenotype correlations have been well examined in detail [72]. Phenotypes of CYP2D6 metabolic capacity related to these polymorphisms have been divided into extensive, poor, and ultrarapid metabolizers (EM, PM, and UM) according to enzymatic activity. The PM phenotype, with no CYP2D6 being expressed, is caused by total gene deletion or single nucleotide polymorphisms in the gene that are inherited in an autosomal recessive manner. In the PM phenotype, CYP2D6 substrates are metabolized very slowly, resulting in unexpectedly high plasma drug concentrations [72] that can produce adverse drug reactions even at a conventional dose [8, 73]. In contrast, the UM phenotype, reflecting the presence of additional copies of a functional CYP2D6 gene, shows an accelerated rate of drug metabolism that requires a higher dose than usually recommended to achieve therapeutic plasma drug concentrations [74-76]. This phenotype may contribute to refractoriness in schizophrenia or depression [71, 72, 77]. The reported distribution for debrisoquine metabolic ratio in northern European Caucasians and corresponding genotypes is shown in Figure 2.

Phenotypes for CYP2D6 metabolic capacity differ in prevalence between ethnic populations depending on the distribution of polymorphisms of the gene. Prevalence of the PM phenotype varies between 6% to 10% in European Caucasians, while it is only about 1% in Far Easterners (Chinese, Koreans, and Japanese). The *3 and *4 alleles, which together with gene deletion (the *5 allele) account for most occurrences of the PM phenotype in Caucasians, are very uncommon in eastern Asia. Instead, the *10 allele, which encodes an unstable enzyme with decreased catalytic activity, is predominant in this region. As a result, the clear bimodal distribution for debrisoquine metabolic ratio shown in Figure 2 is not observed in Japanese; instead, distribution of debrisoquine metabolic ratio shifts to the right, and on average Chinese, Koreans, and Japanese show lower CYP2D6 metabolic capacity than European Caucasians [9, 78, 79].

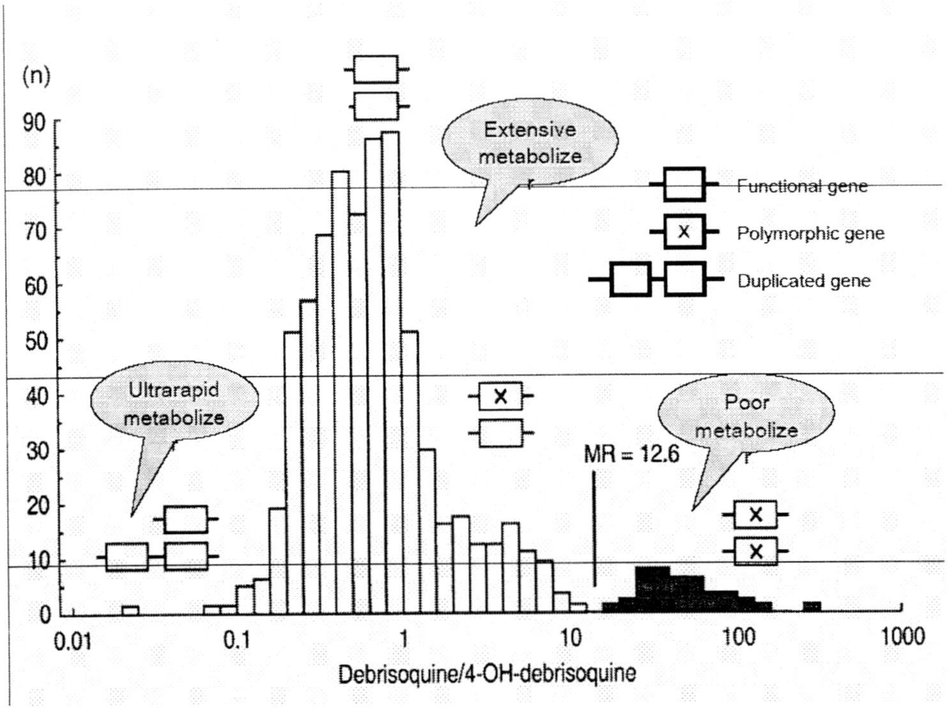

Figure 2. Distribution of the urinary debrisoquine/4-hydroxy-debrisoquine metabolic ratio (MR; from 757 Swedish subjects [72]). The MR of 12.6 is the antimode between extensive (unfilled columns) and poor metabolizers (filled columns). Debrisoquine is a CYP2D6 probe drug, and the relationship between the MR and CYP2D6 genotypes are shown. Reproduced with permission

We have reported two NMS patients who were homozygous for the *10 allele, speculating that NMS occurrence may be related to that genotype [80]. This hypothesis had been supported by studies of other adverse reactions to neuroleptics [81-83]; Ohmori et al. [82] and Kapitany et al. [83] respectively demonstrated possible associations of the *10 allele or PM alleles of the CYP2D6 gene with tardive dyskinesia, respectively. To examine the possible association between unstable CYP2D6 activity and NMS, we compared the frequency of *10 mutations between NMS patients and controls, obtaining negative results [84]. Iwahashi et al. [85] examined the Arg296Cys mutation in the CYP2D6 gene in eight patients with a history of NMS, but could not demonstrate an association between Arg296Cys and the syndrome. The Arg296Cys mutation has been observed in several polymorphic alleles, and the effect of this mutation itself on phenotype is not clear. Otani et al. [86] examined drug oxidation capacity in five patients with a history of NMS, including familial cases that they had reported [42]. CYP2D6 and CYP2C19 probe drugs were used; the patients showed a normal oxidation capacity. Therefore, genetically determined drug oxidation seems unlikely to be a definite contributor to development of NMS. However, in our own pilot study, the deletion genotype of CYP2D6 (involving at least one *5 allele) is showed increased frequency among NMS patients (unpublished data); this point warrants further investigation.

NMS and Drug Targets

As intense dopaminergic blockade generally is accepted as a key component in the pathogenesis of NMS, many investigations have focused on the central dopaminergic system, especially DRD2. This system is related to positive symptoms of schizophrenia, including hallucinations and delusions, as well as to the therapeutic effect of neuroleptics against such symptoms.

The DRD2 gene, which consists of 8 exons, is located at 11q22-23. Schematic presentations of DRD2 and its polymorphisms are shown in Figure 3. When Ram et al. [87] examined the entire coding sequence of DRD2 in 12 patients with a history of NMS, including siblings previously reported by Otani et al. [42], they found Pro310Ser polymorphism in exon 7 in a sporadic case. However, since control subjects were not studied, no conclusion could be reached as to whether the polymorphism affects NMS. This polymorphism is so rare among Japanese that the author has not tried to replicate the study with Japanese patients. Recently, Suzuki et al. [88] reported a possible association between *Taq*I A polymorphism (designated as an A1 or A2 allele) of the DRD2 gene and NMS in Japanese patients. *Taq*I A polymorphism is situated in the untranslated region of the DRD_2 gene, approximately 10 kb downstream from the coding exons. *Taq*I A polymorphism is believed to affect D2 receptor gene regulation. In neuroimaging studies, the A1 allele was associated with reduced DRD2 binding in the striatum, which suggests a relationship of the polymorphism to neuroleptic responsiveness and psychiatric symptoms [89-92]. In clinical studies, *Taq*I A polymorphism was associated with early therapeutic responses to neuroleptics such as nemonapride [94], haloperidol [95], and bromperidol [95], and with enhanced prolactin responses to neuroleptics [95, 96]. Although A1 allele frequency was found to be significantly elevated in 15 patients with NMS [88], this association between *Taq*I A polymorphism and NMS was not replicated in our own recent study of a larger number of NMS patients (49 Japanese subjects) [97]. When we performed systematic screening for genetic polymorphisms of the D2 receptor in NMS patients, we noted an increased frequency of the -141C del allele (-141C ins/del polymorphism) in NMS patients [97]; -141C ins/del polymorphism also is thought to affect D2 receptor gene expression. In an *in vitro* experiment, promoter activity was decreased in del allele constructs compared to that in constructs with the ins allele [99], although some *in vivo* studies did not support a relationship [92, 100].

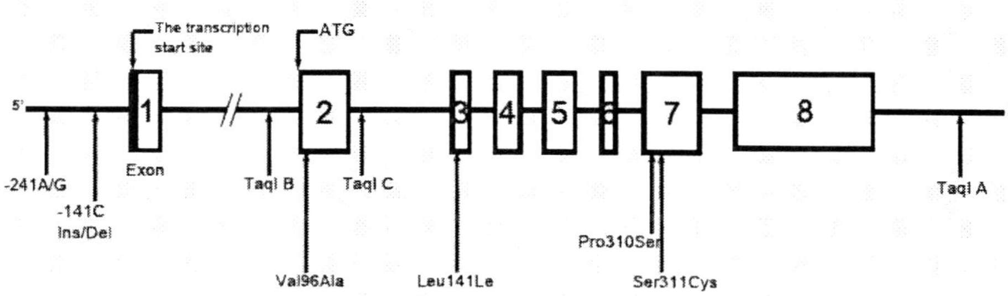

Figure 3. Schematic overview of the dopamine D2 receptor gene and single nucleotide polymorphisms

The author's group has performed a haplotype analysis, finding the A2 (*Taq*I A polymorphisms)-Ins (-141C ins/del)-Ser (Ser311Cys) haplotype to be more prevalent in NMS patients [98].

The serotonergic system mediates various physiologic responses through serotonin receptors and a transporter. The author considered parallels between NMS and another severe adverse reaction to psychotropic drugs, serotonin syndrome, which is caused by exaggerated serotonergic function [101, 102]. Serotonin syndrome clinically resembles NMS, showing hyperpyrexia, restlessness, diaphoresis, myoclonus, hyperreflexia, tremor, and incoordination, and some cases of serotonin syndrome indeed may have been misinterpreted as NMS [56]. Some investigators have pointed out that serotonin syndrome and NMS appear to share common elements of pathophysiology [56, 57]. Hypothesizing that the serotonergic system could be involved in the onset or pathophysiology of NMS, our group examined the influence of serotonin receptor gene polymorphisms on NMS occurrence. Specifically, frequencies of polymorphisms in the 5HT1A (Arg219Leu) and 5HT2A (Thr25Asn and His452Tyr) receptor genes were compared between patients with NMS and neuroleptic-treated schizophrenic patients who had no history of NMS. No polymorphic allele was detected in any NMS patient [103].

Future Prospectives

The present survey of pharmacogenetic studies in NMS underscored the difficulties of research in NMS. Sufficient numbers of subjects are difficult to attain in this relatively rare condition, and clinical researchers are unlikely to encounter familial cases with NMS in their daily practice. These limitations restrict study methodology and possibly may distort data analysis. When performing or assessing association studies, one also needs to consider the appropriateness of the control group. Psychiatrists must intervene immediately in treatment of NMS, which may delay or preclude functional imaging of the brain during the acute phase. Polypharmacy and insufficient therapeutic drug monitoring also can be obstacles to pharmacogenetic investigation. Table 4 lists genetic studies of NMS that have been performed to date. Genetic predisposition toward NMS has been examined mainly with controlled association studies, and some candidate polymorphisms warrant further consideration. However, even these positive findings remain far from practical application. More detailed studies and studies with a sufficiently large scale to attain the required statistical power will be needed.

In future studies, researchers should focus on detailed clinical information, rather than on stringency of diagnostic criteria for the syndrome. If anything, larger samples of NMS and related conditions (such as incomplete NMS, serotonin syndrome, rhabdomyolysis, and elevated plasma creatine kinase) with sufficient available clinical information should be fully examined. NMS might be heterogeneous, with common characteristic symptoms but differing causes and early mechanisms, considering the variety of possible clinical pictures. NMS and related conditions also may represent different parts of a spectrum of adverse reactions to antipsychotic agents. Reconsideration of the entity of NMS now is needed, and these efforts will require accumulation of genetic information together with detailed clinical data concerning patients with NMS and related conditions.

Table 4. Summary of genetic association studies on neuroleptic malignant syndrome

Gene	Polymorphism/ Mutation	Population	Sample size (n)	Results	Reference
Dopamine D2 receptor	-141C Ins/Del	Japanese	15	n.d.	Suzuki et al. (2001)[88]
		Japanese	32	s.d.	Kishida et al. (2004)[98]
	Pro310Ser	Caucasian, Black Japanese	12	Detected in a single case	Ram et al. (1995)[87]
	Pro311Ser	Japanese	15	n.d.	Suzuki et al. (2001)[88]
		Japanese	32	n.d.	Kishida et al. (2004)[98]
	TaqI A	Japanese	15	s.d.	Suzuki et al. (2001)[88]
		Japanese	32	n.d.	Kishida et al. (2004)[98]
D3 receptor	Ser9Gly	Japanese	17	n.d.	Mihara et al. (2003) [104]
		Japanese	36	n.d.	Kishida, Kawanishi, unpublished data
Serotonin 1A receptor	Arg219Leu	Japanese	29	n.d.	Kawanishi et al. (1998)[103]
2A receptor	Thr25Asn, His452Tyr	Japanese	29	n.d.	Kawanishi et al. (1998)[103]
CYP2D6	Arg296Cys	Japanese	8	n.d.	Iwahashi et al. (1999)[85]
	*3, *4	Japanese	24	n.d.	Kawanishi et al. (1997)[105]
	*10	Japanese	36	n.d.	Kawanishi et al. (2000)[84]
RYR1	Arg163Cys, Gly248Arg, Gly341Arg, Ile403Met, Arg614Cys, Arg2434His	Japanese	10	Not detected in any case.	Miyatake et al. (1996)[54]

n.d.: nonsignificant difference from controls
s.d.: significant difference from controls

References

[1] Leucht S, Pitschel-Walz G, Abraham D,: Efficacy and extrapyramidal side-effects of the new antipsychotics olanzapine, quetiapine, risperidone, and sertindole compared to conventional antipsychotic and placebo. A meta-analysis of randomized controlled trials. *Schizophr Res*, 35, 51-68, 1999.

[2] Wetterling T.Bodyweight gain with atypical antipsychotics: a comparative review. *Drug saf*, 24, 59-73, 2001.

[3] Henderson DC: Atypical antipsychotic-induced diabetes mellitus: how strong is the evidence?*CNS drugs*, 16, 77-89, 2002.
[4] Alvir JM, Lieberman JA, Safferman AZ, schwimmer JL, Schaaf JA: Clozapine-induced agranulocytosis: incidence and risk factors in the United States. *N Eng J Med*, 329, 162-167, 1993.
[5] Lazarou J, Pomeranz BH, Corey PN. Incidence of adverse drug reactions in hospitalized patients: a meta-analysis of prospective studies. *JAMA* 1989; 279: 1200-1205.
[6] Masellis M, Basile VS, Özdemir V, Meltzer HY, Macciardi FM, Kennedy JL: Pharmacogenetics of antipsychotic treatment: lessons learned from clozapine. *Biol Psychiatry* 2000; 47: 252-266.
[7] Veenstra-VanderWeele J, Anderson GM, Cook Jr EH. Pharmacogenetics and the serotonin system: initial studies and future directions. *Eur J Pharmacol* 2000; 410: 165-181.
[8] Ingelman-Sundberg M. Pharmacogenetics: an opportunity for a safer and more efficient pharmacotherapy. *J Int Med* 2001; 250: 186-200.
[9] Pacifici GM, Pelkonen O, editors. *Interindividual variability in drug metabolism in humans*. London: Taylor and Francis, 2001.
[10] Caroff SN, Mann SC. Neuroleptic malignant syndrome. *Med Clin North Am* 1993; 77: 185-202.
[11] Ayd FJ. Fatal hyperpyrexia during chlorpromazine therapy. *J Clin Exp Psychopath* 1956; 17: 189.
[12] Delay J, Pichot P, Lemperiere T, Elissalde B, Peigne F: Un neuroleptique majeur non phenothiazinique et non reserpinique, l'haloperidol, dans le traitement des psychoses. *Ann Med Psychol* 1960; 18: 145-152.
[13] Delay J, Deniker P, editors. Drug-induced extrapyramidal syndrome. In: Vinken PJ, Bruyn GW, editors. *Handbook of clinical neurology: Diseases of the basal ganglia.* Amsterdam: North-Holland Publishing Company, 1968: 248-66.
[14] Shalev A, Hermesh H, Munitz H. Mortality from neuroleptic malignant syndrome. *J Clin Psychiatry* 1989; 50: 18-25.
[15] Adityanjee, Mathews T, Aderibigbe YA.: Proposed research diagnostic criteria for neuroleptic malignant syndrome. *Int J Neuropsychopharmacol* 1999; 2: 129-144.
[16] Pope GH, Keck PE, McElroy SL. Frequency and presentation of neuroleptic malignant syndrome in a large psychiatric hospital. *Am J Psychiatry* 1986; 143: 1227-1233.
[17] Adityanjee, Aderibigbe YA, Mathews T. Epidemiology of neuroleptic malignant syndrome. *Clin Neuropharmacol* 1999; 22: 151-158.
[18] Yamawaki S. *Pathogenesis, diagnosis and therapy of neuroleptic malignant syndrome.* Tokyo: Shinkoh Igaku Shuppan; 1989.
[19] Tanaka K, Akechi T, Yamazaki M, Hayashi R, Nishiwaki Y, Uchitomi Y. Neuroleptic malignant syndrome during haloperidol treatment in a cacer patient: a case report. *Support Care Cancer*, 6, 536-538, 1998.
[20] Russell CS, Lang C, McCambridge M, Calhoun B: Neuroleptic malignant syndrome in pregnancy. *Obstet Gynecol* 2001; 98: 906-8.

[21] Onose M, Kawanishi C, Onishi H, Yamada T, Itoh M, KOsaka K, Taguchi J, Fujisawa S, Kanamori H: Neuroleptic malignant syndrome following bone marrow transplantation. *Bone Marrow Transplant* 2002; 29: 803-4.

[22] Hasan S, Buckley P. Novel antipsychotics and the neuroleptic malignant syndrome: a review and critique. *Am J Psychiatry* 1998; 155: 1113-1116.

[23] Caroff SN, Mann SC, Campbell EC. Atypical antipsychotics and neuroleptic malignant syndrome. *Psychiatric Ann* 2000; 30: 314-321.

[24] Sakkas P, Davis JM, Janicak PG, Wang ZY: Drug treatment of the neuroleptic malignant syndrome. *Psychopharmacol Bull*, 27, 381-384, 1991.

[25] Addonizio G, Susman VL, Roth SD. Neuroleptic malignant syndrome: review and analysis of 115 cases. *Biol Psychiatry* 1987; 22: 1004-20.

[26] Kontaxakis VP, Christodoulou GN, Markidis MP, Havaki-Kontaxaki BJ: Treatment of a mild form of neuroleptic malignant syndrome with oral diazepam. *Acta Psychiatr Scand* 1988; 78: 396-398.

[27] Miyaoka H, Shishikura K, Otsubo T, Muramatsu D, Kamijima K: Diazepam-responsive neuroleptic malignant syndrome: a diagnostic subtype? *Am J Psychiatry* 1997;154: 882.

[28] Yamawaki S, Yanagawa K. Possible central effect of dantrolene sodium in neuroleptic malignant syndrome. *J Clin Psychopharmacol* 1986; 6: 378-379.

[29] Caroff SN, Mann SC, Keck PE, Francis A: Residual catatonic state following neuroleptic malignant syndrome. *J Clin Psychoparmacol* 2000; 20: 257-259.

[30] American Psychiatric Association: Task force on electroconvulsive therapy: the practice of electroconvulsive therapy: recommendations for treatment, training and privileging, second edition. *APA*, Washington DC, 2001.

[31] Itoh H, Ohtsuka N, Ogita K yagi G, Miura S, Koga Y: Malignant neuroleptic syndrome: its present status in Japan and clinical problems. *Folia Psychiatr Neurol Jpn* 1977; 31: 565-576.

[32] Shalev A, Munitz H. The neuroleptic malignant syndrome: agent and host interaction. *Acta Psychiatr Scand* 1986; 73: 337-47.

[33] Keck PE Jr, Pope HG Jr, Cohen BM, McElroy SL, Nierenberger AA: Risk factors for neuroleptic malignant syndrome: A case-control study. *Arch Gen Psychiatry* 1989; 46: 914-8.

[34] Sachdev P, Mason C, Hadzi-Pavlovic D. Case-control study of neuroleptic malignant syndrome. *Am J Psychiatry* 1997; 154: 1156-1158.

[35] Berardi D, Amore M, Keck PE Jr, Troia M, Dell'Atti M: Clinical and pharmacologic risk factors for neuroleptic malignant syndrome: a case-control study. *Biol Psychiatry* 1998; 44: 748-754.

[36] Caroff SN, Mann SC, McCarthy M, Naser J, Rynn M, Morrison M: Acute infectious encephalitis complicated by neuroleptic malignant syndrome. *J Clin Psychopharmacol* 1998; 18: 349-51.

[37] Caroff SN, Mann SC. Neuroleptic Malignant Syndrome. *Psychopharmacol Bull* 1988; 24: 25-9.

[38] Wells AJ, Sommi RW, Crismon L. Neuroleptic malignant syndrome: case report and literature review. *Drug Intell Clin Pharm* 1988; 22: 475-80.

[39] Lazarus AL, Moore KE, Spinner NB. Recurrent neuroleptic malignant syndrome associated with inv dup (15) and mental retardation. *Clin Genet* 1991; 39: 65-67.

[40] Mahendran R, Winslow M, Lim D. Recurrent neuroleptic malignant syndrome. *Aust NZ J Psychiatry* 2000; 34: 699-700.

[41] Deuschl G, Oepen G and Hermle L. Neuroleptic malignant syndrome: Observations on altered consciousness. *Pharmacopsychiatry* 1987; 20: 168-170.

[42] Otani K, Horiuchi M, Kondo T, Kaneko S, Fukushima Y: Is the predisposition to neuroleptic malignant syndrome genetically transmitted? *Br J Psychiatry* 1991; 158: 850-3.

[43] Manor I, Hermesh H, Munitz H, Weizman A: Neuroleptic malignant syndrome with gangliosidosis type II. *Biol Psychiatry* 1997; 41: 1222-4.

[44] Seeman P, Lee T, Chau-Wong M, Wong K: Antipsychotic drug doses and neuroleptics/dopamine receptors, *Nature*, 1976, 261, 717-719.

[45] Nemecek D, Rastogi-Cruz D, Csernansky JG: Atropinism may precipitate neuroleptic malignant syndrome during treatment of clozapine. *Am J Psychiatry*, 150, 1561. 1993.

[46] Young C: A case of neuroleptic malignant syndrome and serotonin disturbance. *J Clin Psychopharmacol* 1997; 17: 65-66.

[47] Nishijima K, Ishiguro T. Neuroleptic malignant syndrome: a study of CSF monoamine metabolism. *Biol Psychiatry* 1990; 27: 280-288.

[48] Jauss M, Krack P, Franz M, Klett R, Bauer R, Gallhofer B, Dorndorf W: Imaging of dopamine receptors with [^{123}I] Iodobenzamide single-photon emission-computed tomography in neurolptic malignant syndrome. *Mov Dis*, 11, 726-726, 1996.

[49] Iwabuchi K, Amano N, Yokoi S, Yagishita S, Saito A, Nagatomo H, Matsushita M: Two autopsied cases of neuroleptic malignant syndrome with the irreversible brain damage and myogenic muscular atrophy. *Shinkei Kennkyu no Shinpo* (Japanese), 1989; 33: 674-84.

[50] Lee S, Merriam A, Kim T-S, Liebling M, Dickson DW, Moore GR: Cerebellar degeneration in neuroleptic malignant syndrome: neurologic findings and review of the literature concerning heat-related nervous system injury. *J neurol Neurosurg Psychiatry* 1989; 52: 387-391.

[51] Wappler F. Malignant hyperthermia. *Eur J Anaesthesiol* 2001; 18: 632-652.

[52] Adnet PJ, Krivosic-Horber RM, Adamantidis MM, Haudecoeur G, Adnet-Bonte CA, Saulnier F, Dupuis BA: The association between the neuroleptic malignant syndrome and malignant hyperthermia. *Acta Anaesthesiol Scand* 1989; 33: 676-680.

[53] McCarthy TV, Quane KA, Lynch PJ. Ryanodine receptor mutations in malignant hyperthermia and central core disease. *Hum Mutat*, 2000; 15: 410-7.

[54] Miyatake R, Iwahashi K, Matsushita M, Nakamura K, Suwaki H: No association between the neuroleptic malignant syndrome and mutations in the RYR 1 gene associated malignant hyperthermia. *J Neurol Sci* 1996; 143: 161-5.

[55] Portel L, Hilbert G, Gruson D, Favier JC, Gbikpi-Benissan G, Cardinaud JP: Malignant hyperthermia and neuroleptic malignant syndrome in a patient during treatment for acute asthma. *Acta Anaesthesiol Scand* 1999; 43: 107-10.

[56] Heyland D, Sauve M. Neuroleptic malignant syndrome. *Can Med Assoc J* 1991; 145: 817-819.

[57] Ames D, Wirshing WC. Ecstasy, the serotonin syndrome, and neuroleptic malignant syndrome: a possible link? *JAMA* 1993; 269: 869.

[58] Daras M, Kakkouras L, Tuchman AJ, Koppel BS: Rhabdomyolysis and hyperthermia after cocaine abuse: a variant of the neuroleptic malignant syndrome? *Acta Neurol Scand* 1995; 92: 161-165.

[59] Gurrera R. Sympathoadrenal hyperactivity and the etiology of neuroleptic malignant syndrome. *Am J Psychiatry* 1999; 156: 169-80.

[60] Weinhold P, Wegner JT, Kane JM: Familial occurrence of tardive dyskinesia. *J Clin Psychiatry*, 42, 165-166, 1981.

[61] Yassa R, Annanth J: Familial tardive dyskinesia. *Am J Psychiatry*, 138, 1618-1619, 1981.

[62] Youssef H, Lyster G, Youssef F: Familial psychosis and vulnerability to tardive dyskinesia. *Int Clin Psychopharmacol*, 4, 323-328, 1989.

[63] Scordo MG, Spina E: Cytochrome P450 polymorphisms and response to antipsychotic therapy. *Pharmacogenomics*, 3, 201-218, 2002.

[64] Eichhammer P, Albus M, Borrmann-Hasseenbach M, Schoeler A, Putzhammer A, Frick U, Klein HE, Rohrmeier T: Association of dopamine D3-receptor gene variants with neuroleptic induced akathisia in schizophrenic patients: a generalization of Steen's study on DRD3 and tardive dyskinesia. *Am J Med Genet*, 96, 187-191, 2000.

[65] Dettling M, Cascorbi I: Genetic determinants of clozapine-induced agranulocytosis: recent results of HLA subtyping in a non-Jewish Caucasian sample. *Arch Gen Psychiatry*, 58, 93-94, 2001.

[66] Ellingrod VL, Miller D, Schultz SK, Wehring H, Arndt S: CYP2D6 polymorphisms and atypical antipsychotic weight gain. *Psychiatric Genet*, 12, 55-58, 2002.

[67] Reynolds GP, Zhang ZJ, Zhang XB: Association of antipsychotic drug-induced weight gain with a 5-HT2C receptor gene polymorphism. *Lancet*, 359, 2086-2087.

[68] Ohmori O, Shinkai T, Hori H, Matsumoto C, Nakamura J: A perspective on molecular genetic studies of tardive dyskinesia: one clue for individualized antipsychotic drug therapy. *Prog Neuro-psychopharmacol Biol Psychiatry*, 27, 581-586, 2003.

[69] Lotrich FE, Pollock BG, Ferrell RE: Polymorphism of the serotonin transporter: implication for use of selective serotonin reuptake inhibitors. *Am J Pharmacogenomics*, 1, 153-164, 2001.

[70] Arranz MJ, Munro J, Birkett J, Bolonna A, Mancama D, Sodhi M, Lesch KP, Meyer JF, Sham P, Collier DA, Murray RM, Kerwin RW: Pharmacogenetic prediction of clozapine response. *Lancet*, 355, 1615-1616, 2000.

[71] Kawanishi C, Lundgren S, Agren H, Bertilsson L: Increased incidence of CYP2D6 gene duplication in patients with persistent mood disorders: ultrarapid metabolism of antidepressants as a cause of nonresponse. *A pilot study. Eur J Clin Pharmacol*, 59, 803-807, 2004.

[72] Bertilsson L, Dahl M-L, Dalén P, et al. Molecular genetics of CYP2D6: Clinical relevance with focus on psychotropic drugs. *Br J Clin Pharmacol* 2002; 53: 111-122.

[73] Mayer UA. Pharmacogenetics and adverse drug reactions. *Lancet* 2000; 356: 1667-71.

[74] Bertilsson L, Dahl ML, Sjöqvist F, Aberg-Wistedt A, Humble M, Johansson I, Lundqvist E, Ingelman-Sundberg M: Molecular basis for rational megaprescribing in ultrarapid hydroxylation of debrisoquine. *Lancet* 1993; 341: 63.

[75] Johansson I, Lundqvist E, Bertilsson L, Dahl ML, Sjöqvist F, Ingelman-Sundberg M: Inherited amplification of an active gene in the cytochrome P450 CYP2D locus as a cause of ultrarapid metabolism of debrisoquine. *Proc Natl Acad Sci USA* 1993; 90: 11825-9.

[76] Dahl M-L, Johansson I, Bertilsson L, Ingelman-Sundberg M Sjöqvist F: Ultrarapid hydroxylation of debrisoquine in a Swedish population: analysis of the molecular genetic basis. *J Pharmacol Exp Ther* 1995; 274: 516-20.

[77] Kawanishi C, Furuno T, Kishida I Matsumura T, Kosaka K: A patient with treatment-resistant schizophrenia and CYP2D6 gene duplication. *Clin Genet*, 61, 152-154, 2002.

[78] Roh HK, Dahl M-L, Johansson I, Ingelman-Sundberg M, Cha YN, Bertilsson L: Debrisoquine and S-mephenytoin hydroxylation phenotypes and genotypes in a Korean population. *Pharmacogenet* 1996; 6: 441-7.

[79] Nishida Y, Fukuda T, Yamamoto I, Azuma J: CYP2D6 genotypes in a Japanese population: low frequencies of CYP2D6 gene duplication but high frequency of CYP2D6*10. *Pharmacogenet* 2000; 10: 567-70.

[80] Kawanishi C, Shimoda Y, Fujimaki J, Onishi H, Suzuki K, Hanihara T, Sugiyama N, Kosaka K: Mutation involving cytochrome P450IID6 in two Japanese patients with neuroleptic malignant syndrome. *J Neurol Sci* 1998; 160: 102-104.

[81] Andreassen OA, MacEwan T, Gulbrandsen AK, McCreadie RG, Steen VM: Non-functional CYP2D6 alleles and risk for neuroleptic-induced movement disorders in schizophrenic patients. *Psychopharmacol* 1997; 131: 174-179.

[82] Ohmori O, Suzuki T, Kojima H, Shinkai T, Terao T, Mita T, Abe K: Tardive dyskinesia and debrisoquine 4-hydroxylase genotype in Japanese schizophrenics. *Schizophrenia Res* 1998; 32: 107-113.

[83] Kapitany T, Meszaros K, Lenzinger E, Schindler SD, Barnas C, Fuchs K, SieghartW, Aschauer HN, Kasper S: Genetic polymorphisms for drug metabolism and tardive dyskinesia in schizophrenia. *Schizophrenia Res* 1998; 32: 101-6.

[84] Kawanishi C, Furuno T, Onishi H Sugiyama N, Suzuki K, Matsumura T, Ishigami T, Kosaka K: Lack of association in Japanese patients between neuroleptic malignant syndrome and a debrisoquine 4-hydroxylase genotype with low enzyme activity. *Psychiatric Genet* 2000; 10: 145-7.

[85] Iwahashi K, Yoshihara E, Nakamura K, Ameno K, Watanabe M, Tsuneoka Y, Ichikawa Y, Igarashi K: CYP2D6 HhaI genotype and the neuroleptic malignant syndrome. *Neuropsychobiol* 1999; 39: 33-37.

[86] Otani K, Kaneko S, Fukushima Y, Chiba K, Ishizaki T: NMS and genetic drug oxidation. *Br J Psychiatry* 1991; 159: 595-596.

[87] Ram A, Cao Q, Keck PE Jr, Pope HG Jr, Otani K, Addonizio G, McElroy SL, Kaneko S, Redlichova M, Gershon ES, Gejman PV: Structural change in dopamine D2 receptor gene in a patient with neuroleptic malignant syndrome. *Am J Med Genet* 1995; 60: 228-230.

[88] Suzuki A, Kondo T, Otani K, Mihara K, Yasui-Furukori N, Sano A, Koshiro K, Kaneko S: Association of the TaqI A polymorphism of the dopamine D(2) receptor gene with predisposition to neuroleptic malignant syndrome. *Am J Psychiatry* 2001; 158: 1714-1716.

[89] Thompson J, Thomas N, Singleton A, Piggott M, Lloyd S, Perry EK, Morris CM, Perry RH, Ferrier IN, Court JA: D2 dopamine receptor gene (DRD2) TaqI A polymorphism: reduced dopamine D2 receptor binding in the human striatum associated with the A1 allele. *Pharmacogenet* 1997; 7: 479-84.

[90] Noble EP. The D_2 dopamine receptor gene: a review of association studies in alcoholism and phenotypes. *Alcohol* 1998; 16: 33-45.

[91] Pohjalainen T, Rinne JO, Någren K, Lehikoinen P, Anttila K, Syvälahti EKG, Hietala J. The A1 allele of the human D2 dopamine receptor gene predicts low D2 receptor availability in healthy volunteers. *Mol Psychiatry* 1998; 3: 256-260.

[92] Jönsson EG, öthen MM, Grünhage F, Farde L, Nakashima Y, Propping P, Sedvall GC. Polymorphisms in the dopamine D2 receptor gene and their relationships to striatal dopamine receptor density of healthy volunteers. *Mol Psychiatry* 1999; 4: 290-296.

[93] Suzuki A, Mihara K, Kondo T, Tanaka T, Nagashima U, Otani K, Kaneko S: The relationship between dopamine D2 receptor polymorphism at the Taq1 A locus and therapeutic response to nemonapride, a selective dopamine antagonist, in schizophrenic patients. *Pharmacogenet* 2000; 10: 335-41.

[94] Schäfer M, Rujescu D, Giegling I, Guntermann A, Erfurth A, Bondy B, Möller HJ: Association of short-term response to haloperidol treatment with a polymorphism in the dopamine D2 receptor gene. *Am J Psychiatry* 2001; 158: 802-4.

[95] Mihara K, Suzuki A, Kondo T, Yasui-Furukori N, Ono S, Otani K, Kaneko S, Inoue Y: Relationship between Taq1A dopamine D2 receptor (DRD2) polymorphism and prolactin response to bromperidol. *Am J Med Genet* 2001; 105: 271-274.

[96] Mihara K, Kondo T, Suzuki A, Yasui N, Furukori H, Nagashima U, Ono S, Kaneko S, Otani K, Inoue Y: Prolactin response to nemonapride, a selective antagonist for D2 like dopamine receptors, in schizophrenic patients in relation to Taq1A polymorphism of DRD2 gene. *Psychopharmacol* 2000; 149: 246-250.

[97] Kishida I, Kawanishi C, Furuno T, Matsumura T, Hasegawa H, Sugiyama N, Suzuki K, Yamada Y, Kosaka K: Lack of association in Japanese patients between neuroleptic malignant syndrome and the TaqI A polymorphism of the dopamine D2 receptor gene. *Psychiatric Genet*, 2003, 13, 55-57.

[98] Kishida I, Kawanishi C, Furuno T, Kato D, Ishigami T, Kosaka K: Association in Japanese patients between neuroleptic malignant syndrome and functional polymorphisms of the dopamine D2 receptor gene. *Mol Psychiatry*, 9, 293-298, 2004.

[99] Arinami T, Gao M, Hamaguchi H, Toru M: A functional polymorphism in the promoter region of the dopamine D2 receptor gene is associated with schizophrenia. *Hum Mol Genet* 1997; 6: 577-582.

[100] Pohjalainen T, Någren K, Syvälahti EKG, Hietala J. The dopamine D_2 receptor 5'-flanking variant, $^{-141}$C *Ins/Del*, is not associated with reduced dopamine D_2 receptor density *in vivo*. *Pharmacogenetics* 1999; 9: 505-509.

[101] Insel TR, Roy BF, Cohen RM, Murphy DL: Possible development of the serotonin syndrome in man. *Am J Psychiatry* 1982; 139: 954-955.

[102] Sternbach H. The serotonin syndrome. *Am J Psychiatry* 1991; 148: 705-713.

[103] Kawanishi C, Hanihara T, Shimoda Y, Suzuki K, Sugiyama N, Onishi H, Miyakawa T, Yamada Y, Kosaka K: Lack of association between neuroleptic malignant syndrome and polymorphisms in the 5-HT1A and 5-HT2A receptor genes. *Am J Psychiatry* 1998; 155: 1275-1277.

[104] Mihara K, Kondo T, Suzuki A, Yasui-Furukori N, Ono S, Sano A, Koshir K, Otani K, Kaneko S: Relationship between functional dopamine D2 and D3 receptor gene polymorphisms and neuroleptic malignant syndrome. *Am J Med Genet* 2003; 117B: 57-60.

[105] Kawanishi C, Hanihara T, Maruyama Y, Matsumura T, Onishi H, Inoue K, Sugiyama N, Suzuki K, Yamada Y, Kosaka K: Neuroleptic malignant syndrome and hydroxylase gene mutations: no association with CYP2D6A or CYP2D6B. *Psychiatric Genet* 1997; 7: 127-129.

In: New Research on Pharmacogenetics
Editors: Linda P. Barnes, pp. 103-122
ISBN: 1-60021-056-2

Chapter IV

Genetic Detection of Antimicrobial Resistance Determinants in Gram-Positive Cocci

Toshinobu Horii
Division of Bacteriology, Department of Microbiology and Immunology,
Tottori University School of Medicine,
86 Nishi, Yonago 683-8503, Japan

Abstract

Antimicrobial resistance is a clinical problem in treating bacterial infections. Antimicrobial-resistant Gram-positive cocci include methicillin-resistant *Staphylococcus aureus* (MRSA), methicillin-resistant coagulase-negative staphylococci (MRCNS), penicillin-resistant *Streptococcus pneumoniae* (PRSP), and vancomycin-resistant enterococci (VRE). MRSA and VRE also are recognized as important nosocomial pathogens. Spread of antimicrobial resistance determinants by gene transfer can cause emergence of antimicrobial-resistant Gram-positive cocci (horizontal spread).

MRSA produces penicillin-binding protein (PBP)2' (PBP2a) encoded by the *mecA* gene, which confers resistance to all β-lactams. MRCNS, similarly resistant, also produce PBP2'. MRSA can show concurrent resistance to fluoroquinolones and/or aminoglycosides. Fluoroquinolone resistance is determined mainly by mutations within the *gyrAB* and *grlAB* genes respectively encoding subunits of DNA gyrase and those of DNA topoisomerase IV, or by increased expression of the *norA* gene encoding a drug efflux protein, NorA. Fluoroquinolone resistance is associated with mutations in specific regions of the *gyrAB* and *grlAB* genes termed quinolone resistance-determining regions (QRDRs). Aminoglycoside resistance is conferred by aminoglycoside-modifying enzymes (AMEs) encoded by the *aac(6')-aph(2")*, *ant(4')-I*, and *aph(3')-III* genes.

Among *S. pneumoniae*, prevalence of isolates resistant to β-lactams such as penicillins and cephems, macrolides, and fluoroquinolones has increased worldwide. *S. pneumoniae* resistant to β-lactams emerged through recombination events between the PBP genes of *S. pneumoniae* and those of closely related species. PRSP has multiple alterations in PBPs, which are associated with a mosaic of PBP gene alleles. Resistance of *S. pneumoniae* to macrolides involves target site modification by a 23S rRNA-methylating enzyme encoded by the *ermB* gene and an efflux pump formed by membrane-associated proteins encoded by the *mefA* gene.

Enterococcus faecalis and *Enterococcus faecium* resistant to glycopeptides such as vancomycin and teicoplanin are referred to as VRE, which attain glycopeptide resistance in association with acquisition of *van* gene clusters located in a conjugative element. Genotypes include *vanA*, *vanB*, and *vanD*. VRE synthesize peptidoglycan precursors with pentapeptide side chains terminating in D-Ala-D-Lac, to which glycopeptides bind more poorly than that to D-Ala-D-Ala. Synthesis of D-Ala- D-Lac depsipeptide is catalyzed by VanA, VanB, and VanD ligases respectively encoded by the *vanA*, *vanB*, and *vanD* genes. Antimicrobial therapy for VRE infections is difficult since VRE can develop concurrent resistance to penicillins and aminoglycosides.

We can reliably detect these antibiotic resistance determinants by advanced genetic techniques based mainly on polymerase chain reactions (PCR), DNA-DNA hybridization, and nucleotide sequencing. Antimicrobial resistance determinants detected by PCR with or without DNA-DNA hybridization include the *mecA* gene in MRSA and MRCNS, the PBP genes and the *mefA* and *ermB* genes in *S. pneumoniae*, the *van* genes in VRE, and the AME genes in *S. aureus* and enterococci. Fluoroquinolone resistance of *S. aureus* and *S. pneumoniae* commonly is determined by nucleotide sequencing in the regions (QRDRs) coding for DNA gyrase and topoisomerase IV. Genetic methods, including new methods such as real-time PCR and DNA microarray systems, should guide antimicrobial therapy against infections caused by Gram-positive cocci by early prediction of antimicrobial susceptibility patterns of the isolate. Moreover, information regarding these genotypic traits will contribute identification of nosocomial infections caused by antimicrobial-resistant Gram-positive cocci.

1. Introduction

Bacterial resistance to antimicrobials is a major cause of failure treating infections [1]. Frequency and diversity of infections with antimicrobial-resistant bacteria have increased worldwide during the past few decades [2]. In 2000, the World Health Organization (WHO) warned that overuse of antimicrobials in industrialized countries, underuse of efficacious antimicrobials in developing countries, misdiagnosis of infections, defensive and unnecessary prescribing, increased traffic in counterfeit antimicrobial compounds in developing countries, and use of large amounts of antimicrobials in food production and the agricultural industry are exacerbating the problem, as are clinicians, pharmacists, and patients who are uniformed about the nature of bacterial resistance [3]. Emergence and increases of antimicrobial-resistant bacteria have been attributed to a combination of microbial characteristics, selection pressure from antimicrobial use, and social and technical changes that enhance transmission of resistance factors among organisms [2, 3].

Resistance mechanisms in microorganisms include four strategies: inactivation of antimicrobials [e.g., β-lactamases and aminoglycoside-modifying enzymes (AMEs)]; mutational change of antimicrobial targets [e.g., alterations in penicillin-binding proteins (PBPs), DNA gyrase, or topoisomerase IV; and ribosomal modifications]; acquisition of a new, insensitive target [e.g., altered PBPs such as PBP2' (PBP2a) in methicillin-resistant *Staphylococcus aureus* (MRSA), and altered cell-wall target sites in vancomycin-resistant enterococci (VRE)]; and acquisition of active efflux or a permeability mutation affecting influx or efflux systems (Table 1). Among Gram-positive cocci, antimicrobial resistance generally is acquired by mutational changes such as point and mosaic mutations in the bacterial genome or by acquisition of determinants conferring antimicrobial resistance [2, 4-7]. The determinants can be spread horizontally by means of inter- and intra-species modalities of gene transfer such as conjugation, transduction, and transformation [2, 6]. Interestingly, a mosaic of PBP gene alleles of *Streptococcus pneumoniae* has arisen through intra-species recombination [4, 5]. Recently, acquisition by *S. aureus* of the *vanA* gene via plasmids from eterococci to result in vancomycin-resistant *S. aureus* (VRSA) has been realized as an emerging problem [8].

Overall, nosocomial infections caused by antimicrobial-resistant Gram-positive cocci have become a major clinical concern [2]. The organisms include MRSA, VRE, and *Clostridium difficile* [2, 9].

Development of molecular microbiology and genetics has provided methods for rapid detection of these antimicrobial resistance determinants by means of polymerase chain reactions (PCR), real-time PCR, DNA-DNA hybridization, nucleotide sequencing, and DNA microarray systems (Table 1). Antimicrobial therapy against infections with antimicrobial-resistant Gram-positive cocci should benefit from such rapid and convenient detection of resistance determinants that can predict antimicrobial susceptibility patterns of the pathogen. Moreover, information regarding these genotypic traits should contribute to ongoing identification of nosocomial infections caused by antimicrobial-resistant Gram-positive cocci. The present review will focus on genetic determination of antimicrobial resistance in Gram-positive cocci.

2. Antimicrobial Resistance in *S. aureus*

S. aureus causes a variety of diseases. Some are caused by exotoxin production, such as toxic shock and staphylococcal scalded skin syndrome, and others by direct tissue invasion and systemic dissemination, such as bacteremia, meningitis, skin and soft tissue infections, and abscesses [10]. Resistance to β-lactams, fluoroquinolones, and aminoglycosides in *S. aureus* has emerged as a clinical challenge [11, 12]. MRSA is the leading cause of nosocomial infections and is an increasing concern in community practice as well; indeed, MRSA is a major nosocomial pathogen in hospital settings worldwide [13], while prevalence of MRSA in individuals with infections acquired outside hospitals has increased [14]. Another emerging problem is threatening appearance of VRSA [8, 11].

Coagulase-negative staphylococci (CNS), which cause both nosocomial and community-acquired infections [15, 16], also constitute an important reservoir of β-lactam resistance [17, 18].

Table 1. Mechanisms and genetic detection of antimicrobial resistance in Gram-positive cocci

	Bacteria	Antimicrobial	Resistance gene	Gene product	Method for genetic detection	Reference
1	*Staphylococcus aureus*	β-Lactam	*bla*	β-Lactamase	PCR, multiplex PCR	[19]
2			*mecA*	PBP2' (PBP2a)	PCR, multiplex PCR, DNA-DNA hybridization, real-time PCR, DNA microarray system	[19-23, 38]
3		Fluoroquinolone	*grlA*, *grlB*	Topoisomerase IV	Nucleotide sequencing, DNA microarray system	[25-29, 37, 38]
4			*gyrA*, *gyrB*	DNA gyrase	Nucleotide sequencing, DNA microarray system	[27-30, 37, 38]
5			*norA*	Efflux protein	Nucleotide sequencing	[31-36]
6		Aminoglycoside	*aac(6')-aph(2")*, *ant(4')-I*, *aph(3')-III*	AMEs	PCR, multiplex PCR, DNA-DNA hybridization	[12, 19, 40, 41]
7		Mupirocin	*ileS-2*	Isoleucyl t-RNA synthetase	PCR, multiplex PCR	[22, 45]
8		Linezolid	23S rRNA gene	(23S rRNA)	Nucleotide sequencing	[49]
9	*Streptococcus pneumoniae*	β-Lactam	*pbp*	PBP	PCR, semi-nested PCR, multiplex PCR, real-time PCR	[62, 66, 67]
10		Macrolide	*mefA*	Efflux protein	PCR, multiplex PCR	[53, 63, 68]
11			*ermB*	23S rRNA methylase	PCR, multiplex PCR	[53, 63, 68]
12			L4 and 23S rRNA gene	(L4 and 23S rRNA)	Nucleotide sequencing	[75]
13		Fluoroquinolone	*parC*, *parE*	Topoisomerase IV	Nucleotide sequencing	[27, 69, 78, 80, 81]
14			*gyrA*, *gyrB*	DNA gyrase	Nucleotide sequencing	[27, 69, 78, 80, 81]
15			*pmrA*	Efflux protein	Nucleotide sequencing	[82]
16	Enterococci	β-Lactam	*bla*	β-Lactamase	PCR	[89]
17			*pbp5*	PBP5	Nucleotide sequencing, real-time PCR	[85-87]
18		Aminoglycoside	*aac(6')-aph(2")*	AME	Multiplex PCR	[90]
19		Glycopeptide	*vanA*, *vanB*, *vanD*	VanA, VanB, VanD ligases (catalyze synthesis of D-Ala-D-Lac depsipeptide)	PCR, real-time PCR	[88-90]

AME = aminoglycoside-modifying enzymes, PBP = penicillin-binding protein, PCR = polymerase chain reaction.

2.1. β-Lactams

Mechanisms of β-lactam resistance in *S. aureus* include production of plasmid-mediated β-lactamase encoded by the *bla* gene and PBP2' encoded by the chromosomally located *mecA* gene [11]. The β-lactamase hydrolyzes β-lactam rings of penicillins and related drugs, which is termed penicillinase [11].

More than 90% of *S. aureus* isolates from clinical settings produce the β-lactamase [11]. The *bla* gene in *S. aureus* can be detected by PCR-based methods [19]. Methicillin resistance requires the presence of the *mecA* gene [11]. Production of PBP2' results in resistance to all β-lactams because of its uniformly low affinity for these agents [11]. CNS harboring the *mecA* determinant have been reported [17, 18]. Presence of the *mecA* gene can be detected by methods based on PCR with or without DNA-DNA hybridization in MRSA and methicillin-resistant CNS (MRCNS) [17-23].

2.2. Fluoroquinolones

Fluoroquinolone resistance in *S. aureus* can emerge shortly after these drugs were introduced [24]. Fluoroquinolone resistance in *S. aureus* is conferred by three main mechanisms. The first includes mutations within the *gyrA* and *gyrB* genes, which encode subunits of DNA gyrase, an established target of fluoroquinolone action [25-29]. The second involves analogous resistance-conferring mutations in the *grlA* and *grlB* genes, which encode subunits of topoisomerase IV, another target of fluoroquinolones [27-30]. Mutations associated with increased resistance to fluoroquinolones have been documented in specific regions of the *gyrA*, *gyrB*, *grlA*, and *grlB* genes, which are referred to as quinolone resistance-determining regions (QRDRs) [27]. The third mechanism of resistance involves increased expression of the *norA* gene, which encodes a drug efflux protein, NorA, and/or mutations in the *norA* coding region [31-36]. NorA is a membrane-associated protein that actively transports norfloxacin and other hydrophilic fluoroquinolones out of bacterial cells, effectively decreasing the intracellular concentration of the drug [31, 32, 34].

To determine fluoroquinolone resistance by genetic methods in *S. aureus*, nucleotide sequencing of the QRDRs is performed [37]. In *S. aureus*, patterns of amino acid mutations in the QRDRs can predict fluoroquinolone resistance (Table 2) [37]. Recently a DNA microarray system has been developed for rapid detection of fluoroquinolone and β-lactam resistance in combination [38]. To detect point mutations in the QRDRs by a method of sequencing by hybridization, and the *mecA* gene by reverse dot blot hybridization, the PCR products were hybridized with the synthesized oligonucleotide probes on a three-dimensional microarray, PamChip® (PamGene International, Hertogenbosch, Netherlands; Fig. 1). Hybridization and fluorescence detection were totally performed with the FD10 microarray system (Olympus, Tokyo, Japan; Fig. 2).

Table 2. Mutations in the quinolone resistance-determining regions of GrlA, GrlB, GyrA, and GyrB and the corresponding MICs in clinical isolates of levofloxacin-resistant MRSA [37]

Strain	PFGE Genotype	Mutation				MIC (µg/ml)			
		GrlA	GrlB	GyrA	GyrB	Norfloxacin	Levofloxacin	Gatifloxacin	Sitafloxacin
HU2000-156	F	Ser80Phe	Pro451Ser	Ser84Leu	-	>128	32	8	2
HU2000-063	D	Ser80Tyr, Glu84Lys	-	Ser84Leu	-	>128	32	8	1
HU2000-064	I	Asp79Val, Ser80Tyr	-	Ser84Leu	-	>128	16	8	2
HU2000-136	B-I	Ser80Tyr	-	Ser84Leu	-	128	8	2	0.5
HU2000-091	C	Asp79Val, Ser80Phe	-	Glu88Lys	-	64	8	2	0.5
HU2000-092	A-I	Ser80Phe	-	Glu88Lys	-	64	8	2	0.5

PFGE=pulsed-field gel electrophoresis.

2.3. Aminoglycosides

A major mechanism of aminoglycoside resistance in *S. aureus* is inactivation of aminoglycosides by AMEs that catalyze acetylation, phosphorylation, and/or adenylation [12, 39-41]. The most common AMEs include acetyltransferase (AAC)(6')-phosphotransferase (APH)(2"), which inactivates gentamicin, kanamycin, tobramycin, and amikacin [12, 40, 41]; nucleotidyltransferase (ANT)(4'), which inactivates kanamycin and tobramycin [12, 41]; and APH(3'), which inactivates kanamycin and amikacin [12, 41]. Arbekacin is an aminoglycoside used in Japan only for MRSA infections. It has been reported that 3% to 7% of MRSA showed arbekacin resistance [12, 42]. The major mechanism of arbekacin resistance is production of AAC(6')-APH(2"), which modifies arbekacin by simultaneous acetylation and phosphorylation [12]. To determine aminoglycoside resistance, the presence of the *aac(6')-aph(2")*, *ant(4')-I*, and *aph(3')-III* genes, which encode respectively AAC(6')-APH(2"), ANT(4'), and APH(3'), can be detected by PCR methods with or without DNA-DNA hybridization [12, 19, 40, 41].

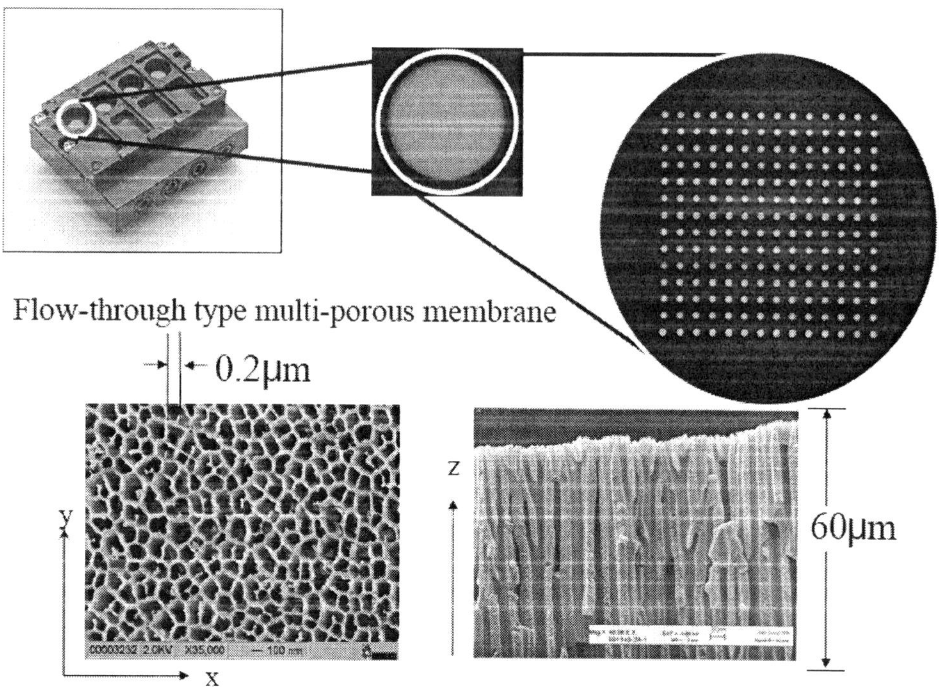

Figure 1. PamChip® microarray

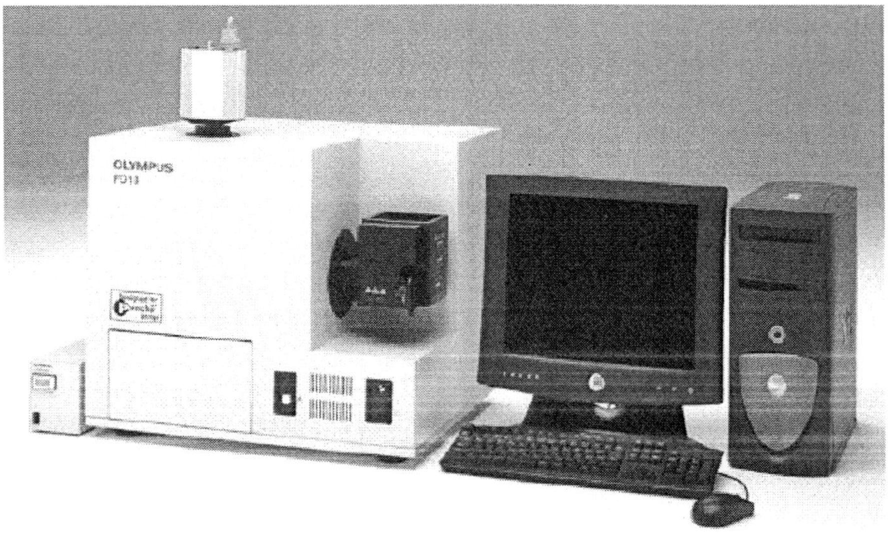

Figure 2. FD10 microarray system

2.4. Mupirocin

Mupirocin (pseudomonic acid A), which inhibits bacterial growth by binding isoleucyl tRNA-synthetase encoded by the *ileS* gene, is used mainly as a topical agent to reduce spread of MRSA. However, low concentrations of mupirocin may contribute to mupirocin resistance in MRSA [43], and increasing mupirocin resistance among *S. aureus* isolates is a matter of concern. Mupirocin resistance usually is mediated by a conjugative plasmid-associated *ileS-2* gene encoding an additional isoleucyl t-RNA-synthetase that is not bound by mupirocin [44, 45]. To detect mupirocin resistance, the *ileS-2* gene is detected by PCR-based methods [22, 45].

2.5. Glycopeptides

Another emerging problem is the appearance of VRSA. In June 2002, the first clinical isolate of VRSA was obtained from the tip and the exit site of a catheter of a Michigan patient with diabetes, peripheral vascular disease, and chronic renal failure [8]. This isolate showed resistance to vancomycin (MIC, >128 μg/ml) and teicoplanin (MIC, 32 μg/ml) by the broth microdilution method [8]. In September 2002, a second isolate of VRSA obtained from culture of a chronic foot ulcer of a patient in Pennsylvania showed resistance to vancomycin (MIC, 32 μg/ml) by the broth microdilution method [46]. Recently, a third isolate of VRSA obtained in March 2004 from a urine culture from a resident of a New York long-term care facility showed MIC for vancomycin of 64 μg/ml by the broth microdilution method [47]. These VRSA isolates were resistant to β-lactams but susceptible to antimicrobials such as linezolid, quinupristin-dalfopristin, and trimethoprim-sulfamethoxazole [8, 46, 47]. All three isolates contained the *vanA* gene, conferring vancomycin resistance, and the *mecA* gene [8,

46, 47]. The presence of the *vanA* gene in these VRSA suggests that the resistance determinant was acquired from VRE [8, 46].

2.6. Others

Linezolid is active against *S. aureus*, including MRSA and VRSA. However, linezolid resistance in MRSA has been reported in a patient with dialysis-related peritonitis and another with empyema [48, 49]. Linezolid resistance was conferred by mutations in the central loop of domain V of 23S rRNA in both cases [48, 49]. To detect linezolid resistance, the 23S rRNA gene was amplified by PCR and the amplified products were sequenced [49]. Additionally, resistance to quinupristin-dalfopriostin has been reported in French hospitals, although rarely in *S. aureus* isolates [50].

Antimicrobial Resistance in *S. pneumoniae*

S. pneumoniae is a common pathogen in community-acquired respiratory infections, acute sinusitis, acute otitis media, acute exacerbations of chronic bronchitis, and invasive infections such as meningitis and bacteremia. To date, a number of surveillance studies [51-54] have demonstrated an ongoing worldwide increase in resistance to antimicrobials among *S. pneumoniae*, especially to β-lactams and macrolides, and to a lesser degree, fluoroquinolones.

3.1. β-Lactams

Prevalence of penicillin-resistant *S. pneumoniae* (PRSP) is increasing [55-57]. PRSP is defined as an isolate with MIC for benzylpenicillin of ≥ 2 μg/ml, in accordance with the Clinical and Laboratory Standards Institute (CLSI) criteria (formerly National Committee for Clinical Laboratory Standards [NCCLS]) [58]. *S. pneumoniae* resistant to β-lactams, including penicillins and cephems, originated through recombinatory events between the PBP genes of *S. pneumoniae* and closely related species [59-61]. Production of altered PBPs, particularly PBP1A and PBP2B, and emergence of PBP2X, have been reported to be the cause of this resistance [59, 61-63]. Alterations in the PBPs lead to decreased affinity between the PBPs and β-lactams [64]. Sequence polymorphisms in the *pbp2b* gene resulted in decreased susceptibility to penicillins [65]. PCR-based determination of β-lactam resistance has been reported [62, 66, 67]; semi-nested PCR based on amplification of the *pbp2b* gene derived from PRSP was capable of differentiating PRSP from penicillin-susceptible *S. pneumoniae* (PSSP) [66], while PCR targeting the *pbp2b* gene derived from PSSP amplified the gene in some isolates of PRSP as well as PSSP [62]. As a rapid assay for specific determination of the *pbp2b* gene derived from PSSP, real-time PCR-hybridization has been developed [67]. PRSP shows various susceptibility patterns to β-lactams, especially to cephems, because of varied alterations in PBPs [59, 62]. Therefore, susceptibility to specific β-lactams among PRSP may be difficult to predict using PCR-based methods alone.

3.2. Macrolides, Lincosamides, Streptogramins, and Ketolides

Increasing prevalence of macrolide resistance in *S. pneumoniae* is another important problem [52, 53, 68]. The most common mechanisms of macrolide resistance described in *S. pneumoniae* include ribosomal modification and active efflux [69, 70]. Ribosomal modifications are mainly the result of production of a 23S rRNA methylase encoded by the *ermB* gene [69, 70]. Alterations of 23S rRNA confer resistance to macrolides, lincosamides, and streptogramins (MLS) [71]. Production of an efflux pump is another common cause of macrolide resistance in *S. pneumoniae* [70]. Membrane-associated proteins encoded by the *mefA* gene form the pump [70]. The active efflux system conveys resistance to 14- and 15-membered macrolides but not to 16-membered macrolides and lincosamides, this pattern is referred to as M resistance [69, 70]. A number of studies have shown an unexpected prevalence of the *ermB* and *mefA* genes, resulting in a rapid increase in macrolide-resistant *S. pneumoniae* [53,68]. Recent studies have shown that 56% to 88% and 19% to 60% of clinical isolates carried the *mefA* and *ermB* genes, respectively [68, 72-74]. Macrolide resistance attributable to the *mefA* or *ermB* genes was found frequently in penicillin-susceptible *S. pneumoniae* (PSSP), penicillin-intermediate *S. pneumoniae* (PISP), and PRSP (Table 3) [63]. PCR-based methods have been proposed to detect macrolide resistance determinants of the *ermB* and *mefA* genes [53, 63, 68]. Recently, ribosomal protein mutations in L4 and 23S rRNA that led to macrolide resistance in clinical isolates of *S. pneumoniae* have been described as new mechanisms [75].

A ketolide, telithromycin, is active against *S. pneumoniae*, including macrolide-resistant isolates, *ermB*-positive isolates with MLS resistance, and *mefA*-positive isolates with M resistance [63, 71]. Recently, however, emergence and prevalence of resistant isolates of *S. pneumoniae* to telithromycin (MIC, $\geq$ 1 μg/ml) has been reported from Taiwan, although resistance mechanisms remain unknown at present [77].

Table 3. Frequency of the *mefA*$^+$ and *ermB*$^+$ isolates in penicillin-susceptible, penicillin-intermediate, and penicillin-resistant *S. pneumoniae* [63]

Isolate (n)	Number (and percent) of isolates	
	mefA$^+$	*ermB*$^+$
Penicillin-susceptible *S. pneumoniae* (13)	1 (7.7%)	7 (53.8%)
Penicillin-intermedite *S. pneumoniae* (14)	6 (42.9%)	4 (28.6%)
Penicillin-resistant *S. pneumoniae* (11)	6 (54.5%)	5 (45.5%)

3.3. Fluoroquinolones

Although prevalence of fluoroquinolone resistance is relatively low in *S. pneumoniae*, increases in resistance to fluoroquinolones such as ciprofloxacin and ofloxacin recently have been reported worldwide [52, 69, 78, 79]. Major mechanisms of fluoroquinolone resistance in *S. pneumoniae* include target modification and active efflux [69, 78]. Target modification involves alterations in ParC and ParE, which are subunits of topoisomerase IV encoded by the *parC* and *parE* genes respectively, and in GyrA and GyrB, which are subunits of DNA gyrase encoded by the *gyrA* and *gyrB* genes respectively [27, 69, 78, 80]. Most clinical isolates of *S. pneumoniae* showing resistance to fluoroquinolones have amino acid alterations either in ParC alone or in both ParC and GyrA [27, 69, 78, 80]. To a lesser extent, additional alterations in ParE and GyrB have been reported [78, 80]. Genetic detection of fluoroquinolone resistance commonly is performed by determination of nucleotide sequences in the QRDRs of the *parC*, *parE*, *gyrA*, and *gyrB* genes according to those defined in *Escherichia coli* [80]. However, recent studies have suggested that mutations conferring fluoroquinolone resistance in *S. pneumoniae* may exist outside of the QRDRs of the *parC* and *gyrA* genes [81].

Additionally, fluoroquinolone resistance in *S. pneumoniae* can occur on the basis of active efflux, which is mediated by a membrane-associated protein, PmrA [27, 82].

4. Antimicrobial Resistance in Enterococci

Enterococci are part of the normal gut flora (intestinal colonizers). Most enterococcal infections occur in hospitalized patients and include urinary tract infections, bacteremia, endocarditis, intra-abdominal and pelvic infections, and wound infections. In general, cephems and carbapenems are less active against enterococci than penicillins. Enterococci can acquire resistance to ampicillin, aminoglycosides, and glycopeptides [83]. Ampicillin resistance is conferred by production of β-lactamase or altered PBPs [84]. Increased prevalence of ampicillin resistance arising from mutations within the *pbp5* gene that decrease the binding affinity of PBP5 for ampicillin represents a clinical problem in *Enterococcus faecium* [84, 85]. Alterations of PBP5 have been detected by determination of nucleotide sequences and PCR-based methods [83, 86, 87]. A transposon-mediated PBP5, which was associated with β-lactam resistance, was reported in *E. faecium* [88]. Production of β-lactamase has been reported almost exclusively in *Enterococcus faecalis* [84]. The β-lactamase gene found in enterococci is related to the *S. aureus* β-lactamase operon in most cases [84, 89]. Enterococci resistant to aminoglycosides, including gentamicin, have acquired AMEs such as AAC(6')-APH(2") [83, 90].

VRE are *E. faecalis* and *E. faecium* that are resistant to glycopeptides such as vancomycin and teicoplanin. Glycopeptide resistance in these enterococci is associated with acquisition of *van* gene clusters, located on a conjugative element [83]. Genotypes include *vanA*, *vanB*, and *vanD* (Table 4) [83, 91, 92]. The *vanA* gene cluster, which often is plasmid-borne, confers high-level resistance to both vancomycin and teicoplanin [83]. The *vanB* gene cluster confers inducible resistance to vancomycin but not to teicoplanin [83]. The *vanA* and *vanB* genes can be transferred to other microorganisms [83]. The *vanD* gene cluster confers inducible or moderate constitutive degrees of vancomycin and teicoplanin resistance [83]. VRE synthesize peptidoglycan precursors with pentapeptide side chains terminating with D-Ala-D-Lac, which exhibit less binding affinity for glycopeptides than is shown by side chains terminating with inherent D-Ala-D-Ala [83]. The synthesis of D-Ala-D-Lac depsipeptide is catalyzed by VanA, VanB, and VanD ligases, which are encoded by the *vanA*, *vanB*, and *vanD* genes respectively [83]. To date, PCR-based methods have been used to identify the *vanA* and *vanB* genes [93-95]. Recently a real-time PCR method, the LightCycler *vanA/vanB* detection assay (Roche Diagnostics, Tokyo, Japan) was developed and applied to detection of vancomycin resistance from direct swab specimens [90].

Table 4. Genetic traits of glycopeptide resistance in vancomycin-resistant enterococci [97]

	Genotype		
	vanA	*vanB*	*vanD*
Vancomycin resistance	Inducible, High-level resistance	Constitutive, inducible, Low- to high-level resistance	High-level resistance
Teicoplanin resistance	Inducible, High-level resistance	Susceptible	Low-level resistance
Gene location	Transposon, plasmid	Transposon, plasmid	Chromosome
Transfer of gene elements	Transferable	Transferable	Non-transferable
Peptidoglycan terminus	D-Ala-D-Lac	D-Ala-D-Lac	D-Ala-D-Lac
Species	*E. faecium*, *E. faecalis*	*E. faecium*, *E. faecalis*	*E. faecium*

Resistance of *E. faecium* to quinupristin/dalfopristin has been found clinically, especially in Europe [96]. Although resistance of *E. faecium* during therapy has been rare in clinical trials, concern exists that quinupristin/dalfopristin-resistant *E. faecium* may emerge and spread [96]. The *satA* gene has been reported to be associated with quinupristin/dalfopristin resistance [96].

5. Conclusion(s)

Developments in molecular microbiology and genetics as applied to clinical microbiology now permit rapid and reliable detection of antimicrobial resistance determinants in Gram-positive cocci such as *S. aureus*, CNS, *S. pneumoniae*, and enterococci. Genetic detection generally is based on PCR, DNA-DNA hybridization, and nucleotide sequencing methods. Newly developed techniques have become available for rapid and convenient determination of antimicrobial resistance, including real-time PCR and DNA micoarray systems. These molecular methods should provide rapid, reliable guidance to clinicians concerning antimicrobial therapy. A number of determinants of antimicrobial resistance in Gram-positive cocci now can be detected rapidly and conveniently using these genetic methods. Therefore, antimicrobial susceptibility patterns of the causative pathogen can be predicted early. Moreover, such information can help to identify nosocomial infections caused by antimicrobial-resistant Gram-positive cocci.

References

[1] Jones, R. N. and Phaller, M. A. (1998). Bacterial resistance; a worldwide problem. *Diagn. Microbiol. Infect. Dis.*, 31, 379-388.

[2] Dzidic, S. and Bedeković, V. (2003). Horizontal gene transfer-emerging multidrug resistance in hospital bacteria. *Acta Pharmacol. Sin.*, 24, 519-526.

[3] World Health Organization. (2000). *Overcoming antimicrobial resistance:* World Health Organization Report on Infectious Diseases. Geneva, Switzerland: WHO.

[4] Laible, G., Spratt, B. G. and Hakenbeck, R. (1991). Interspecies recombinational events during the evolution of altered PBP2x genes in penicillin-resistant *Streptococcus pneumoniae*. *Mol. Microbiol.*, 5, 1993-2002.

[5] Dowson, C. G., Coffey, T. J., Kell, C. and Whiley, R. A. (1993). Evolution of penicillin resistance in *Streptococcus pneumoniae*; the role of *Streptococcus mitis* in the formation of a low affinity PBP2B in *S. pneumoniae*. *Mol. Microbiol.*, 9, 635-643.

[6] Berger-Bächi, B. (2002). Resistance mechanisms of Gram-positive bacteria. *Int. J. Med. Microbiol.*, 292, 27-35.

[7] Normark, B. H. and Normark S. (2002). Evolution and spread of antibiotic resistance. *J. Intern. Med.*, 252, 91-106.

[8] Centers for Disease Control and Prevention. (2002). *Staphylococcus aureus* resistant to vancomycin – United States, 2002. *Morb. Mort. Wkly. Rep.*, 51, 565-567.

[9] Amyes, G. S. B. and Gemmell, C. G. (1997). Antibiotic resistance. *J. Med. Microbiol.*, 46, 436-470.

[10] Lowy, F. D. (1998). *Staphylococcus aureus* infections. *N. Engl. J. Med.*, 339, 520-532.

[11] Lowy, F. D. (2003). Antimicrobial resistance: the example of *Staphylococcus aureus*. *J. Clin. Invest.*, 111, 1265-1273.

[12] Ida, T., Okamoto, R., Shimauchi, C., Okubo, T., Kuga, A. and Inoue, M. (2001). Identification of aminoglycoside-modifying enzymes by susceptibility testing: epidemiology of methicillin-resistant *Staphylococcus aureus* in Japan. *J. Clin. Microbiol.*, 39, 3115-3121.

[13] Brumfitt, W. and Hamilton-Miller, J. (1989). Methicillin-resistant *Staphylococcus aureus*. *N. Engl. J. Med.*, 320, 1188-1195.

[14] Centers for Disease Control and Prevention. (2000). Four pediatric deaths from community-acquired methicillin-resistant *Staphylococcus aureus* – Minnesota and North Dakota 1997-1999. *Morb. Mort. Wkly. Rep.*, 48, 707-710.

[15] National Nosocomial Infections Surveillance System. (1996). National Nosocomial Infections Surveillance System (NNIS) report, data summary from October 1986-April 1996, issued May 1996. *Am. J. Infect. Control.*, 24, 380-388.

[16] Weinstein, M. P., Towns, M. L., Quartey, S. M., Mirrett, S, Reimer, L. G., Parmigiani, G. and Reller, L. B. (1997). The clinical significance of positive blood cultures in the 1990s: a prospective comprehensive evaluation of the microbiology, epidemiology, and outcome of bacteremia and fungemia in adults. *Clin. Inefect. Dis.*, 24, 584-602.

[17] Suzuki, E., Hiramatsu, K. and Yokota, T. (1992). Survey of methicillin-resistant clinical strains of coagulase-negative staphylococci for *mecA* gene distribution. *Antimicrob. Agents Chemother.*, 36, 429-434.

[18] Horii, T., Suzuki, Y., Kimura, T., Kanno, T. and Maekawa, M. (2001). Intravenous catheter-related septic shock caused by Staphylococcus sciuri and Escherichia vulneris. *Scand. J. Infect. Dis.*, 33, 929-931.

[19] Martineau, F., Picard, F. J., Lansac, N., Ménard, C., Roy, P. H., Ouellette, M. and Bergeron, M. G. (2000). Correlation between the resistance genotype determined by multiplex PCR assays and the antibiotic susceptibility patterns of *Staphylococcus aureus* and *Staphylococcus epidermidis*. *Antimicrob. Agnets Chemother.*, 44, 231-238.

[20] Shimaoka, M., Yoh, M., Segawa, A., Takarada, Y., Yamamoto, K. and Honda, T. (1994). Development of enzyme-labeled oligonucleotide probe for detection of *mecA* gene in methicillin-resistant *Staphylococcus aureus*. *J. Clin. Microbiol.*, 32, 1866-1869.

[21] Kolbert, C. P., Connolly, J. E., Lee, M. J. and Persing, D. H. (1995). Detection of the Staphylococcal *mecA* gene by chemiluminescent DNA hybridization. *J. Clin. Microbiol.*, 33, 2179-2182.

[22] Perez-Roth, E., Claverie-Martin, F., Villar, J. and Mendez-Alvarez, S. (2001). Multiplex PCR for simultaneous identification of *Staphylococcus aureus* and detection of methicillin and mupirocin resistance. *J. Clin. Microbiol.*, 39, 4037-4041.

[23] Huletsky, A., Giroux, R., Rossbach, V., Gagnon, M., Vaillancourt, M., Bernier, M., Gagnon, F., Truchon, K., Bastien, M., Picard, F. J., van Belkum, A., Ouellette, M., Roy, P. H. and Bergeron, M. G. (2004). New real-time PCR assay for rapid detection of methicillin-resistant *Staphylococcus aureus* directly from specimens containing a mixture of staphylococci. *J. Clin. Microbiol.*, 42, 1875-1884.

[24] Hooper, D. C. (2001). Emerging mechanisms of fluoroquinolone resistance. *Emerg. Infect. Dis.*, 7, 337-341.

[25] Hooper, D. C. (1991). Mode of action of the new quinolones: new data. *Eur. J. Clin. Microbiol. Infect. Dis.*, 10, 223-231.

[26] Ito, H., Yoshida, H., Bogaki-Shonai, M., Niga, T., Hattori, H. and Nakamura, S. (1994). Quinolone resistance mutations in the DNA gyrase *gyrA* and *gyrB* genes of *Staphylococcus aureus*. *Antimicrob. Agents Chemother.*, 38, 2014-2023.

[27] Piddock, L. J. V. (1998). Mechanisms of fluoroquinolone resistance: an update 1994-1998. *Drugs*, 58 (*Suppl 2*), 11-18.

[28] Schmitz, F.-J., Jones, M. E., Hofmann, B., Hansen, B., Scheuring, S., Luckefahr, M., Fluit, A. C., Verhoef, J., Haddings, U., Heinz, H.-P. and Kohrer, K. (1998). Characterization of *grlA*, *grlB*, *gyrA*, and *gyrB* mutations in 116 unrelated isolates of *Staphylococcus aureus* and effects of mutations on ciprofloxacin MIC. *Antimicrob. Agents Chemother.*, 42, 1249-1252.

[29] Takahashi, H., Kikuchi, T., Shoji, S., Fujimura, S., Lutfor, A. B., Tokue, Y., Nukiwa, T. and Watanabe, A. (1998). Characterization of *gyrA*, *gyrB*, *grlA* and *grlB* mutations

in fluoroquinolone-resistant clinical isolates of *Staphylococcus aureus*. *J. Antimicrob. Chemother.*, 41, 49-57.

[30] Ferrero, L., Cameron, B., Manse, B., Lagneaux, D., Crouzet, J., Famechon, A. and Blanche, F. (1994). Cloning and primary structure of *Staphylococcus aureus* DNA topoisomerase IV: a primary target of fluoroquinolone. *Mol. Microbiol.*, 13, 641-653.

[31] Yoshida, H., Bogaki, M., Nakamura, S., Ubukata, K. and Konno, M. (1990). Nucleotide sequence and characterization of the *Staphylococcus aureus norA* gene, which confers resistance to quinolones. *J. Bacteriol.*, 172, 6942-6949.

[32] Kaatz, G. W., Seo, S. M. and Ruble, C. A. (1993). Efflux-mediated fluoroquinolone resistance in *Staphylococcus aureus*. *Antimicrob. Agents Chemother.*, 37, 1086-1094.

[33] Ng, E. Y., Trucksis, M. and Hooper, D. C. (1994). Quinolone resistance mediated by *norA*: physiologic characterization and relationship to *flqB*, a quinolone resistance locus on *Staphylococcus aureus* chromosome. *Antimicrob. Agents Chemother.*, 38, 1345-1355.

[34] Kaatz, G. W. and Seo, S. M. (1995). Inducible NorA-mediated multidrug resistance in *Staphylococcus aureus*. *Antimicrob. Agents Chemother.*, 39, 2650-2655.

[35] Schmitz, F.-J., Hertel, B., Hofmann, B., Scheuring, S., Verhoef, J., Fluit, A. C., Heinz, H.-P., Kohrer, K. and Jones, M. E. (1998). Relationship between mutations in the coding and promoter regions of the *norA* genes in 42 unrelated clinical isolates of *Staphylococcus aureus* and the MICs of norfloxacin for these strains. *J. Antimicrob. Chemother.*, 42, 561-563.

[36] Jones, M. E., Boenink, N. M., Verhoef, J., Kohrer, K. and Schmitz, F.-J. (2000). Multiple mutations conferring ciprofloxacin resistance in *Staphylococcus aureus* demonstrate long-term stability in an antibiotic-free environment. *J. Antimicrob. Chemother.*, 45, 353-356.

[37] Horii, T., Suzuki, Y., Monji, A., Morita, M., Muramatsu, H., Kondo, Y., Doi, M., Takeshita, A., Kanno, T. and Maekawa, M. (2003). Detection of mutations in quinolone resistance-determining regions in levofloxacin- and methicillin-resistant *Staphylococcus aureus*: effects of the mutations on fluoroquinolone MICs. *Diagn. Microbiol. Infect. Dis.*, 46, 139-145.

[38] Nagaoka, T., Horii, T., Satoh, T., Ito, T., Monji, A., Takeshita, A. and Maekawa, M. (2005). Use of a three-dimensional microarray system for detection of levofloxacin resistance and the *mecA* gene in *Staphylococcus aureus*. *J. Clin. Microbiol.*, 43, 5187-5194.

[39] Gray, G. S. and Fitch, W. M. (1984). Evolution of antibiotic resistance genes: the DNA sequence of a kanamycin resistance gene from *Staphylococcus aureus*. *Mol. Biol. Evol.*, 1, 57-66.

[40] Rouch, D. A., Byrne, M. E., Kong, Y. C. and Skurray, R. A. (1987). The *aacA-aphD* gentamicin and kanamycin resistance determinant of Tn*4001* from *Staphylococcus aureus*: expression and nucleotide sequence analysis. *J. Gen. Microbiol.*, 133, 3039-3052.

[41] Udo, E. E. and Dashti, A. A. (2000). Detection of genes encoding aminoglycoside-modifying enzymes in staphylococci by polymerase chain reaction and dot blot hybridization. *Int. J. Antimicrob. Agents*, 13, 273-279.

[42] Fujimura, S., Tokue, Y., Takahashi, H., Kobayashi, T., Gomi, K., Abe, T., Nukiwa, T. and Watanabe, A. (2000). Novel arbekacin- and amikacin-modifying enzyme of methicilli-resistant *Staphylococcus aureus*. *FEMS Microbiol. Lett.*, 190, 299-303.

[43] Watanabe, H., Masaki, H., Asoh, N., Watanabe, K., Oishi, K., Kobayashi, S., Sato, A., Sugita, R., Nagatake, T. (2001). Low concentrations of mupirocin in the pharynx following intranasal application may contribute to mupirocin resistance in methicillin-resistant *Staphylococcus aureus*. *J. Clin. Microbiol.*, 39, 3775-3777.

[44] Bastos, M. C., Mondino, P. J., Azevedo, M. L., Santos, K. R. and Giambiagi-deMarval, M. (1999). Molecular characterization and transfer among *Staphylococcus* strains of a plasmid conferring high-level resistance to mupirocin. *Eur. J. Clin. Microbiol. Infect. Dis.*, 18, 393-398.

[45] Perez-Roth, E., Claverie-Martin, F., Villar, J. and Mendez-Alvarez, S. (2001). Multiplex PCR for simultaneous identification of *Staphylococcus aureus* and detection of methicillin and mupirocin resistance. *J. Clin. Microbiol.*, 39, 4037-4041.

[46] Centers for Disease Control and Prevention. (2002). Vancomycin-resistant *Staphylococcus aureus* – Pennsylvania, 2002. *Morb. Mort. Wkly. Rep.*, 51, 902.

[47] Centers for Disease Control and Prevention. (2004). Brief report: vancomycin-resistant *Staphylococcus aureus* – New York, 2004. *Morb. Mort. Wkly. Rep.*, 53, 322-323.

[48] Tsiodras, S., Gold, H. S., Sakoulas, G., Eliopoulos, G. M., Wennersten, C., Venkataraman, L., Moellering, R. C. and Forraro, M. J. (2001). Linezolid resistance in a clinical isolate of *Staphylococcus aureus*. *Lancet*, 358, 207-208.

[49] Wilson, P., Andrews, J. A., Charlesworth, R., Walesby, R., Singer, M., Farrell, D. J. and Robbins, M. (2003). Linezolid resistance in clinical isolates of *Staphylococcus aureus*. *J. Antimicrob. Chemother.*, 51, 186-188.

[50] Hershberger, E., Donabedian, S., Konstantinou, K. and Zervos, J. (2004). Quinupristin-dalfopristin resistance in gram-positive bacteria: mechanism of resistance and epidemiology. *Clin. Infect. Dis.*, 38, 92-98.

[51] Butler, J. C., Hofmann, J., Cetron, M. S., Elliott, J. A., Facklam, R. R. and Breiman, R. F. (1996). The continued emergence of drug-resistant *Streptococcus pneumoniae* in the United States: an update from the Centers for Disease Control and Prevention's Pneumococcal Sentinel Surveillance System. *J. Infect. Dis.*, 174, 986-993.

[52] Doern, G. V., Pfaller, M. A., Kugler, K., Freeman, J. and Jones, R. N. (1998). Prevalence of antimicrobial resistance among respiratory tract isolates of *Streptococcus pneumoniae* in North America: 1997 results from the SENTRY antimicrobial surveillance program. *Clin. Infect. Dis.*, 27, 764-770.

[53] Shortridge, V. D., Doern, G. V., Brueggemann, A. B., Beyer, J. M. and Flamm, R. K. (1999). Prevalence of macrolide resistance mechanisms in *Streptococcus pneumoniae* isolates from a multicenter antibiotic resistance surveillance study conducted in the United States in 1994-1995. *Clin. Infect. Dis.*, 29, 1186-1188.

[54] Schito, G. C., Debbia, E. A. and Marchese, A. (2000). The evolving threat of antibiotic resistance in Europe: new data from Alexander Project. *J. Antimicrob. Chemothe.*, 46, 3-9.

[55] Baquero, F., Martinez-Beltran, J. and Loza, E. (1991). A review of antibiotic resistance patterns in *Streptococcus pneumoniae* in Europe. *J. Antimicrob. Chemother.*, 28, 31-38.

[56] Hofmann, J., Cetron, M. S., Farley, M. M. and Baughman, W. S. (1995). The prevalence of drug-resistant *Streptococcus pneumoniae* in Atlanta. *N. Engl. J. Med.*, 333, 481-486.

[57] Leggiadro, R. J. (2000). Penicillin-nonsusceptible pneumococcus. *Int. J. Antimicrob. Agents*, 14, 123-127.

[58] Clinical and Laboratory Standards Institute. (2006). *Methods for Dilution Antimicrobial Susceptibility Tests for Bacterial that Grow Aerobically* (seventh edition): Approved Standard M7-A7. Wayne, PA: CLSI.

[59] Hakenbeck, R., Tarpay, M. and Tomasz, A. (1980). Multiple changes of penicillin-binding proteins in penicillin-resistant clinical isolates of *Streptococcus pneumoniae*. *Antimicrob. Agents Chemother.*, 17, 364-371.

[60] Dowson, C. G., Hutchinson, A., Woodford, N., Johnson, A. P., George, R. C. and Spratt, B. G. (1990). Penicillin-resistant viridans streptococci have obtained altered penicillin-binding protein genes from penicillin-resistant strains of *Streptococcus pneumoniae*. *Proc. Natl. Acad. Sci. USA.*, 87, 5858-5862.

[61] Dowson, C. G., Coffey, T. J., Kell, C. and Whiley, R. A. (1993). Evolution of penicillin resistance in *Streptococcus pneumoniae*; the role of *Streptococcus mitis* in the formation of a low affinity PBP2B in *S. pneumoniae*. *Mol. Microbiol.*, 9, 635-643.

[62] Ubukata, K., Asahi, Y., Yamane, A. and Konno, M. (1996). Combinational detection of autolysin and penicillin-binding protein 2B genes of *Streptococcus pneumoniae*. *J. Clin. Microbiol.*, 34, 592-596.

[63] Kimura, T., Horii, T., Morita, M., Muramatsu, H., Kanno, T. and Maekawa, M. (2003). Detection of macrolide resistance in *Streptococcus pneumoniae*. *Chemother.*, 49, 56-61.

[64] Markiewicz, Z and Tomasz, A. (1989). Variation in penicillin-binding protein patterns of penicillin-resistant clinical isolates of pneumococci. *J. Clin. Microbiol.*, 27, 405-410.

[65] Smith, A. M. and Klugman, K. P. (1995). Alterations in penicillin-binding protein 2B from penicillin-resistant wild-type strains *of Streptococcus pneumoniae*. *Antimicrob. Agents Chemother.*, 39, 859-867.

[66] du Plessis, M., Smith, A. M. and Klugman, K. P. (1998). Rapid detection of penicillin-resistant *Streptococcus pneumoniae* in cerebrospinal fluid by a seminested-PCR strategy. *J. Clin. Mucrobiol.*, 36, 453-457.

[67] Kearns, A. M., Graham, C., Burdess, D., Heatherington, J. and Freeman, R. (2002). Rapid real-time PCR for determination of penicillin susceptibility in pneumococcal meningitis, including culture-negative cases. *J. Clin. Microbiol.*, 40, 682-684.

[68] Gay, K., Baughman, W., Miller, Y., Jackson, D., Whitney, C. G., Schuchat, A., Farley, M. M., Tenover, F. and Stephens, D. S. (2000). The emergence of *Streptococcus pneumoniae* resistant to macrolide antimicrobial agents: a 6-year population-based assessment. *J. Infect. Dis.*, 182, 1417-1424.

[69] Appelbaum, P. C. (2002). Resistance among *Streptococcus pneumoniae*: implications for drug selection. *Clin. Infect. Dis.*, 34, 1613-1620.

[70] Edelstein, P. H. (2004). Pneumococcal resistance to macrolides, lincosamides, ketolides, and streptogramin B agents: molecular mechanisms and resistance phenotypes. *Clin. Infect. Dis.*, 38 (suppl. 4), S322-S-327.

[71] Leclercq, R. and Courvalin, P. (1991). Bacterial resistance to macrolide, lincosamide, and streptogramin antibiotics by target modification. *Antimicrob. Agents Chemother.*, 35, 1267-1272.

[72] Nishijima, T., Saito, Y., Aoki, A., Toriya, M., Toyonaga, Y. and Fujii, R. (1999). Distribution of *mefE* and *ermB* genes in macrolide-resistant strains of *Streptococcus pneumoniae* and their variable susceptibility to various antibiotics. *J. Antimicrob. Chemother.*, 43, 637-643.

[73] Luna, V. A., Coates, P., Eady, E. A., Cova, J. H., Nguyen, T. T. H. and Roberts, M. C. (1999). A variety of gram-positive bacteria carry mobile *mef* genes. *J. Antimicrob. Chemother.*, 44, 19-25.

[74] Waites, K., Johnson, C., Gray, B., Edwards, K., Crain, M. and Benjamin, W. Jr. (2000). Use of clindamycin disks to detect macrolide resistance mediated by *ermB* and *mefE* in *Streptococcus pneumoniae* isolates from adults and children. *J. Clin. Microbiol.*, 38, 1731-1734.

[75] Tait-Kamradt, A., Davies, T., Appelbaum, P. C., Depardieu, F., Courvalin, P., Petitpas, J., Wondrack, L., Walker, A., Jacobs, M. R. and Sutcliffe, J. (2000). Two new mechanisms of macrolide resistance in clinical strains of *Streptococcus pneumoniae* from Eastern Europe and North America. *Antimicrob. Agents Chemother.*, 44, 3395-3401.

[76] Felmingham, D. (2001). Microbiological profiles of telithromycin, the first ketolide antimicrobial. *Clin. Microbiol. Infect.*, 7 (Suppl. 3), 2-10.

[77] Hsueh, P.-R., Teng, L.-J., Wu, T.-L., Yang, D., Huang, W.-K., Shyr, J.-M., Chuang, Y.-C., Wan, J.-H., Yan, J.-J., Lu, J.-J., Wu, J.-J., Ko, W.-C., Chang, F.-Y., Yang, Y.-C., Lau, Y.-J., Liu, Y.-C., Lee, C.-M., Leu, H.-S., Liu, C.-Y. and Luh, K.-T. (2003). Telithromycin- and fluoroquinolone-resistant *Streptococcus pneumoniae* in Taiwan with high prevalence of resistance to macrolides and β-lactams: SMART program 2001 data. *Antimicrob. Agents Chemother.*, 47, 2145-2151.

[78] Eliopoulos, G. M. (2004). Quinolone resistance mechanisms in pneumococci. *Clin. Infect. Dis.*, 38 (suppl. 4), S350-S356.

[79] Hooper, D. C. (2002). Fluoroquinolone resistance among Gram-positive cocci. *Lancet Infect. Dis.*, 2, 530-538.

[80] Pan, X. S., Ambler, J., Mehtar, S. and Fisher, L. M. (1996). Involvement of topoisomerase IV and DNA gyrase as ciprofloxacin targets in *Streptococcus pneumoniae*. *Antimicrob. Agents Chemother.*, 40, 2321-2326.

[81] Smith, H. J., Nichol, K. A., Hoban, D. J. and Zhanel, G. G. (2002). Dual activity of fluoroquinolones against *Streptococcus pneumoniae*: the facts behind the claims. *J. Antimicrob. Chemother.*, 49, 893-895.

[82] Gill, M. J., Brenwald, N. P. and Wise, R. (1999). Identification of an efflux pump gene, *pmrA*, associated with fluoroquinolone resistance in *Streptococcus pneumoniae*. *Antimicrob. Agents Chemother.*, 43, 187-189.

[83] Berber-Bächi, B. (2002). Resistance mechanisms of Gram-positive bacteria. *Int. J. Med. Microbiol.*, 292, 27-35.

[84] Rice, L. B. (2001). Emergence of vancomycin-resistant enterococci. *Emerg. Infect. Dis.*, 7, 183-187.

[85] Rybkine, T., Mainardi, J.-L., Sougakoff, W., Collatz, E. and Gutmann, L. (1998). Penicillin-binding protein 5 sequence alterations in clinical isolates of *Enterococcus faecium* with different levels of β-lactam resistance. *J. Infect. Dis.*, 178, 159-163.

[86] El Amin, N., Lund, B., Tjernlund, A., Lundberg, C., Jalakas, K. and Wretlind, B. (2001). Mechanisms of resistance to imipenem in imipenem-resistant, ampicillin-sensitive *Enterococcus faecium*. APMIS, 109, 791-796.

[87] Mohn, S. C., Ulvik, A., Jureen, R., Willems, R. J. L., Top, J., Leavis, H., Harthug, S. and Langeland, N. (2004). Duplex real-time PCR assay for rapid detection of ampicillin-resistant *Enterococcus faecium*. *Antimicrob. Agents Chemother.*, 48, 556-560.

[88] Carias, L. L., Rudin, S. D., Donskey, C. J. and Rice, L. B. (1998). Genetic linkage and cotransfer of a novel, *vanB*-containing transposon (Tn*5382*) and a low-affinity penicillin-binding protein 5 gene in a clinical vancomycin-resistant *Enterococcus faecium* isolate. *J. Bacteriol.*, 180, 4426-4434.

[89] Okamoto, R., Okubo, T. and Inoue, M. (1996). Detection of genes regulating β-lactamase production in *Enterococcus faecalis* and *Staphylococcus aureus*. *Antimicrob. Agents Chemother.*, 40, 2550-2554.

[90] Kobayashi, N., Alam, M., Nishimoto, Y., Urasawa, S., Uehara, N. and Watanabe, N. (2001). Distribution of aminoglycoside resistance genes in recent clinical isolates of *Enterococcus faecalis*, *Enterococcus faecium* and *Enterococcus avium*. *Epidemiol. Infect.*, 126, 197-204.

[91] Arthur, M. and Quintiliani, R. (2001). Regulation of VanA- and VanB-type glycopeptide resistance in enterococci. *Antimicrob. Agents Chemother.*, 45, 375-381.

[92] Casadewall, B., Reynolds, P. E. and Courvalin, P. (2001). Regulation of expression of the *vanD* glycopeptide resistance gene cluster from *Enterococcus faecium* BM4339. *J. Bacteriol.*, 183, 3436-3446.

[93] Dutka-Malen, S., Evans, S. and Courvalin, P. (1995). Detection of glycopeptide resistance genotypes and identification to the species level of clinically relevant enterococci by PCR. *J. Clin. Microbiol.*, 33, 24-27.

[94] Satake, S., Clark, N., Rimland, D., Nolte, F. S. and Tenover, F. C. (2004). Detection of vancomycin-resistant enterococci in fecal samples by PCR. *J. Clin. Microbiol.*, 35, 2325-2330.

[95] Sloan, L. M., Uhl, J. R., Vetter, E. A., Schleck, C. D., Harmsen, W. S., Manahan, J., Thompson, R. L., Rosenblatt, J. E. and Cockerill, F. R. (2004). Comparison of the Roche LightCycler *vanA/vanB* detection assay and culture for detection of vancomycin-resistant enterococci from perianal swabs. *J. Clin. Microbiol.*, 42, 2636-2643.

[96] Thal, L. A. and Zervos, M. J. (1999). Occurrence and epidemiology of resistance to virginiamycin and streptogramins. *J. Antimicrob. Chemother.*, 43, 171-176.

[97] DeLisle, S. and Perl, T. M. (2003). Vancomycin-resistant enterococci. A road map on how to prevent the emergence and transmission of antimicrobial resistance. *Chest*, 123, 504S-518S.

In: New Research on Pharmacogenetics
Editors: Linda P. Barnes, pp. 123-584

ISBN: 1-60021-056-2

Chapter V

A Special Bibliography

AAOHN J. 2005 Dec;53(12):529-33. Related Articles, Links Health and employment practices: ethical, legal, and social implications of advances in toxicogenomics. Weinstein M, Widenor M, Hecker S. Labor Education Research Center, University of Oregon, Eugene, USA. Advances in toxicogenomics research may allow the identification of individuals who may be hyper-susceptible to occupational exposures and could create a shift from population to individual-based risk assessment in occupational health. Although many states have passed legislation to prevent the misuse of genetic information in employment, there is no general federal protection from the use of genetic information after a conditional offer of employment. Occupational health professionals have a crucial role in shaping future guidelines governing the use of genetic information in employment. Publication Types: Review

AAPS J. 2005 Jun 23;7(1):E134-40. Related Articles, Links Comment in: AAPS J. 2005;7(1):E141-2. A stochastic version of corticosteriod pharmacogenomic model. Qi X. National Pharmaceutical Engineering Research Center, No. 1111 Zhongshanbeiyi Road, Shanghai 200437, China. xiaohong.qi@andrx.com The purpose of this study was to develop a stochastic version of corticosteriod fifth generation pharmacogenomic model. The Gillespie algorithm was used to generate the independent time courses of the receptor messenger RNA (mRNA). Initial parameters for the stochastic simulation were adapted from the study by Jin et al. The result obtained from the proposed stochastic model showed an overall agreement with the deterministic fifth generation model. This study suggested that because the stochastic model takes into account the "noise" nature of gene regulation, it would have potential application in pharmacogenomic modeling.

AAPS J. 2005;7(1):E141-2. Related Articles, Links Comment on: AAPS J. 2005;7(1):E134-40. Commentary: stochastic phenomena in pharmacokinetic, pharmacodynamic and pharmacogenomic models. Siegel RA, Ramanathan M. Departments of Pharmaceutics and Biomedical Engineering, University of Minnesota, Minneapolis, MN, USA. siege017@umn.edu Publication Types: Comment

AAPS PharmSci. 2003 Nov 5;5(4):E29. Related Articles, Links Pharmacogenomics of multigenic diseases: sex-specific differences in disease and treatment outcome. Pinsonneault J, Sadee W. Ohio State University Program in Pharmacogenomics, Ohio State University, Columbus OH 43210, USA. Numerous genetic variations have been shown to affect disease susceptibility and drug response. Pharmacogenomics aims at improving therapy on the basis of genetic information for each individual patient. Furthermore, sex chromosomes broadly determine biological differences between males and females. Consequently, substantial sex differences exist in phenotypic manifestation of disease and treatment response. This review discusses the role of sex in coronary artery disease, schizophrenia, and depression--complex multigenic disorders with considerable sex differences in frequency and presentation. Moreover, genetic factors underlying disease and drug response appear to differ between male and female patients. This appears to result at least in part from different physiological effects exerted by sex hormones such that polymorphisms in susceptibility genes may have physiological relevance only in males or females. However, few examples have been discovered to play a role in complex multigenic diseases, and the mechanistic basis of genetic variants as sex-dependent susceptibility factors has yet to be explored. Therefore, pharmacogenomic studies must consider sex differences in an effort to optimize individual drug therapy.

Account Res. 2004 Jul-Dec;11(3-4):161-82. Related Articles, Links Ethics and research assessing the relative roles of genes and the environment. DeCamp M, Sugarman J. Duke University Medical Scientist Training Program, School of Medicine, Durham, NC, USA. Research on the interaction of genes and the environment is revealing that many human diseases have both genetic and environmental components. Even traditional "environmental" diseases, such as infections, appear to interact with genetic components in the human host. Environmental genetics research will inevitably increase understanding of individual susceptibilities to toxic exposures in the environment and harmful side effects of medications; therefore, it has great promise for improving the prevention and treatment of human diseases. However, realizing the benefits of this research requires careful attention to ethical issues that are particularly relevant in this context. This article reviews some of the most pressing issues related to research design and methods, as well as from the application of research results (e.g., workplace genetic screening and legal toxic torts, personal medical responsibility, and the relationship between genetics and public health measures). Publication Types: Review

Acta Gastroenterol Belg. 2005 Apr-Jun;68(2):233-6. Related Articles, Links Is HBV genotyping of clinical relevance? Verschuere V, Yap PS, Fevery J. Hepatology, UZ Gasthuisberg, B-3000 Leuven, Belgium. The hepatitis B virus, as is the case of the hepatitis C virus, can be categorized in several genotypes. The genotyping of HBV is based on the nucleotide sequence divergence encoding the amino acids constituting the HBV surface proteins. Since the genotype of the hepatitis C virus is shown to be related to epidemiology and response to interferon therapy, one wonders whether this also holds for the hepatitis B virus. HBV genotypes clearly are found to be different in various geographical areas of infection. In Europe, genotypes A and D are predominant, whereas in Asian patients genotypes B and C are more frequent, and in the Middle-East the genotype D. Data concerning the clinical relevance are less clear but it seems that in Europe, the genotype A has a higher HBeAg clearance rate and a better outcome. In Asia, genotype B (and especially the genotype Bj) is associated with a higher HBeAg clearance and with less development of cirrhosis and HCC. The impact on spontaneous or therapy induced viral resolution is not yet clearly identified. Further evaluation in different countries is needed to delineate the impact of the genotype relative to other factors such as age at infection, level of serum transaminases and viral load, on the course of infection, complication, outcome of treatment and prognosis. Publication Types: Review

Acta Neurol Scand Suppl. 2005;181:47-51. Related Articles, Links The role of genetics and ethnicity in epilepsy management. Scheffer IE. Department of Medicine and Paediatrics, The University of Melbourne, Epilepsy Research Centre, Melbourne, Vic., Australia. scheffer@unimelb.edu.au Recent exciting developments in epilepsy genetics have led to significant insights into the mechanisms underlying seizure disorders. Success in epilepsy genetics research to date has resulted from identification of genes responsible for rare monogenic disorders, the majority encoding either voltage- or ligand-gated ion channels. For some conditions, such as benign familial neonatal seizures, an understanding of the underlying genetics is helpful in predicting prognosis. However, for other disorders, such as autosomal dominant nocturnal frontal lobe epilepsy, phenotypic severity is determined by factors other than the major dominant nicotinic subunit mutation found in some families. Further complexity arises when single-gene mutations give rise to heterogeneous phenotypes, as typically occur with generalized epilepsy with febrile seizures plus. Another area of increasing genetic endeavour, pharmacogenetics will allow tailoring of antiepileptic medication for each patient. Pharmacogenetics explores genetic polymorphisms in genes coding for drug-metabolizing enzymes, receptors and transporters. Polymorphisms have been identified that result in marked ethnic and interindividual differences in response to treatment. With further understanding of the impact of these differences, pharmacogenetic screening is likely to guide the management of epilepsy in the future.

Acta Pharmacol Sin. 2005 Mar;26(3):302-6. Related Articles, Links Exo+ proofreading polymerases mediate genetic analysis and its application in biomedical studies. Liao DF, Chen LL, Peng CY, Zhang J, Li K. Division of Pharmacogenomics, SNP Institute, School of Life Science, Nanhua University, Hengyang 421001, China. Polymerases with a proofreading function in their internal 3' to 5' exonuclease possess high fidelity for DNA replication both in vivo and in vitro. The obstacle facing Exo+ polymerases for single nucleotide polymorphism (SNP) detection could be bypassed by using primer-3'-termini modification. This hypothesis has been well tested using three types of modified allele specific primers with: 3' labeling, 3' to 5' exonuclease resistance, and 3' dehydroxylation. Accordingly, three new SNP assaying methods have been developed to carry out genome-wide genotyping, taking advantage of the enzymatic properties of Exo+ polymerases. These new mutation detection assays are widely adaptable to a variety of platforms, including multi-well plate and microarray technologies. Application of Exo+ polymerases to genetic analysis, including genotyping that is mostly relevant to pharma-cogenetics, high-fidelity gene expression profiling, rare mutation detection and mutation load assay, will help to accelerate the pace of personalized medicine. In this review paper, we will first introduce three new assays that we have recently developed, and then describe a number of their applications in pharmacogenetics and in other biomedical studies. Publication Types: Review

Adv Anat Pathol. 2004 Jul;11(4):211-20. Related Articles, Links Pharmacogenomics. Ross JS, Schenkein DP, Kashala O, Linette GP, Stec J, Symmans WF, Pusztai L, Hortobagyi GN. Division of Molecular Medicine, Millennium Pharmaceuticals, Inc, Cambridge, Massachusetts, USA. rossj@mail.amc.edu The discovery of the human genome and subsequent expansion of proteomics research combined with emerging technologies such as functional imaging, biosensors and sophisticated computational biology are producing unprecedented changes in today's healthcare. The expanding knowledge of the molecular basis of cancer has shown that significant differences in gene expression patterns can guide therapy not only for neoplastic conditions, but also for a variety of diseases including inflammatory disorders, cardiovascular disease and neurodegenerative processes. As a result, the fields of pharmacogenetics and pharmacogenomics have emerged as potential new testing platforms for the individualized management of patients. An individual's response to a drug is the complex interaction of both genetic and non-genetic factors. Genetic variants in the drug target itself, disease pathway genes, or drug metabolizing enzymes may all be used as predictors of drug efficacy or toxicity. In oncology, the SNP technology has focused on detecting the predisposition for cancer, predicting of toxic responses to drugs and selecting the best individual and combinations of anti-cancer drugs. Pharmacogenomics involves the application of whole genome technologies (e.g., gene and protein expression data) for the prediction of the sensitivity or resistance of an individual's disease to a single or group of drugs. Genomic microarrays and transcriptional profiling have the ability to generate hundreds of thousands of data points requiring sophisticated and complex information systems necessary for accurate and useful data analysis. This technique has generated a wealth of new information in the fields of leukemia/lymphoma, and solid tumor classification and prediction of metastasis, drug and biomarker target discovery and pharmacogenomic drug efficacy testing. Publication Types: Review

Adv Appl Microbiol. 2004;56:379-401. Related Articles, Links Current issues in genetic toxicology testing for microbiologists. Mortelmans K, Rupa DS. Toxicology and Pharmacology Laboratory Biosciences Division, SRI International Menlo Park, California 94025, USA. kristien.mortelmans@sri.com Publication Types: Review

Adv Neurol. 2006;97:389-98. Related Articles, Links Polygenic epilepsy. Ferraro TN, Buono RJ. Center for Neurobiology and Behavior, Department of Psychiatry, University of Pennsylvania School of Medicine, Philadelphia, Pennsylvania, USA. Current perspective on the etiology of common forms of epilepsy reflects clinical and preclinical data that document a complex determinism involving multiple gene variations and environmental influences. This multifactorial architecture precludes effective use of conventional types of genetic analysis and requires application of alternative methods. Presently, such methods are based on candidate gene studies, and it is likely that these approaches will continue to be useful in the near term. Long-range strategies will combine traditional linkage methods with single nucleotide polymorphism gene maps and will seek to collect data on a genomic scale in the search for gene variation that influences both the development of epilepsy and the response to antiepileptic medication. Such studies will require large numbers of patients and controls and also valid, standardized clinical criteria for parsing patients into phenotypic categories. Animal models will continue to provide clues regarding potentially important candidate genes and can also be used in a reverse-translational manner to confirm and study the effects of gene variation that is identified in humans. In the end, genetic research approaches to common forms of human epilepsy will enhance understanding of underlying neurobiological mechanisms, and through this understanding will come new treatment options, new molecular markers to improve current diagnostic criteria, and new genetic tests for predicting drug efficacy in patients with epilepsy. Publication Types: Review

Ageing Res Rev. 2004 Apr;3(2):153-69. Related Articles, Links The pharmacogenomics of Alzheimer's disease. Crentsil V. The Committee on Clinical Pharmacology and Pharmacogenomics, The University of Chicago, 5841 S. Maryland Avenue, MC 2115 Chicago, IL, USA. vcrentsi@medince.bsd.uchicago.edu Alzheimer's disease (AD) is a neurodegenerative disorder mostly affecting geriatric patients worldwide. The high emotional and economic impact of AD on patients, families, and the society has made AD one of the paramount geriatric syndromes. Efforts to find disease-modifying therapy have not yet been rewarding. Despite our increasing appreciation of the role of genetics in AD pathogenesis, pharmacogenomic approaches to uncover drug targets have not been extensively explored. The current knowledge of the genetics of both familial and non-familial (sporadic) AD, and the emerging data on the effect of Apolipoprotein E (ApoE) alleles on the response to AD therapeutic agents, is evidence that the potential utility of pharmacogenomics may not be limited to the familial AD (FAD) but provide answers for AD as a whole. The apparent inability of presently available drugs to alter the course of AD could be a signal that it is time to change the way we think about AD therapeutics. Copyright 2003 Elsevier Ireland Ltd. Publication Types: Review

Ageing Res Rev. 2005 Nov;4(4):548-63. Epub 2005 Oct 21. Related Articles, Links Discovering causes and cures for cancer from gene expression analysis. Weeraratna AT. Laboratory of Immunology, National Institutes of Health, National Institute on Aging, Gerontology Research Center, 5600 Nathan Shock Drive, Box 21, Baltimore, MD 21224, USA. weerarat@grc.nia.nih.gov Tumorigenesis is governed by a series of complex genetic and epigenetic changes. Both mechanisms can result in either the silencing or aberrant expression of messages in a cell. Gene expression profiling techniques such as the serial analysis of gene expression (SAGE) or microarray analysis can provide global overviews of these changes, as well identify key genes and pathways involved in this process. This review outlines the current roles of these techniques in cancer research, and how they may contribute to finding not only mechanisms of this disease, but potential targets for therapy. Publication Types: Review

AHIP Cover. 2005 Mar-Apr;46(2):14-7. Related Articles, Links The future of genomics: hope or hype? Arp D.

AIDS Patient Care STDS. 2004 May;18(5):259-73. Related Articles, Links Preventing and managing antiretroviral drug resistance. Kuritzkes DR. Harvard Medical School, Brigham and Women's Hospital, Boston, Massachusetts, USA. dkuritzkes@partners.org Development of resistance to antiretroviral drugs (ARVs) is a major impediment to optimum treatment of HIV-1 infection. Although resistance testing can help to select subsequent regimens when virologic failure occurs, cross-resistance, which affects all classes of ARVs, may make it more difficult to achieve optimum control of HIV. We have known for some time that our first choice of antiretroviral therapy offers the best chance to control HIV replication and that initial therapy should be selected with an eye on future options. Potency is the first line of defense against the development of resistance. Other factors that affect resistance development include: tolerability, potential for optimum adherence, and genetic and pharmacologic barriers to development of resistance. If resistance emerges, only a single drug may be affected initially, and a rapid change in ARVs may preserve the efficacy of other components. One cautionary note is that we can no longer assume that a patient's HIV is fully susceptible to all ARVs even in the initial regimen. Transmission of drug-resistant HIV means that the genetic composition may be that of an "experienced" virus with reduced susceptibility to ARVs. Resistance testing at the time of transmission is most likely to reveal this resistance, but over time the dominant genetic pattern may revert to wild-type, and be missed by resistance testing. Because "archived" resistant HIV may emerge quickly once treatment is initiated, we need to keep this in mind when selecting initial therapy. Publication Types: Review

AIDS Read. 2004 Sep;14(9):462-3. Related Articles, Links XV International AIDS Conference: science versus political science. Laurence J. Publication Types: Congresses Editorial

AIDS Rev. 2005 Apr-Jun;7(2):103-12. Related Articles, Links Pharmacogenetics in HIV therapy. Rodriguez-Novoa S, Barreiro P, Jimenez-Nacher I, Rendon A, Soriano V. Pharmacokinetic Unit, Hospital Carlos III, Madrid, Spain. Administration of standard doses of most antiretroviral drugs results in significant variations in plasma drug concentrations among different individuals, as well as different rates of drug-associated toxicity. The reasons for the large interindividual variability in drug levels are multifactorial, and involve differences in gender metabolism, concomitant medications, drug compliance, underlying diseases, and genetic factors. Pharmacogenetics is the discipline that analyses the genetic basis for the interindividual variation in the body disposition of drugs. One of the main goals is to give grounds to individualized therapy. The majority of pharmacogenetic traits so far have involved drug metabolism. An example of this is the inherited variation in the pharmacokinetics and pharmacodynamics of drugs such as hydralazine or isoniazid. This variation is due to polymorphisms in the N-acetyltransferase-2 (NAT2) gene, which may split the population into three categories: slow, intermediate, and fast metabolizers. Pharmacogenetic studies conducted so far with antiretrovirals have focused on metabolizing enzymes and transporter proteins in the cell membrane. Herein, we review the genetic polymorphisms known to be associated with altered pharmacokinetics of antiretrovirals, which may influence the efficacy and toxicity of these drugs. Publication Types: Review

AIDS Treat News. 2004 Mar 26;(399):6. Related Articles, Links Abacavir hypersensitivity reaction predicted by genetic test. [No authors listed] Researchers in Australia found an accurate test to predict who cannot tolerate Ziagen (abacavir). This is still a research test, not in general use. Publication Types: Newspaper Article

AIDS. 2004 Dec 3;18(18):2391-400. Related Articles, Links Pharmacogenetics of efavirenz and central nervous system side effects: an Adult AIDS Clinical Trials Group study. Haas DW, Ribaudo HJ, Kim RB, Tierney C, Wilkinson GR, Gulick RM, Clifford DB, Hulgan T, Marzolini C, Acosta EP. Program for Human Genetics, Vanderbilt University School of Medicine, 345 24th Avenue North, Nashville, TN 37203, USA. david.w.haas@vanderbilt.edu OBJECTIVES: Efavirenz is an effective antiretroviral agent, but central nervous system side effects occur commonly, and population (racial) differences in pharmacokinetics and response have been reported. Efavirenz is metabolized by cytochrome P4502B6 (CYP2B6). We investigated whether polymorphisms in CYP2B6, CYP3A4, CYP3A5, and MDR1 were associated with efavirenz central nervous system side effects and pharmacokinetics. DESIGN: Twenty-four week cohort from a randomized study. METHODS: Adult AIDS Clinical Trials Group study A5097s examined relationships between central nervous system side effects and efavirenz plasma concentration-time profiles in HIV-infected subjects. Efavirenz plasma pharmacokinetics were estimated by a population-based method. Central nervous system symptoms were assessed by questionnaires and neuropsychological testing. RESULTS: Study subjects included 89 (57%) European-Americans, 50 (32%) African-Americans, and 15 (10%) Hispanics. The CYP2B6 T/T genotype at position 516 (GlnHis) was more common in African-Americans (20%) than in European-Americans (3%), and was associated with greater efavirenz plasma exposure ($P < 0.0001$). The median efavirenz [area-under-the-curve] (0-24 h) according to G/G, G/T, and T/T genotype was 44 ($n = 78$), 60 ($n = 60$), and 130 ($n = 14$) mug.h/ml, respectively ($P < 0.0001$). The CYP2B6 G516T genotype was also associated with central nervous system symptoms at week 1 ($P = 0.036$). Analysis of DNA from other subjects confirmed population differences in frequency of the G516T variant. No associations were apparent with the other polymorphisms studied. CONCLUSIONS: A CYP2B6 allelic variant that is more common in African-Americans than in Europeans-Americans was associated with significantly greater efavirenz plasma exposure during HIV therapy. Inter-individual differences in metabolism may, in part, explain susceptibility to efavirenz central nervous system side effects. Publication Types: Clinical Trial Randomized Controlled Trial

AIDS. 2005 Jun 10;19(9):975-7. Related Articles, Links Comment on: AIDS. 2005

Jun 10;19(9):871-7. Toward genetic rationalization of antiretroviral therapy for HIV. Schwartz DH, Iyengar S. Publication Types: Comment Editorial

Alcohol. 2004 Jan;32(1):37-43. Related Articles, Links Workshop on Alcohol Use and Health Disparities 2002: a call to arms. Russo D, Purohit V, Foudin L, Salin M. Biomedical Research Branch/Division of Basic Research, National Institute on Alcohol Abuse and Alcoholism, National Institutes of Health, 6000 Executive Boulevard, Suite 402, Bethesda MD 20892-7003, USA. drusso@mail.nih.gov The National Institute on Alcohol Abuse and Alcoholism (NIAAA) of the National Institutes of Health (NIH) sponsored a "Workshop on Alcohol Use and Health Disparities 2002: A Call to Arms," on December 5, 2002, in Bethesda, Maryland, USA. This workshop was part of the NIAAA/NIH comprehensive strategic plan to reduce, and ultimately eliminate, health disparities. Eleven topics were addressed: (1). biomedical risk factors that may contribute to disparities in the toxic effects of alcohol; (2). alcohol and gene-environment interactions that affect the health of diverse groups; (3). alcohol pharmacogenetics in Mexican-Americans; (4). determinants of risk for alcoholism in minority populations; (5). consideration of population groups in linkage-disequilibrium studies to identify genes associated with alcohol dependence; (6). interaction between alcohol dependence and African-American ethnicity in disordered sleep, nocturnal cytokines, and immunity; (7). disparities of brain functional reserve capacity affecting brain morbidity related to substance abuse; (8). alcohol and pregnancy disparities; (9). role of alcohol in cancer risk disparities; (10). ethnic diversity in alcoholic cardiomyopathy; and (11). postmenopausal health disparities. On the basis of these presentations, seven conclusions emerged: (1). Genetic variations in alcohol-metabolizing enzymes exist in various populations. (2). These enzymes play a role in the variation in health effect outcomes seen in different populations, owing to alcohol consumption. (3). Differences between and among population groups can be critically important for the design and interpretation of studies in genetics. These include differences in expression of phenotype, in locus heterogeneity, in risk alleles, and in population structure. (4). Incidence rates for fetal alcohol syndrome and fetal alcohol spectrum disorders are greater in African-Americans and Native-Americans than in Caucasians. Genetic polymorphisms, nutrition, and other factors may account for these differences. (5). The highest mortality rate for cirrhosis has been found in white Hispanic men. (6). Mexican-Americans have a low frequency of the protective alleles ADH1B(*)2 and ALDH2(*)2 and a relatively high frequency of CYP2E1 c2, which is associated with early onset alcoholism. (7). The incidence rate for cancer is greater for African-Americans than for Caucasians, and part of the higher risk may be attributed to heavier drinking. Publication Types: Consensus Development Conference Consensus Development Conference, NIH Review

Altern Lab Anim. 2004 Dec;32(6):625-9. Related Articles, Links INVITOX 2004: 13th Workshop of the European Society of Toxicology In Vitro, organised in cooperation with the Scandinavian Society for Cell Toxicology. Kolman A. Department of Molecular Biology and Functional Genomics, Stockholm University, 106 91 Stockholm, Sweden. ada.kolman@telia.com INVITOX 2004, the 13th Workshop of the European Society of Toxicology In Vitro, was held on 8-11 September 2004, in Zegrze, Poland, in cooperation with the Scandinavian Society for Cell Toxicology. The workshop was attended by 112 participants from 19 countries. The programme included 11 main sessions and two round table discussions. The lectures of the invited speakers, together with short oral presentations and posters, covered the most important aspects of current research in the field of in vitro toxicology. ECVAM's strategies for the replacement of animal testing for toxic chemicals by alternative test systems were discussed. Publication Types: Congresses

Altern Med Rev. 2005 Jun;10(2):81-2. Related Articles, Links Color blind, or just plain blind? Czap A. Publication Types: Editorial

Am Fam Physician. 2004 Nov 1;70(9):1637, 1642. Related Articles, Links Genomics and the family physician: realizing the potential. Collins F. Publication Types: Editorial

Am J Cardiol. 2005 Nov 7;96(9A):65K-70K; discussion 34K-35K. Epub 2005 Oct 21. Related Articles, Links Pharmacogenomics of statin responsiveness. Kajinami K, Akao H, Polisecki E, Schaefer EJ. Department of Cardiology, Kanazawa Medical University, Daigaku Uchinada, Japan. Kajinami@kanazawa-med.ac.jp Statins are widely prescribed and are established as first-line therapy for the primary and secondary prevention of coronary artery disease. However, the benefit of treatment varies between patients. Genetic variation can contribute to interindividual variations in clinical efficacy of drug therapy, and significant progress has been made in identifying common genetic polymorphisms that influence responsiveness to statin therapy. To date, >30 candidate genes related to pharmacokinetics and pharmacodynamics of statins have been investigated as potential determinants of drug responsiveness in terms of low-density lipoprotein cholesterol lowering. Genetic variation at gene loci that affect intestinal cholesterol absorption include apolipoprotein (apo) E; adenosine triphosphate-binding cassette transporter G5 and G8; cholesterol production, such as 3-hydroxy-3-methylglutaryl coenzyme A reductase; and lipoprotein catabolism, such as apoB and the low-density lipoprotein receptor, all may play a role in modulating responsivesness as well genes involved in metabolism of statins such as cytochrome P450. However, there is considerable variation in results reported, and the data suggest that combined analysis of multiple genetic variants in several genes, all of which have possible functional significance, is more likely to give significant results than single gene studies in small sample populations. In the future, pharmacogenomic studies with a greater number of participants (>2,000 participants) should provide a better picture as to who is most likely and who is least likely to benefit from statin therapy. Publication Types: Review

Am J Cardiol. 2006 Mar 15;97(6):843-50. Epub 2006 Jan 27. Related Articles, Links Phenotypic predictors of response to simvastatin therapy among African-Americans and caucasians: the cholesterol and pharmacogenetics (CAP) study. Simon JA, Lin F, Hulley SB, Blanche PJ, Waters D, Shiboski S, Rotter JI, Nickerson DA, Yang H, Saad M, Krauss RM. General Internal Medicine Section, Medical Service, Veterans Affairs Medical Center, San Francisco, California, USA. jasimon@itsa.ucsf.edu Although statins are effective lipid-lowering agents, the phenotypic and demographic predictors of such lowering have been less well examined. We enrolled 944 African-American and white men and women who completed an open-label, 6-week pharmacogenetics trial of 40 mg of simvastatin. The phenotypic and demographic variables were examined as predictors of the change in lipids and lipoproteins using linear regression analysis. On average, treatment with simvastatin lowered low-density lipoprotein (LDL) cholesterol by 54 mg/dl and increased high-density lipoprotein (HDL) cholesterol by 2 mg/dl. Compared with African-Americans, whites had a 3-mg/dl greater LDL reduction and a 1-mg/dl higher HDL elevation, independent of other variables, including baseline lipoprotein levels ($p < 0.01$). Multivariate analyses revealed moderate subgroup differences, with older participants having a larger decrease in LDL cholesterol and apolipoprotein B levels compared with younger participants ($p < 0.001$), women having larger increases in HDL than men ($p < 0.01$), nonsmokers having larger decreases in LDL and triglyceride levels compared with smokers ($p < 0.05$), those with hypertension having smaller decreases in apolipoprotein B than those without hypertension ($p < 0.05$), and those with a larger waist circumference having a diminished lowering of triglycerides in response to treatment with simvastatin ($p < 0.01$). In conclusion, treatment with simvastatin produced favorable lipid and lipoprotein changes among all participants. The magnitude of the lipid and lipoprotein responses, however, differed among participants according to a number of phenotypic and demographic characteristics.

Am J Clin Pathol. 2004 Oct;122(4):598-609. Related Articles, Links Targeted therapies for cancer 2004. Ross JS, Schenkein DP, Pietrusko R, Rolfe M, Linette GP, Stec J, Stagliano NE, Ginsburg GS, Symmans WF, Pusztai L, Hortobagyi GN. Department of Pathology and Laboratory Medicine, Albany Medical College, NY 12208, USA. The regulatory agency approvals in the United States and Europe of imatinib mesylate (Gleevec) for patients with bcr/abl-positive chronic myelogenous leukemia, cetuximab (Erbitux) for patients with epidermal growth factor receptor overexpressing metastatic colorectal cancer, the antiangiogenesis agent bevacizumab (Avastin), and the proteasome inhibitor bortezomib (Velcade)--and the considerable public interest in new anticancer drugs that take advantage of specific genetic defects that render the malignant cells more likely to respond to specific treatment--are driving a new era of integrated diagnostics and therapeutics. The recent discovery of a drug response predicting activating mutation in the epidermal growth factor receptor gene for patients with non-small cell lung cancer treated with gefitinib (Iressa) has intensified this interest. In this review, the history of targeted anticancer therapies is highlighted, with focus on the development of molecular diagnostics for hematologic malignancies and the emergence of trastuzumab (Herceptin), an antibody-based targeted therapy for HER-2/neu overexpressing metastatic breast cancer: The potential of pharmacogenomic strategies and the use of high-density genomic microarrays to classify and select therapy for cancer are briefly considered. This review also considers the widely held view that, in the next 5 to 10 years, the clinical application of molecular diagnostics will further revolutionize the drug discovery and development process;

customize the selection, dosing, route of administration of existing and new therapeutic agents; and truly personalize medical care for cancer patients.
Publication Types: Review

Am J Clin Pathol. 2005 Dec;124 Suppl:S29-41. Related Articles, Links Pharmacogenomics and clinical biomarkers in drug discovery and development. Ross JS, Symmans WF, Pusztai L, Hortobagyi GN. Department of Pathology and Laboratory Medicine, Albany Medical College, NY 12208, USA. The fields of pathology and clinical pharmacology are in an era of rapid evolution, reflecting continuous technological advancements in molecular diagnostics focused on improving drug efficacy and reducing toxicity. The discovery and refinement of the human genome sequence, further understanding of epigenetic events, and the expansion of proteomics research combined with emerging technologies such as functional imaging, biosensors, and sophisticated computational biology are having an unprecedented impact on the pharmaceutical industry. This review focuses on the discovery and development of DNA-based gene sequence tests and RNA-based gene expression profiles as applied to the prediction of response, resistance, and toxicity of both new and existing anticancer, cardiovascular, and anti-inflammatory drugs. This review will also consider the potential of emerging biomarkers designed to assist in the clinical development of these agents.
Publication Types: Review

Am J Geriatr Psychiatry. 2005 Dec;13(12):1027-40. Related Articles, Links Looking forward in geriatric anxiety and depression: implications of basic science for the future. Gershenfeld HK, Philibert RA, Boehm GW. Departments of Psychiatry and Integrative Biology, University of Texas Southwestern Medical Center/ NC6.530, 5323 Harry Hines Blvd., Dallas, TX 75390-9070, USA. Howard.Gershenfeld@UTSouthwestern.edu Major depression and anxiety are common psychiatric illnesses whose etiology remains incompletely understood. This review highlights progress in understanding the etiology of these illnesses through genetic strategies and looks forward to their impact on geriatric psychiatry. We briefly address three broad domains of progress, namely 1) genetic approaches to etiology, including linkage and association studies, pharmacogenetics ("personalized medicine"), and gene x environment interactions; 2) mechanisms of thyroid and testosterone action via nuclear receptors, given these hormones' status as possible augmenters of antidepressants; and 3) the role of the neuroimmune system as a contributor to the stress response. Genetic strategies offer one path for converting correlational findings into causal pathways while complementing studies of a gene's function at the molecular, cellular, network, and whole-organismal levels. Neuroendocrine supplementation (thyroid and testosterone) has a long history and tradition. A molecular understanding of nuclear receptor pathways and their coactivators, the mediator complex proteins, provides a rationale for improved targeting of hormonal action in a tissue-selective manner, yielding drugs with improved safety and efficacy. Neural-immune interactions in psychiatric illness remain tantalizing topics. Research suggests that cytokine pathways may contribute to the maintenance or susceptibility to stress, anxiety, and depressive disorders. The reciprocal and recursive interactions among basic science, drug discovery, and clinical science will continue to provide hopeful themes for improving the lives of patients with treatment-refractive psychiatric illness.

Am J Health Syst Pharm. 2004 Nov 15;61(22):2380-8. Related Articles, Links Pharmacotherapy, pharmacogenomics, and the future of alcohol dependence treatment, Part 2. Kenna GA, McGeary JE, Swift RM. Center for Alcohol and Addiction Studies, Brown University, Providence, RI, USA. george_kenna@brown.edu PURPOSE: The neurobiological basis of alcohol dependence, established pharmacotherapies for alcohol dependence, pharmacotherapies under investigation, and obstacles to treatment are discussed. SUMMARY: Alcohol binds to hydrophobic pockets of proteins, changing their three-dimensional structure and their function. Proteins that are particularly sensitive to alcohol include ion channels, neurotransmitter receptors, and enzymes involved in signal transduction. Established pharmacologic treatments, notably disulfiram and naltrexone, combined with behavioral therapies, may reduce the amount of drinking, the risk of relapse, the number of days of drinking, and craving in some alcohol-dependent individuals. For many patients, however, these treatments are not effective. Recent advances in molecular and behavior genetics are guiding the development of new drugs; these efforts seek to identify pharmacologic pathways relevant to alcohol dependence and to more effectively match treatments to individuals according to their genetic characteristics. Efficacy and safety concerns for acamprosate have been satisfied; the drug was recently released for marketing in the United States. Medications such as sertraline, ondansetron, topiramate, and aripiprazole represent novel lines of research and are currently being tested for use in the treatment of alcoholism. Even with more efficacious medications, however, a transformation must occur in how alcoholism treatment is viewed, not only by the public but also by clinicians. CONCLUSION: In addition to existing drug treatments for alcohol dependence, many other medications are under investigation, particularly for specific types of alcoholism. Pharmacogenomics is expected to play an important role in this research effort. Publication Types: Review

Am J Health Syst Pharm. 2005 Jun 15;62(12):1226. Related Articles, Links Scientists focus on pharmacogenomics at FDA Science Forum. Young D. Publication Types: News

Am J Hum Genet. 2004 Dec;75(6):1059-69. Epub 2004 Oct 18. Related Articles, Links CYP3A variation and the evolution of salt-sensitivity variants. Thompson EE, Kuttab-Boulos H, Witonsky D, Yang L, Roe BA, Di Rienzo A. Committee on Genetics and Department of Human Genetics, University of Chicago, Chicago, IL, USA. Members of the cytochrome P450 3A subfamily catalyze the metabolism of endogenous substrates, environmental carcinogens, and clinically important exogenous compounds, such as prescription drugs and therapeutic agents. In particular, the CYP3A4 and CYP3A5 genes play an especially important role in pharmacogenetics, since they metabolize >50% of the drugs on the market. However, known genetic variants at these two loci are not sufficient to account for the observed phenotypic variability in drug response. We used a comparative genomics approach to identify conserved coding and noncoding regions at these genes and resequenced them in three ethnically diverse human populations. We show that remarkable interpopulation differences exist with regard to frequency spectrum and haplotype structure. The non-African samples are characterized by a marked excess of rare variants and the presence of a homogeneous group of long-range haplotypes at high frequency. The CYP3A5*1/*3 polymorphism, which is likely to influence salt and water retention and risk for salt-sensitive hypertension, was genotyped in >1,000 individuals from 52 worldwide population samples. The results reveal an unusual geographic pattern whereby the CYP3A5*3 frequency shows extreme variation across human populations and is significantly correlated with distance from the equator. Furthermore, we show that an unlinked variant, AGT M235T, previously implicated in hypertension and pre-eclampsia, exhibits a similar geographic distribution and is significantly correlated in frequency with CYP3A5*1/*3. Taken together, these results suggest that variants that influence salt homeostasis were the targets of a shared selective pressure that resulted from an environmental variable correlated with latitude.

Am J Infect Control. 2004 Jun;32(4):215-9. Related Articles, Links Dissemination of nosocomial multiple-aminoglycoside-resistant Staphylococcus aureus caused by horizontal transfer of the resistance determinant (aacA/aphD) and clonal spread of resistant strains. Udou T. Department of Clinical Microbiology, School of Health Sciences, University of Occupational and Environmental Health, Kitakyushu, Japan. BACKGROUND: The multiple-aminoglycoside-resistant gene aacA/aphD exists as a transposable genetic element (Tn4001) in gram-positive cocci. Here we describe our retrospective investigation of the mechanism responsible for the dissemination of Tn4001 among staphylococci present in clinical isolates collected in our university hospital. At its peak, about 80% of the total isolates of methicillin-resistant Staphylococcus aureus showed multiple-aminoglycoside resistance, and all harbored aacA/aphD. METHODS: Clonal relatedness was analyzed by pulsed field gel electrophoresis after SmaI endonuclease digestion of the genomic DNA from isolates collected in 1991 and 1997. To detect Tn4001 on the chromosome and conjugative plasmids, specific sequences from aacA/aphD and the insertion sequence IS256, whose inverted sequence flanks aacA/aphD, were amplified by polymerase chain reaction. RESULTS: Pulsed field gel electrophoresis of genomic DNA, plasmid analysis, and polymerase chain reaction detection of the resistance determinant all indicated the presence of disseminated clones that had survived among hospitalized patients through acquisition of conjugative plasmids harboring aacA/aphD. Furthermore, aacA/aphD also disseminated among nosocomial strains other than S aureus as a consequence of the self-transferability of Tn4001. CONCLUSIONS: The nosocomial prevalence of multiple-aminoglycoside-resistant staphylococci is the result of both horizontal and interspecific transfer of aacA/aphD and the clonal spread and survival of resistant strains.

Am J Kidney Dis. 2005 Dec;46(6):1129-39. Related Articles, Links Pharmacology. Perazella MA, Parikh C. Section of Nephrology, Yale University School of Medicine, New Haven, CT 06520-8029, USA. mark.perazella@yale.edu Publication Types: Review

Am J Law Med. 2005;31(2-3):365-80. Related Articles, Links Potential interactions of the Orphan Drug Act and pharmacogenomics:

a flood of orphan drugs and abuses? Loughnot D.

Am J Manag Care. 2004 Jul;10(7 Pt 1):425-32. Related Articles, Links Genetic testing and pharmacogenomics: issues for determining the impact to healthcare delivery and costs. Phillips KA, Veenstra DL, Ramsey SD, Van Bebber SL, Sakowski J. Program in Pharmacogenomics and Population Screening, School of Pharmacy, Institute for Health Policy Studies, and UCSF Comprehensive Cancer Center, University of California, San Francisco, 94143, USA. kathryn@itsa.ucsf.edu OBJECTIVES: To determine the potential impact of genetic testing and pharmacogenomics on healthcare delivery and costs. STUDY DESIGN: Literature review. METHODS: We examined 3 examples: (1) BRCA1/2 testing for breast cancer risk, (2) HER2/neu overexpression testing to guide drug treatment in women with breast cancer, and (3) CYP2C9 testing before the use of the anticoagulant warfarin. We discussed each genetic testing example from the perspective of the patient, provider, insurer, industry, government, and society. RESULTS: The expanded use of genetic information offers many potential clinical benefits, but also many economic challenges. One of those challenges will be managing the impact of genetic testing on healthcare delivery and costs. CONCLUSIONS: Systematic, evidence-based technology assessments and economic evaluations will have to be used to guide the incorporation of genomics into clinical practice. More research also will be needed to assess patient preferences and willingness to pay for genomic technologies; how providers can assess and use genomic technologies; and how the industry, insurers, and government can best balance the relevant costs and benefits. Publication Types: Review

Am J Med. 2005 Dec;118(12):1323-30. Related Articles, Links Progression of chronic kidney disease: can it be prevented or arrested? Jaber BL, Madias NE. Department of Medicine, Tufts University School of Medicine, Caritas St. Elizabeth's Medical Center, Boston, Mass 02135, USA. Chronic kidney disease constitutes a highly prevalent health problem worldwide. Left untreated, it progresses inexorably to greater levels of severity at variable rates. The morbid impact of chronic kidney disease is heightened by its role as risk factor for cardiovascular disease. In the past two decades, considerable gains have been realized in retarding progression of chronic kidney disease by emphasizing blood pressure control and blockade of the renin-angiotensin system. Notwithstanding, the therapeutic goal of preventing or arresting chronic kidney disease progression remains unfulfilled. Currently attainable rates of decrease in glomerular filtration rate remain at 2 to 8 mL/min/y depending on the underlying disease. It is now believed that to achieve optimal therapeutic targets (proteinuria of <500 mg/day and decrease in glomerular filtration rate of 1 mL/min/y, the average age-related decline) we must introduce novel strategies and a multifaceted approach to treatment that interrupts multiple mechanisms of progression. To this end, and wherever relevant, new approaches to cause-specific treatment must be applied, such as targeted immunosuppression, intensive glycemic control, gene therapy, and enzyme replacement therapy. Furthermore, in all chronic kidney disease, we must interfere more effectively with the multitude of common mechanisms of progression.

Established or putative, such approaches include aggressive blood pressure control; advanced renin-angiotensin system blockade; cytokine modulation and antifibrotic therapy; aldosterone blockade; endothelin blockade, nitric oxide modulation and vasopeptidase inhibition; antioxidant therapy; statin therapy; glycosaminoglycan therapy; anemia therapy; dietary restrictions; lifestyle changes; and pharmacogenomic profiling. Such a concerted, multifaceted approach to management might indeed prevent or arrest progression of chronic kidney disease, or even achieve regression of chronic kidney disease. Publication Types: Review

Am J Nurs. 2004 May;104(5):60-70; quiz 71. Related Articles, Links Comment in: Am J Nurs. 2004 Aug;104(8):16. Medication selection by genotype: How genetics is changing drug prescribing and efficacy. Prows CA, Prows DR. Department of Patient Services, Division of Nursing, Cincinnati Children's Hospital Medical Center, Cincinnati, OH 45229-3039, USA. cindy.prows@cchmc.org Publication Types: Review

Am J Pharmacogenomics. 2004;4(2):73-82. Related Articles, Links Population genomics of drug response. Halapi E, Stefansson K, Hakonarson H. deCODE genetics, Inc., Reykjavik, Iceland. Genetic diversity contributes to both disease susceptibility and variability in response to drugs. However, it has proven difficult to isolate genes that underlie common complex disease, and genetic variations that influence clinical responses to drugs remain largely uncovered. The candidate gene approach to uncover genetic variations that contribute to disease susceptibility or variations in response to common drugs has not met expectations. Although the sib-pair linkage approach has certain theoretical advantages in dealing with common/complex disease, success has been slow in coming. Meanwhile family studies including siblings, cousins and second cousins, and studies in well-defined founder populations, have increasingly gained popularity and enabled scientists to map and isolate genes for common complex disease, such as schizophrenia and asthma. The latter method has generated new hope that this approach may also be effective in mapping genes that regulate drug response. Indeed, there is compelling evidence that corticosteroid sensitivity is a mapable trait in patients with asthma. Collectively, these studies support the value of leveraging information available within population-based data systems to map and isolate genes for common complex disease and drug response. Publication Types: Review

Am J Pharmacogenomics. 2004;4(3):141-50. Related Articles, Links HIV pharmacogenomics: closer to personalized therapy? Payne DA, Bryant BJ; AACC Pharmacogenomic Committee. Department of Pathology, University of Texas Medical Branch, Galveston, Texas 77555-0743, USA. dpayne@utmb.edu Pharmacogenomics classically focuses on host nuclear genetic polymorphisms that can be used to predict adverse drug reactions (ADRs). Because ADRs are defined as any noxious, unintended, and undesired drug effects, loss of efficacy due to the development of antiretroviral drug resistance and both acute and cumulative adverse effects of antiretroviral therapy can be considered ADRs. In order to address these types of antiretroviral-associated ADRs, pharmacogenomic testing methods have expanded to include molecular assays that characterize extranuclear genetic material (e.g. HIV and mitochondrial genomes), as well as the host nuclear genetic material. Recent molecular advances permit high resolution resistance testing that detects loss of therapeutic efficacy through the use of phenotypic, genotypic and/or virtual phenotypic resistance testing. These assays use complex technical and interpretative methods to improve the therapeutic efficacy of antiretroviral therapy. The resistance assays demonstrate the utility of pharmacogenomic testing for patients undergoing lifelong and complex antiretroviral therapies. Future applications of antiretroviral-directed pharmacogenomic tests range from quantitative detection of mitochondrial depletion as an early surrogate marker for drug toxicity, to qualitative analysis of host immune haplotypes, and metabolic/transporter genetic polymorphisms for predicting disease progression.In summary, pharmacogenomic testing for HIV-positive patients provides proof of principle that these tests can be used clinically to improve outcomes for patients undergoing complex and sustained drug regimens. Publication Types: Review

Am J Pharmacogenomics. 2004;4(3):151-60. Related Articles, Links Pharmacogenetics of antihypertensive drug responses. Schwartz GL, Turner ST. Department of Internal Medicine, Mayo Clinic and Foundation, Rochester, Minnesota 55905, USA. gschwartz@mayo.edu The blood pressure (BP) response to any single antihypertensive drug is characterized by marked interindividual variation, and the known predictors of response are of limited value in identifying the optimum drug for an individual patient. Analysis of genetic variation has the potential to improve our understanding of determinants of antihypertensive drug response in order to individualize drug selection. Genetic variation can influence both pharmacokinetic and pharmacodynamic mechanisms underlying variation in drug response.Classic pharmacogenetic investigations have identified variations in single genes that have a large effect on antihypertensive drug metabolism and are inherited in a Mendelian fashion. These include a polymorphism in the CYP2D6 gene, encoding a cytochrome p450 family member involved in phase I drug metabolism, and polymorphisms in genes encoding enzymes involved in phase II drug metabolism, including N-acetyltransferase (NAT2), catechol-O-methyltransferase (COMT), and phenol sulfotransferase (P-PST, SULT1A1). Although these polymorphisms have major effects on the pharmacokinetic profiles of both commonly used antihypertensive drugs such as metoprolol (CYP2D6), and lesser used drugs such as hydralazine (NAT2), methyldopa (COMT), and minoxidil (SULT1A1), they have not been shown to influence variation in the antihypertensive effect of these drugs at conventional doses. Interest is now focused on identifying genetic polymorphisms that influence the pharmacodynamic determinants of antihypertensive response. Using a candidate gene approach, such polymorphisms have been identified in genes encoding alpha-adducin (ADD1), subunits of G-proteins (GNB3 and GNAS1), the beta(1)-adrenergic receptor (ADRB1), endothelial nitric oxide synthase (NOS3), and components of the renin-angiotensin-aldosterone system (angiotensinogen [AGT], angiotensin converting enzyme [ACE], the angiotensin type I receptor [AGTR1], and aldosterone synthase [CYP11B2]). These polymorphisms have been shown to influence the BP response to diuretics (ADD1, GNB3, NOS3, and ACE), beta-blockers (GNAS1 and ADRB1), ACE inhibitors (AGT, ACE, and AGTR1), angiotensin receptor blockers (ACE and CYP11B2), and clonidine (GNB3).An emerging consensus from these studies is that single gene effects on antihypertensive drug responses are small, and even the combined effects of all presently known polymorphisms do not account for enough variation in response to be clinically useful. New genome-wide scanning techniques may lead to the identification of genes previously unsuspected of influencing drug response. Additional requirements for pharmacogenetic approaches to become clinically useful are the characterization of the effects of haplotypes and multi-locus genotypes on drug response, and consideration of gene-by-environment interactions. Such studies will require huge sample sizes and novel statistical methods, but the theoretical and technical framework is in place to make this possible. Publication Types: Review

Am J Pharmacogenomics. 2004;4(5):293-8. Related Articles, Links Human genetics and responses to influenza vaccination: clinical implications. Lambkin R, Novelli P, Oxford J, Gelder C. Department of Medical Microbiology and Retroscreen Virology, Queen Mary's School of Medicine and Dentistry, London, England. r.lambkin@retroscreen.com Influenza A and B viruses are negative-strand RNA viruses that cause regular outbreaks of respiratory disease and substantially impact on morbidity and mortality. Our primary defense against the influenza virus infection is provided by neutralizing antibodies that inhibit the function of the virus surface coat proteins hemagglutinin and neuraminidase. Production of these antibodies by B lymphocytes requires help from CD4+ T cells. The most commonly used vaccines against the influenza virus comprise purified preparations of hemagglutinin and neuraminidase, and are designed to induce a protective neutralizing antibody response. Because of regular antigenic change in these proteins (drift and shift mutation), the vaccines have to be administered on an annual basis. Current defense strategies center on prophylactic vaccination of those individuals who are considered to be most at risk from the serious complications of infection (principally individuals aged >65 years and those with chronic respiratory, cardiac, or metabolic disease).The clinical effectiveness of influenza virus vaccination is dependent on several vaccine-related factors, including the quantity of hemagglutinin within the vaccine, the number of doses administered, and the route of immunization. In addition, the immunocompetence of the recipient, their previous exposure to influenza virus and influenza virus vaccines, and the closeness of the match between the vaccine and circulating influenza virus strains, all influence the serologic response to vaccination.However, even when these vaccines are administered to young fit adults a proportion of individuals do not mount a significant serologic response to the vaccine. It is not clear whether these nonresponding individuals are genetically pre-programmed to be nonresponders or whether failure to respond to the vaccine is a random event. There is good evidence that nonresponsiveness to hepatitis B vaccine, another purified protein vaccine, is at least partially modulated by an individual's human leucocyte antigen (HLA) alleles. Because CD4+ T cells, which control the neutralizing antibody response to influenza virus, recognize antigens in association with HLA class II molecules, we recently conducted a small study to investigate whether there was any association between HLA class II molecules and nonresponsiveness to influenza virus vaccination. This work revealed that the HLA-DRB1*0701 allele was over represented among persons who fail to mount a neutralizing antibody response. This preliminary finding is important because it potentially identifies a group who may not be protected by current vaccination strategies. Further investigation into the role of HLA polymorphisms and nonresponse to influenza virus vaccination, and vaccination against viruses in general, is clearly required. Publication Types: Review

Am J Pharmacogenomics. 2005;5(1):1-20. Related Articles, Links The epidemiologic approach to pharmacogenomics. Little J, Sharp L, Khoury MJ, Bradley L, Gwinn M. Department of Epidemiology and Community Medicine, University of Ottawa, 451 Smyth Rd, Ottawa, Ontario K1H 8M5, Canada. jlittle@uottawa.ca The epidemiologic approach enables the systematic evaluation of potential improvements in the safety and efficacy of drug treatment which might result from targeting treatment on the basis of genomic information. The main epidemiologic designs are the randomized control trial, the cohort study, and the case-control study, and derivatives of these proposed for investigating gene-environment interactions. However, no one design is ideal for every situation, and methodological issues, notably selection bias, information bias, confounding and chance, all play a part in determining which study design is best for a given situation. There is also a need to employ a range of different designs to establish a portfolio of evidence about specific gene-drug interactions.In view of the complexity of gene-drug interactions, pooling of data across studies is likely to be needed in order to have adequate statistical power to test hypotheses. We suggest that there may be opportunities (i) to exploit samples from trials already completed to investigate possible gene-drug interactions; (ii) to consider the use of the case-only design nested within randomized controlled trials as a possible means of reducing genotyping costs when dichotomous outcomes are being investigated; and (iii) to make use of population-based disease registries that can be linked with tissue samples, treatment information and death records, to investigate gene-treatment interactions in survival. Publication Types: Review

Am J Pharmacogenomics. 2005;5(1):21-33. Related Articles, Links Pharmacogenomics of fluorouracil, irinotecan, and oxaliplatin in hepatic metastases of colorectal cancer: clinical implications. Lentz F, Tran A, Rey E, Pons G, Treluyer JM. Service de Pharmacologie, Hopital Saint Vincent de Paul, avenue Denfert-Rochereau, Paris, 75014, France. Hepatic metastases occur in about half of patients with colorectal cancer. Since hepatic metastases are often not accessible for surgery, chemotherapy of metastases is important. The most commonly used chemotherapy drugs for hepatic metastases are fluorouracil, irinotecan, and oxaliplatin. Several enzymes are known to be involved in the catabolism and anabolism of these drugs, and the activity of these enzymes varies greatly between individuals. The causes of this variation include genetic polymorphisms, different regulation between normal and cancer tissue, and the influence of chemotherapy on enzyme expression. The varying enzyme activity may have an important effect on the outcome of chemotherapy. Several studies confirm the influence of the activity of thymidylate synthase, thymidine phosphorylase and dihydropyrimidine dehydrogenase on the outcome of fluorouracil therapy for colorectal cancer, with higher enzyme activities predicting lower treatment efficacy. Although fewer studies are available regarding therapy of hepatic metastases, the same relationship between thymidylate synthase activity and outcome of fluorouracil therapy observed for primary colorectal cancer was found. For the other two enzymes, only a few studies are available, but the results indicate similarly that higher enzyme activity seems to be disadvantageous. The enzymes responsible for the activation, metabolism and mechanism of action of irinotecan, namely carboxylesterase 2, cytochrome P450 (CYP) 3A4, uridine diphosphate glucuronosyltransferase isoform 1A1 (UGT1A1), and topoisomerase-I, also exhibit variable interindividual activity. Thus, there may be an association between enzyme activity and response to therapy. For instance, in patients with colorectal cancer, higher enzyme activity of topoisomerase-I seems to be predictive of a better response to irinotecan. CYP3A4 and UGT1A1 activity levels might be predictive of irinotecan toxicity rather than efficacy. The degradation of oxaliplatin is independent of potentially varying enzyme activity, but for this drug, the DNA repair enzyme ERCC1 may influence the survival time after chemotherapy. Taken together, the available data indicate the importance of the different enzyme activities on the outcome of chemotherapy of hepatic metastases in colorectal cancer. More information is needed, especially for the newer drugs irinotecan and oxaliplatin. However, the existing data are very promising in respect to the potential to guide dose and drug selection for more efficient and less toxic chemotherapy of hepatic metastases. Publication Types: Review

Am J Pharmacogenomics. 2005;5(1):35-43. Related Articles, Links Advances in myeloma genetics and prospects for pharmacogenomic testing in multiple myeloma. Claudio JO, Stewart AK. Department of Medical Oncology, Princess Margaret Hospital, Toronto, Ontario, Canada Pharmacogenomic studies in multiple myeloma, a neoplasia of clonally expanded malignant bone marrow plasma cells, are helping to set the stage for individualized therapy. Although relatively few in numbers, these studies are already providing new therapeutic targets and avenues for drug discoveries as well as contributing to novel prognostic markers in multiple myeloma. High-throughput mutation screening of the kinome promises to identify further novel targets for therapy. Genetics and gene expression profiling technology have improved molecular-based patient stratification and prognostic staging, expanded knowledge of the molecular mechanism of chemotherapeutic agents, and provided a better understanding of myeloma bone disease. The use of pharmacogenomic strategies in myeloma is thus already changing medical practice. Publication Types: Review

Am J Pharmacogenomics. 2005;5(1):53-62. Related Articles, Links Pharmacogenomics and the drug discovery pipeline: when should it be implemented? Penny MA, McHale D. Clinical Pharmacogenomics, Pfizer Global Research and Development, Sandwich Laboratories (ipc 746), Sandwich, Kent, Ramsgate Road, CT13 9NJ, UK. michelle.penny@pfizer.com One of the key factors in developing improved medicines lies in understanding the molecular basis of the complex diseases we treat. Investigation of genetic associations with disease utilizing advances in linkage disequilibrium-based whole genome association strategies will provide novel targets for therapy and define relevant pathways contributing to disease pathogenesis. Genetic studies in conjunction with gene expression, proteomic, and metabonomic analyses provide a powerful tool to identify molecular subtypes of disease. Using these molecular data, pharmacogenomics has the potential to impact on the drug discovery and development process at many stages of the pipeline, contributing to both target identification and increased confidence in the therapeutic rationale. This is exemplified by the identified association of 5-lipoxygenase-activating protein (ALOX5AP/FLAP) with increased risk of myocardial infarction, and of the chemokine receptor 5 (CCR5) with HIV infection and therapy. Pharmacogenomics has already been used in oncology to demonstrate that molecular data facilitates assessment of disease heterogeneity, and thus identification of molecular markers of response to drugs such as imatinib mesylate (Gleevec) and trastuzumab (Herceptin).Knowledge of genetic variation in a target allows early assessment of the clinical significance of polymorphism through the appropriate design of preclinical studies and use of relevant animal models. A focussed pharmacogenomic strategy at the preclinical phase of drug development will produce data to inform the pharmacogenomic plan for exploratory and full development of compounds. Opportunities post-approval show the value of large well-characterized data sets for a systematic assessment of the contribution of genetic determinants to adverse drug reactions and efficacy. The availability of genomic samples in large phase IV trials also provides a valuable resource for further understanding the molecular basis of disease heterogeneity, providing data that feeds back into the drug discovery process in target identification and validation for the next generation of improved medicines. Publication Types: Review

Am J Pharmacogenomics. 2005;5(3):141-8. Related Articles, Links Applying proteomics in clinical trials: assessing the potential and practical limitations in ovarian cancer. Tchabo NE, Liel MS, Kohn EC. Laboratory of Pathology, Molecular Signaling Section Center for Cancer Research, National Cancer Institute, Bethesda, Maryland 20892, USA. Ovarian cancer is the leading cause of death from gynecologic malignancies among American women and the fourth most frequent cause of death from cancer in women in Europe and the US. Despite appropriate surgical and chemotherapeutic intervention, the 5-year survival in patients with metastatic cancer remains poor. Currently available screening methods, including CA125, additional biomarkers, and transvaginal ultrasound lack the necessary sensitivity and specificity to provide accurate and cost-efficient screening for the general population or the ability to assess who will benefit most from each treatment. These limitations have prompted the study of proteomic technology and its application in ovarian cancer diagnostics. Proteomics is the study of molecules in the functional protein pathways of normal or diseased states. Clinical trials are currently being conducted to assess the sensitivity and specificity of serum proteomic patterns and additional clinical trials are designed to evaluate the effects of molecularly targeted agents on protein signaling pathways in human subjects. Overcoming both scientific and practical limitations will lead to increased knowledge of deranged protein networks in cancer cells. Clinical trials in proteomics may result in improved early detection, better monitoring, new drugs and molecularly targeted therapeutics, and individualized therapies. Publication Types: Review

Am J Pharmacogenomics. 2005;5(3):149-60. Related Articles, Links Genetics and epigenetics in major psychiatric disorders: dilemmas, achievements, applications, and future scope. Abdolmaleky HM, Thiagalingam S, Wilcox M. Department of Psychiatry, Harvard Medical School at Massachusetts Mental Health Center, Boston, Massachusetts, USA. sayed_abdolmaleky@hms.harvard.edu No specific gene has been identified for any major psychiatric disorder, including schizophrenia, in spite of strong evidence supporting a genetic basis for these complex and devastating disorders. There are several likely reasons for this failure, ranging from poor study design with low statistical power to genetic mechanisms such as polygenic inheritance, epigenetic interactions, and pleiotropy. Most study designs currently in use are inadequate to uncover these mechanisms. However, to date, genetic studies have provided some valuable insight into the causes and potential therapies for psychiatric disorders. There is a growing body of evidence suggesting that the understanding of the genetic etiology of psychiatric illnesses, including schizophrenia, will be more successful with integrative approaches considering both genetic and epigenetic factors. For example, several genes including those encoding dopamine receptors (DRD2, DRD3, and DRD4), serotonin receptor 2A (HTR2A) and catechol-O-methyltransferase (COMT) have been implicated in the etiology of schizophrenia and related disorders through meta-analyses and large, multicenter studies. There is also growing evidence for the role of DRD1, NMDA receptor genes (GRIN1, GRIN2A, GRIN2B), brain-derived neurotrophic factor (BDNF), and dopamine transporter (SLC6A3) in both schizophrenia and bipolar disorder. Recent studies have indicated that epigenetic modification of reelin (RELN), BDNF, and the DRD2 promoters confer susceptibility to clinical psychiatric conditions. Pharmacologic therapy of psychiatric disorders will likely be more effective once the molecular pathogenesis is known. For example, the hypoactive alleles of DRD2 and the hyperactive alleles of COMT, which degrade the dopamine in the synaptic cleft, are associated with schizophrenia. It is likely that insufficient dopaminergic transmission in the frontal lobe plays a role in the development of negative symptoms associated with this disorder. Antipsychotic therapies with a partial dopamine D2 receptor agonist effect may be a plausible alternative to current therapies, and would be effective in symptom reduction in psychotic individuals. It is also possible that therapies employing dopamine D1/D2 receptor agonists or COMT inhibitors will be beneficial for patients with negative symptoms in schizophrenia and bipolar disorder. The complex etiology of schizophrenia, and other psychiatric disorders, warrants the consideration of both genetic and epigenetic systems and the careful design of experiments to illumine the genetic mechanisms conferring liability for these disorders and the benefit of existing and new therapies. Publication Types: Review

Am J Pharmacogenomics. 2005;5(3):161-71. Related Articles, Links Preclinical drug safety analysis by chemogenomic profiling in the liver. Fielden MR, Pearson C, Brennan R, Kolaja KL. Iconix

Pharmaceuticals, Mountain View, California 94043, USA. The economic hurdles of drug development and the emergence of genomic technologies such as chemogenomics are combining to shift the existing paradigms in preclinical drug development. Today, the information gleaned from high content molecular data has begun to augment traditional approaches to the assessment of drug safety. The optimal approach is a hybrid strategy employing chemogenomic data and gene expression-based biomarkers of drug efficacy and toxicity to supplement low content and insensitive methods for risk assessment and mechanistic evaluation of drug candidates. Large reference databases of chemogenomic data are essential to the derivation and validation of accurate and predictive gene expression biomarkers. An example of the development of a predictive biomarker for hepatic bile duct hyperplasia is described herein. As gene expression technologies improve, biomarkers will achieve higher throughput, and become more cost effective and increasingly accurate. This will elevate the value of chemogenomics in drug development, shift attrition to earlier in the process, and reduce the overall cost of drug development. Over the past 2 to 3 years, the transition of chemogenomics from a research tool to a decision-making tool has begun and regulatory agencies are anxiously awaiting implementation of this technology to make faster and more informed evaluations of potential drugs. Publication Types: Review

Am J Pharmacogenomics. 2005;5(3):173-90. Related Articles, Links Oncogenes as novel targets for cancer therapy (part I): growth factors and protein tyrosine kinases. Zhang Z, Li M, Rayburn ER, Hill DL, Zhang R, Wang H. Department of Pharmacology and Toxicology, and Division of Clinical Pharmacology, University of Alabama at Birmingham, Birmingham, Alabama 35294-0019, USA. In the past 10 years, progress made in cancer biology, genetics, and biotechnology has led to a major transition in cancer drug design and development. There has been a change from an emphasis on non-specific, cytotoxic agents to specific, molecular-based therapeutics. Mechanism-based therapy is designed to act on cellular and molecular targets that are causally involved in the formation, growth, and progression of human cancers. These agents, which may have greater selectivity for cancer versus normal cells, and which may produce better anti-tumor efficacy and lower host toxicity, can be small molecules, natural or engineered peptides, proteins, antibodies, or synthetic nucleic acids (e.g. antisense oligonucleotides, ribozymes, and siRNAs). Novel targets are identified and validated by state-of-the-art approaches, including high-throughput screening, combinatorial chemistry, and gene expression arrays, which increase the speed and efficiency of drug discovery and development. Examples of oncogene-based, molecular therapeutics that show promising clinical activity include trastuzumab (Herceptin), imatinib (Gleevec), and gefitinib (Iressa). However, the full potential of oncogenes as novel targets for cancer therapy has not been realized and many challenges remain, from the validation of novel targets, to the design of specific agents, to the evaluation of these agents in both preclinical and clinical settings. In maximizing the benefits of molecular therapeutics in monotherapy or combination therapy of cancer, it is necessary to have an understanding of the underlying molecular abnormalities and mechanisms involved. This is the first part of a four-part review in which we discuss progress made in the last decade as it relates to the discovery of novel oncogenes and signal transduction pathways, in the context of their potential as targets for cancer therapy. This part delineates the latest discoveries about the potential use of growth factors and protein tyrosine kinases as targets for therapy. Later parts focus on intermediate signaling pathways, transcription factors, and proteins involved in cell cycle, DNA damage, and apoptotic pathways. Publication Types: Review

Am J Pharmacogenomics. 2005;5(3):191-5. Related Articles, Links CYP3A5 genotype is associated with diagnosis of hypertension in elderly patients: data from the DEBATE Study. Kivisto KT, Niemi M, Schaeffeler E, Pitkala K, Tilvis R, Fromm MF, Schwab M, Lang F, Eichelbaum M, Strandberg T. Dr Margarete Fischer-Bosch Institute of Clinical Pharmacology, Stuttgart, Germany. kari.kivisto@ikp-stuttgart.de OBJECTIVE: The aim of this study was to address the presently controversial question of whether cytochrome P450 (CYP) 3A5 polymorphism is associated with hypertension. METHOD: We studied 373 elderly (age > or =75 years) Finnish (Caucasian) patients from the ongoing DEBATE (Drugs and Evidence Based Medicine in the Elderly) trial. The patients were classified into those with a history of hypertension (n = 229) and those without a history of hypertension (n = 144) on the basis of a detailed questionnaire on each patient's medical history and an interview. The patients were genotyped for the CYP3A5 6986A/G single nucleotide polymorphism (SNP) [CYP3A5*1/*3 alleles]. RESULTS: The proportion of individuals with the CYP3A5*1/*3 genotype, i.e. CYP3A5 expressors, was significantly higher among patients with a diagnosis of hypertension than among patients without (18.3% vs 9.0%, p = 0.016). The corresponding odds ratio was 2.26 (95% CI 1.17, 4.38). The allele and genotype frequencies for the two control SNPs, ABCB1 (MDR1) 3435C/T and SLCO1B1 521T/C, did not differ between the two groups. CONCLUSION: This work lends support to the theory that the polymorphic CYP3A5 enzyme may be involved in regulation of blood pressure. The possible role of CYP3A5 as a genetic contributor to hypertension susceptibility warrants further study. Publication Types: Clinical Trial

Am J Pharmacogenomics. 2005;5(3):197-205. Related Articles, Links Comparison of linear weighting schemes for perfect match and mismatch gene expression levels from microarray data. Beasley TM, Holt JK, Allison DB. Section on Statistical Genetics, Department of Biostatistics, University of Alabama at Birmingham, Birmingham, Alabama 35294, USA. BACKGROUND: Data analytic approaches to Affymetrix microarray data include: (a) a covariate model, in which the observed signal is some estimated linear function of perfect match (PM) and mismatch (MM) signals; (b) a difference model [PM-MM]; and (c) a PM-only model, in which MM data is not utilized. METHODS: By decomposing the correlations among the variables in the statistical model and making certain assumptions, we theoretically derive the statistical model that reflects the actual gene expression level under a variety of conditions expected in microarray data. RESULTS AND CONCLUSION: When modeling non-systematic variation, the covariate model provides maximum flexibility and often reflects the actual gene expression levels better than the difference model. However, the PM-only model demonstrates superior power in an overwhelming majority of realistic situations, which provides theoretical support for the current trend to employ PM-only models in microarray data analyzes.

Am J Pharmacogenomics. 2005;5(5):303-15. Related Articles, Links Pharmacodiagnostic testing in breast cancer: focus on HER2 and trastuzumab therapy. Bartlett JM. Section of Surgical and Translational Research, Division of Cancer, Department of Surgery, Sciences and Molecular Pathology, Endocrine Cancer Group, Glasgow Royal Infirmary, University of Glasgow, Glasgow, Scotland. J.M.Bartlett@clinmed.gla.ac.uk Pharmacogenomics is defined as research into inherited genetic variations that determine an individual's response to therapeutic agents. In oncology, pharmacogenomics based on somatic molecular alterations inherited by subsequent cancer cell generations forms the basis of molecular targeting of novel therapeutic agents. What has emerged from clinical experience with such agents is the need for appropriate pharmacodiagnostic approaches to ensure the drugs are correctly targeted. Given the broad range of pharmacogenomic agents currently under evaluation for cancer therapy, it appears that a rapid extension of pharmacodiagnostic profiling will be required in the next 5-10 years, if not sooner. If this is to be successfully achieved, lessons learned in the past, particularly during the development of HER2 (ERBB2) testing for directing trastuzumab therapy in breast cancer, may provide a valuable framework for the development of future pharmacodiagnostic assays system. This article reviews the biological and clinical rationale for targeting breast cancer with trastuzumab and the steps taken to validate and improve pharmacodiagnostic procedures for testing tumor HER2 protein expression and HER2 gene amplification. Attention is given to quality assurance and reproducibility of testing approaches and the optimal selection of patients for response to trastuzumab. This approach serves as a paradigm for the future development of pharmacodiagnostic tests in oncology. Publication Types: Review

Am J Pharmacogenomics. 2005;5(6):345-55. Related Articles, Links The Personalized Medicine Coalition: goals and strategies. Abrahams E, Ginsburg GS, Silver M. Personalized Medicine Coalition, Washington, DC 20005, USA. eabrahams@personalizedmedicinecoalition.org The concept of personalized medicine--that medical care can be tailored to the genomic and molecular profile of the individual--has repercussions that extend far beyond the technology that makes it possible. The adoption of personalized medicine will require changes in healthcare infrastructure, diagnostics and therapeutics business models, reimbursement policy from government and private payers, and a different approach to regulatory oversight. Personalized medicine will shift medical practices upstream from the reactive treatment of disease, to proactive healthcare management including screening, early treatment, and prevention, and will alter the roles of both physician and patient. It will create a greater reliance on electronic medical records and decision support systems in an industry that has a long history of resistance to information technology. Personalized medicine requires a systems approach to implementation. But in a healthcare economy that is highly decentralized and market driven, it is incumbent upon the stakeholders themselves to advocate for a consistent set of policies and legislation that pave the way for the adoption of personalized medicine. To address this need, the Personalized Medicine Coalition (PMC) was formed as a nonprofit umbrella organization of pharmaceutical, biotechnology, diagnostic, and information technology companies, healthcare providers and payers, patient advocacy groups, industry policy organizations, major academic institutions, and government agencies. The PMC provides a structure for achieving consensus positions among these stakeholders on crucial public policy issues, a role which will be vital to translating personalized medicine into widespread clinical practice. In this article, we outline the goals of the PMC, and the strategies it will take to foster communication, debate, and consensus on issues such as genetic discrimination, the reimbursement structures for pharmacogenomic drugs and diagnostics, regulation, physician training and medical school curricula, and public education.

Am J Pharmacogenomics. 2005;5(6):365-86. Related Articles, Links Antimycotic drug discovery in the age of genomics. Cleary JD, Walker LA, Hawke RL. Department of Pharmacy Practice and Medicine, University of Mississippi, Jackson, Mississippi 39216, USA. jcleary@medicine.umsmed.edu Genomic-based methodologies are increasingly used at all stages of drug development. The most extensive applications have occurred in early drug discovery stages due to advances in technologies that allow for automated synthesis and characterization of organic compounds, and for high-throughput screening of these molecules against known drug targets. The adaptation of genomic-based methodologies in later stages of drug development presents a more difficult task. In this review we describe how genomics can be used to identify previously uncharacterized pharmacologic actions that provide a basis for the development of new classes of antimycotic agents or for adverse event aversion. Clinically, novel antimycotics are gravely needed. This review provides a perspective on new technologies that will bridge the gap between drug discovery and development that may enable more rapid access to new antimycotic agents. Publication Types: Review

Am J Psychiatry. 2004 Aug;161(8):1324-33. Related Articles, Links Gender differences in the prescribing of antipsychotic drugs. Seeman MV. Centre for Addiction and Mental Health, Department of Psychiatry, University of Toronto, 250 College St., Toronto, Ont., Canada, M5T 1R8. mary.seeman@utoronto.ca OBJECTIVE: The aim of this article is to offer recommendations and rationale for gender-specific antipsychotic treatment. METHOD: The author summarizes reviews of recent literature in psychiatric clinical trials, pharmacology, drug safety, toxicology, obstetrics and gynecology, and pediatrics. RESULTS: The pharmacokinetics and pharmacodynamics of antipsychotic drugs differ in women and men and are influenced by gender-specific factors such as body build, diet, smoking, concurrent medication, exercise, substance use, and hormonal transitions. In general, and for some drugs in particular, women require lower doses in order to stay well. Because preliminary drug testing is not done in pregnant women, the issue of effective dosing during pregnancy is unstudied, and safety for fetuses and nursing infants may not become evident until a drug is widely used. Specific adverse effects on issues crucial to women (e.g., parenting) have not been well studied, but some side effects, such as weight gain, passivity, hypotension, and hyperprolactinemia, are reported to be particularly problematic for women. Some serious side effects are more often seen among women than among men. CONCLUSIONS: Optimal maintenance regimens of antipsychotics for women and men are not the same. Publication Types: Review

Am J Psychiatry. 2004 Jul;161(7):1308-9; author reply 1309. Related Articles, Links Comment on: Am J Psychiatry. 2003 Oct;160(10):1830-5. Genetics in pharmacokinetics? Hartter S. Publication Types: Comment Letter

Am J Psychiatry. 2004 May;161(5):780-96. Related Articles, Links Pharmacogenetics of psychotropic drug response. Malhotra AK, Murphy GM Jr, Kennedy JL. Department of Psychiatry Research, Zucker Hillside Hospital, 75-59 263rd St., Glen Oaks, NY 11004, USA. malhotra@lij.edu OBJECTIVE: Molecular genetic approaches provide a novel method of dissecting the heterogeneity of psychotropic drug response. These pharmacogenetic strategies offer the prospect of identifying biological predictors of psychotropic drug response and could provide the means of determining the molecular substrates of drug efficacy and drug-induced adverse events. METHOD: The authors discuss methods issues in executing pharmacogenetic studies, review the first generation of pharmacogenetic studies of psychotropic drug response, and consider future directions for this rapidly evolving field. RESULTS: Pharmacogenetics has been most commonly used in studies of antipsychotic drug efficacy, antidepressant drug response, and drug-induced adverse effects. Data from antipsychotic drug studies indicate that polymorphisms within the serotonin 2A and dopamine receptor 2 genes may influence drug efficacy in schizophrenia. Moreover, a growing body of data suggests a relationship between the serotonin transporter gene and clinical effects of the selective serotonin reuptake inhibitors used to treat depression. A significant relationship between genetic variation in the cytochrome P450 system and drug-induced adverse effects may exist for certain medications. Finally, a number of independent studies point to a significant effect of a dopamine D(3) receptor polymorphism on susceptibility to tardive dyskinesia. CONCLUSIONS: Initial research into the pharmacogenetics of psychotropic drug response suggests that specific genes may influence phenotypes associated with psychotropic drug administration. These results remain preliminary and will require further replication and validation. New developments in molecular biology, human genomic information, statistical methods, and bioinformatics are ongoing and could pave the way for the next generation of pharmacogenetic studies in psychiatry. Publication Types: Review

Am J Psychiatry. 2004 Sep;161(9):1575-80. Related Articles, Links Prediction of antidepressant response to milnacipran by norepinephrine transporter gene polymorphisms. Yoshida K, Takahashi H, Higuchi H, Kamata M, Ito K, Sato K, Naito S, Shimizu T, Itoh K, Inoue K, Suzuki T, Nemeroff CB. Department of Psychiatry and Behavioral Sciences, Emory University School of Medicine, USA. cxw01076@nifty.com OBJECTIVE: With a multitude of antidepressants available, predictors of response to different classes of antidepressants are of considerable interest. The purpose of the present study was to determine whether norepinephrine transporter gene (NET) and serotonin transporter gene (5-HTT) polymorphisms are associated with the antidepressant response to milnacipran, a dual serotonin/norepinephrine reuptake inhibitor. METHOD: Ninety-six Japanese patients with major depressive disorder were treated with milnacipran, 50-100 mg/day, for 6 weeks. Severity of depression was assessed with the Montgomery-Asberg Depression Rating Scale. Assessments were carried out at baseline and at 1, 2, 4, and 6 weeks of treatment. The method of polymerase chain reaction was used to determine allelic variants. RESULTS: Eighty patients completed the study. The presence of the T allele of the NET T-182C polymorphism was associated with a superior antidepressant response, whereas the A/A genotype of the NET G1287A polymorphism was associated with a slower onset of therapeutic response. In contrast, no influence of 5-HTT polymorphisms on the antidepressant response to milnacipran was detected. CONCLUSIONS: The results suggest that NET but not 5-HTT polymorphisms in part determine the antidepressant response to milnacipran.

Am J Psychiatry. 2005 Aug;162(8):1423-31. Related Articles, Links Anticraving medications for relapse prevention: a possible new class of psychoactive medications. O'Brien CP. University of Pennsylvania/Philadelphia VA Medical Center, Philadelphia, PA 19104-6178, USA. obrien@mail.trc.upenn.edu Psychiatrists have gradually developed a list of medications that are effective in the treatment of addictive disorders. Although alcoholism has received the most attention, nicotine, heroin, and cocaine have all been shown to be influenced by heredity. Of course, the immediate goal is the reduction of drug craving and the prevention of relapse to compulsive drug taking. A medication that can aid in the maintenance of the opiate-free state is naltrexone, a specific opiate antagonist. Naltrexone is also a good example of an anticraving medication used in the treatment of alcoholism. Clinicians currently have two types of medication to aid in the treatment of tobacco use disorder, arguably the most important addiction. Bupropion and nicotine replacement can be given in a coordinated fashion to provide the best available results. At present, no medication is approved by the Food and Drug Administration for the indication of cocaine addiction. Recently, however, five different medications, already approved for other purposes, have been found to be effective among cocaine addicts. Despite clinical trials that show benefit, anticraving medications are not well known and are underused by clinicians. Addiction is a heterogeneous condition, with variability in reactivity to the drug of abuse and to the medications available to treat it. Recent developments in pharmacogenetics may result in improved selection of medications based on genotype. Publication Types: Review

Am J Psychiatry. 2005 Aug;162(8):1441-51. Related Articles, Links Pharmacotherapy and pharmacogenetics of nicotine dependence. Berrettini WH, Lerman CE. Center for Neurobiology and Behavior, Department of Psychiatry, University of Pennsylvania School of Medicine, Clinical Research Bldg., Room 111, 415 Curie Blvd., Philadelphia, PA 19104, USA. wadeb@mail.med.upenn.edu The authors review recent advances in the pharmacotherapy and pharmacogenetics of nicotine dependence. Despite the negative health consequences of smoking, approximately 23% of adults in the United States are daily tobacco smokers and approximately 13% are nicotine dependent.

Data for development of new medications for nicotine dependence are likely to come from animal models of the reinforcing value of nicotine, studies to identify proteins in transgenic rodents, and pharmacological studies of nicotine withdrawal. The initial pharmacogenetic studies of pharmacotherapies approved by the United States Food and Drug Administration for treatment of nicotine dependence-nicotine replacement (nicotine gum, nicotine nasal spray, and transdermal nicotine) and bupropion-have identified candidate alleles at the dopamine D2 receptor gene and mu opioid receptor gene that may predict therapeutic response. Because no one medication is likely to be safe and efficacious for a majority of persons with nicotine dependence, it will be useful to develop genetics-based methods and other tools to predict therapeutic response in subgroups of nicotine-dependent persons. Publication Types: Review

Am J Public Health. 2005 Dec;95(12):2133-8. Epub 2005 Oct 27. Related Articles, Links Racializing drug design: implications of pharmacogenomics for health disparities. Lee SS. Stanford Center for Biomedical Ethics, Stanford University, Palo Alto, CA 94304, USA. sandra.lee@stanford.edu Current practices of using "race" in pharmacogenomics research demands consideration of the ethical and social implications for understandings of group difference and for efforts to eliminate health disparities. This discussion focuses on an "infrastructure of racialization" created by current trajectories of research on genetic differences among racially identified groups, the use of race as a proxy for risk in clinical practice, and increasing interest in new market niches by the pharmaceutical industry. The confluence of these factors has resulted in the conflation of genes, disease, and race. I argue that public investment in pharmacogenomics requires careful consideration of current inequities in health status and social and ethical concerns over reifying race and issues of distributive justice.

Am J Respir Crit Care Med. 2004 Sep 15;170(6):683-90. Epub 2004 Jun 23. Related Articles, Links Future research directions in asthma: an NHLBI Working Group report. Busse W, Banks-Schlegel S, Noel P, Ortega H, Taggart V, Elias J; NHLBI Working Group. Department of Medicine, University of Wisconsin Hospital and Clinics, Madison, USA. Over the last 20 years, the prevalence of asthma has nearly doubled and now affects 8-10% of the population in the United States. Asthma also remains a major illness in terms of morbidity and suffering, and is the leading cause of hospitalizations in children under 15 years of age. Because asthma poses a lifelong burden to patients and society, efforts to increase the understanding of its pathogenesis are a key factor leading to its control and cure. Consequently, the National Heart, Lung, and Blood Institute (NHLBI) convened a Working Group of extramural experts, entitled "Future Research Directions in Asthma," on April 9-10, 2003, to identify research areas of greatest promise and opportunity in the field of asthma. The priority areas identified for research in asthma include: (1) innate immunity, adaptive immunity, and tolerance; (2) mechanisms and consequences of persistent asthma and asthma exacerbations; (3) airway remodeling: clinical consequences and reversibility (clinical relevance and resolution); (4) genetics/gene-environment interactions, pharmacogenetics; (5) intervention/prevention/therapeutics; and

(6) vascular basis of asthma. Publication Types: Consensus Development Conference Consensus Development Conference, NIH Review

Am J Respir Crit Care Med. 2005 Jul 1;172(1):12-8. Epub 2005 Mar 18. Related Articles, Links How pharmacogenomics will play a role in the management of asthma. Wechsler ME, Israel E. Pulmonary and Critical Care Division, Brigham and Women's Hospital, 75 Francis Street, Boston, MA 02115, USA. Publication Types: Review

Am J Respir Crit Care Med. 2005 Mar 15;171(6):535-6. Related Articles, Links Comment on: Am J Respir Crit Care Med. 2005 Mar 15;171(6):563-70. Pharmacogenetics and ethnicity: more complexities of personalized prescribing. Hall IP. Publication Types: Comment Editorial

Am J Transplant. 2004 Jun;4(6):843. Related Articles, Links Comment on: Am J Transplant. 2004 Jun;4(6):914-9. Pharmacogenomics and transplantation: where are we? Frassetto LA, Benet LZ. Publication Types: Comment Editorial

Am J Transplant. 2004 Jun;4(6):914-9. Related Articles, Links Comment in: Am J Transplant. 2004 Jun;4(6):843. The influence of pharmacogenetics on the time to achieve target tacrolimus concentrations after kidney transplantation. MacPhee IA, Fredericks S, Tai T, Syrris P, Carter ND, Johnston A, Goldberg L, Holt DW. Cellular and Molecular Medicine-Renal Medicine, St. George's Hospital Medical School, London, UK. imacphee@sghms.ac.uk Previously, we reported that, at 3 months after renal transplantation, individuals with CYP3AP1 genotype CYP3AP1*1 (linked to CYP3A5*1 and strongly associated with expression of CYP3A5) required twofold higher doses of tacrolimus to achieve target blood concentrations than individuals with the genotype CYP3AP1*3/*3 (CYP3A5 nonexpressors). This study assesses the relationship between concentration-controlled dosing during the early period after transplantation, the time to achieve target concentrations and genotype in 178 renal transplant recipients (CYP3AP1*1/*3 or *1/*1: n = 53, CYP3AP1*3/*3: n = 125). Patients with CYP3AP1*1/*3 or *1/*1 had lower mean tacrolimus concentrations during the first week (Median 13.5 vs. 18.5 microg/L, $p < 0.0001$) with significant delay in achieving target concentrations (15-20 microg/L during week 1, then 10-15 microg/L). More CYP3AP1*3/*3 patients had tacrolimus concentrations above target during the first week (73.6% vs. 35.8%, $p = 0.003$). There was no difference in the rate of biopsy-confirmed acute rejection, but rejection occurred earlier in the CYP3AP1*1/*3 or *1/*1 group (median 7 d vs. 13 d, $p = 0.005$). In conclusion, an initial dosing regimen for tacrolimus based on knowledge of the CYP3AP1 genotype and subsequently guided by concentration measurements has the potential to increase the proportion of patients achieving target blood concentrations early after transplantation.

Am J Vet Res. 2004 Nov;65(11):1573-9. Related Articles, Links Evaluation of haplotypes associated with copper toxicosis in Bedlington Terriers in Australia. Hyun C, Lavulo LT, Filippich LJ. School of Veterinary Science, University of Queensland, Brisbane, QLD 4072, Australia. OBJECTIVE: To evaluate the haplotype distribution associated with the copper toxicosis gene and the segregation of the mutated allele in a Bedlington Terrier population in Australia.

ANIMALS: 131 Bedlington Terriers. PROCEDURE: Samples of DNA and RNA were obtained from each dog. Genetic status of each dog was evaluated by use of the DNA markers C04107; single nucleotide polymorphism (SNP), which was adjacent to exon 2 of Murr1; and a deletion marker for exon 2. A subgroup of the study population was evaluated by use of biochemical and histologic techniques to elucidate the correlation between genotype and phenotype. RESULTS: We identified a recombination between the C04107 marker and Murr1 and a variation in a nucleotide in the splice site of exon 2 in our Bedlington Terrier cohort. Furthermore, we identified a novel haplotype associated with copper toxicosis in this cohort. CONCLUSIONS AND CLINICAL RELEVANCE: Our findings indicate that the deletion of exon 2 was not the sole cause of copper toxicosis, although only exon 2 deletion of Murr1 has been responsible for copper toxicosis in Bedlington Terriers. Although we failed to find a novel mutation in our cohort, we identified an affected dog family with an intact exon 2. Furthermore, we found that an SNP in the 5' splicing site of exon 2 may or may not be associated with a novel mutation of the Murr1 gene or other genes. Loss of linkage between the C04107 marker and the Murr1 gene was also identified in a certain family of dogs.

An Pediatr (Barc). 2006 Mar;64(3):221-3. Related Articles, Links [Pharmacogenetics in the treatment of asthma.] [Article in Spanish] Telleria Orriols J, Blanco Quiros A. Area de Pediatria de la Universidad de Valladolid. Instituto de Biologia y Genetica Molecular (IBGM). Universidad de Valladolid. CSIC. Espana.

Anal Biochem. 2005 Feb 15;337(2):256-61. Related Articles, Links Erratum in: Anal Biochem. 2005 Aug 15;343(2):359. High-throughput detection of multiple genetic polymorphisms influencing drug metabolism with mismatch primers in allele-specific polymerase chain reaction. Ishiguro A, Kubota T, Soya Y, Sasaki H, Yagyu O, Takarada Y, Iga T. Department of Pharmacy, University of Tokyo Hospital, Faculty of Medicine, Tokyo, 113-8655, Japan. Because of genetic polymorphisms of drug-metabolizing enzyme genes, the activities of the enzymes in humans vary widely and alter the metabolism of commonly used clinical agents. Severe adverse effects or resistance to therapy may result. We have developed a rapid and high-throughput genotyping method for detecting polymorphisms of the drug-metabolizing enzyme genes CYP2C9*3, CYP2C19*2, *3, CYP2D6*2, *4, *10, *14, *21, NAT2*5, *6, *7, and TPMT*3 using allele-specific polymerase chain reaction (PCR) with mismatch primers (ASPCR-MP) and CYP2D6*5, *36, and CYP2D6xN using stepdown PCR with detection by SYBR Green I. We analyzed genomic DNA from 139 Japanese volunteers. Identical genotyping results were obtained by using ASPCR-MP, stepdown PCR, and conventional PCR. We found that the methods clearly differentiate three specific profiles with no overlap in the signals. Moreover, both ASPCR-MP and stepdown PCR for genotyping took less than 3-4h. To our knowledge, this is the first report of successful simultaneous detection of multiple genetic polymorphisms with point mutations using ASPCR-MP or multiple genetic polymorphisms with large structural alterations using stepdown PCR. In conclusion, ASPCR-MP and stepdown PCR appear to be suitable for large clinical and epidemiological studies as methods that enable highly sensitive genotyping and yield a high-throughput.

Anesteziol Reanimatol. 2005 Mar-Apr;(2):4-11. Related Articles, Links [Man's metabolic passport is the basis of new strategy in pharmacology] [Article in Russian] Piruzian LA. Publication Types: Editorial

Anesthesiology. 2005 Mar;102(3):494-5. Related Articles, Links Comment on: Anesthesiology. 2005 Mar;102(3):663-71. Anesthesia and the human genome project: the quest for accurate prediction of drug responses. Allen PD. Publication Types: Comment Editorial

Anesthesiology. 2005 Mar;102(3):543-9. Related Articles, Links The impact of pharmacogenomics on postoperative nausea and vomiting: do CYP2D6 allele copy number and polymorphisms affect the success or failure of ondansetron prophylaxis? Candiotti KA, Birnbach DJ, Lubarsky DA, Nhuch F, Kamat A, Koch WH, Nikoloff M, Wu L, Andrews D. Department of Anesthesiology, Perioperative Medicine and Pain Management, University of Miami School of Medicine, Florida 33101, USA. kcandiotti@miami.edu BACKGROUND: Some patients treated with ondansetron for postoperative nausea and vomiting do not respond to therapy. One possible mechanism for this failure is ultrarapid drug metabolism via the cytochrome P-450 system, specifically the enzyme 2D6 (CYP2D6). Ultrarapid metabolism is seen in patients with multiple functional copies (>/= 3) of the CYP2D6 allele. This study was designed to determine whether patients who were given prophylactic ondansetron and had multiple CYP2D6 alleles had an increased rate of postoperative nausea and vomiting. METHODS: Two hundred fifty female patients undergoing standardized general anesthesia were given 4 mg ondansetron 30 min before extubation. Patients were observed for symptoms of nausea and vomiting. DNA was extracted from blood in all patients and was analyzed by using a gene-specific probe to determine the CYP2D6 gene copy number and genotyped by polymerase chain reaction amplification with a custom oligonucleotide microarray to determine the specific CYP2D6 genotypes. RESULTS: Eighty-eight patients experienced nausea, and 37 of those patients also had vomiting. In patients with one, two, or three CYP2D6 copies, the incidences of vomiting were 3 in 33 (27%), 27 in 198 (14%), and 7 in 23 (30%), respectively. The incidence of vomiting in subjects with three CYP2D6 copies was significantly different from those with two copies, but not from those with one copy. When analyzed by genotype, the incidences of vomiting in poor, intermediate, extensive, and ultrarapid metabolizers were 1 in 12 (8%), 5 in 30 (17%), 26 in 176 (15%), and 5 in 11 (45%), respectively ($P < 0.01$ vs. all other groups). There were no differences between groups in the incidence of nausea based on CYP2D6 copy number or genotype. CONCLUSIONS: Patients with three copies of the CYP2D6 gene, a genotype consistent with ultrarapid metabolism, or both have an increased incidence of ondansetron failure for the prevention of postoperative vomiting but not nausea.

Anesthesiology. 2005 Mar;102(3):550-6. Related Articles, Links Pharmacogenetic determinants of human liver microsomal alfentanil metabolism and the role of cytochrome P450 3A5. Klees TM, Sheffels P, Thummel KE, Kharasch ED. Norwegian University of Science and Technology, Trondheim, Norway. BACKGROUND: There is considerable unexplained interindividual variability in the clearance of alfentanil. Alfentanil undergoes extensive metabolism by cytochrome P4503A4 (CYP3A4). CYP3A5 is structurally similar to CYP3A4 and metabolizes most CYP3A4 substrates but is polymorphically expressed. Livers with the CYP3A5*1 allele contain higher amounts of the native CYP3A5 protein than livers homozygous for the mutant CYP3A5*3 allele. This investigation tested the hypothesis that alfentanil is a substrate for CYP3A5 and that CYP3A5 pharmacogenetic variability influences human liver alfentanil metabolism. METHODS: Alfentanil metabolism to noralfentanil and N-phenylpropionamide was determined in microsomes from two groups of human livers, characterized for CYP3A4 and CYP3A5 protein content: low CYP3A5 (2.0-5.2% of total CYP3A, n = 10) and high CYP3A5 (46-76% of total CYP3A, n = 10). Mean CYP3A4 content was the same in both groups. The effects of the CYP3A inhibitors troleandomycin and ketoconazole, the latter being more potent toward CYP3A4, on alfentanil metabolism were also determined. RESULTS: In the low versus high CYP3A5 livers, respectively, noralfentanil formation was 77 +/- 31 versus 255 +/- 170 pmol . min . mg, N-phenylpropionamide formation was 8.0 +/- 3.1 versus 20.5 +/- 14.0 pmol . min . mg, and the metabolite ratio was 9.5 +/- 0.4 versus 12.7 +/- 1.4 ($P < 0.05$ for all). There was a poor correlation between alfentanil metabolism and CYP3A4 content but an excellent correlation when CYP3A5 (i.e., total CYP3A content) was considered ($r = 0.81$, $P < 0.0001$). Troleandomycin inhibited alfentanil metabolism similarly in the low and high CYP3A5 livers; ketoconazole inhibition was less in the high CYP3A5 livers. CONCLUSION: In microsomes from human livers expressing the CYP3A5*1 allele and containing higher amounts of CYP3A5 protein, compared with those with the CYP3A5*3 allele and little CYP3A5, there was greater alfentanil metabolism, metabolite ratios more closely resembled those for expressed CYP3A5, and inhibitors with differing CYP3A4 and CYP3A5 selectivities had effects resembling those for expressed CYP3A5. Therefore, alfentanil is metabolized by human liver microsomal CYP3A5 in addition to CYP3A4, and pharmacogenetic variability in CYP3A5 expression significantly influences human liver alfentanil metabolism in vitro. Further investigation is warranted to assess whether the CYP3A5 polymorphism is a factor in the interindividual variability of alfentanil metabolism and clearance in vivo.

Anesthesiology. 2005 Mar;102(3):663-71. Related Articles, Links Comment in: Anesthesiology. 2005 Mar;102(3):494-5. Anesthesiology. 2005 Nov;103(5):1099; author reply 1101. Anesthesiology. 2005 Nov;103(5):1100; author reply 1101. Pharmacogenetics of anesthetic and analgesic agents. Palmer SN, Giesecke NM, Body SC, Shernan SK, Fox AA, Collard CD. Department of Cardiovascular Anesthesia, Texas Heart Institute, St. Luke's Episcopal Hospital, Houston 77030, USA. Predicting a patient's response to a particular drug has long been a goal of clinicians. Rapid advances in molecular biology have enabled researchers to identify associations between an individual's genetic profile and drug response. Pharmacogenetics is the study of the molecular mechanisms that underlie individual differences in drug metabolism, efficacy, and side effects. The pharmacogenetics of commonly used anesthetic and analgesic agents are reviewed. Publication Types: Review

Anesthesiology. 2005 Nov;103(5):1099; author reply 1101. Related Articles, Links Comment on: Anesthesiology. 2005 Mar;102(3):663-71. Pharmacogenetics of anesthetic and analgesic agents: CYP2D6 genetic variations. Stamer UM, Stuber F. Publication Types: Comment Letter

Anesthesiology. 2005 Nov;103(5):1100; author reply 1101. Related Articles, Links Comment on: Anesthesiology. 2005 Mar;102(3):663-71. The practicality and need for genetic testing for malignant hyperthermia. Brandom BW, Muldoon SM. Publication Types: Comment Letter

Ann Biol Clin (Paris). 2004 Sep-Oct;62(5):499-511. Related Articles, Links [Pharmacogenetics or the promise of a personalized medicine: variability in drug metabolism and transport] [Article in French] Allorge D, Loriot MA. Laboratoire de biochimie et de biologie moleculaire, Hopital Calmette, CHRU de Lille et EA2679, Faculte de medecine / pole recherche, Lille. dallorge@univ-lille2.fr There is much variability in the manner individuals respond to drugs, such that the management of some drugs is problematic. In France, the incidence of hospital admissions related to adverse drug reactions is estimated to be 3.2 %, at an annual cost of over 300 millions euros. Genetic factors affecting the pharmacokinetics and pharmacodynamics of drugs partly explain interindividual variability in drug response. Pharmacogenetic focuses on the molecular mechanisms involved in drug response, and its ultimate goal is the optimisation of drug treatments, both in terms of efficacy and safety. Numerous polymorphisms in genes encoding drug-metabolising enzymes, transporters and receptors have been described and their consequences on disposition and effect of a substantial number of medications have been elucidated. This review focuses on variability of drug metabolism and transport to define the objectives of pharmacogenetics, the molecular bases of interindividual variation in drug response and the methods used for the evaluation of the individual risk of drug failure or toxicity. Some clinical applications of pharmacogenetics have already been developed in routine medicine resulting in significant improvement in patient treatment. The clinical validation of an increasing number of pharmacogenetic tests, as well as the development of new highly efficient technologies for genotyping (real-time PCR, DNA chips) should further promote pharmacogenetics in clinical practice and lead to the development of a patient-tailored drug therapy. Publication Types: Review

Ann Clin Biochem. 2004 Jul;41(Pt 4):260-2. Related Articles, Links Comment on: Ann Clin Biochem. 2004 Jul;41(Pt 4):294-302. Ann Clin Biochem. 2004 Jul;41(Pt 4):303-8. The drugs don't work: pharmacogenomics--clinical biochemistry's future? Hallworth MJ. Department of Clinical Biochemistry, Royal Shrewsbury Hospital, Mytton Oak Road, Shrewsbury SY3 8XQ, UK. Publication Types: Comment

Ann Clin Biochem. 2004 Jul;41(Pt 4):294-302. Related Articles, Links Comment in: Ann Clin Biochem. 2004 Jul;41(Pt 4):260-2. Thiopurine methyltransferase: should it be measured before commencing thiopurine drug therapy? Sanderson J, Ansari A, Marinaki T, Duley J. Departments of Purine Research and Gastroenterology, Guy's and St Thomas' Hospitals, London SE1 7EH, UK. jeremy.sanderson@gstt.sthames.nhs.uk Thiopurines [azathioprine (AZA), 6-

mercaptopurine (6-MP) and thioguanine (6-TG)] have a well-established role as immunosuppressive agents in a variety of chronic inflammatory conditions, haematological neoplasia and in transplant rejection. Despite good overall clinical response rates, particularly when used as steroid sparing agents, adverse effects are a limiting problem leading to withdrawal in up to a quarter of patients. Severe myelosuppression is the most serious toxicity occurring early or occasionally later during treatment. An understanding of the competing pathways involved in the metabolism of thiopurines has important implications for predicting some of the more severe toxicity seen with these drugs. Thiopurine methyl transferase (TPMT) is an enzyme catalysing the methylation of 6-MP, competing with xanthine oxidase (XO) and hypoxanthine guanine phosphoribosyl transferase (HGPRT) to determine the amount of 6-MP metabolised to cytotoxic thioguanine nucleotides. Allelic polymorphisms in the TPMT gene predict the activity of the enzyme such that 1 in 10 of the population are heterozygous and have approximately 50% of normal activity, whilst 1 in 300 are completely deficient. As a result, these individuals are at high risk of severe myelosuppression. Conversely, individuals with very high levels of TPMT activity are hyper-methylators in whom clinical response is less likely. Prior knowledge of TPMT status avoids exposure of individuals with zero TPMT to potentially fatal treatment with AZA or 6-MP and provides one of the best examples of predictive pharmacogenetics in therapeutics. This article reviews literature on the role of TPMT measurement prior to treatment with thiopurines and provides some guidance to the use of TPMT as a guide to tailoring thiopurine therapy. Publication Types: Review

Ann Fr Anesth Reanim. 2003 Dec;22 Spec No 1:48-52. Related Articles, Links [Can genetics guide or modify the management of severe sepsis?] [Article in French] Mira JP, Charpentier J. Service de reanimation medicale, CHU Cochin Port-Royal, 27, rue du Faubourg-Saint-Jacques, 75679 Paris cedex 14, France. Publication Types: Review

Ann Hum Biol. 2005 Sep-Oct;32(5):574-84. Related Articles, Links Indian ethnic populations characterized by dopamine (D4) receptor VNTR polymorphism. Ghosh A, Seshadri M. Low Level Radiation Studies Section, Biosciences Group, Bhabha Atomic Research Centre, Trombay, Mumbai 400 085, India. anugh@magnum.barc.ernet.in BACKGROUND: The human dopamine receptor D4 gene (DRD4) contains a 48-bp tandem repeat in exon 3 and shows alleles varying between repeats 2 and 11. The gene shows a high level of expression in the prefrontal cortex of the brain and association of particular alleles of this locus with various neuropsychiatric and personality disorders have been reported. OBJECTIVE: The present study reports allele frequency distribution at the DRD4 variable number tandem repeat (VNTR) locus among five ethnic populations of India. This background information is fundamental to the field of pharmacogenetics for disease susceptibility and association studies. SUBJECTS AND METHODS: Three hundred and thirty two healthy unrelated adult individuals belonging to five ethnic groups: Konkanastha Brahmins, Marathas, Ezhavas, Nairs and Muslims, have been typed. Genomic DNA, extracted from peripheral blood, was PCR amplified using a two-enzyme system. The use of ALF Express DNA sequencer was found to be helpful for large-scale population genotyping. Statistical analysis was performed using the POPGENE and DISPAN programs. RESULTS: A total of eight alleles ranging from repeat 2 to repeat 9 were observed. Allele 4 was the predominant allele among all the five populations, consistent with the data on other world populations. A rare allele 9 was detected exclusively among Marathas. The observed heterozygosity was low, ranging from 0.38 to 0.54 while other parameters like Polymorphism Information Content (PIC) and Power of Discrimination (PD) showed moderate values. The populations were in genetic equilibrium when tested under Hardy-Weinberg expectations. CONCLUSION: The allele frequency estimates for DRD4 provided here will contribute towards developing an informative database for this functionally relevant locus. This will prove useful when studying the association between genetic factors and pathogenesis of disease in Indian populations and will address the concern of biased results of association due to population admixtures.

Ann Hum Genet. 2004 Nov;68(Pt 6):563-73. Related Articles, Links Erratum in: Ann Hum Genet. 2005 Jul;69(Pt 4):499. Linkage disequilibrium and haplotype architecture for two ABC transporter genes (ABCC1 and ABCG2) in Chinese population: implications for pharmacogenomic association studies. Wang H, Hao B, Zhou K, Chen X, Wu S, Zhou G, Zhu Y, He F. Laboratory of Systems Biology, Beijing Institute of Radiation Medicine, Beijing 100850 PR China. Information about linkage disequilibrium (LD) patterns and haplotype structures for candidate genes is instructive for the design and analysis of genetic association studies for complex diseases and drug response. ABCC1 and ABCG2 are genes coding for two multidrug resistance (MDR) associated transporters; they are also related to some pathophysiological traits. To pinpoint the LD profiles of these MDR genes in Chinese, we systemically screened 27 unrelated individuals for single nucleotide polymorphisms (SNPs) in the coding and regulatory regions of these genes, and thereby characterized their haplotype structures. Despite marked variations in haplotype diversity, LD pattern and intragenic recombination intensity between the two genes, both loci could be partitioned into several LD blocks, in which a modest number of haplotypes accounted for a high fraction of the sampled chromosomes. We concluded that each locus has its own genomic LD profile, but that they still share a common segmental LD architecture with low haplotype diversity. Our data will benefit genetic association studies of complex traits and drug response possibly related to these genes.

Ann Oncol. 2004;15 Suppl 4:iv173-7. Related Articles, Links Pharmacogenomics and colorectal cancer. Lenz HJ. Division of Medical Oncology, University of Southern California/Norris Comprehensive Cancer Center, Keck School of Medicine, Los Angeles, USA. Publication Types: Review

Ann Oncol. 2005;16 Suppl 2:ii240-5. Related Articles, Links State of the art in mesothelioma. Scagliotti GV, Novello S. University of Turin, Department of Clinical and Biological Sciences, S. Luigi Hospital, Orbassano (Torino), Italy. Publication Types: Review

Ann Pathol. 2003 Dec;23(6):623-32. Related Articles, Links [Small but high throughput: how "tissue-microarrays" became a favorite tool for pathologists and scientists] [Article in French] Jacquemier J, Ginestier C, Charafe-Jauffret E, Bertucci F, Bege T,

Geneix J, Birnbaum D. Departement d'Oncologie Moleculaire, Institut Paoli-Calmettes, 232 Bd de Sainte Marguerite, 13273 Marseille Cedex 9, France. jacquemierj@marseille.Fnclcc.fr Progress in the knowledge of molecular genetics and availability of high-throughput technologies offer the opportunity to identify new diagnostic and prognostic markers and new therapeutic targets in human cancer. The recently developed "tIssue microarrays" (TMA) technology allows parallel molecular profiling of clinical samples. Using this technique and immunohistochemistry (IHC), fluorescence in situ hybridisation (FISH), or RNA in situ hybridisation (ISH), the pathologist is now able to perform unprecedented large-scale analyses. The advantages are significant: large number of cases assessed simultaneously for numerous markers, processed in identical conditions, from reduced amount of archival tIssues, with an excellent correlation with standard methods, and a reduction in cost and time. This Article provides a short review of this technology, and points out several aspects of the TMA construction and its applications for clinical research.

Ann Pharm Fr. 2005 Mar;63(2):114-6. Related Articles, Links [New tools for preclinical pharmaceutic research] [Article in French] Tartar A. Faculte de pharmacie de Lille, rue du Professeur Laguesse, F59045 Lille Cedex. Despite constantly growing expenditures for pharmaceutical research, which have double in the last ten years, the number of new drugs marketed in the world has continued to decline. The last decade has nevertheless seen a series of major methodological advances in the fields including pharmacogenomics, pharamcogenetics, high-flow screening, and structural biology, all considered to contribute to the discovery of "drugs of the future". Systemic screening of compound banks has become the starting point for nearly all drug research. It is nevertheless only the first step towards a drug (typically lasting a few months compared with ten years before the final drug is marketed). For a compound to passe from a leading screening compound to a marketed drug, its often contradictory properties (solubility, permeability, duration of action, activity, selectivity, absence of toxicity) must undergo a long multidimensional optimization process. The development of easily interpreted low-cost in vitro tests allow prediction of these properties without animal experimentation, greatly facilitating the multidisciplinary process. Publication Types: Congresses

Ann Pharmacother. 2006 Mar 6; [Epub ahead of print] Related Articles, Links Discordance Between Availability of Pharmacogenetics Studies and Pharmacogenetics-Based Prescribing Information for the Top 200 Drugs (April). Zineh I, Pebanco GD, Aquilante CL, Gerhard T, Beitelshees AL, Beasley BN, Hartzema AG. College of Pharmacy, Department of Pharmacy Practice and Center for Pharmacogenomics, University of Florida, Gainesville, FL. BACKGROUND: Despite growing numbers of pharmacogenetics studies, little pharmacogenetics-based prescribing information is available to practitioners. It is possible that the lack of prescribing data for commonly used drugs is due to a paucity of evidence-based pharmacogenetics literature for these agents. OBJECTIVE: To investigate the relationship between pharmacogenetics prescribing data in drug package inserts (PIs) and pharmacogenetics research literature for agents represented in the top 200 prescribed drugs for 2003. METHODS: A PubMed search (to August

7, 2004) was performed to identify pharmacogenetics studies relevant to the top 200 drugs. These data were compared with PIs for drugs in the top 200 list that contained pharmacogenetics prescribing information. RESULTS: Pharmacogenetics data in the literature were available for 71.3% of the top 200 drugs. The gene involved coded for a drug-metabolizing enzyme in 34.5% of the literature sampled. The remaining 65.5% of the pharmacogenetics studies contained information largely related to genetic variability in target proteins and drug transporters. Three drugs with PIs containing pharmacogenetics prescribing information deemed to be useful to guide therapy were in the top 200 list (celecoxib, fluoxetine, pantoprazole). There was no consensus on the strength of association between genetic variability and drug response for these agents. CONCLUSIONS: The lack of specific pharmacogenetics-based prescribing information in PIs for commonly used drugs does not seem to be related to a paucity of pharmacogenetics data in the research literature. Rather, other factors including, but not limited to, the uncertain clinical relevance of genetic associations may make practical prescribing recommendations difficult. y publisher]

Ann Rheum Dis. 2004 Nov;63 Suppl 2:ii25-ii27. Related Articles, Links Pharmacogenetics in the rheumatic diseases. Cronstein BN. New York University School of Medicine, 550 First Ave., New York, NY 10016, USA. cronsb01@med.nyu.edu Publication Types: Review

Ann Rheum Dis. 2005 May;64(5):793-4. Related Articles, Links Polymorphism at position -308 of the tumour necrosis factor alpha gene and rheumatoid arthritis pharmacogenetics. Fonseca JE, Carvalho T, Cruz M, Nero P, Sobral M, Mourao AF, Cavaleiro J, Ligeiro D, Abreu I, Carmo-Fonseca M, Branco JC. Publication Types: Letter

Annu Rev Genomics Hum Genet. 2004;5:1-14. Related Articles, Links Genetic testing in primary care. Burke W. Department of Medical History and Ethics, University of Washington , Seattle, Washington 98195-7120, USA. wburke@u.washington.edu Rapid advances in genetic research are leading to an expanding array of genetic tests. Primary care providers will increasingly be challenged to identify patients whose symptoms, physical findings, or family history indicate the need for genetic testing, and to determine how to use genetic information most effectively to improve disease prevention. In addressing these challenges, practitioners will need to consider the range of different uses of genetic testing, including diagnosis in symptomatic and asymptomatic people, risk assessment, reproductive decision-making, and population screening. They will need a set of core skills and knowledge to evaluate family history and to recognize clinical findings that indicate genetic risk. At the same time, the primary care perspective will contribute to the evaluation of appropriate uses of genetic testing. A partnership between medical genetics and primary care will help to ensure the development of effective policies, educational tools, and practice guidelines for the coming era of genomic health care. Publication Types: Review

Annu Rev Med. 2006;57:119-37. Related Articles, Links Pharmacogenomics and individualized drug therapy. Eichelbaum M, Ingelman-Sundberg M, Evans WE. Dr. Margarete Fischer-Bosch-Institute of

Clinical Pharmacology, Auerbachstr. 112, D-70376 Stuttgart, Germany. michel.eichelbaum@ikp-stuttgart.de Pharmacogenetics deals with inherited differences in the response to drugs. The best-recognized examples are genetic polymorphisms of drug-metabolizing enzymes, which affect about 30% of all drugs. Loss of function of thiopurine S-methyltransferase (TPMT) results in severe and life-threatening hematopoietic toxicity if patients receive standard doses of mercaptopurine and azathioprine. Gene duplication of cytochrome P4502D6 (CYP2D6), which metabolizes many antidepressants, has been identified as a mechanism of poor response in the treatment of depression. There is also a growing list of genetic polymorphisms in drug targets that have been shown to influence drug response. A major limitation that has heretofore moderated the use of pharmacogenetic testing in the clinical setting is the lack of prospective clinical trials demonstrating that such testing can improve the benefit/risk ratio of drug therapy.

Annu Rev Pharmacol Toxicol. 2005;45:477-94. Related Articles, Links Clinical and toxicological relevance of CYP2C9: drug-drug interactions and pharmacogenetics. Rettie AE, Jones JP. Department of Medicinal Chemistry, University of Washington, Seattle, Washington 98195, USA. rettie@u.washington.edu CYP2C9 is a major cytochrome P450 enzyme that is involved in the metabolic clearance of a wide variety of therapeutic agents, including nonsteroidal antiinflammatories, oral anticoagulants, and oral hypoglycemics. Disruption of CYP2C9 activity by metabolic inhibition or pharmacogenetic variability underlies many of the adverse drug reactions that are associated with the enzyme. CYP2C9 is also the first human P450 to be crystallized, and the structural basis for its substrate and inhibitor selectivity is becoming increasingly clear. New, ultrapotent inhibitors of CYP2C9 have been synthesised that aid in the development of quantitative structure-activity relationship (QSAR) models to facilitate drug redesign, and extensive resequencing of the gene and studies of its regulation will undoubtedly help us understand interindividual variability in drug response and toxicity controlled by this enzyme. Publication Types: Review

Annu Rev Pharmacol Toxicol. 2006;46:317-53. Related Articles, Links Pharmacogenomics of acute leukemia. Cheok MH, Lugthart S, Evans WE. St. Jude Children's Research Hospital, Department of Pharmaceutical Sciences, Memphis, TN 38105, USA. meyling.cheok@stjude.org Over the past four decades, treatment of acute leukemia in children has made remarkable progress, from this disease being lethal to now achieving cure rates of 80% for acute lymphoblastic leukemia and 45% for acute myeloid leukemia. This progress is largely owed to the optimization of existing treatment modalities rather than the discovery of new agents. However, the annual number of patients with leukemia who experience relapse after initial therapy remains greater than that of new cases of most childhood cancers. The aim of pharmacogenetics is to develop strategies to personalize medications and tailor treatment regimens to individual patients, with the goal of enhancing efficacy and safety through better understanding of the person's genetic makeup. In this review, we summarize recent pharmacogenomic studies related to the treatment of pediatric acute leukemia. These include work using candidate-gene approaches, as well as genome-wide studies using haplotype mapping and gene expression profiling. These strategies illustrate the promise of pharmacogenomics to further advance the treatment of human cancers, with childhood leukemia serving as a paradigm.

Anticancer Drugs. 2005 Oct;16(9):923-33. Related Articles, Links Genetic determinants of cancer drug efficacy and toxicity: practical considerations and perspectives. Candelaria M, Taja-Chayeb L, Arce-Salinas C, Vidal-Millan S, Serrano-Olvera A, Duenas-Gonzalez A. Division of Clinical Research, Instituto Nacional de Cancerologia, UNAM, Tlalpan, Mexico. myrnac@prodigy.net.mx Drug-metabolizing enzymes are responsible for the activation or detoxification of cytotoxic drugs. Allelic variants are present with a variable frequency in different populations around the world and have an important role in the therapeutic index of such drugs. It is known that polymorphisms in thiopurine methyltransferase and dihydropyrimidine dehydrogenase have been associated with altered drug metabolism and increased risk of severe toxicity from 6-mercaptopurine and 5-fluorouracil, respectively. Additionally, a variant number of dinucleotide-repeat sequences in the promotor for uridine 5'-diphosphate glucuronosyltransferase 1A1 influences the glucuronidation of SN-38, the active metabolite of irinotecan, which is associated with severe toxicity, including diarrhea and neutropenia. In the same way, polymorphisms in thymidylate synthase have been associated with pyrimidine-associated toxicity and also with response to chemotherapy. The examples shown in this review demonstrate the usefulness of pre-screening patients for well-characterized polymorphism to identify the best-tolerated and most-effective treatment. Publication Types: Review

Arch Dis Child. 2004 Jul;89(7):598-603. Related Articles, Links Unravelling the complex genetics of inflammatory bowel disease. Russell RK, Wilson DC, Satsangi J. Gastrointestinal Unit, University of Edinburgh, Department of Medical Sciences, Edinburgh, UK . richardkrussell71@hotmail.com The rapid pace of progress in molecular genetics over the past 15 years--since the seminal description of the polymerase chain reaction--has led to the identification of the genes involved in many single gene disorders. These successes in the laboratory have already led directly to clinical applications in diagnosis, pharmacogenetics, and the development of new therapies. Progress in unravelling the genetics of complex diseases has been less straightforward. However, real excitement has followed the identification of the NOD 2/CARD 15 gene as an important determinant of susceptibility to Crohn's disease.(1,)(2) Not only has this finding provided a proof of principle for the technique of genome-wide scanning in complex disorders, but the discovery also has given real insight into the primary pathophysiology involved in chronic inflammatory bowel disease. The background to this discovery and its implications form the basis for the present article. Publication Types: Review

Arch Dis Child. 2005 Jun;90(6):551-3. Related Articles, Links Comment on: Arch Dis Child. 2005 Jun;90(6):614-8. Isoniazid treatment of children: can genetics help guide treatment? Cranswick N, Mulholland K. Royal Children's Hospital and Murdoch Children's Research Institute, University of Melbourne, Australia. Publication Types: Comment Review

Arch Gen Psychiatry. 2004 Nov;61(11):1163-9. Related Articles, Links Effects of the serotonin transporter gene promoter polymorphism on mirtazapine and paroxetine efficacy and adverse events in geriatric major depression. Murphy GM Jr, Hollander SB, Rodrigues HE, Kremer C, Schatzberg AF. Neuroscience Research Laboratories, Department of Psychiatry and Behavioral Sciences, Stanford University School of Medicine, Stanford, Calif, USA. BACKGROUND: The "long/short"polymorphism (5HTTLPR) in the promoter of the serotonin transporter gene (SLC6A4) has been proposed as a pharmacogenetic marker for antidepressant efficacy. Some but not all studies have found that the short form of 5HTTLPR (S allele) results in decreased efficacy of selective serotonin reuptake inhibitors. OBJECTIVE: To determine if the 5HTTLPR polymorphism influences the efficacy and tolerability of mirtazapine and paroxetine hydrochloride, 2 frequently prescribed antidepressants with differing pharmacologic profiles, in geriatric depression. DESIGN: Double-blind, randomized 8-week study. SETTING: Eighteen academic and private outpatient clinics. PATIENTS: We evaluated 246 cognitively intact patients 65 years or older with major depression. INTERVENTIONS: Antidepressant therapy with 15 to 45 mg/d of mirtazapine (n = 124) or 20 to 40 mg/d of paroxetine (n = 122). MAIN OUTCOME MEASURES: The Hamilton Depression Rating Scale-17 and Geriatric Depression Scale, severity of adverse events and dosing compliance indexes, and discontinuations due to adverse events. Outcome measures were stratified according to 5HTTLPR genotypes. RESULTS: Geriatric Depression Scale scores indicated that S allele carriers treated with paroxetine showed a small impairment in antidepressant response. Among mirtazapine-treated patients, there was little indication that the 5HTTLPR genotype affected antidepressant efficacy. However, the 5HTTLPR polymorphism had a dramatic effect on adverse events. Among paroxetine-treated subjects, S allele carriers experienced more severe adverse events during the course of the study, achieved significantly lower final daily doses, and had more discontinuations at days 14, 21, 28, 42, and 49. Surprisingly, among mirtazapine-treated subjects, S allele carriers had fewer discontinuations due to adverse events, experienced less severe adverse events, and achieved higher final daily doses. CONCLUSIONS: These results support the hypothesis that the S allele of 5HTTLPR at the SLC6A4 locus is associated with a poor outcome after treatment with selective serotonin reuptake inhibitors. However, the major effect was on the tolerability of these drugs rather than efficacy. Results from mirtazapine-treated patients indicate that the effect of this polymorphism on outcome may depend on the mechanism of antidepressant action. Publication Types: Clinical Trial Randomized Controlled Trial

Arch Intern Med. 2005 Nov 14;165(20):2331-6. Related Articles, Links Implications of pharmacogenomics for drug development and clinical practice. Ginsburg GS, Konstance RP, Allsbrook JS, Schulman KA. Department of Medicine, School of Medicine, Center for Genomic Medicine, Institute for Genome Sciences and Policy, Duke University, Durham, NC, USA. Pharmacogenomics is likely to be among the first clinical applications of the Human Genome Project and is certain to have an enormous impact on the clinical practice of medicine. Herein, we discuss the potential implications of pharmacogenomics on the drug development process, including drug safety, productivity, market segmentation, market expansion, differentiation, and personalized health care. We also review 3 challenges facing the translation of pharmacogenomics into clinical practice: dependence on information technology, limited health care financing, and the scientific uncertainty surrounding validation of specific applications of the technology. To our knowledge, there is currently no formal agenda to promote and cultivate innovation, to develop progressive information technology, or to obtain the financing that would be required to advance the use of pharmacogenomic technologies in patient care. Although the potential of these technologies is driving change in the development of clinical sciences, it remains to be seen which health care systems level needs will be addressed. Publication Types: Review

Arch Mal Coeur Vaiss. 2006 Jan;99 Spec No 1(1):23-8. Related Articles, Links [The best of thrombosis in 2005] [Article in French] Helft G. Institut de cardiologie, Groupe hospitalier La Pitie-Salpetriere, 47, boulevard de l'Hopital, 75651 Paris. gerard.helft@psl.ap-hop-paris.fr The year 2005 was rich in new information. Many articles were published on antithrombotic therapy, the key stone in the management of several cardiovascular diseases which are the cardiologists' "daily bread". Antithrombotic treatment is essential in the treatment of patients undergoing interventional coronary procedures. The loading dose of 300 mg clopidogrel has been questioned. The ARMYDA-2 trial showed that a loading dose of 600 mg of clopidogrel administered 4 to 8 hours before coronary angioplasty significantly reduced the number of peri-procedural myocardial infarctions without increasing the risk of bleeding complications. Other molecules such as prasugrel could provide an alternative to treatment with clopidogrel. The results of a phase 2 trial (JUMBO-TIMI 26) comparing clopidogrel and prasugrel have opened the way for a large scale phase 3 trial which is currently under way. In myocardial infarction, the CLARITY-TIMI 28 trial showed that patients under 75 years of age with acute myocardial infarction of less than 12 hours duration treated with aspirin and thrombolytic therapy had better results with respect to the combined criteria of patency of the culprit artery and ischaemic complications with the addition of clopidogrel. In the CREATE trial, patients with acute myocardial infarction had a lower mortality and recurrence of infarction without significantly increasing the risk of stroke with reviparin. The development of ximelagatran has been held up by a potentially serious hepato-toxicity. Two large-scale trials were published this year, one in atrial fibrillation and the other in venous thrombosis. In the former, the hypothesis of non-inferiority compared with well conducted oral anticoagulation with coumadine was supported and, in the latter, the hypothesis of non-inferiority compared with treatment with enoxaparin followed by warfarin was also confirmed despite a higher number of coronary events in the xinelagatran group. Another study which merits a citation showed that in patients with a previous history of aspirin-induced bleeding ulcers, the association of low dose aspirin and a proton pump inhibitor was superior to the prescription of clopidogrel in the prevention of recurrent bleeding. A study of the pharmacogenetics of coumadine and the variability of its dosage was also a valuable contribution. In the field of management of bleeding, a study demonstrated the potential benefits of treatment with VIIa recombinant factor.

Arch Pathol Lab Med. 2004 Dec;128(12):1330-3. Related Articles, Links Adding pharmacogenetics to the clinical laboratory: narrow therapeutic index medications as a place to start. Bukaveckas BL. Publication Types: Editorial

Arch Pathol Lab Med. 2004 Dec;128(12):1360-3. Related Articles, Links Effect of polymorphisms in the cytochrome P450 CYP2C9 gene on warfarin anticoagulation. Adcock DM, Koftan C, Crisan D, Kiechle FL. Esoterix Coagulation, Aurora, Colo 80014, USA. dot.adcock@esoterix.com CONTEXT: Warfarin is a widely used anticoagulant with efficacy in treatment and prevention of thrombosis. Patient management, however, is difficult because of interindividual variation in response to standard doses due to significant differences in metabolic rates. Warfarin metabolism is under genetic control, involving primarily the CYP2C9 gene encoding the enzyme that catalyzes the conversion of warfarin to inactive metabolites. OBJECTIVE: Several polymorphisms of CYP2C9 have been reported; the variant alleles *2 and *3 have decreased enzymatic activity. The objective of this case study is to investigate the relationship between CYP2C9 genotype and warfarin anticoagulation. DESIGN: A case of deep vein thrombosis treated with the standard warfarin dose is investigated for intensity of anticoagulation and CYP2C9 genotype; the case illustrates the relationship between CYP2C9 variant and overanticoagulation with subsequent bleeding complication. RESULTS: The patient's genotype, CYP2C9*1*3, correlated with an exaggerated anticoagulant response during the initiation of warfarin therapy at standard dose, and a bleeding episode ensued. Based on heterozygosity for the *3 variant allele, it was recommended that the patient be maintained on a low-dose warfarin regimen. CONCLUSIONS: The practical implications of identifying genetic risk factors that lead to overanticoagulation are multiple. Genotype knowledge of the CYP2C9 variant alleles may help the clinician to individualize warfarin therapy with the ultimate goals of shortening the initial period of induction therapy, reaching a stable maintenance dose earlier, and minimizing bleeding complications in patients who are high responders and need lower warfarin doses.

Arch Pediatr. 2004 May;11(5):489-92. Related Articles, Links [Cutaneous drug reactions: pharmacogenetic news] [Article in French] Buffard V, Roujeau JC. Service de dermatologie, hopital Henri-Mondor, Creteil, France. valerie.buffard@hmn.ap-hop-paris.fr Identifying genetic factors in severe drug eruption should improve efficacy and safety of drug prescription. The first pharmacogenetic studies concerned the polymorphism of genes encoding drug metabolism enzymes (especially for sulfamides reactions in AIDS and anticonvulsants reactions). Recent studies did not confirm the role of genotypic variation in metabolism enzymes in drug reaction. Genes controlling immune response are another research issue. Certain MHC phenotypes are linked to a higher risk of toxidermy, such as in abacavir hypersensitivity or fixed drug eruption. Indeed, severe drug eruptions seem to be linked to a specific immune response controlled by T lymphocytes. Publication Types: Review

Arerugi. 2004 Oct;53(10):1062-5. Related Articles, Links [Personalized medicine: current status] [Article in Japanese] Tsujimoto G. Department of Genomic Drug Discovery Science, Graduate School of Pharmaceutical Sciences, Kyoto University. gtsuji@pharm.kyoto-u.ac.jp Publication Types: Review

Arthritis Rheum. 2004 Jul;50(7):2202-10. Related Articles, Links Cytochrome P450 pharmacogenetics as a predictor of toxicity and clinical response to pulse cyclophosphamide in lupus nephritis. Takada K, Arefayene M, Desta Z, Yarboro CH, Boumpas DT, Balow JE, Flockhart DA, Illei GG. National Institute of Arthritis and Musculoskeletal and Skin Diseases, NIH, Bethesda, Maryland 20892, USA. OBJECTIVE: Pulse cyclophosphamide is the treatment of choice for severe lupus nephritis. However, not all patients respond to this therapy, and gonadal toxicity is of particular concern. Cyclophosphamide is a prodrug that requires activation by cytochrome P450 (CYP) enzymes. We conducted a retrospective cohort study to test whether genetic polymorphisms of these enzymes are associated with the toxicity of, and clinical response to, cyclophosphamide in patients with lupus nephritis. METHODS: Sixty-two patients with proliferative lupus nephritis treated with cyclophosphamide were genotyped for common variant alleles of CYP2B6, 2C19, 2C9, and 3A5. We examined the association between these genotypes and the following clinical end points: development of premature ovarian failure, end-stage renal disease (ESRD), doubling of serum creatinine level, and achievement of complete renal response. RESULTS: The observed frequencies of the variant alleles CYP2B6*5, CYP2C19*2, CYP2C9*2, and CYP3A5*3 were 12.1%, 25.0%, 4.0%, and 75.8%, respectively. Patients who were either heterozygous or homozygous for CYP2C19*2 had a significantly lower risk of developing premature ovarian failure (relative risk 0.10; 95% confidence interval 0.02-0.52), after adjustment for age and total number of cyclophosphamide pulses received. In a survival analysis, patients homozygous for CYP2B6*5 (n = 3) or CYP2C19*2 (n = 4) had a higher probability of reaching ESRD (P = 0.0005) and of doubling the creatinine level (P = 0.0005) as well as a trend toward a lower probability of achieving a complete renal response (P = 0.051). CONCLUSION: Determination of selected cytochrome P450 enzyme genotypes may be valuable for predicting the risk of premature ovarian failure in lupus nephritis patients treated with cyclophosphamide. The association of these genotypes with renal response needs further validation.

Arthritis Rheum. 2005 May;52(5):1349-59. Related Articles, Links Pharmacogenetics and rheumatology: Molecular mechanisms contributing to variability in drug response. Asanuma Y, Xie HG, Stein CM. Vanderbilt University School of Medicine, Nashville, Tennessee, USA. Publication Types: Review

Arzneimittelforschung. 2004;54(6):307-13. Related Articles, Links [Clinical-pharmacological aspects to accelerate the development process from the preclinical to the clinical phase/2nd communication: promising strategies] [Article in German] Kuhlmann J. Bayer HealthCare AG, Pharma Research Center, Institute of Clinical Pharmacology, Wuppertal, Germany. jochen.kuhlmann@bayerhealthcare.com To improve the transition from research to development a critical evaluation of the individual project by research and disease area teams is required to include input from pharmacology, toxicology, pharmacokinetics, galenics, clinical pharmacology, clinical as well as regulatory experts and marketing. Decisions on the individual development strategy should be made prior to the start of development and all projects should be reviewed at predefined stages throughout the product development life cycle. This ensures consistency of decision-making not only during the development of individual products but throughout the entire development pipeline. Studies in the exploratory stage of drug development should be designed for decision making in contrast to later clinical trials in the confirmatory stage that require power for proof-of-safety and proof-of-efficacy. The more thorough and profound studies have been carried out during this exploratory stage of drug development, the earlier a decision can be made on the continuation or discontinuation of further development, thus saving development time and money and assessing and considerably reducing the risk for the patients and increasing the success rate of the project in the later confirmatory effectiveness trial with an adequate number of subjects receiving the new therapy under typical conditions of use. Strategies which may be helpful to improve the quality of decisions in drug discovery and drug development are: discovery experiments should be done to critically evaluate the compound, the "killer" experiments should be done as early as possible, continuous effort on preclinical disease models is necessary to improve predictability of efficacy in patients ("humanized" research): genomic technology should be used to identify novel, disease-related targets and to characterise preclinical test systems, improvement of knowledge and experience concerning the relevance of new technologies for the clinical picture, genotyping of clinical trial patients to select patient groups which are likely to respond to treatment (pharmacogenomics), modelling and simulation of preclinical and clinical trials, integration of pharmacokinetic and pharmacodynamic principles into drug development, assessment of the interaction potential (CYP-450, trasporter proteins and others), increasing use of biomarker/surrogate marker for rapid clinical feedback, involvement of the target population as soon as possible, applying statistical data analysis techniques for proving effectiveness, co-operation with high quality centers. To reach this goal clinical pharmacology must be fully integrated in the whole process from the candidate selection to its positioning within the market. Publication Types: Review

Assay Drug Dev Technol. 2002 Nov;1(1 Pt 1):49-59. Related Articles, Links Cytochrome p450 genotyping by multiplexed real-time dna sequencing with pyrosequencing technology. Eriksson S, Berg LM, Wadelius M, Alderborn A. Pyrosequencing AB, Uppsala, Sweden. Individual differences in xenobiotic metabolism influence the therapeutic value of many drugs and are of major concern during the development of new drug candidates. A number of polymorphic cytochrome p450 enzymes account for a significant part of this variation. A better understanding of these genetic factors would be of value for drug development, as well as clinical practice. To fulfill the goal of a personalized medicine, methods for simple and accurate assessment of cytochrome p450 genes are required. We report on the development of multiplex assays for genotyping of the cytochrome p450 drug-metabolizing enzymes CYP2D6, CYP2C9, and CYP2C19 with Pyrosequencing technology. Eleven variable positions, representing 12 of the most frequent alleles, were scored: CYP2D6 alleles *2, *3, *4, *6, *7, *8, and *14, CYP2C19 alleles *2, *3, and *4, and CYP2C9 alleles *2 and *3. Four multiplex Pyrosequencing reactions per patient sample were performed to cover these positions, using either simplex or multiplex

PCR for amplification of target DNA sequences. Unequivocal genotypes were obtained for all patient samples, and the results were validated by comparing with results obtained using PCR-RFLP. For positions addressed with both methods, the results were in complete agreement. Pyrosequencing technology offers a highly automated, rapid, and accurate method for identification of cytochrome p450 alleles, which is suitable for pharmacogenomic research, as well as for routine assessment of patient genotypes.

Assay Drug Dev Technol. 2003 Apr;1(2):317-26. Related Articles, Links Polymorphisms of adrenergic receptors: variations on a theme. Liggett SB. Department of Medicine, University of Cincinnati College of Medicine, Cincinnati, Ohio, USA. stephen.liggett@uc.edu Recent studies have revealed that most of the adrenergic receptor genes are polymorphic, leading to changes in the amino sequence of the encoded receptor. The variations occur in multiple functional regions of the receptors, and appear as haplotypes with other coding and noncoding polymorphisms in their genes. The consequences of such genetic variability have been explored in recombinant cell-based systems and in human studies. Adrenergic receptor polymorphisms have been shown to alter receptor binding, G-protein coupling, regulation, and expression compared with their allelic counterparts. Here, the genetic and molecular characterization of these polymorphisms is reviewed, as well as their potential impact on pharmacogenetics, disease risk, and disease modification. Publication Types: Review

Atherosclerosis. 2004 Dec;177(2):219-34. Related Articles, Links Pharmacogenetics of HMG-CoA reductase inhibitors: exploring the potential for genotype-based individualization of coronary heart disease management. Kajinami K, Takekoshi N, Brousseau ME, Schaefer EJ. Department of Cardiology, Kanazawa Medical University, 1-1 Daigaku, Uchinada 920-0293, Japan. kajinami@kanazawa-med.ac.jp Despite the benefit of statin therapy in the prevention of coronary heart disease, a considerable inter-individual variation exists in its response. It is well recognized that genetic variation can contribute to differences in drug disposition and, consequently, clinical efficacy at the population level. Pharmacogenetics, exploring genetic polymorphisms that influence response to drug therapy, may one day allow the clinician to customize treatment strategies for patients in order to improve the success rate of drug therapies. To date, 41 studies have investigated the relationships between common genetic variants and response to statin therapy in terms of lipid effects and clinical outcomes; 16 candidate genes involved in lipoprotein metabolism and 3 in pharmacokinetics. APOE is the most extensively studied locus, and absolute difference in LDL cholesterol reduction across genotypes remained 3-6%. Moreover, none of the associations was striking enough to justify genetic analysis in clinical practice. Reported data have suggested that larger studies (>1000 participants) or combination analyses with >2 different polymorphisms would enable us to find clinically or biologically meaningful difference, which could be assumed as >10% absolute difference, and that genes influencing cholesterol biosynthesis in the liver, such as ABCG5/G8, CYP7A1, HMGCR, would be good candidates for future studies. Publication Types: Review

Atherosclerosis. 2005 Feb;178(2):331-8. Related Articles, Links Gender-specific effects of estrogen receptor alpha gene haplotype on high-density lipoprotein cholesterol response to atorvastatin: interaction with apolipoprotein AI gene polymorphism. Kajinami K, Brousseau ME, Lamon-Fava S, Ordovas JM, Schaefer EJ. Lipid Research Laboratory, Division of Endocrinology Metabolism and Molecular Biology, Tufts-New England Medical Center, Boston, MA, USA. kajinami@kanazawa-med.ac.jp Statins can modestly raise the levels of HDL cholesterol and apolipoprotein A-I (APOA1). Recently, associations between polymorphisms in the estrogen receptor alpha (ESR1) and the HDL cholesterol response to hormone replacement therapy were reported. To test the hypothesis that common polymorphisms in ESR1 and APOA1 genes are associated with the response to statin therapy, two ESR1 (PvuII and XbaI) and two APOA1 (G-75A and +83) polymorphisms were examined in 338 hypercholesterolemic patients treated with atorvastatin 10mg. The ESR1 PvuII-XbaI+ haplotype was significantly, and independently, associated with a greater response of HDL raising in women (+13% versus +7%, p=0.010) but not in men (+9% versus +7%, p=0.248). Effects of the APOA1+83 variant allele on HDL cholesterol response also differed significantly by gender (p=0.012). The APOA1+83 variant allele was associated with higher basal LDL cholesterol levels in men as well, but not in women. Finally, significant interactions were observed between the ESR1 PvuII-XbaI+ haplotype and the APOA1+83 variant allele regarding both HDL (p=0.042) and LDL (p=0.031) cholesterol responses. In conclusion, the ESR1 haplotype was associated with a greater HDL-raising to atorvastatin in a gender-specific manner, and the interactions between ESR1 and APOA1 genotypes regarding HDL and LDL cholesterol response were also gender specific. Publication Types: Clinical Trial Multicenter Study Randomized Controlled Trial

Aust N Z J Psychiatry. 2004 Jul;38(7):483-9. Related Articles, Links The emerging role of pharmacogenetics: implications for clinical psychiatry. Ng CH, Schweitzer I, Norman T, Easteal S. The Melbourne Clinic, Department of Psychiatry, University of Melbourne, Victoria, Australia. cng@unimelb.edu.au OBJECTIVE: This article aims to review the implications of pharmacogenetics for clinical psychiatry; these are discussed in the context of environmental and sociocultural factors. METHOD: A selective literature review was conducted using Medline search and other relevant references available to the authors. RESULTS: The individual differences in therapeutic and adverse effects of psychotropic drugs are largely determined by genetic factors. Recent advances in pharmacogenetics have highlighted the potential utility in predicting metabolic phenotypes, risks for side-effects and likelihood of drug response for the individual patient. CONCLUSIONS: Genotyping, especially for drug metabolizing enzymes, could enable more rational, cost-effective and optimal prescribing in future psychopharmacotherapy. Although the advances of pharmacogenetics may have many benefits in clinical practice, the importance of non-genetic factors must also be considered as cultural and environmental factors significantly impinge on response to medications. To clarify the extent pharmacogenetics can be adopted in clinical practice to predict drug response in patients from diverse backgrounds, further studies in different ethnic groups and clinical settings are required. Publication Types: Review

Best Pract Res Clin Gastroenterol. 2004 Jun;18(3):597-609. Related Articles, Links Pharmacogenetics of inflammatory bowel disease. Mascheretti S, Croucher PJ, Schreiber S. 1st Department of Medicine, Christian-Albrechts-Universtitat Kiel, Schittenhelmstr. 12, Kiel D-24105, Germany. The therapeutic efficacy and toxicity of many commonly employed drugs show interindividual variations that relate to several factors, including genetic variability in drug-metabolizing enzymes, transporters or targets. The study of the genetic determinants influencing interindividual variations in drug response is known as pharmacogenetics. The ability to identify, through preliminary genetic screening, the patients most likely to respond positively to a medication should facilitate the best choice of treatment for each patient; drugs likely to exhibit low efficacy or to give negative side-effects can be avoided. Among the medications used for inflammatory bowel disease, the best studied pharmacogenetically is azathioprine. The hematopoietic toxicity of azathioprine is due to single nucleotide polymorphisms in the thiopurine S-methyltransferase enzyme. Additionally, likely gene targets have been investigated to predict the response to glucocorticoids and infliximab, a monoclonal antibody against tumour necrosis factor that induces remission in approximately 30-40% of patients. However, no genetic predictor of response has been identified in either case. Publication Types: Review

Best Pract Res Clin Haematol. 2005;18(4):537-52. Related Articles, Links Gene expression profiling and multiple myeloma. Shaughnessy J Jr, Zhan F, Barlogie B, Stewart AK. Donna D. and Donald M. Lambert Laboratory of Myeloma Genetics, Myeloma Institute for Research and Therapy University of Arkansas for Medical Sciences, Little Rock, AR, USA. Gene expression profiling is a powerful tool through which the biology of multiple myeloma can be dissected. We will describe in this chapter how early studies using this technology have provided meaningful insights into myeloma biology, have led to the identification of new therapeutic targets, and have identified powerful prognostic and pharmacogenomic markers. Specifically, we will demonstrate that gene expression profiling can be used to segregate myeloma patients into prognostic categories within which known IgH translocation signatures can be readily defined. We also show that expression signatures can identify patients with chromosome 13 deletion. Finally, we demonstrate that global gene expression signatures can be distilled to short lists of three genes or more which together impart clinical outcome information, which is significantly more powerful than any previously defined prognostic tool. Expression profiling has also led to the identification of a number of new therapeutic targets not only in myeloma cell survival but also in the pathogenesis of the osteolysis which is a hallmark of this disease. Publication Types: Review

Best Pract Res Clin Rheumatol. 2004 Apr;18(2):233-47. Related Articles, Links Pharmacogenetics of disease-modifying anti-rheumatic drugs. Tanaka E, Taniguchi A, Urano W, Yamanaka H, Kamatani N. Institute of Rheumatology, Tokyo Women's Medical University, 10-22 Kawada-cho, Shinjuku-ku, Tokyo 162-0054, Japan. e-tanaka@tkg.att.ne.jp The outcome of treatment with disease-modifying anti-rheumatic drugs (DMARDs) in rheumatoid arthritis (RA) patients is considerably variable and is also unpredictable. It would be useful clinically if physicians were able to predict responses to DMARDs prior to their administration. One possible cause of differences in efficacy and adverse drug reactions is genetic variation in how individuals metabolize drugs. Based on pharmacogenetics, tailor-made drug therapy, also called personalized drug therapy or individual drug therapy, will be possible with analysis of genetic polymorphism, such as single nucleotide polymorphism (SNP), and analysis of haplotype and diplotype configuration. Several studies of the correlation between the genetic polymorphism of enzymes metabolizing several DMARDs and efficacy or adverse drug reactions have already been reported, suggesting that pharmacogenetics will be applicable to the treatment of RA in the near future. Publication Types: Review

Biochem Biophys Res Commun. 2004 Dec 10;325(2):426-33. Related Articles, Links Aggresome formation and pharmacogenetics: sulfotransferase 1A3 as a model system. Wang L, Yee VC, Weinshilboum RM. Department of Molecular Pharmacology and Experimental Therapeutics, Mayo Medical School-Mayo Clinic-Mayo Foundation, Rochester, MN 55905, USA. A common cause for pharmacogenetic alteration in drug response is genetic variation in encoded amino acid sequence. We have used the catecholamine and drug-metabolizing enzyme sulfotransferase (SULT)1A3 to create an artificial model system to study mechanisms-especially possible aggresome formation-by which genetic alteration in amino acid sequence might influence function. Specifically, we created a double variant SULT1A3 allozyme that included the naturally occurring Asn234 polymorphism plus an additional Trp172Arg mutation. Analysis of the SULT1A3 X-ray crystal structure had indicated that the Trp172Arg mutation might destabilize the protein's structure. Expression of SULT1A3 Arg172,Asn234 in COS-1 cells resulted in undetectable enzyme activity and a virtual lack of enzyme protein. Rabbit reticulocyte lysate degradation studies showed that the double variant allozyme was degraded much more rapidly than was wild type SULT1A3 by a ubiquitin-proteasome-dependent process. In addition, after expression in COS-1 cells, the double variant allozyme localized to aggresomes, a process not previously described or studied in pharmacogenetics. Therefore, the alteration of only one or two amino acids can lead to decreased levels of protein as a result of both aggresome formation and accelerated degradation. The possible role of aggresome formation in pharmacogenetics should be evaluated in naturally occurring systems with inherited alteration in encoded amino acid sequence.

Biochem Biophys Res Commun. 2004 Sep 3;321(4):870-8. Related Articles, Links Human SULT1A3 pharmacogenetics: gene duplication and functional genomic studies. Hildebrandt MA, Salavaggione OE, Martin YN, Flynn HC, Jalal S, Wieben ED, Weinshilboum RM. Department of Molecular Pharmacology, Mayo Clinic College of Medicine, Mayo Foundation, Rochester, MN 55905, USA. Sulfotransferase (SULT) 1A3 catalyzes the sulfate conjugation of catecholamines. Inheritance is an important factor responsible for individual variation in SULT1A3 activity, and gene resequencing studies have shown the presence of one functionally significant SULT1A3 nonsynonymous cSNP. However, following completion of the Human Genome Project, it appeared that SULT1A3 might be duplicated. We used specific PCR-based assays and fluorescence in situ hybridization to verify that 2 SULT1A3 genes-SULT1A3 and SULT1A4-were present on chromosome 16 in all human DNA samples studied. Furthermore, reanalysis of previous gene resequencing data confirmed the presence of the SULT1A3 SNPs identified previously, but also revealed 11 novel polymorphisms, including 3 nonsynonymous cSNPs. Functional genomic studies showed that two of those cSNPs, C302T, and C302A, resulted in decreased enzyme activity without striking changes in substrate kinetics but with parallel changes in levels of immunoreactive protein. In addition, RT-PCR revealed that both SULT1A3 and SULT1A4 can be transcriptionally active. The duplication of SULT1A3 will have to be taken into account in future efforts to understand individual variation in SULT1A3 activity or properties.

Biochem Pharmacol. 2005 Oct 1;70(7):1096-103. Related Articles, Links CYP2C-catalyzed delta9-tetrahydrocannabinol metabolism: kinetics, pharmacogenetics and interaction with phenytoin. Bland TM, Haining RL, Tracy TS, Callery PS. Department of Basic Pharmaceutical Sciences, School of Pharmacy, P.O. Box 9530, West Virginia University, 1 Medical Center Drive, Morgantown, WV 26506, USA. Delta9-tetrahydrocannabinol (delta9-THC), the primary psychoactive constituent of marijuana, is subject to first pass hepatic metabolism primarily by hydroxylation to yield active and inactive oxygenated products. The primary metabolite is formed via oxidation of the allylic methyl group to yield 11-hydroxy-delta9-THC, which is oxidized further to 11-nor-9-carboxy-delta9-THC. The hydroxylation is thought to be mediated by CYP2C9. The present study was designed to address the kinetics and pharmacogenetics of CYP2C-mediated metabolism of (delta9)-THC by studying its metabolism in human liver microsomes and expressed enzymes. Expressed CYP2C9.1 exhibited high affinity for the hydroxylation of delta9-THC (apparent Km, 2 microM), similar to that observed in human liver microsomes (apparent Km 0.8 microM). In contrast, the calculated intrinsic clearance (apparent Vm/Km) for CYP2C9.2 and CYP2C9.3 was approximately 30% that of the wild type, CYP2C9.1. Given the high affinity of CYP2C9 for the hydroxylation of delta9-THC, we evaluated the potential for an interaction between delta9-THC, 11-hydroxy-delta9-THC, or 11-nor-9-carboxy-delta9-THC and the CYP2C9 substrate, phenytoin. Surprisingly, delta9-THC increased the rate of phenytoin hydroxylation in human liver microsomes and expressed CYP2C9 enzyme. Similar increases in rate were observed with co-incubation of 11-hydroxy-delta9-THC and 11-nor-9-carboxy-delta9-THC with phenytoin. These in vitro data suggest the potential for an interaction from the concomitant administration of delta9-THC and phenytoin that could result in decreased phenytoin concentrations in vivo.

Biochim Biophys Acta. 2006 Mar;1760(3):301-9. Epub 2005 Dec 20. Related Articles, Links Dictyostelium discoideum to human cells: Pharmacogenetic studies demonstrate a role for sphingolipids in chemoresistance. Alexander S, Min J, Alexander H. Division of Biological Sciences, 303 Tucker Hall, University of Missouri, Columbia, MO 65211-7400, USA. Resistance to chemotherapy is a major obstacle for the treatment of cancer and a subject of extensive research. Numerous mechanisms of drug resistance have been proposed, and they differ for different drugs. Nevertheless, it is clear that our understanding of this important problem is still incomplete, and that new targets for modulating therapy still await discovery. The attractive biology and the availability of powerful molecular techniques have made the cellular slime mold Dictyostelium discoideum, a powerful non-mammalian model for drug target discovery, and the problem of drug resistance. To understand the molecular basis of chemoresistance to the widely used drug cisplatin, both genetic and pharmacological approaches have been applied to this versatile experimental system. These studies have resulted in the identification of novel molecular pathways which can be used to increase the efficacy of cisplatin, and brought attention to the role of sphingolipids in mediating the cellular response to chemotherapeutic drugs. In the following review, we will describe the history and utility of D. discoideum in pharmacogenetics, and discuss recent studies which focus attention on the role of sphingolipids in chemotherapy and chemoresistance.

Bioethics. 2004 Aug;18(4):303-21. Related Articles, Links Tailor-made pharmacotherapy: future developments and ethical challenges in the field of pharmacogenomics. van Delden J, Bolt I, Kalis A, Derijks J, Leufkens H. Julius Center for Health Sciences, University Medical Center Utrecht, HP Str. 6. 131, PO Box 85500, 3508 GA Utrecht, The Netherlands. J.J.M.vanDelden@umcutrecht.nl Pharmacogenomics is the study of the myriad interactions between genes and pharmacotherapy. Developments in pharmacogenomics have changed and will affect pharmaceutical research, drug development and the practice of medicine in a significant way. In this article, we make an inventory of the ethical implications that might arise as a result of possible developments in pharmacogenomics and investigate whether the present ethical framework will be able to adequately answer arising questions. We think that many of the questions related to the consequences of pharmacogenomics are answerable along the lines of present ethical thinking. We also believe, however, that many 'changes of degree' may result in a 'change of kind.' We therefore think that pharmacogenomics may potentially have such a profound influence on scientific research and the pharmaceutical industry, the practice of medicine and society at large, that this will generate its own unique dynamic, which will require new ethical research. We suggest that the notion of 'responsibility' will be a major focus of such research.

Bioethics. 2004 Aug;18(4):322-42. Related Articles, Links Tailored medicine: whom will it fit? The ethics of patient and disease stratification. Smart A, Martin P, Parker M. Oxford Genetics Knowledge Park, The Ethox Centre, Division of Public Health and Primary Health Care, University of Oxford, Old Road Campus, Headington, Oxford, OX3 7LF, UK. andrew.smart@ethox.ox.ac.uk A key selling point of pharmacogenetics is the genetic stratification of either patients or diseases in order to target the prescribing of medicine. The hope is that genetically 'tailored' medicines will replace the current 'one-size-fits-all' paradigm of drug development and usage. This paper is concerned with the relationship between difference and justice in the use of pharmacogenetics. This new technology, which facilitates the identification and use of difference, has, we shall argue, the potential to lead to injustice either by the inappropriate use of difference or through the inappropriate failure to use difference. We build on empirical data from a detailed study of the range of options for the development of pharmacogenetics to present a consideration of the ethical issues that surround patient and disease stratification. In it we explore the ways in which the use of pharmacogenetics may lead to the creation of new, genetically stratified, forms of difference and new forms of injustice based on these divisions. We also examine the ways in which existing forms of difference and social stratification may interact with the use of pharmacogenetics. In conclusion, we suggest how an understanding of these ethical issues could usefully inform future policy discussions.

Bioethics. 2004 Aug;18(4):344-60. Related Articles, Links Pharmacogenetic testing, informed consent and the problem of secondary information. Netzer C, Biller-Andorno N. Institut fur Humangenetik, Universitat Bonn, Germany. cnetzer@web.de Numerous benefits for patients have been predicted if prescribing decisions were routinely accompanied by pharmacogenetic testing. So far, little attention has been paid to the possibility that the routine application of this new technology could result in considerable harm to patients. This article emphasises that pharmacogenetic testing shares both the opportunities and the pitfalls with 'conventional' disease-genetic testing. It demonstrates that performing pharmacogenetic tests as well as interpreting the results are extraordinarily complex issues requiring a high level of expertise. It further argues that pharmacogenetic testing can have a huge impact on clinical decisions and may influence the therapeutic strategy as well as the clinical monitoring of a patient. This view challenges the predominant paradigm that pharmacogenetic testing will predict patients' responses to medicines, but that it will not provide any other significant disease-specific predictive information about the patient or family members. The article also questions published proposals to reduce the consent procedure for pharmacogenetic testing to a simple statement that the physician wishes to test a sample of the patient's DNA to see if a drug will be safe or whether it will work, and presents an alternative model that is better suited to protect patient's interests and to obtain meaningful informed consent. The paper concludes by outlining conditions for the application of pharmacogenetic testing in clinical practice in a way that can make full use of its potential benefits while minimising possible harm to patients and their families.

Bioethics. 2004 Aug;18(4):361-78. Related Articles, Links Ethical implications of pharmacogenetics--do slippery slope arguments matter? Schubert L. Tuebingen University, Wilhelmstr. 19, 72074 Tuebingen, Germany. lilian.schubert@uni-tuebingen.de Pharmacogenetics is a rapidly expanding area of research exploring the relationship between inter-individual genetic variation and drug response, with the goal of developing genetically optimised therapies. Slippery slope arguments claim that a particular action should be rejected (or supported) because it might be the first step onto a slippery slope leading to undesirable (or desirable) consequences. In this article, several slippery slope arguments relevant to the context of pharmacogenetics are evaluated under consideration of underlying reasons for their popularity. The author concludes that although the examined arguments are unconvincing as slippery slope arguments, they do matter in this context. While positive slippery slope arguments serve as a driving force to fuel the development of pharmacogenetics, their negative counterparts play an important role to sensitise policy makers and the public to potential problems.

Bioethics. 2004 Aug;18(4):iii-viii. Related Articles, Links Pharmacogenetics: ethical issues. Sutrop M. Centre for Ethics, University of Tartu, Estonia. msutrop@ut.ee Publication Types: Editorial

Bioinformatics. 2004 Sep 22;20(14):2315-6. Epub 2004 Apr 1. Related Articles, Links PedSplit: pedigree management for stratified analysis. Lanktree MB, VanderBeek L, Macciardi FM, Kennedy JL. Neurogenetics Section, Centre for Addiction and Mental Health, Department of Psychiatry, University of Toronto, 250 College Street, Toronto M5T 1R8, Canada. SUMMARY: PedSplit facilitates pedigree management for gene-gene interaction and sex specific tests for increased homogeneity within subgroups. PedSplit also provides a simple approach for calculating haplotype relative risk and generating internal 'controls'. AVAILABILITY: Executables, C++ source code and documentation for PedSplit can be downloaded from http://www.pharmacogenetics.ca in the links and software section.

Bioinformatics. 2005 Aug 1;21(15):3286-93. Epub 2005 May 26. Related Articles, Links A latent variable model for chemogenomic profiling. Flaherty P, Giaever G, Kumm J, Jordan MI, Arkin AP. Department of Electrical Engineering and Computer Science, University of California, Berkeley, CA 94720, USA. flaherty@berkeley.edu MOTIVATION: In haploinsufficiency profiling data, pleiotropic genes are often misclassified by clustering algorithms that impose the constraint that a gene or experiment belong to only one cluster. We have developed a general probabilistic model that clusters genes and experiments without requiring that a given gene or drug only appear in one cluster. The model also incorporates the functional annotation of known genes to guide the clustering procedure. RESULTS: We applied our model to the clustering of 79 chemogenomic experiments in yeast. Known pleiotropic genes PDR5 and MAL11 are more accurately represented by the model than by a clustering procedure that requires genes to belong to a single cluster. Drugs such as miconazole and fenpropimorph that have different targets but similar off-target genes are clustered more accurately by the model-based framework. We show that this model is useful for summarizing the relationship among treatments and genes affected by those treatments in a compendium of microarray profiles. AVAILABILITY: Supplementary information and computer code at http://genomics.lbl.gov/llda. Publication Types: Evaluation Studies

Biol Pharm Bull. 2004 Jul;27(7):939-48. Related Articles, Links Pharmacogenomics of drug transporters: a new approach to functional analysis of the genetic polymorphisms of ABCB1 (P-glycoprotein/MDR1). Ishikawa T, Onishi Y, Hirano H, Oosumi K, Nagakura M, Tarui S. Department of Biomolecular Engineering, Graduate School of Bioscience and Biotechnology, Tokyo Institute of Technology, Yokohama, Japan. tishikaw@bio.titech.ac.jp In the 21st century, emerging genomic technologies (i.e., bioinformatics, functional genomics, and pharmacogenomics) are shifting the paradigm of drug discovery research and improving the strategy of medical care for patients. In order to realize the personalized medicine, it is critically important to understand molecular mechanisms underlying inter-individual differences in the drug response, namely, pharmacological effect vs. side effect. Evidence is now accumulating to strongly suggest that drug transporters are one of the determinant factors governing the pharmacokinetic profile of drugs. Effort has been made to identify genetic variation in drug transporter genes. In particular, genetic variations of the human ABCB1 (P-glycoprotein/MDR1) gene have been most extensively studied. Hitherto more than fifty single nucleotide polymorphisms (SNPs) and insertion/deletion polymorphisms in the ABCB1 gene have been reported. However, at the present time, information is still limited with respect to the actual effect of those genetic polymorphisms on the function of ABCB1. In this context, we have undertaken functional analyses of ABCB1 polymorphisms. To quantify the impact of genetic polymorphisms on the substrate specificity of ABCB1, we have developed a high-speed screening system and a new structure-activity relationship (SAR) analysis method. This review addresses functional aspects of the genetic polymorphism of ABCB1 and provides the standard method to evaluate the effect of polymorphisms on the function. Publication Types: Review

Biol Psychiatry. 2004 Apr 15;55(8):785-8. Related Articles, Links Comprehensive strategies to study neuronal function in transgenic animal models. Carter DA. School of Biosciences, Cardiff University, PO Box 911, Museum Avenue, Cardiff CF10 3US, Wales, UK. In the last 20 years of transgenic research, transgenic technology has been developed and refined to provide a seemingly comprehensive range of experimental approaches to questions of neuronal gene function; however, parallel developments in other technologies, such as whole genome sequencing and microarray analysis of gene expression, has meant that the questions have gotten harder. The complexity of neuronal systems and the difficulty of modeling neurologic diseases in rodents also present considerable challenges to molecular neuroscientists. Future functional genomic studies of brain and behavior will involve the full range of available transgenic methods and the incorporation of new technologies, including RNA interference.

Biol Psychiatry. 2005 Jun 1;57(11):1367-73. Epub 2005 Jan 5. Related Articles, Links Attention-deficit/hyperactivity disorder pharmacogenomics. McGough JJ. Neuropsychiatric Institute and David Geffen School of Medicine at University of California-Los Angeles, Los Angeles, California 90095, USA. jmcgough@mednet.ucla.edu Although the efficacy of medications for attention-deficit/hyperactivity disorder (ADHD) is well demonstrated in clinical trials, substantial numbers of patients fail to remain on therapy, and there is tremendous variability in tolerability and treatment acceptance. The emerging science of pharmacogenomics seeks to identify patterns of genetic variation that will direct individually tailored treatment regimens and enhance long-term adherence. For this review, existing studies in ADHD pharmacogenomics were reviewed to assess current knowledge and provide a basis for planning future research. Twelve studies were identified. The majority investigated the role of candidate genes in predicting clinical response to methylphenidate. The most frequently studied is DAT1, although findings are inconsistent, with the 10-repeat polymorphism predicting both increased and decreased symptom reduction in various reports. Other candidates include DRD4, DRD5, DBH, 5HTT, SNAP-25, and COMT. One study was based on quantitative trait analyses in a genome-wide scan. Although interest in ADHD pharmacogenomics is encouraging, preliminary studies have been limited by small sample sizes, inconsistent research designs, retrospective reports, and a focus on symptom response. Future studies should emphasize large, prospective trials, assess multiple medications in individual subjects, and consider a full range of pharmacodynamic and pharmacokinetic outcomes. Publication Types: Review

Biomed Chromatogr. 2004 Dec;18(10):759-84. Related Articles, Links Simultaneous chiral analyses of multiple analytes: case studies, implications and method development considerations. Srinivas NR. Drug Development, Discovery Research, Dr Reddy's Laboratories, Bollaram Road, Miyapur, Hyderabad 500 049, India. nrsrinivas@drreddys.com The field of chiral separations had a modest beginning some two decades ago. However, due to rapid technological advancement coupled with simultaneous availability of innovative chiral stationary phases and novel chiral derivatization agents, the field of chiral separations has now totally outpaced many other separation fields. Keeping pace with rapid changes in the field of chiral separations, investigators continue to add stereoselective pharmacokinetic, pharmacodynamic, pharmacologic and toxicological data of new and/or marketed racemic compounds to the literature. Examination of the evolution of chiral separations suggests that in the beginning many investigators attempted to separate and quantify a single pair of enantiomers, adopting either direct (separation made on a chiral stationary phase) or indirect (separation made following precolumn conversion of enantiomers to corresponding diastereomers) approaches. However, more recent trends in chiral separations suggest that investigators are attempting to separate and quantify multiple pairs of enantiomers with available technologies. Added to this, some interesting trends have been observed in many of the recently reported chiral applications, including preferences regarding internal standard selection, mobile phase contents and composition, sorting out issues with mass spectrometric detection, determination of elution order, analytical manipulations of metabolite(s) without reference standards and addressing some specificity-related issues. This review mainly focuses on chiral separations involving multiple chiral analytes and attempts to justify the need for such chiral separations involving multiple analytes. In this context, several cases studies are described on the utility and applicability of such chiral separations under discrete headings to provide an account to the readership on the implications of such tasks. The topics of case studies covered in this review include: (a) therapy markers--differentiation from drug abuse and/or applicability in forensics; (b) role in pharmacogenetic/polymorphic evaluation; (c) monitoring and understanding the role of parent and active metabolite(s) in clinical and preclinical investigations; (d) exploration on the pharmacokinetic utility of an active chiral metabolite vis-a-vis the racemic parent moiety; (e) understanding the chirality play in delineating peculiar toxic effects; (f) exploration of chiral inversion phenomenon, and understanding the role of stereoselective metabolism. For the further benefit of readership, some select examples (n = 19) of the separation of multiple chiral analytes with appropriate information on chromatography, detection system, validation parameters and applicable conclusion are also provided. Finally, the review covers some useful considerations for method development involving multiple chiral analytes. Copyright 2004 John Wiley and Sons, Ltd. Publication Types: Review

Biosci Rep. 2005 Oct-Dec;25(5-6):289-97. Related Articles, Links Chemical genetics: Drug screens in Zebrafish. den Hertog J. Hubrecht Laboratory, Netherlands Institute for Developmental Biology, Uppsalalaan 8, 3584, Utrecht, CT, The Netherlands. hertog@niob.knaw.nl High throughput chemical genetic screens for compounds with specific biological activity in a whole organism are feasible using zebrafish embryos. At least two medium to large scale drug screens have been carried out to date, leading to the identification of compounds that disturb zebrafish development. Chemical genetics using zebrafish embryos may become an important step in the discovery of drugs and their targets. Publication Types: Review

Biotechniques. 2005 Oct;39(4):563-4. Related Articles, Links Applying technologies towards safe and effective medicines. Roses AD. GlaxoSmithKline, Research Triangle Park, NC 27709, USA. allen.d.roses@gsk.com

Biotechniques. 2005 Oct;39(4):565-8. Related Articles, Links Pharmacogenetics and pharmacogenomics in oncology therapeutic antibody development. Yan L, Beckman RA. Hematology and Oncology, Clinical Research and Development, Centocor Research and Development, Inc, Wayne, PA 19087, USA. LYan2@cntus.jnj.com Pharmacogenetics and pharmacogenomics are keys to the success of personalized medicine, prescribing drugs based on a patient's individual genetic and biological profile. In this review, we will focus on the application of pharmacogenetics and pharmacogenomics in developing monoclonal antibody (MAb) therapeutics in oncology. The significance of pharmacogenomics in MAb therapeutics is highlighted by the association between polymorphisms in Fc receptors and clinical response to anti-CD20 MAb rituximab (Rituxan) or anti-ganglioside GD2 MAb 3F8, as well as the potential link between polymorphisms in HER2 and cardiac toxicity in patients treated with the anti-HER2 MAb trastuzumab (Herceptin). The dependence on gene copy number or expression levels of HER2 and epidermal growth factor receptor (EGFR) for therapeutic efficacy of trastuzumab and cetuximab (Erbitux), respectively, supports the importance of selecting suitable patient populations based on their pharmacogenetic profile. In addition, a better understanding of target mutation status and biological consequences will benefit MAAb development and may guide clinical development and use of these innovative therapeutics. The application of pharmacogenetics and pharmacogenomics in developing MAb therapeutics will be largely dependent on the discovery of novel surrogate biomarkers and identification of disease- and therapeutics-relevant polymorphisms. Challenges and opportunities in biomarker discovery and validation, and in implementing clinical pharmacogenetics and pharmacogenomics in oncology MAb development and clinical practice will also be discussed.

Biotechniques. 2005 Oct;39(4):571-4. Related Articles, Links Development of a PCR-based strategy for CYP2D6 genotyping including gene multiplication of worldwide potential use. Dorado P, Caceres MC, Pozo-Guisado E, Wong ML, Licinio J, Llerena A. University of Beira Interior, Covilha, Portugal. There is growing consensus on the potential use of pharmacogenetics in clinical practice, and hopes have been expressed for application to the improvement of global health. However, two major challenges may lead to widening the "biotechnological gap" between the developing and the industrial world;first the unaffordability of some current technologies for poorer countries, and second the necessity of analyzing all described alleles for every clinical case due to the inability to predict the ethnic group of a given patient. Because of its role in the metabolism of a number of drugs, cytochrome P450 2D6 (CYP2D6) is an excellent candidate for use in the optimization of drug therapy. CYP2D6 is a highly polymorphic gene locus with more than 50 variant alleles, and subjects can be classified as poor metabolizers (PM), extensive metabolizers (EM), or ultrarapid metabolizers (UM) of a given CYP2D6 substrate. Several strategies and methods for CYP2D6 genotyping exist. Some, however, are expensive and laborious. The aim of this study was to design a PCR-based genotyping methodology to allow rapid, straightforward, and inexpensive identification of 90%-95% of CYP2D6 PM or UM genotypes for routine clinical use, independent of the individual's ethnic group. CYP2D6 is amplified in initial extra long PCRs (XL-PCRs), which subsequently undergo fragment-length polymorphism analysis for the determination of carriers of CYP2D6 allelic variants. The same XL-PCRs are also used for the determination of CYP2D6 multiplication and 2D6*5 allele (abolished activity). The application of this new strategy for the detection of CYP2D6 mutated alleles and multiplications to routine clinical analysis will enable the PM and UM phenotypes to be predicted and identified at a reasonable cost in a large number of individuals at most locations.

Biotechniques. 2005 Oct;39(4):577-82. Related Articles, Links Clinical applications of microarray-based diagnostic tests. Wu L, Williams PM, Koch WH. Roche Molecular Diagnostics, Pleasanton, CA 94588, USA. Nearly 15 years have passed since the possibility of analyzing nucleic acid analytes in a massively parallel fashion was proposed using the then new concept of microarrays. A decade ago, proof of principle demonstration projects established the use of high density microarrays to genotype multiple polymorphisms within a large gene [cystic fibrosis transmembrance regulator (CFTR)], to rapidly analyze DNA sequences by hybridization and to ascertain differential gene expression of the entire genome of an organism. The use of microarrays has had an explosive influence on the rate at which new biological information can be learned, including in a nonhypothesis driven manner. The past decade has also seen these research tools applied increasingly to questions of clinical and medical relevance. Genotyping drug metabolizing enzyme genes, resequencing important tumor suppressor genes, and classifying neoplastic disease by differential gene expression profiles are but a few of the many possibilities to provide clinically useful information using microarray-based diagnostic tests.

Biotechniques. 2005 Oct;39(4):583-8. Related Articles, Links BeadArray-based solutions for enabling the promise of pharmacogenomics. Fan JB, Hu SX, Craumer WC, Barker DL. Illumina, San Diego, CA 92121, USA. A "one-size-fits-all" approach continues to characterize today's healthcare paradigm. But emergent rules, information, genomics tools, and economics are driving a fundamental and inevitable shift to a more personalized world of medicine. In this new world, the interests of insurers, regulators, suppliers, healthcare providers, and most important, patients, will have converged. The new goal will be the right treatment for the right individual at the right time. In this world, personalized medicine, through pharmacogenomics (PGx), will be the new healthcare paradigm. We will briefly examine healthcare trends and current opportunities for PGx development. We will then demonstrate how microarray technologies-among them bead-based approaches-have emerged as a key enabler for bringing home the promise of PGx.

BJOG. 2005 Mar;112 Suppl 1:97-102. Related Articles, Links Genetic factors in preterm birth--the future. Esplin MS, Varner MW. Department of Obstetrics and Gynecology, University of Utah School of Medicine, 30 North 1900 East, Salt Lake City, UT 84132, USA. The genetic regulation of common biological functions has redundant control mechanisms, and it is unlikely that a single marker will ever be identified that will be both highly sensitive and specific. It is more likely that combinations of gene and/or protein markers, perhaps also combined with obstetric family histories, will be required to achieve the goal of a truly sensitive and specific screening profile for spontaneous preterm labour and preterm birth. The rapidly evolving disciplines of genomics and proteomics are now beginning to be applied to the study of spontaneous preterm labour and preterm birth. These techniques are able to measure multiple markers (in the thousands) in a biological sample and, given the likely presence of biological changes that precede by weeks or even months the clinical manifestations of the disease, are ideally suited to the evaluation of spontaneous preterm labour and preterm birth. Over the next few years, these technologies will hasten a deeper understanding of the pathophysiology of spontaneous preterm labour, discover novel target molecules and diagnostic biomarkers and ultimately aid in formulating more effective interventions to prevent preterm birth. Pharmacogenomics is another rapidly evolving discipline that holds great promise for the treatment and prevention of spontaneous preterm labour and preterm birth. Because spontaneous preterm labour is a final common pathway for multiple aetiologies, there remains no reason why any single therapy will work optimally for all women. As patient-specific pharmacogenomic profiles are developed, it will be possible to develop patient-specific treatment regimens. Beyond that, it may become possible to identify those women who are, or are not, destined to labour spontaneously and give birth remote from term and to institute patient-specific preventive measures. Spontaneous preterm labour and preterm birth remains a syndrome, with a final common pathway for multiple aetiologies. As a result, no single explanation, marker or treatment is likely to be 100% sensitive, specific or successful. It is also clear, however, that there is a genetic predisposition in many cases of spontaneous preterm labour. Over the next few years, several recently developed diagnostic mechanisms, and others that have yet to evolve, will hold a greater potential than ever before to unlock the secrets of the genetic predisposition to spontaneous preterm labour and its underlying causes. An improved understanding of these mechanisms will allow clinicians to employ therapies that will be optimally effective for individual women and their unborn babies. Eventually, these advances could be applied to the presymptomatic prevention of spontaneous preterm labour. It is the intent of this manuscript to review the current status of these new technologies and disciplines and to speculate on their applications in the intermediate future. Publication Types: Review

Blood Coagul Fibrinolysis. 2004 Jul;15(5):427-33. Related Articles, Links 807 C/T Polymorphism of the glycoprotein Ia gene and pharmacogenetic modulation of platelet response to dual antiplatelet treatment. Angiolillo DJ, Fernandez-Ortiz A, Bernardo E, Ramirez C, Escaned J, Moreno R, Hernandez-Antolin R, Sabate M, Trabetti E, Pignatti PF, Macaya C. Cardiovascular Institute, San Carlos University Hospital, Madrid, Spain. dominickjangiolillo@hotmail.com Glycoprotein (GP) Ia/IIa is a major platelet-collagen receptor playing a key role in thrombosis following collagen exposure. The 807 C/T polymorphism of the GP Ia gene (ITGA2) has been associated with platelet GP Ia/IIa receptor expression, having T-allele carriers, increased receptor density and thrombotic risk. The aim of the study was to assess the role of the 807 C/T polymorphism on modulating platelet function in patients undergoing coronary stenting receiving a 300 mg clopidogrel loading dose. Platelet aggregation was assessed in 44 patients by light transmittance aggregometry following adenosine diphosphate and collagen stimuli at baseline, and 10 min, 4 h and 24 h after clopidogrel front loading. The T allele was found in 73% of patients. Clopidogrel reduced adenosine diphosphate-induced platelet aggregation ($P < 0.01$), which was similar in carriers and non-carriers of the T allele throughout the study ($P = 0.73$). Clopidogrel reduced collagen-induced platelet aggregation only in non-carriers of the T allele ($P = 0.03$), which resulted in an increase in T allele carriers during the overall study ($P = 0.04$). In conclusion, the T allele of the GP Ia gene modulates platelet aggregation and clopidogrel antiplatelet effects, suggesting an enhanced reactivity to fibrillar collagens (exposed during coronary stenting) in T allele carriers and might contribute to an increased thrombotic risk in these patients. Copyright 2004 Lippincott Williams and Wilkins

Blood Coagul Fibrinolysis. 2005 Sep;16(6):389-98. Related Articles, Links Pharmacogenetics of oral anticoagulants. Rojas JC, Aguilar B, Rodriguez-Maldonado E, Collados MT. Center for Research and Extension in Health Sciences, Instituto Tecnologico y de Estudios Superiores de Monterrey, Nuevo Leon, Mexico. The use of oral anticoagulants (OA) is problematic due to its association with hemorrhagic complications. OA metabolism relies on the CYP2C9 complex. Genetic variations compromising metabolic competence of this complex may explain the risk of excessive and hazardous anticoagulation. A pharmacogenetics-based approach to this issue could be beneficial for choosing adequate dose and duration of treatment, in addition to having a better understanding of pharmacological interactions to which OA are susceptible. However, evidence from several basic and clinical studies indicates that both a complicated system of regulation of expression of multiple genes and the influence of a wide variety of epigenetic factors could be responsible for adverse drug reactions associated with the use of OA. Emphasis on understanding the gene-environment interactions could attain new paths to facilitate the use of these important drugs in the quotidian clinical practice. Publication Types: Review

Blood. 2004 Nov 1;104(9):2867-72. Epub 2004 Jul 15. Related Articles, Links Variable sensitivity of FLT3 activation loop mutations to the small molecule tyrosine kinase inhibitor MLN518. Clark JJ, Cools J, Curley DP, Yu JC, Lokker NA, Giese NA, Gilliland DG. Division of Hematology/Oncology, Brigham and Women's Hospital, 75 Francis St, Boston, MA 02115, USA. Jennifer_Clark@dfci.harvard.edu FLT3 is constitutively activated by internal tandem duplications (ITDs) in the juxtamembrane domain or by activation loop mutations in acute myeloid leukemia (AML). We tested the sensitivity of 8 activation loop mutations to the small molecule FLT3 inhibitor, MLN518. Each FLT3 activation loop mutant, including D835Y, D835A, D835E, D835H, D835N, D835V, D835del, and I836del, transformed Ba/F3 cells to factor-independent proliferation and had constitutive tyrosine kinase activation, as assessed by FLT3 autophosphorylation and activation of downstream effectors, including STAT5 and ERK. MLN518 inhibited FLT3 autophosphorylation and phosphorylation of STAT5 and ERK in FLT3-ITD-transformed Ba/F3 cells with an IC(50) (50% inhibition of cell viability) of approximately 500 nM. However, there was a broad spectrum of sensitivity among the 8 activation loop mutants, with IC(50) ranging from approximately 500 nM to more than 10 microM for the inhibition of phosphorylation of FLT3, STAT5, and ERK. The relative sensitivity of the mutants to MLN518 in biochemical assays correlated with the cellular IC(50) for cytokine-independent proliferation of FLT3-transformed Ba/F3 cells in the presence of MLN518. Thus, certain activation loop mutations in FLT3 simultaneously confer resistance to small molecule inhibitors. These findings have implications for the evaluation of responses in clinical trials with FLT3 inhibitors and provide a strategy to screen for compounds that can overcome resistance.

Blood. 2005 Aug 15;106(4):1503-4; author reply 1504-5. Related Articles, Links Comment on: Blood. 2004 Jun 1;103(11):4028-35. Dose-response relationship and pharmacogenetics of anti-RhD monoclonal antibodies. Ternant D, Ohresser M, Thomas C, Cartron G, Watier H, Paintaud G. Publication Types: Comment Letter

Blood. 2005 Jun 15;105(12):4752-8. Epub 2005 Feb 15. Related Articles, Links Pharmacogenetics of outcome in children with acute lymphoblastic leukemia. Rocha JC, Cheng C, Liu W, Kishi S, Das S, Cook EH, Sandlund JT, Rubnitz J, Ribeiro R, Campana D, Pui CH, Evans WE, Relling MV. Department of Pharmaceutical Sciences, Saint Jude Children's Research Hospital of the University of Tennessee, Memphis 38105-2794, USA. Acquired genetic characteristics of acute lymphoblastic leukemia (ALL) cells are used to individualize therapy, whereas germ line genetic characteristics generally are not. We determined whether ALL outcome was related to 16 genetic polymorphisms affecting the pharmacodynamics of antileukemic agents. Of 246 children, 116 were treated on the lower-risk (LR) and 130 on the higher-risk (HR) arms of a St Jude protocol. Patients in the HR group with the glutathione S-transferase (GSTM1) non-null genotype had greater risk of hematologic relapse (P = .03), which was further increased by the thymidylate synthetase (TYMS) 3/3 genotype (P = .03). These genotypes remained predictive in multivariate analyses (P < .001 and .003, respectively). No genotypes were predictive in the LR arm. Expression of these 2 genes in ALL blasts was lower in those with low-activity genotypes. For central nervous system relapse, among the HR group, the vitamin D receptor start site (P = .02) and intron 8 genotypes (P = .04) predisposed, whereas for LR patients the TYMS 3/3 genotype predisposed (P = .04). The GSTM1 non-null and TYMS 3/3 genotypes are plausibly linked to drug resistance. Polymorphisms interact to influence antileukemic outcome and represent determinants of response that can be used to optimize therapy. Publication Types: Clinical Trial

Blood. 2005 Oct 1;106(7):2329-33. Epub 2005 Jun 9. Related Articles, Links The impact of CYP2C9 and VKORC1 genetic polymorphism and patient characteristics upon warfarin dose requirements: proposal for a new dosing regimen. Sconce EA, Khan TI, Wynne HA, Avery P, Monkhouse L, King BP, Wood P, Kesteven P, Daly AK, Kamali F. School of Clinical and Laboratory Sciences, University of Newcastle, Newcastle Upon Tyne, United Kingdom. Current dosing algorithms do not account for genetic and environmental factors for warfarin dose determinations. This study investigated the contribution of age, CYP2C9 and VKORC1 genotype, and body size to warfarin-dose requirements. Studied were 297 patients with stable anticoagulation with a target international normalized ratio (INR) of 2.0 to 3.0. Genetic analyses for CYP2C9 (*2 and *3 alleles) and VKORC1 (-1639 polymorphism) were performed and venous INR and plasma R- and S-warfarin concentrations determined. The mean warfarin daily dose requirement was highest in CYP2C9 homozygous wild-type patients, compared with those with the variant *2 and *3 alleles (P < .001) and highest in patients with the VKORC1 (position -1639) GG genotype compared with those with the GA genotype and the AA genotype (P < .001). Mean warfarin daily dose requirements fell by 0.5 to 0.7 mg per decade between the ages of 20 to 90 years. Age, height, and CYP2C9 genotype significantly contributed to S-warfarin and total warfarin clearance, whereas only age and body size significantly contributed to R-warfarin clearance. The multivariate regression model including the variables of age, CYP2C9 and VKORC1 genotype, and height produced the best model for estimating warfarin dose (R2 = 55%). Based upon the data, a new warfarin dosing regimen has been developed. The validity of the dosing regimen was confirmed in a second cohort of patients on warfarin therapy.

BMC Bioinformatics. 2005 Dec 1;6 Suppl 4:S6. Related Articles, Links MicroGen: a MIAME compliant web system for microarray experiment information and workflow management. Burgarella S, Cattaneo D, Pinciroli F, Masseroli M. Bioengineering Department, Politecnico di Milano, Piazza Leonardo da Vinci 32, 20133 Milan, Italy. sarah_burgarella@virgilio.it BACKGROUND: Improvements of bio-nano-technologies and biomolecular techniques have led to increasing production of high-throughput experimental data. Spotted cDNA microarray is one of the most diffuse technologies, used in single research laboratories and in biotechnology service facilities. Although they are routinely performed, spotted microarray experiments are complex procedures entailing several experimental steps and actors with different technical skills and roles. During an experiment, involved actors, who can also be located in a distance, need to access and share specific experiment information according to their roles. Furthermore, complete information describing all experimental steps must be orderly collected to allow subsequent correct interpretation of experimental results. RESULTS: We developed MicroGen, a web system for managing information and workflow in the production pipeline of spotted microarray experiments. It is constituted of a core multi-database system able to store all data completely characterizing different spotted microarray experiments according to the Minimum Information About Microarray Experiments (MIAME) standard, and of an intuitive and user-friendly web interface able to support the collaborative work required among multidisciplinary actors and roles involved in spotted microarray experiment production. MicroGen supports six types of user roles: the researcher who designs and requests the experiment, the spotting operator, the hybridisation operator, the image processing operator, the system administrator, and the generic public user who can access the unrestricted part of the system to get information about MicroGen services. CONCLUSION: MicroGen represents a MIAME compliant information system that enables managing workflow and supporting collaborative work in spotted microarray experiment production.

BMC Cardiovasc Disord. 2004 Sep 28;4(1):16. Related Articles, Links Single nucleotide polymorphisms in the apolipoprotein B and low density lipoprotein receptor genes affect response to antihypertensive treatment. Liljedahl U, Lind L, Kurland L, Berglund L, Kahan T, Syvanen AC. Department of Medical Sciences, Uppsala University, Uppsala University Hospital, Entrance 70, 3rd floor, 751 85 Uppsala, Sweden. Ulrika.Liljedahl@medsci.uu.se BACKGROUND: Dyslipidemia has been associated with hypertension. The present study explored if polymorphisms in genes encoding proteins in lipid metabolism could be used as predictors for the individual response to antihypertensive treatment. METHODS: Ten single nucleotide polymorphisms (SNP) in genes related to lipid metabolism were analysed by a microarray based minisequencing system in DNA samples from ninety-seven hypertensive subjects randomised to treatment with either 150 mg of the angiotensin II type 1 receptor blocker irbesartan or 50 mg of the beta1-adrenergic receptor blocker atenolol for twelve weeks. RESULTS: The reduction in blood pressure was similar in both treatment groups. The SNP C711T in the apolipoprotein B gene was associated with the blood pressure response to irbesartan with an average reduction of 19 mmHg in the individuals carrying the C-allele, but not to atenolol. The C16730T polymorphism in the low density lipoprotein receptor gene predicted the change in systolic blood pressure in the atenolol group with an average reduction of 14 mmHg in the individuals carrying the C-allele. CONCLUSIONS: Polymorphisms in genes encoding proteins in the lipid metabolism are associated with the response to antihypertensive treatment in a drug specific pattern. These results highlight the potential use of pharmacogenetics as a guide for individualised antihypertensive treatment, and also the role of lipids in blood pressure control.

BMC Genet. 2004 May 11;5:9. Related Articles, Links Interval estimation of genetic susceptibility for retrospective case-control studies. Zaykin DV, Meng Z, Ghosh SK. Department of Population Genetics, GlaxoSmithKline Inc, Research Triangle Park NC 27709, USA. dmitri.v.zaykin@gsk.com BACKGROUND: This article describes classical and Bayesian interval estimation of genetic susceptibility based on random samples with pre-specified numbers of unrelated cases and controls. RESULTS: Frequencies of genotypes in cases and controls can be estimated directly from retrospective case-control data. On the other hand, genetic susceptibility defined as the expected proportion of cases among individuals with a particular genotype depends on the population proportion of cases (prevalence). Given this design, prevalence is an external parameter and hence the susceptibility cannot be estimated based on only the observed data. Interval estimation of susceptibility that can incorporate uncertainty in prevalence values is explored from both classical and Bayesian perspective. Similarity between classical and Bayesian interval estimates in terms of frequentist coverage probabilities for this problem allows an appealing interpretation of classical intervals as bounds for genetic susceptibility. In addition, it is observed that both the asymptotic classical and Bayesian interval estimates have comparable average length. These interval estimates serve as a very good approximation to the "exact" (finite sample) Bayesian interval estimates. Extension from genotypic to allelic susceptibility intervals shows dependency on phenotype-induced deviations from Hardy-Weinberg equilibrium. CONCLUSIONS: The suggested classical and Bayesian interval estimates appear to perform reasonably well. Generally, the use of exact Bayesian interval estimation method is recommended for genetic susceptibility, however the asymptotic classical and approximate Bayesian methods are adequate for sample sizes of at least 50 cases and controls.

BMC Med Genet. 2004 Dec 9;5:27. Related Articles, Links Neural network analysis in pharmacogenetics of mood disorders. Serretti A, Smeraldi E. Istituto Scientifico Universitario Ospedale San Raffaele, Department of Neuropsychiatric Sciences, Milano, Italy. serretti.alessandro@hsr.it BACKGROUND: The increasing number of available genotypes for genetic studies in humans requires more advanced techniques of analysis. We previously reported significant univariate associations between gene polymorphisms and antidepressant response in mood disorders. However the combined analysis of multiple gene polymorphisms and clinical variables requires the use of non linear methods. METHODS: In the present study we tested a neural network strategy for a combined analysis of two gene polymorphisms. A Multi Layer Perceptron model showed the best performance and was therefore selected over the other networks. One hundred and twenty one depressed inpatients treated with fluvoxamine in the context of previously reported pharmacogenetic studies were included. The polymorphism in the transcriptional control region upstream of the 5HTT coding sequence (SERTPR) and in the Tryptophan Hydroxylase (TPH) gene were analysed simultaneously. RESULTS: A multi layer perceptron network composed by 1 hidden layer with 7 nodes was chosen. 77.5 % of responders and 51.2% of non responders were correctly classified (ROC area = 0.731-- empirical p value = 0.0082). Finally, we performed a comparison with traditional techniques. A discriminant function analysis correctly classified 34.1 % of responders and 68.1 % of non responders (F = 8.16 p = 0.0005). CONCLUSIONS: Overall, our findings suggest that neural networks may be a valid technique for the analysis of gene polymorphisms in pharmacogenetic studies. The complex interactions modelled through NN may be eventually applied at the clinical level for the individualized therapy.

BMC Med Genet. 2004 Sep 10;5:23. Related Articles, Links What is the impact of the ACE gene insertion/deletion (I/D) polymorphism on the clinical effectiveness and adverse events of ACE inhibitors?--Protocol of a systematic review. Scharplatz M, Puhan MA, Steurer J, Bachmann LM. Horten Centre, University of Zurich, Switzerland. madlaina.scharplatz@usz.ch BACKGROUND: The Angiotensin Converting Enzyme (ACE) insertion/deletion (I/D) polymorphism has received much attention in pharmacogenetic research because observed variations in response to ACE inhibitors might be associated with this polymorphism. Pharmacogenetic testing raises the hope to individualise ACE inhibitor therapy in order to optimise its effectiveness and to reduce adverse effects for genetically different subgroups. However, the extent of its effect modification in patients treated with ACE inhibitors remains inconclusive. Therefore our objective is to quantify the effect modification of the insertion/deletion polymorphism of the angiotensin converting enzyme gene on any surrogate and clinically relevant parameters in patients with cardiovascular diseases, diabetes, renal transplantation and/or renal failure. METHODS: Systematic Review. We will perform literature searches in six electronic databases to identify randomised controlled trials comparing the effectiveness and occurrence of adverse events of ACE inhibitor therapy against placebo or any active treatment stratified by the I/D gene polymorphism. In addition, authors of trials, experts in pharmacogenetics and pharmaceutical companies will be contacted for further published or unpublished data. Hand searching will be accomplished by reviewing the reference lists of all included studies. The methodological quality of included papers will be assessed. Data analyses will be performed in clinically and methodologically cogent subgroups. The results of the quantitative assessment will be pooled statistically where appropriate to produce an estimate of the differences in the effect of ACE inhibitors observed between the three ACE genotypes. DISCUSSION: This protocol describes a strategy to quantify the effect modification of the ACE polymorphism on ACE inhibitors in relevant clinical domains using meta-epidemiological research methods. The results may provide evidence for the usefulness of pharmacogenetic testing for individualised ACE inhibitor therapy. Publication Types: Review

BMJ. 2004 Jul 3;329(7456):4-6. Related Articles, Links Pharmacogenetics--expectations and reality. Tucker G. Publication Types: Editorial

BMJ. 2004 Jun 19;328(7454):1482-6. Related Articles, Links Criteria influencing the clinical uptake of pharmacogenomic strategies. Shah J. Department of Social Policy, London School of Economics and Political Science, London WC2A 2AE. jai.shah-alumni@lse.ac.uk Publication Types: Review

BMJ. 2004 Oct 23;329(7472):966-8. Related Articles, Links Comment in: BMJ. 2004 Dec 4;329(7478):1346. Individual response to treatment: is it a valid assumption? Senn S. Department of Statistics, University of Glasgow, Glasgow G12 8QQ. stephen@stats.gla.ac.uk Publication Types: Review

BMJ. 2005 Feb 12;330(7487):352. Related Articles, Links Comment on: BMJ. 2005 Feb 12;330(7487):350-1. Testing patients to allow tailored drug treatment. Leman P, Greene S. University of Western Australia, Emergency Department, Royal Perth Hospital, Perth, WA, Australia. peter.leman@health.wa.gov.au Publication Types: Comment

BMJ. 2005 Jun 25;330(7506):1508; author reply 1508. Related Articles, Links Comment on: BMJ. 2005 May 7;330(7499):1036-7. Pharmacogenetics and ethnically targeted therapies: racial drugs need to be put in context. Kahn JD. Publication Types: Comment Letter

BMJ. 2005 May 7;330(7499):1036-7. Related Articles, Links Comment in: BMJ. 2005 Jun 25;330(7506):1508; author reply 1508. Pharmacogenetics and ethnically targeted therapies. Rahemtulla T, Bhopal R. Publication Types: Editorial

BMJ. 2005 Nov 19;331(7526):1202. Related Articles, Links Comment on: BMJ. 2005 Nov 5;331(7524):1035-6. Adjuvant trastuzumab for breast cancer: advent of pharmacogenetics raises many issues. Thornton H. Publication Types: Comment Letter

BMJ. 2005 Sep 24;331(7518):656. Related Articles, Links Royal Society predicts that personalised medicines are still decades away. Mayor S. Publication Types: News

Br J Anaesth. 2004 Sep;93(3):440-50. Epub 2004 Jun 25. Related Articles, Links Comment in: Br J Anaesth. 2005 Dec;95(6):728. Principles of pharmacogenetics--implications for the anaesthetist. Iohom G, Fitzgerald D, Cunningham AJ. Department of Anaesthesia and Intensive Care Medicine, Beaumont Hospital, Dublin 9, Ireland. Publication Types: Review

Br J Anaesth. 2005 Dec;95(6):728. Related Articles, Links Comment on: Br J Anaesth. 2004 Sep;93(3):440-50. Re: Iohom G, Fitzgerald D, Cunningham AJ. Principles of pharmacogenetics--implications for the anaesthetist. Br J Anaesth 2004; 93: 440-50. Iohom G, Fitzgerald D, Cunningham AJ. Publication Types: Comment

Br J Cancer. 2004 Aug 16;91(4):678-82. Related Articles, Links UGT1A1 gene variations and irinotecan treatment in patients with metastatic colorectal cancer. Marcuello E, Altes A, Menoyo A, Del Rio E, Gomez-Pardo M, Baiget M. Department of Medical Oncology, Hospital de la Santa Creu i Sant Pau. Avda. S. Antoni M Claret 167, 08025 Barcelona, Spain. SN-38 is the active metabolite of irinotecan and it is metabolised through conjugation by uridine diphosphate glucuronosyl transferase (UGT1A1). The major toxicity of irinotecan therapy is diarrhoea, which has been related to the enzymatic activity of UGT1A1. We examined the influence of the UGT1A1 gene promoter polymorphism in the toxicity profile, in the response rate and in the overall survival (OS) in 95 patients with metastatic colorectal cancer treated with an irinotecan-containing chemotherapy. Genotypes were determined by analysing the sequence of TATA box of UGT1A1 of genomic DNA from the patients. Clinical parameters and genotypes were compared by univariate and multivariate statistical methods. The more frequent adverse effects were asthenia (34 patients), diarrhoea (29 patients) and neutropenia (20 patients). Severe diarrhoea was observed in 7/10 homozygous (70%) and 15/45 heterozygous (33%) in comparison to 7/40 (17%) wild-type patients (P=0.005). These results maintained the statistical significance in logistic regression analysis (P=0.01) after adjustment for other clinical relevant variables. The presence of severe haematological toxicity increased from wild-type patients to UGT1A1(*)28 homozygotes, but without achieving statistical significance. No relationship was found between the UGT1A1(*)28 genotypes and infection, nausea or mucositis. In univariate studies, patients with the UGT1A1(*)28 polymorphism showed a trend to a poorer OS (P=0.09). In the multivariate analysis, the genotype was not related to clinical response or to OS. The role of the UGT1A1 genotype as a predictor of toxicity in cancer patients receiving irinotecan demands the performance of a randomized trial to ascertain whether genotype-adjusted dosages of the drug can help to establish safe and effective doses not only for patients with the UGT1A1(*)28 homozygous genotype but also for those with the most common UGT1A1 6/6 or 6/7 genotype. Publication Types: Clinical Trial

Br J Cancer. 2005 Jul 11;93(1):35-40. Related Articles, Links Prolonged fixed dose rate infusion of gemcitabine with autologous haemopoietic support in advanced pancreatic adenocarcinoma. Bengala C, Guarneri V, Giovannetti E, Lencioni M, Fontana E, Mey V, Fontana A, Boggi U, Del Chiaro M, Danesi R, Ricci S, Mosca F, Del Tacca M, Conte PF. Department of Oncology and Hematology, Division of Medical Oncology, University of Modena and Reggio Emilia, Via del Pozzo71, Modena 41100, Modena, Italy. bengala.carmelo@policlinico.mo.it This study aimed to define the maximum-tolerated dose (MTD) of fixed dose rate (FDR) of gemcitabine (2'-2'-difluorodeoxycitidine) infusion with circulating haemopoietic progenitor support and to evaluate the activity of the treatment. Secondary end points were pharmacokinetic of gemcitabine and difluorodeoxyuridina (dFdU) measured at first course and the activity andexpression profile of cytidine deaminase (CdA) on circulating mononuclear cells. Patients with advanced pancreatic carcinoma received escalating dose of gemcitabine 10 mg m(-2) min(-1) every 2 weeks with circulating haemopoietic progenitor support. First dose level was 3000 mg m(-2) and the doses were increased by 500 mg m(-2) until MTD. In all, 23 patients were enrolled. Toxicities were mild or moderate; the only patient treated at 7000 mg m(-2) died because of toxicity; therefore; the MTD was established at 6500 mg m(-2). The overall response rate was 22.2%. The AUC of gemcitabine showed a dose-dependent increase, while the AUC of dFdU reached a plateau at 4500 mg m(-2). A significant relationship was found between the AUC of dFdU and CdA expression and activity (P<0.05). Moreover, progression rate and survival were significantly related to CdA expression and activity levels. The activity of high-dose gemcitabine is not superior to that reported with less intensive FDR schedules. The predictive role of CdA expression and activity on outcome deserves further investigation.

Br J Clin Pharmacol. 2004 Dec;58(6):601-8. Related Articles, Links The use of pharmacokinetic and pharmacodynamic data in the assessment of drug safety in early drug development. Walker DK. Department of Pharmacokinetics, Dynamics and Metabolism, Pfizer Global Research and Development, Sandwich, Kent CT13 9NJ, UK. don_walker@sandwich.pfizer.com The pharmaceutical industry continues to look for ways to reduce drug candidate attrition throughout the drug discovery and development process. A significant cause of attrition is due to safety issues arising either as a result of animal toxicity testing or in the clinical programme itself. A factor in the assessment of safety during early drug development is the pharmacokinetic profile of the compound. This allows safety data to be considered in the light of systemic drug exposure and therefore permits a quantitative assessment. This is particularly applicable when assessing the risk of a new chemical entity (NCE) in relation to safety parameters such as QT interval prolongation, where free plasma concentrations have been shown to be predictive of this property in relation to potency in preclinical testing. Prior to actual human exposure it is therefore important to be able to predict reliably the pharmacokinetic behaviour of an NCE in order to place such safety findings into a quantitative risk context. The emerging science of pharmacogenetics is likely to further our ability to assess the risk of NCEs to populations and individuals due to genetic variance. The drug metabolizing enzyme CYP2D6 has been recognized as providing the potential to result in widely differing systemic drug exposure in the patient population due to polymorphic expression. Further knowledge is likely to add to our understanding of population differences in exposure and response and aid in the identification of risk factors. One potential strategy for improving the effectiveness of the drug discovery process is to obtain clinical pharmacokinetic data more rapidly in order to assess more accurately the potential for both efficacy and safety of an NCE. Whilst procedures and technologies are available that allow this on the microdose scale, it is important that we recognize potential limitations of these approaches in order that they can be applied beneficially. Publication Types: Review

Br J Clin Pharmacol. 2004 Nov;58(5):452-69. Related Articles, Links Drug development and use in the elderly: search for the right dose and dosing regimen (Parts I and II). Shah RR. Medicines and Healthcare products Regulatory Agency, Market Towers, 1 Nine Elms Lane, Vauxhall, London, UK. rashmi.shah@mhra.gsi.gov.uk Publication Types: Review

Br J Clin Pharmacol. 2004 Nov;58(5):482-7. Related Articles, Links Internet based clinical trial protocols -- as applied to a study of warfarin pharmacogenetics. Lindh JD, Kublickas M, Westgren M, Rane A. Division of Clinical Pharmacology, Karolinksa University Hospital Huddinge, Stockholm, Sweden. jonatan.linh@labmed.ki.se AIMS: To describe and evaluate the use of an Internet-based study protocol in a multicentre study of genetic risk factors in anticoagulant treatment. METHODS: A web-based study protocol, similar to existing anticoagulation medical record systems, was developed for entry of clinical data. It was also supplied with a separate interface for study monitoring. Measures were taken to assure the confidentiality of transferred data. In addition, software modifications were made to enable automated transfer of clinical data from an existing medical record system to the study database.

RESULTS: The system has been in use since March 2002, and at present 39 centres have included 909 patients with a dropout rate of 2.8%. The need for education of participating clinicians has been satisfactorily provided for by means of written instructions and telephone support. CONCLUSIONS: Our study demonstrates the usability of Internet-based data acquisition techniques in a full-scale multicentre clinical trial. The main advantages of such a protocol are automated data validation and standardization, fast data transfer independent of geographical distance, user feedback, synchronization of protocol updates and automatic data formatting facilitating statistical analyses. Safety and accessibility are possibly cumbersome areas and should be addressed duly. Publication Types: Evaluation Studies

Br J Clin Pharmacol. 2005 Jul;60(1):1-4. Related Articles, Links Personalized drug therapy; the genome, the chip and the physician. Lewis LD. Publication Types: Editorial

Br J Clin Pharmacol. 2005 Jun;59(6):670-3. Related Articles, Links How children's responses to drugs differ from adults. Stephenson T. University of Nottingham, Nottingham, UK. terence.stephenson@nottingham.ac.uk Children are not small adults. However, the main thesis of this review will be that children's responses to drugs have much in common with the responses in adults and indeed in other mammals. Often, it is assumed that drug effects differ in children but in reality this perception often arises because the drugs have not been adequately studied in paediatric populations of different ages and with different diseases. There may also be difficulties in measuring small but significant effects because the outcome measures are more difficult to assess in children. In some cases, stage of development can alter the action of, and response to, a drug - a truly age-dependent difference in pharmacodynamics. This may be true of both the desired action and adverse events. Examples are given. Programming by drugs is also a phenomenon almost exclusive to early life, i.e. permanent effects result from a stimulus applied at a sensitive point in development ('critical window'), often in fetal or neonatal life. Again, examples are discussed. Different pathophysiology, different disease variants, different pharmacodynamics, different 'host' response and different adverse drug reactions can all explain why some drugs behave differently in children. However, we need to explore ways to avoid re-inventing the wheel by determining how data from adult animal and human models can help inform research and practice for children. Publication Types: Review

Br J Dermatol. 2005 Nov;153(5):869-73. Related Articles, Links The potential of pharmacogenetics in optimizing the use of methotrexate for psoriasis. Warren RB, Griffiths CE. Department of Dermatology, Royal Liverpool and Broadgreen Hospital, Liverpool L14 3LB, UK. rich1975@aol.com The study of pharmacogenetics will optimize the use of systemic therapies in dermatology. Directed prescription of azathioprine dependent on phenotypic expression of the thiopurine methyltransferase gene is now accepted practice. To some extent other, older drugs have been neglected. We look at the role that pharmacogenetics could play in the use of methotrexate for psoriasis, focusing on known polymorphisms in the folate metabolic pathway. Publication Types: Review

Br J Haematol. 2004 May;125(4):421-34. Related Articles, Links Pharmacogenetic determinants of outcome in acute lymphoblastic leukaemia. Aplenc R, Lange B. Department of Pediatrics, The Children's Hospital of Philadelphia, Philadelphia, PA 19104, USA. raplenc@cceb.med.upenn.edu Present day paediatric co-operative group acute lymphoblastic leukaemia (ALL) protocols cure approximately 80% of patients, a result achieved largely through the use of risk-stratified therapies that employ multiple chemotherapy agents. These risk-based therapies utilize host and leukaemia traits to select the most appropriate therapy. However, these risk-stratified approaches predict therapy response imperfectly and an important fraction of patients experience relapse or therapy-related toxicity. Pharmacogenetics, the study of genetic variations in drug-processing genes and individual responses to drugs, may enable the improved identification of patients at higher risk for either disease relapse or chemotherapy-associated side effects. While the impact of genetic variation in the thiopurine-S-methyltransferase gene on ALL treatment outcome and toxicity has been extensively studied, the role of other polymorphisms remains less well known. This review summarizes current research on the impact of genetic variation in drug-processing genes in paediatric ALL and reviews important methodological and statistical issues presently challenging the field of pharmacogenetics. Publication Types: Review

Br J Pharmacol. 2006 Jan;147 Suppl 1:S89-99. Related Articles, Links Drug metabolism and pharmacogenetics: the British contribution to fields of international significance. Caldwell J. 1Faculty of Medicine, The University of Liverpool, Duncan Building, Daulby Street, Liverpool L69 3GA. The branch of pharmacology we now call 'drug metabolism', the consideration of the enzymes and processess determining the disposition of drugs in the body, emerged in the 1840s on the continent of Europe, but British science made little or no contribution until the 1920s. From this point on, the development of the field through the 20th century was shaped to a very significant extent by a series of influential British workers, whose contributions were of global significance and who can now be seen as fathers of the subject. Since the 1950s, and gaining pace inexorably from the 1970s, the significance of drug metabolism to human therapeutics has been greatly added to by the emergence of pharmacogenetics, clinically important hereditary variation in response to drugs, which underpins the current emphasis on personalised medicine. This review examines the British contributions to both these fields through the lives of seven key contributors and attempts to place their work both in the context of its time and its lasting influence.British Journal of Pharmacology (2006) 147, S89-S99. doi:10.1038/sj.bjp.0706466.

Br J Psychiatry. 2005 Feb;186:91-2. Related Articles, Links Psychiatry and the 'new genetics': hunting for genes for behaviour and drug response. Aitchison KJ, Basu A, McGuffin P, Craig I. Publication Types: Editorial

Braz J Med Biol Res. 2005 Sep;38(9):1389-97. Epub 2005 Aug 26. Related Articles, Links High baseline serum total and LDL cholesterol levels are associated with MDR1 haplotypes in Brazilian hypercholesterolemic individuals of European descent. Rodrigues AC, Rebecchi IM, Bertolami MC, Faludi AA,

Hirata MH, Hirata RD. Departamento de Analises Clinicas e Toxicologicas, Faculdade de Ciencias Farmaceuticas, Universidade de Sao Paulo, Sao Paulo, SP, Brazil. The MDR1 gene encodes the P-glycoprotein, an efflux transporter with broad substrate specificity. P-glycoprotein has raised great interest in pharmacogenetics because it transports a variety of structurally divergent drugs, including lipid-lowering drugs. The synonymous single-nucleotide polymorphism C3435T and the nonsynonymous single-nucleotide polymorphism G2677T/A in MDR1 have been indicated as potential determinants of variability in drug disposition and efficacy. In order to evaluate the effect of G2677T/A and C3435T MDR1 polymorphisms on serum levels of lipids before and after atorvastatin administration, 69 unrelated hypercholesterolemic individuals from Sao Paulo city, Brazil, were selected and treated with 10 mg atorvastatin orally once daily for four weeks. MDR1 polymorphisms were analyzed by PCR-RFLP. C3435T and G2677T polymorphisms were found to be linked. The allelic frequencies for C3435T polymorphism were 0.536 and 0.464 for the 3435C and 3435T alleles, respectively, while for G2677T/A polymorphism allele frequencies were 0.580 for the 2677G allele, 0.384 for the 2677T allele and 0.036 for the 2677A allele. There was no significant relation between atorvastatin response and MDR1 polymorphisms (repeated measures ANOVA; $P > 0.05$). However, haplotype analysis revealed an association between T/T carriers and higher basal serum total (TC) and LDL cholesterol levels (TC: 303 +/- 56, LDL-C: 216 +/- 57 mg/dl, respectively) compared with non-T/T carriers (TC: 278 +/- 28, LDL-C: 189 +/- 24 mg/dl; repeated measures ANOVA/Tukey test; $P < 0.05$). These data indicate that MDR1 polymorphism may have an important contribution to the control of basal serum cholesterol levels in Brazilian hypercholesterolemic individuals of European descent.

Breast Cancer Res. 2004;6(4):148-52. Epub 2004 May 18. Related Articles, Links Report on the 4th European Breast Cancer Conference, Hamburg, Germany, 16-20 March 2004. Senkus-Konefka E, Jassem J. Department of Oncology and Radiotherapy, Medical University of Gdansk, Poland. elsenkus@amg.gda.pl The 4th European Breast Cancer Conference, organized under the auspices of the European Organization for Research and Treatment of Cancer Breast Cancer Group, of the European Breast Cancer Coalition (Europa Donna) and of the European Society of Mastology (EUSOMA), was held in Hamburg, Germany on 16-20 March 2004. The leading theme of the conference was partnership among scientists, clinicians, carers, advocates and patients. The present article provides a brief description of the most important conference presentations on molecular biology, epidemiology, prevention, pathology, diagnosis and treatment at all stages of breast cancer. Publication Types: Congresses

Breast Cancer. 2005;12(2):73-85. Related Articles, Links Development of pharmacogenomic markers to select preoperative chemotherapy for breast cancer. Pusztai L, Symmans FW, Hortobagyi GN. Department of Breast Medical Oncology, University of Texas M. D. Anderson Cancer Center, Houston, TX 77030-4009, USA. lpusztai@mdanderson.org Individualized selection of the most effective adjuvant (or neoadjuvant) chemotherapy for breast cancer based on the molecular characteristics of the tumor could improve the risk:benefit ratio of current therapies. It could also streamline the development of new regimens for those who are unlikely to benefit from existing drugs. It is expected that combinations of markers will be more informative to predict response than any single gene and may yield regimen-specific predictors. Novel molecular analytical tools, particularly transcriptional profiling, provide a method to test this hypothesis. Several small exploratory studies have shown encouraging results. This article reviews recent progress in this field including experience from the breast cancer pharmacogenomic marker discovery program at the Nellie B. Connally Breast Center of the University of Texas M. D. Anderson Cancer Center. This manuscript is based on a presentation that was given during the Presidential Symposium of the annual meeting of the Japanese Breast Cancer Society in 2004. Publication Types: Review

Brief Funct Genomic Proteomic. 2002 Feb;1(1):66-79. Related Articles, Links Pharmacogenetics of cardiovascular drugs. Johnson JA, Humma LM. Center for Pharmacogenomics, University of Florida, USA. johnson@cop.ufl.edu Pharmacogenetics is a field aimed at understanding the genetic contribution to inter-patient variability in drug efficacy and toxicity. Treatment of cardiovascular disease is, in most cases, guided by evidence from well-controlled clinical trials. Given the solid scientific basis for the treatment of most cardiovascular diseases, it is common for patients with a given disease to be treated in essentially the same manner. Thus, the clinical trials have been very informative about treating large groups of patients with a given disease, but are slightly less informative about the treatment of individual patients. Pharmacogenetics and pharmacogenomics have the potential of taking the information derived from large clinical trials and further refining it to select the drugs with the greatest likelihood for benefit, and least likelihood for harm, in individual patients, based on their genetic make-up. In this paper, the current literature on cardiovascular pharmacogenetics is emphasised, and how the use of pharmacogenetic/pharmacogenomic information may be particularly useful in the future in the treatment of cardiovascular diseases is also highlighted. Publication Types: Review

Brief Funct Genomic Proteomic. 2003 Apr;2(1):4-6. Related Articles, Links Comment on: Brief Funct Genomic Proteomic. 2003 Apr;2(1):7-20. Platform technologies for microarray analysis. Freeman T. Publication Types: Comment Editorial

Brief Funct Genomic Proteomic. 2003 Apr;2(1):7-20. Related Articles, Links Comment in: Brief Funct Genomic Proteomic. 2003 Apr;2(1):4-6. Resource and hardware options for microarray-based experimentation. Affara NA. Department of Pathology, University of Cambridge, UK. na106@cam.ac.uk DNA microarray technology permits the study of biological systems and processes on a genome-wide scale. Arrays based on cDNA clones, oligonucleotides and genomic clones have been developed for investigations of gene expression, genetic analysis and genomic changes associated with disease. Over the past 3-4 years, microarrays have become more widely available to the research community. This has occurred through increased commercial availability of custom and generic arrays and the development of robotic equipment that has enabled array printing and analysis facilities to be established in academic research institutions. This brief review examines the public and commercial resources, the microarray fabrication and data capture and analysis equipment currently available to the user. Publication Types: Review

Brief Funct Genomic Proteomic. 2005 Feb;3(4):303-21. Related Articles, Links Expression genomics and drug development: towards predictive pharmacology. Liu ET. Genome Institute of Singapore, 60 Biopolis Street, #02-01, 128672, Singapore. liue@gis.a-star.edu.sg Expression genomics can be defined as the study of the dynamic transciptome and its regulatory elements. Technologies are available that can assess transcripts on a genome-wide scale over time and across many samples. This comprehensive and dynamic database is being used to decipher signalling pathways and to identify new biomarkers and targets. Biomarkers emerging from these studies have prognostic potential and can be used to predict therapeutic outcome. The multiplex nature of this approach not only telescopes the time to discovery, but also allows for detection of complex interactions. Taken together, these capabilities, if carefully used, can speed drug development, enhance the identification of potent drug combinations and identify patient populations that will benefit from these new drugs. Publication Types: Review

Bull Med Ethics. 2004 Dec-2005 Jan;(204):9-11. Related Articles, Links Ethical, legal and social implications of genetic testing. EC Expert Group.

Bundesgesundheitsblatt Gesundheitsforschung Gesundheitsschutz. 2004 May;47(5):487-92. Related Articles, Links [Genetics of depression. Current knowledge and perspectives] [Article in German] Maier W. Universitat Bonn, Bonn. Wolfgang.Maier@ukb.uni-bonn.de Depression is a common disorder (lifetime prevalence nearly 20% in industrialized countries) that presents in two etiologically different forms (unipolar depression, bipolar disorder). Both forms are subject to a genetic influence, which is stronger in bipolar disorder. Unipolar depression is also strongly influenced by nongenetic environmental factors (e. g., traumas, socialization, critical life events). There is strong evidence for a gene-- environmental interaction in unipolar depression. The search for genes was recently very successful in bipolar disorder. There is currently no evidence for disposition genes with strong effects. The prediction of response to selective serotonin-reuptake inhibitors (SSRI) by genetic markers presents currently the best confirmed molecular-genetic findings for unipolar depression. Complicating factors are gene--environmental interaction, only small to modest effects of disposition genes, and putative epigenetic mechanisms. Publication Types: Review

Can J Anaesth. 2005 Oct;52(8):806-21. Related Articles, Links [Genetic polymorphism and drug interactions: their importance in the treatment of pain] [Article in French] Samer CF, Piguet V, Dayer P, Desmeules JA. Service de pharmacologie et toxicologie cliniques et Centre multidisciplinaire d'etude et de traitement de la douleur, Hopitaux Universitaires de Geneve, Geneve, Suisse. Caroline.Samer@hcuge.ch OBJECTIVES: To evaluate the impact of certain genetic polymorphisms on variable responses to analgesics SOURCES: Systematic review, by means of a structured computerized search in the Medline database (1966-

2004). KEY WORDS: pharmacogenetics, polymorphism, cytochrome P450 (CYP), glycoprotein P (P-gp), pain, antalgics, opiates, morphine, codeine, tramadol, non-steroidal anti-inflammatory drugs (NSAID). Articles in English and French were selected. References in relevant articles were also retrieved. MAIN FINDINGS: Most analgesics are metabolized by CYP isoenzymes subject to genetic polymorphism. NSAIDs are metabolized by CYP2C9; opioids described as "weak" (codeine, tramadol), anti-depressants and dextromethorphan are metabolized by CYP2D6 and some "potent" opioids (buprenorphine, methadone or fentanyl) by CYP3A4/5. After the usual doses have been administered, drug toxicity or, on the contrary, therapeutic ineffectiveness may occur, depending on polymorphism and the substance. Drug interactions mimicking genetic defects because of the existence of CYP inhibitors and inducers, also contribute to the variable response to analgesics.Some opioids are substrates of P-gp, a transmembrane transporter also subject to genetic polymorphism. However, P-gp could only play a minor modulating role in man on the central effects of morphine, methadone and fentanyl. CONCLUSION: In the near future, pharmacogenetics should enable us to optimize therapeutics by individualizing our approach to analgesic drugs and making numerous analgesics safer and more effective. The clinical usefulness of these individualized approaches will have to be demonstrated by appropriate pharmacoeconomic studies and analyses. Publication Types: Meta-Analysis Review

Cancer Biol Ther. 2004 Jun;3(6):566-7. Epub 2004 Jun 24. Related Articles, Links Comment on: Cancer Biol Ther. 2004 Jun;3(6):561-5. Pharmacogenomics on gastric cancer. Katoh M, Katoh M. M and M Medical BioInformatics, Narashino, Japan. Gastric cancer is one of most common malignancies in the world. 5-fluoroyracil, CPT-11, TS-1, Paclitaxel and Docetaxel are used as chemotherapeutic agents for advanced gastric cancer, although endoscopic mucosal resection and surgical gastrectomy are potentially curative treatments. Most important problems associated chemotherapeutic agents are side effects and drug resistances. TSG101, implicated in membrane trafficking and transcriptional regulation, is upregulated in gastric cancer with multidrug resistant phenotype. Shen et al reported that transient transfection of TSG101 siRNA reduced the expression level of TSG101 protein as well as resistance to vincristine and adriamycin in gastric cancer cells. Bioinformatics, microarray analyses, SNP typing, and high-throughput functional analyses are applied for pharmacogenomics in the post-genome era. Therapeutics based on the genotyping of each patient is the future goal of personalized medicine (or tailor-made medicine) for gastric cancer. Publication Types: Comment Editorial

Cancer Cell. 2004 Aug;6(2):105-7. Related Articles, Links Comment on: Cancer Cell. 2004 Aug;6(2):129-37. Mining our ABCs: pharmacogenomic approach for evaluating transporter function in cancer drug resistance. Ross DD, Doyle LA. University of Maryland Greenebaum Cancer Center, Program in Experimental Therapeutics, University of Maryland School of Medicine, Departments of Internal Medicine and Pathology, Baltimore, MD 21201 USA. dross@som.umaryland.edu The association of transporter proteins and cancer drug resistance has been known for approximately 25 years, with recent discoveries pointing to an ever-increasing number of ATP binding cassette (ABC) transporter proteins involved with the response of cancer cells to pharmacotherapy. As reported in this issue of Cancer Cell, Szakacs et al. couple quantitative, real-time PCR assays for all 48 human ABC transporters with chemosensitivity information mined from the NCI-60 cancer cell line database. Predictions of transporter involvement in drug effect were validated in selected cases, and furthermore produced novel leads relating ABC transporter expression and chemoresistance or chemosensitivity. Publication Types: Comment

Cancer Chemother Pharmacol. 2004 May;53(5):445-51. Related Articles, Links Dihydropyrimidine dehydrogenase pharmacogenetics in the Taiwanese population. Hsiao HH, Yang MY, Chang JG, Liu YC, Liu TC, Chang CS, Chen TP, Lin SF. Division of Hematology-Oncology, Department of Internal Medicine, Kaohsiung Medical University Hospital, San-Ming District, Kaohsiung, Taiwan. BACKGROUND/PURPOSE: 5-Fluorouracil (5-FU) remains the most frequently used chemotherapy agent in various human cancers. Over 80% of the 5-FU administered is metabolized by dihydropyrimidine dehydrogenase (DPD) in the liver. However, mutations in the DPD gene have been found to be associated with low DPD activity causing severe complications. The aim of this study was to determine the frequency of 11 known mutations in Taiwanese subjects and the relationship between mutation and DPD level. METHODS: Samples from a total of 300 subjects were investigated in this study. The PCR-RFLP method was used to identify 11 mutations of the DPYD gene, including 62G>A, 74A>G, 85T>C (DPYD*9A), 812delT, 1003G>T, 1156G>T, 1627A>G (DPYD*5), 1714C>G, 1897delC (DPYD*3), 2194G>A (DPYD*6), and IVS14+1G>A (DPYD*2A). DPD protein levels were determined using a DPD ELISA kit. RESULTS: Four mutations, including 74A>G, 85T>C (DPYD*9A), 1627A>G (DPYD*5), and 2194G>A (DPYD*6), were found in our 300 samples. The following mutations were not detected: 62G>A, 812delT, 1003G>T, 1156G>T, 1714C>G, 1897delC (DPYD*3), and IVS14+1G>A (DPYD*2A). The phenotype analysis by DPD protein level indicated that the 1627A>G (DPYD*5) mutation was not associated with the DPD protein level and might be a polymorphism in the DPD gene. The DPD level was also not correlated with gender. CONCLUSION: No significant correlations between these 11 mutations and DPD protein level were found indicating that examination of these mutations is insufficient to provide a high-value prediction of the 5-FU pharmacogenetic syndrome in Taiwanese. Genotype and phenotype analysis indicated the 1627A>G (DPYD*5) mutation to be a polymorphism.

Cancer Chemother Pharmacol. 2005 Oct;56(4):351-7. Epub 2005 May 13. Related Articles, Links Metabolic profile of XK469 (2(R)-[4-(7-chloro-2-quinoxalinyl)oxyphenoxy]-propionic acid; NSC698215) in patients and in vitro: low potential for active or toxic metabolites or for drug-drug interactions. Anderson LW, Collins JM, Klecker RW, Katki AG, Parchment RE, Boinpally RR, LoRusso PM, Ivy SP. Food and Drug Administration, WO Bldg 64, Rm 2014, 10903 New Hampshire Avenue, HFD-902, Silver Spring, MD 20993, USA. ANDERSONL@cder.fda.gov As part of an ongoing phase 1 study, we studied the excretion of XK469 and its metabolism in patients and in vitro. Five primary metabolites were identified by HPLC/MS/MS. An oxidized product formed by cytosolic aldehyde oxidase was the predominant species both in urine and human hepatocytes in vitro. Conjugates of XK469 with glycine, taurine, and glucuronic acid, as well as the microsomal product, 4-oxo-XK469, were also found in urine and in vitro, but none were major contributors to the mass balance for XK469 elimination. Based upon the relative concentrations circulating in plasma, systemic exposure to parent drug was 100-fold higher than for the metabolites. Thus, both toxicity and efficacy of XK469 are most likely to be produced by the parent molecule, rather than the metabolites. Urinary recovery of parent drug was low (2% of dose in 24 h), partly because of the long half-life of XK469 (approximately 3 days). In addition, the metabolite profile in urine indicates that only 25% of the XK469-derived material was unchanged drug. Thus, urinary excretion was not a major factor in XK469 elimination. Variations in systemic exposure to XK469 will be strongly influenced by factors that alter the activity of aldehyde oxidase, including pharmacogenetics, enzyme inhibition, and enzyme induction, but no specific modifiers have been reported. The multiday half-life of XK469 hampered our ability to obtain a complete mass balance, and the possibility exists that other routes, such as biliary excretion, may also play a substantial role in XK469 disposition. Publication Types: Clinical Trial Clinical Trial, Phase I

Cancer Epidemiol Biomarkers Prev. 2004 May;13(5):889-93. Related Articles, Links Polymorphisms in PTGS1 (=COX-1) and risk of colorectal polyps. Ulrich CM, Bigler J, Sparks R, Whitton J, Sibert JG, Goode EL, Yasui Y, Potter JD. Cancer Prevention Research Program, Fred Hutchinson Cancer Research Center, 1100 Fairview Avenue N, M4-B402, Seattle, WA 98109-1024, USA. nulrich@fhcrc.org Two isoforms of prostaglandin H synthase (PTGS = COX) are key enzymes in prostaglandin synthesis and primary targets for aspirin and other non-steroidal anti-inflammatory drugs (NSAIDs). Use of aspirin or other NSAIDs is associated with a lower risk and reduced recurrence of colorectal adenomas, established precursors of adenocarcinoma. This study investigated risk of colorectal adenomatous and hyperplastic polyps associated with several polymorphisms in the coding region of PTGS1. Within the Minnesota polyp case-control study, patients with colorectal adenomatous (n = 521) or hyperplastic (n = 194) polyps and n = 621 polyp-free controls were genotyped for four PTGS1 polymorphisms (R8W, L15-L16del, P17L, L237M); these had been predicted to affect protein function based on sequence-homology software. Age- and sex-adjusted odds ratios (ORs) and 95% confidence intervals (CIs) were computed. Whereas there was no appreciable difference in adenoma or hyperplastic polyp risk associated with R8W, P17L, and L237M, an increased risk was observed for individuals heterozygous for the L15-L16del polymorphism (OR = 3.6, 95% CI 1.2-11.2). The variant L15-L16del allele appeared to be associated with a stronger increase in adenoma risk among nonusers of aspirin/other NSAIDs. The reduced risk observed with aspirin/other NSAID use was limited to those wild type for P17L [PP users: OR = 0.6 (0.5-0.8) versus PP nonusers: 1.0 (referent) (P interaction = 0.03)]. To our knowledge, this study represents the first investigation of polymorphisms in PTGS1 and risk of colorectal polyps. The L15-L16del variant allele may result in an increased risk of colorectal adenomas, whereas P17L may be relevant to the pharmacogenetics of aspirin. These preliminary findings require confirmation in larger studies of colorectal neoplasia.

Cancer Epidemiol Biomarkers Prev. 2006 Mar;15(3):502-8. Related Articles, Links Prostacyclin synthase and arachidonate 5-lipoxygenase polymorphisms and risk of colorectal polyps. Poole EM, Bigler J, Whitton J, Sibert JG, Potter JD, Ulrich CM. Cancer Prevention Program, Fred Hutchinson Cancer Research Center, 1100 Fairview Avenue North, M4-B402, Seattle, WA 98109-1024, USA. Prostacyclin synthase (PGIS) and arachidonate 5-lipoxygenase (ALOX5) are enzymes relevant to prostaglandin and leukotriene synthesis, both important pathways for colon cancer risk. We hypothesized that genetic variation altering the function of these enzymes would modify risk of colorectal polyps. In a Minnesota-based case-control study of adenomatous (n = 517) or hyperplastic (n = 192) polyps versus polyp-free controls (n = 618), we investigated the role of promoter repeat polymorphisms in PGIS and ALOX5 as well as ALOX5 -1700 G>A. Having fewer than six repeats on both PGIS alleles (<6R/<6R) was associated with an increased risk of adenomas compared with the 6R/6R (wild-type) genotype (OR, 1.90; 95% CI, 1.09-3.30). Having more repeats (>6R/> or =6R) reduced risk (OR, 0.73; 95% CI, 0.40-1.35; P(trend) = 0.03). In allele-based analyses, fewer repeats were associated with a modestly increased risk of adenomas and perhaps hyperplastic polyps. There were no risk differences for either the ALOX5 VNTR or -1700 G>A polymorphisms. Associations with regular use of aspirin or other nonsteroidal anti-inflammatory drugs (NSAIDs) differed by PGIS genotype. Among individuals with at least one wild-type allele, NSAID use was associated with a decreased risk; however, those with fewer PGIS repeats (<6R/<6R) did not benefit (P(interaction) = 0.06). There was also evidence of an interaction between the COX-2 -765 G>C and ALOX5 -1700 G>A genotypes (P(interaction) = 0.07). The PGIS promoter polymorphism may affect risk of colorectal polyps and modify the effects of NSAID use on polyp risk. A more comprehensive investigation of genetic variability in prostaglandin synthesis in relation to risk of colorectal neoplasia and NSAID pharmacogenetics is warranted.

Cancer J. 2005 Jul-Aug;11(4):314-23. Related Articles, Links Pharmacogenetics and pediatric cancer. Bomgaars L, McLeod HL. Department of Medicine, Baylor College of Medicine, Houston, Texas 77030, USA. lboomgaars@txccc.org The great advances in therapeutic success for childhood cancers have provided the impetus for strategies to avoid serious systemic toxicities from chemotherapy. This review describes the impact of genetic mutations in drug metabolism pathways on the toxicity of anticancer agents. Although many polymorphisms have been related to toxicity in adults, these associations are less well defined in children. The role of genetic polymorphisms in MTHFR, TYMS, TPMT, and UGT1A1 in influencing drug toxicity is reviewed. Better understanding of the pharmacogenetic determinants of drug metabolism or pharmacologic cofactors may allow for prospective identification of potential patients who are at increased risk for toxicity, allowing for dose optimization and resulting in a decrease in toxic risk while maximizing efficacy. Publication Types: Review

Cancer J. 2005 Jul-Aug;11(4):324-30. Related Articles, Links New approaches to drug development in pediatric oncology. Adamson PC, Blaney SM. The Children's Hospital of Philadelphia, University of Pennsylvania School of Medicine, Philadelphia, PA 19104, USA. adamsonp@mail.med.upenn.edu This article reviews the changing paradigm of new drug development for childhood cancer. Although there have been dramatic improvements in the treatment and outcome for childhood cancer over the past 50 years, in some cancers, only limited progress has been made. New strategies to improve the outcome for poor-prognosis tumors and to minimize the long-term sequelae associated with therapy are required. Such strategies include a new pediatric-specific initiative for the preclinical testing of anticancer drugs for childhood malignancies, and ongoing research into the molecular heterogeneity of childhood tumors to facilitate the evaluation of molecularly targeted drugs. In addition, continued investigation into the genetic basis underlying interpatient variability in drug exposure and response is a priority. The goal of these initiatives is to improve the overall outcome for childhood cancer while minimizing the short and long-term sequelae associated with current treatment strategies. Publication Types: Review

Cancer J. 2005 May-Jun;11(3):175-88. Related Articles, Links Tailored therapy of colorectal cancer: results, challenges and future directions. Gasparini G, Longo R, Torino F, Barone C, Toffoli G. Division of Medical Oncology, S. Filippo Neri Hospital, Universita Cattolica del Sacro Cuore, Rome, Italy. gasparini.oncology@tiscalinet.it Colorectal cancer is a leading cause of cancer mortality and morbidity. Despite the recent results of systemic chemotherapy, more than 40% of patients with advanced cancer still do not achieve substantial benefits with cytotoxic agents. Therefore, new tailored strategies are warranted to improve the probability of disease control. The rationale for this approach is based on the identification of the in vivo interactions among patient's characteristics, disease physiopathology, and drug pharmacodynamics and pharmacokinetics.Genomic and proteomic technologies may clarify the mechanisms involved in cancer growth and progression in each single patient and in the molecular basis of interindividual differences of anticancer drugs in terms of efficacy and toxicity. Despite the recent encouraging data, the clinical use of targeted therapy is hampered by several questions, such as: optimal biologic dose and schedule, lack of predictive surrogate biomarkers, and modalities of combination with chemotherapy/radiotherapy. Further efforts are needed to improve the reliability of genomic and proteomic technologies, in particular regarding their standardization and widespread availability. These unsolved issues make tailored therapy an open challenge. Publication Types: Review

Cancer Lett. 2004 May 10;208(1):1-33. Related Articles, Links Common gene polymorphisms, cancer progression and prognosis. Loktionov A. MRC Dunn Human Nutrition Unit, Wellcome Trust/MRC Building, Hills Road, Cambridge CB2 2XY, UK. alex1@supanet.com Neoplastic growth was often regarded as an autonomous process driven by uncontrolled expansion of malignant cell population. This view is now being transformed as it becomes apparent that basically normal regulatory and metabolic mechanisms comprising subcellular processes as well as homo- and heterotypic cell interactions are extensively used by growing tumours throughout all stages of their development. Therefore the role of normal genetic variation emerges as a major factor determining different aspects of neoplastic growth and eventually outcome of the disease. This review is focused on polymorphisms in the genes encoding products acting at post-initiation stages of tumour development. Its four main sections are devoted to gene polymorphisms affecting: (i) growth control at the cellular level (cell proliferation, differentiation and death); (ii) factors involved in tumour invasion and metastasis (immune and inflammatory responses, extracellular matrix remodelling, angiogenesis and cell adhesion); (iii) action of hormones and vitamines on growing tumours; (iv) outcome of cancer therapy (cancer pharmacogenetics). Although active research in this field has been started only recently, some directions (e.g. cancer pharmacogenetics) already demonstrate impressive achievements. At the same time the reliability of results reported by many groups remains questionable mostly due to insufficient statistical power of the studies and often random choice of polymorphisms. It is evident that large studies based upon combined analysis of groups of genes within relevant regulatory and metabolic pathways have a much higher potential value in terms of unravelling prognostically important individual polymorphism profiles. Publication Types: Review

Cancer Lett. 2005 Apr 28;221(2):123-9. Related Articles, Links Glutathione S-transferase genotypes and cancer risk. Parl FF. Department of Pathology and Vanderbilt Ingram Cancer Center, Vanderbilt University Medical Center, Nashville, TN 37232, USA. fritz.parl@vanderbilt.edu Over 500 studies have examined the association of genetic variants of glutathione S-transferases with various malignancies yielding inconsistent results. The genotyping was based on PCR assays that identified the GSTM1 and GSTT1 null (-/-) genotypes but did not distinguish homozygous wild-type +/+ and heterozygous +/- individuals. Complete GSTM1 and GSTT1 genotyping can be accomplished by recently developed assays [Cancer Res. 64 (2004) 1233-1236; Pharmacogenetics 10 (2000) 557-565] that allow the definition of +/+, +/-, and -/- genotypes by separate identification of the respective GSTM1 and GSTT1 wild-type and null alleles. Application of the new GSTM1 assay to a breast cancer case-control study revealed that the relative risk of breast cancer for the +/+ genotype compared to the -/- genotype was 2.83 (95% confidence interval 1.45-5.59; P=0.002), suggesting a protective effect of the GSTM1 deletion [Cancer Res. 64 (2004) 1233-1236]. Regardless of the explanation for the association between the +/+ genotype and increased breast cancer risk, these results warrant application of true GSTM1 and GSTT1 genotyping to additional or previously analyzed groups with breast cancer or other malignancies. Publication Types: Review

Cancer Lett. 2006 Mar 8;234(1):4-33. Epub 2006 Feb 28. Related Articles, Links Implications of genetic polymorphisms in drug transporters for pharmacotherapy. Kerb R. Department of Medical Science, AstraZeneca, RandD, Pepparedsleden 1, SE-43183 Molndal, Sweden. Drug transporters are increasingly recognized as a key determinant of drug disposition and response. It is now widely appreciated that expression of the ATP-dependent efflux transporter, MDR1 (ABCB1, P-glycoprotein), in organs such as the gastrointestinal tract, liver and kidney significantly alters the extent of drug absorption and excretion. Moreover, expression of MDR1 at the level of the blood-brain barrier limits the entry of many drugs into the central nervous system. Given such an important role of MDR1 in the drug disposition process, it is not surprising to see increasing focus on the role of single nucleotide polymorphisms (SNPs) in this transporter as a potential determinant of interindividual variability in drug disposition and pharmacological response. However, drug transport is often the result of the concerted action of efflux and uptake pumps located both in the basolateral and apical membranes of epithelial cells. A growing list of membrane-spanning proteins involved in the in- or outward transport of a large variety of drugs has been recognized and characterized over the past few years in almost all tissues, including organic anion and cation transporters (OAT, OCT, solute carrier family SLC22A), organic anion transport proteins (OATP, solute carrier family SLCO, formerly SLC21A), and MRPs (ABCCs), other members of the ATP-binding cassette family. We are just beginning to appreciate their role for drug delivery and disposition and the contribution of genetic polymorphisms in these transport proteins to interindividual variability in the efficacy and safety for pharmacotherapy. This review summarizes the consequences of inherited differences in drug transport for pharmacotherapy. With the main focus on ABCB1, an update of recent advances is given and clinically relevant examples are used to illustrate how heritable differential drug transport can help to explain individual variability in drug response. The pharmacogenetics of other transporters is briefly introduced.

Cancer Lett. 2006 Mar 8;234(1):90-106. Epub 2005 Dec 15. Related Articles, Links Role of pharmacogenetics in irinotecan therapy. de Jong FA, de Jonge MJ, Verweij J, Mathijssen RH. Department of Medical Oncology, Daniel den Hoed Cancer Center, Erasmus University Medical Center Rotterdam, Groene Hilledijk 301, 3075 EA Rotterdam, The Netherlands. In the treatment of advanced colorectal cancer, irinotecan has become one of the most important drugs, despite its sometimes unpredictable adverse effects. To understand why some patients experience severe adverse effects (diarrhea and neutropenia), while others do not, the metabolic pathways of this drug have to be unraveled in detail. Individual variation in expression of several phase I and phase II metabolizing enzymes and ABC-transporters involved in irinotecan metabolism and excretion, at least partly explains the observed pharmacokinetic interpatient variability. Although the difference in expression-level of these proteins to a certain amount is explained by physiologic and environmental factors, the presence of specific genetic determinants also does influence their expression and function. In this review, the role of genetic polymorphisms in the main enzyme-systems (carboxylesterase, cytochrome P450 3A, and uridine diphosphate-glucuronosyltransferase) and ABC-transporters (ABCB1, ABCC2, and ABCG2) involved in irinotecan metabolism, are discussed. Since at this moment the field of pharmacogenetics and pharmacogenomics is rapidly expanding and simultaneously more rapid and cost-effective screening methods are emerging, a wealth of future data is expected to enrich our knowledge of the genetic basis of irinotecan metabolism. Eventually, this may help to truly individualize the dosing of this (and other) anti-cancer agent(s), using a personal genetic profile of the most relevant enzymes for every patient.

Cancer Sci. 2006 Jan;97(1):16-24. Related Articles, Links Japanese single nucleotide polymorphism database for 267 possible drug-related genes. Iida A, Saito S, Sekine A, Takahashi A, Kamatani N, Nakamura Y. Laboratories for Pharmacogenetics, RIKEN SNP Research Center, c/o Institute of Medical Science, The University of Tokyo, 4-6-1 Shirokanedai, Minato-ku, Tokyo 108-8639, Japan. To establish 'personalized medicines' that can provide the right drug at the appropriate dose for each individual patient on the basis of genetic background, we have been building the infrastructure for a Japanese single nucleotide polymorphism (SNP) database of the genes encoding various enzymes, transporters and receptors that are involved in the metabolism, transportation and action of drugs. We have so far screened a genomic region of 4,068.3 kb, and identified a total of 7,552 genetic variations, including 6,733 SNP and 819 genetic variations of other types among 267 genes in Japanese populations. Interestingly, among the 212 non-synonymous substitutions we found, six would be considered to be nonsense mutations. In this review, we focused on the molecular features of the non-synonymous substitutions and insertion/deletion polymorphisms within coding regions detected in drug-related gene loci. The database established in this study makes us confident of achieving one of our goals, which is establishment of personalized medicine. (Cancer Sci 2006; 97: 16-24). Publication Types: Review

Cancer Treat Rev. 2005 Apr;31(2):90-105. Related Articles, Links Pharmacology of oxaliplatin and the use of pharmacogenomics to individualize therapy. Kweekel DM, Gelderblom H, Guchelaar HJ. Department of Clinical Pharmacy and Toxicology, Leiden University Medical Center, P.O. Box 9600, 2300 RC Leiden, The Netherlands. D.M.Kweekel@lumc.nl Oxaliplatin is a relatively new platinum analogue that is currently used in pharmacotherapy of metastatic colorectal cancer. Its dose-limiting toxicity is sensory neuropathy, which can be modulated by infusion of calcium and magnesium. Oxaliplatin exerts its anti-tumour effects by platinum-adduct formation, binding to cellular proteins and possibly interfering with RNA synthesis as well. If they are not removed from DNA, oxaliplatin adducts are lethal. Cellular defense mechanisms prevent adduct formation (e.g., glutathione-S-transferase) or remove DNA adducts (e.g., nucleotide excision repair). Depending on the activity of necessary enzymes in these cellular defense pathways, oxaliplatin induced damage varies from one individual to another. There is growing evidence that polymorphisms in genes coding for DNA repair enzymes and metabolic inactivation routes contribute to the interindividual differences in anti-tumour efficacy and toxicity of oxaliplatin. Single nucleotide polymorphisms (SNPs) may yield inactive enzymes, or increased gene transcription and hence increased enzyme production. This review covers findings of recent investigations on the associations of SNPs and clinical outcome after oxaliplatin chemotherapy in metastatic colorectal cancer. Publication Types: Review

Cardiovasc Res. 2004 Oct 1;64(1):32-9. Related Articles, Links Pharmacogenomics of heart failure -- focus on drug disposition and action. Cascorbi I, Paul M, Kroemer HK. Department of Pharmacology, Peter Holtz Research Center of Pharmacology and Experimental Therapeutics, Ernst

Moritz Arndt University, Greifswald, Germany. Heart failure represents the composite endpoint of various cardiovascular disorders. Advanced pharmacotherapy resulted in significant improvement of overall survival, however with highly variable outcome, possibly due to genetic modification of drug disposition and action. This review highlights the role of genetic polymorphisms in systems responsible for disposition of drugs, used in heart failure patients (e.g. the polymorphic drug metabolizing enzymes such as cytochrome P450 enzymes, as well as polymorphic ATP-membrane transporters like P-glycoprotein (P-gp)). In addition, genetic variants in physiological systems, being target of drug action, particularly beta-adrenergic receptors, the renin-angiotensin-aldosterone system (RAAS)- and endothelin system, and the endothelial nitrogene monoxide (NO) synthase are reviewed. The current situation in pharmacogenomics of heart failure with respect to drug disposition and action is characterized by multiple studies investigating single components of a complex system. Therefore, overall conclusions regarding treatment and/or outcome of heart failure patients based on individual genetic traits require large prospective trials allowing for simultaneous assessment of multiple genetic variants in different systems. Using advanced screening technologies, such trials can be carried out in the near future. Publication Types: Review

Cardiovasc Res. 2005 Aug 15;67(3):419-25. Related Articles, Links Proarrhythmia as a pharmacogenomic entity: a critical review and formulation of a unifying hypothesis. Roden DM. Department of Medicine, and Oates Institute for Experimental Therapeutics, Vanderbilt University School of Medicine, 532 Medical Research Building I, Nashville, TN 37232, United States. dan.roden@vanderbilt.edu Proarrhythmia represents an extreme example of the phenomenon that drug effects vary widely among individuals. Studies of mechanisms leading to proarrhythmia have had important implications for understanding arrhythmogenesis, rational use of antiarrhythmic therapies, selection of patients for specific therapies, and drug development. In addition, because proarrhythmia often seems to develop in the absence of clear risk predictors, a role for genetics in predisposing to this adverse drug reaction has been postulated. This review presents mechanisms whereby genetic factors may contribute to variable drug responses and describes our current understanding of how these mechanisms play a role in proarrhythmia. A unifying hypothesis is presented: physiologic processes (such as drug elimination or cardiac repolarization) include multiple redundancies, and congenital or acquired absence of such redundancies--due to disease, interacting drugs, or genetic makeup--may confer no baseline phenotype, but nevertheless enhance susceptibility to unusual drug responses. Publication Types: Review

Cas Lek Cesk. 2005;144(2):134-5. Related Articles, Links [Pharmacogenetics from the aspect of the Coordinating Group for Pharmacogenetics of OECD] [Article in Czech] Brdicka R. Laborator molekularni genetiky UHKT, Praha. molgen@uhkt.cz

Cas Lek Cesk. 2006;145(2):148-52; discussion 152-3. Related Articles, Links [Pharmacogenetics of chronic heart failure--beta blockers] [Article in Czech] Vasku A, Spinarova L, Pavkova-Goldbergova M, Spinar J, Soucek M, Vitovec J. Ustav patologicke fyziologie LF MU, Brno.

avasku@med.muni.cz BACKGROUND: Activation of the renin-angiotensin (RAS) cascade and sympathetic nervous systems adversely affect heart failure progression. ACE deletion allele (ACE D) of insertion/deletion polymorphism in the gene coding for angiotensin-1 converting enzyme is associated with increased renin-angiotensin activation. The aim of the study was to test pharmacogenetic associations of I/D ACE genotype with beta blockers therapy in patients with chronic heart failure. METHODS AND RESULTS: A total of 241 patients were included in the study, 63% with betablocker therapy and 37% without it. Using polymerase chain reaction (PCR) method, I/D genotype was detected in 2% agarose electrophoretic gel in UV light. Patients with chronic heart failure and with the II genotype of polymorphism I/D ACE were younger, with more frequent administration of betablockers and diuretics, with less regular administration of aspirin and with lower glycemia and plasma TNFalpha level. A significant difference in genotype distribution and allele frequency between patients with recommended dose and patients without betablockers therapy was proved, when a decrease of the D allele in patients with betablockers had been observed. Contemporary evaluating of AC inhibitor and betablocker therapy, a decrease of ID+DD genotypes in patients with lower than 50% recommended dose compared with the others was found. CONCLUSIONS: In this study, we proved statistically significant interactions between genotypes in I/D ACE polymorphism, betablocker administration, its dosing and pharmacogenetic interaction with ACE inhibitors in patients with chronic heart failure.

Cell Biol Int. 2004;28(11):755-64. Related Articles, Links Cell biology, chemogenomics and chemoproteomics. Gagna CE, Winokur D, Clark Lambert W. Department of Pathology and Laboratory Medicine, University of Medicine and Dentistry of New Jersey-Medical School, 185 S. Orange Avenue, Newark, NJ 07103, USA. dr.c.gagna@att.net The scientific techniques used in molecular biological research and drug discovery have changed dramatically over the past 10 years due to the influence of genomics, proteomics and bioinformatics. Furthermore, genomics and functional genomics are now merging into a new scientific approach called chemogenomics. Advancements in the study of molecular cell biology are dependent upon "omics" researchers realizing the importance of and using the experimental tools currently available to cell biologists. For example, novel microscopic techniques utilizing advanced computer imaging allow for the examination of live specimens in a fourth dimension, viz., time. Yet, molecular biologists have not taken full advantage of these and other traditional and novel cell biology techniques for the further advancement of genomic and proteomic-oriented research. The application of traditional and novel cellular biological techniques will enhance the science of genomics. The authors hypothesize that a stronger interdisciplinary approach must be taken between cell biology (and its closely related fields) and genomics, proteomics and bio-chemoinformatics. Since there is a lot of confusion regarding many of the "omics" definitions, this article also clarifies some of the basic terminology used in genomics, and related fields. It also reviews the current status and future potential of chemogenomics and its relationship to cell biology. The authors also discuss and expand upon the differences between chemogenomics and the relatively new term--chemoproteomics. We conclude that the advances in cell biology methods and approaches and their adoption by "omics" researchers will allow scientists to maximize our knowledge about life. Publication Types: Review

Cell Metab. 2005 Dec;2(6):349-60. Related Articles, Links Mouse phenogenomics: the fast track to "systems metabolism". Argmann CA, Chambon P, Auwerx J. Institut de Genetique et de Biologie Moleculaire et Cellulaire, Centre National de la Recherche Scientifique/Institut Nationale de la Sante et de la Recherche Medicale/Universite Louis Pasteur, 67404 Illkirch, France. With the completion of the many genomes, genetics is positioned to meet physiology. In this review, we summarize the coming of "systems metabolism" in mammals through the use of the mouse, as a model system to study metabolism. Building on mouse genetics with increasingly sophisticated clinical and molecular phenotyping strategies has enabled scientists to now tackle complex biomedical questions, such as those related to the pathogenesis of the common metabolic disorders. The ultimate goal of such strategies will be to mimic human metabolism with the click of a mouse. Publication Types: Review

Chang Gung Med J. 2005 Apr;28(4):201-11. Related Articles, Links Clinical bioinformatics. Chang PL. Division of Urology, Department of Surgery and Bioinformatics Center, Chang Gung Memorial Hospital, Taipei, Taiwan. henryc@cgmh.org.tw Clinical bioinformatics provides biological and medical information to allow for individualized healthcare. In this review, we describe the uses of clinical bioinformatics. After the analysis of the complete human genome sequences, clinical bioinformatics enables researchers to search online biological databases and use the biological information in their medical practices. The data obtained from using microarray is extremely complicated. In clinical bioinformatics, selecting appropriate software to analyze the microarray data for medical decision making is crucial. Proteomics strategy tools usually focus on similarity searches, structure prediction, and protein modeling. In clinical bioinformatics, the proteomic data only have meaning if they are integrated with clinical data. In pharmacogenomics, clinical bioinformatics includes elaborate studies of bioinformatics tools and various facets of proteomics related to drug target identification and clinical validation. Using clinical bioinformatics, researchers apply computational and high-throughput experimental techniques to cancer research and systems biology. Meanwhile, researchers of bioinformatics and medical information have incorporated clinical bioinformatics to improve health care, using biological and medical information. Using the high volume of biological information from clinical bioinformatics will contribute to changes in practice standards in the healthcare system. We believe that clinical bioinformatics provides benefits of improving healthcare, disease prevention and health maintenance as we move toward the era of personalized medicine. Publication Types: Review

Chem Biol Interact. 2004 Nov 1;150(1):71-85. Related Articles, Links Toxicogenomics in drug discovery: from preclinical studies to clinical trials. Yang Y, Blomme EA, Waring JF. Department of Cellular and Molecular Toxicology, Abbott Laboratories, 100 Abbott Park Road, Abbott Park, IL 60064-6123, USA. Gene expression analysis applied to toxicology studies, also referred to as toxicogenomics, is rapidly being embraced by the pharmaceutical industry as a useful tool to identify safer drugs in a quicker, more cost-effective manner. Studies have already demonstrated the benefits of applying gene expression profiling towards drug safety evaluation, both for identifying mechanisms underlying toxicity, as well as for providing a means to identify safety liabilities early in the drug discovery process. Furthermore, toxicogenomics has the potential to better identify and assess adverse drug reactions of new drug candidates or marketed products in humans. While much still remains to be learned about the relevance and the application of gene expression changes in human toxicology, the next few years should see gene expression technologies applied to more stages and more programs of the drug discovery and development process. This review will focus on how toxicogenomics can or has been applied in drug discovery and development, and will discuss some of the challenges that still remain. Publication Types: Review

Chem Biol. 2004 Feb;11(2):161-71. Related Articles, Links Toxicogenomics in predictive toxicology in drug development. Suter L, Babiss LE, Wheeldon EB. Department of Non-Clinical Drug Safety, F Hoffmann-La Roche, Ltd., 4070 Basel, Switzerland. laura.suter-dick@roche.com The goal of toxicology is the assessment of possible risk to man. An emerging technology with the potential to have a major impact on risk assessment is toxicogenomics. In this review, we provide an overview of the many possibilities for toxicogenomics including technology platforms, data interpretation, and regulatory perspective and we give examples of toxicogenomics investigations. Toxicogenomics is a powerful tool for compound classification, for mechanistic studies, and for the detection of toxicity markers. Thus, toxicogenomics helps in the extrapolation of findings across species and increases predictability. Biomarkers are valuable in the evaluation of compounds at earlier development phases, improving clinical candidate selection. Caution regarding the interpretation of the results is still necessary. Nevertheless, toxicogenomics will accelerate preclinical safety assessments and improve the prediction of toxic liabilities, as well as of potential risk accumulation for drug-drug or drug-disease interactions. Publication Types: Review

Chem Immunol Allergy. 2004;84:1-35. Related Articles, Links Genetics. Holloway JW, Holgate ST. Human Genetics, Southampton General Hospital, University of Southampton, Southampton, UK. j.w.holloway@soton.ac.uk Publication Types: Review

Chem Immunol Allergy. 2005;87:145-53. Related Articles, Links Mast cell beta2-adrenoceptors. Kay LJ, Peachell PT. Molecular Pharmacology, University of Sheffield, The Royal Hallamshire Hospital, Sheffield, UK. The human lung mast cell is a crucial effector cell in the mediation of asthma. Activation of mast cells by allergens, and other insults, leads to the elaboration of a wide variety of autacoids that cause bronchoconstriction and promote inflammation. Of the drugs that are used to treat asthma, only bronchodilator beta2-adrenoceptor agonists are effective at inhibiting the elaboration of mediators from mast cells. Both short- and long-acting beta2-adrenoceptor agonists are effective inhibitors of mast cells although there are differences in the degree of inhibitory activity attained with a given agonist. Human lung mast cells express a homogeneous population of beta2-adrenoceptors. However, the density of beta2-adrenoceptors differs from preparation to preparation and this may influence the extent to which agonists stabilise mast cell activity. Tolerance to the mast cell-stabilising activity of beta2-adrenoceptor agonists can be readily demonstrated. As a generalisation, agonists that are more effective inhibitors of mediator release also induce greater levels of tolerance although weaker agonists induce greater levels of tolerance than might be expected. However, the extent of tolerance does not correlate with the degree of beta2-adrenoceptor loss. The inhibitory activity of agonists and the extent of tolerance observed may be influenced by genetic polymorphisms in the gene for the beta2-adrenoceptor. Publication Types: Review

Chem Res Toxicol. 2005 Mar;18(3):403-14. Related Articles, Links Advances in toxicogenomics. Hayes KR, Bradfield CA. The McArdle Laboratory for Cancer Research, University of Wisconsin Medical School, Madison, Wisconsin 53706, USA. Publication Types: Review

Circulation. 2004 Oct 5;110(14):2066-71. Related Articles, Links Genetic basis of atherosclerosis: part II: clinical implications. Lusis AJ, Fogelman AM, Fonarow GC. Division of Cardiology, David Geffen School of Medicine at University of California, Los Angeles, USA. jlusis@mednet.ucla.edu. Publication Types: Review

Circulation. 2005 Dec 13;112(24):3754-62. Epub 2005 Dec 5. Related Articles, Links NAD(P)H oxidase and multidrug resistance protein genetic polymorphisms are associated with doxorubicin-induced cardiotoxicity. Wojnowski L, Kulle B, Schirmer M, Schluter G, Schmidt A, Rosenberger A, Vonhof S, Bickeboller H, Toliat MR, Suk EK, Tzvetkov M, Kruger A, Seifert S, Kloess M, Hahn H, Loeffler M, Nurnberg P, Pfreundschuh M, Trumper L, Brockmoller J, Hasenfuss G. Department of Pharmacology, University Mainz, D-55101 Mainz, Germany. Wojnowski@uni-mainz.de BACKGROUND: A significant number of patients treated with anthracyclines develop cardiotoxicity (anthracycline-induced cardiotoxicity [ACT]), mainly presenting as arrhythmias (acute ACT) or congestive heart failure (chronic ACT). There are no data on pharmacogenomic predictors of ACT. METHODS AND RESULTS: We genotyped participants of the German non-Hodgkin lymphoma study (NHL-B) who were followed up for the development of heart failure for a median of >3 years. Single-nucleotide polymorphisms (SNPs) were selected from 82 genes with conceivable relevance to ACT. Of 1697 patients, 55 developed acute and 54 developed chronic ACT (cumulative incidence of either form, 3.2%). We detected 5 significant associations with polymorphisms of the NAD(P)H oxidase and doxorubicin efflux transporters. Chronic ACT was associated with a variant of the NAD(P)H oxidase subunit NCF4 (rs1883112, -212A-->G; symbols with right-pointing arrows, as edited?' odds ratio [OR], 2.5; 95% CI, 1.3 to 5.0). Acute ACT was associated with the His72Tyr polymorphism in the p22phox subunit (rs4673, OR, 2.0; 95% CI, 1.0 to 3.9) and with the variant 7508T-->A (rs13058338; OR, 2.6; 95% CI, 1.3 to 5.1) of the RAC2 subunit of the same enzyme. In agreement with these results, mice deficient in NAD(P)H oxidase activity, unlike wild-type mice, were resistant to chronic doxorubicin treatment.

In addition, acute ACT was associated with the Gly671Val variant of the doxorubicin efflux transporter multidrug resistance protein 1 (MRP1) (OR, 3.6; 95% CI, 1.6 to 8.4) and with the Val1188Glu-Cys1515Tyr (rs8187694-rs8187710) haplotype of the functionally similar MRP2 (OR, 2.3; 95% CI, 1.0 to 5.4). Polymorphisms in adrenergic receptors previously demonstrated to be predictive of heart failure were not associated with ACT. CONCLUSIONS: Genetic variants in doxorubicin transport and free radical metabolism may modulate the individual risk to develop ACT. Publication Types: Multicenter Study

Circulation. 2005 Jun 28;111(25):3374-83. Epub 2005 Jun 20. Related Articles, Links Pharmacogenetic association of the angiotensin-converting enzyme insertion/deletion polymorphism on blood pressure and cardiovascular risk in relation to antihypertensive treatment: the Genetics of Hypertension-Associated Treatment (GenHAT) study. Arnett DK, Davis BR, Ford CE, Boerwinkle E, Leiendecker-Foster C, Miller MB, Black H, Eckfeldt JH. University of Minnesota, Division of Epidemiology, Minneapolis, USA. arnett@ms.soph.uab.edu BACKGROUND: Previous studies have reported that blood pressure response to antihypertensive medications is influenced by genetic variation in the renin-angiotensin-aldosterone system, but no clinical trails have tested whether the ACE insertion/deletion (I/D) polymorphism modifies the association between the type of medication and multiple cardiovascular and renal phenotypes. METHODS AND RESULTS: We used a double-blind, active-controlled randomized trial of antihypertensive treatment that included hypertensives > or =55 years of age with > or =1 risk factor for cardiovascular disease. ACE I/D genotypes were determined in 37 939 participants randomized to chlorthalidone, amlodipine, lisinopril, or doxazosin treatments and followed up for 4 to 8 years. Primary outcomes included fatal coronary heart disease (CHD) and/or nonfatal myocardial infarction. Secondary outcomes included stroke, all-cause mortality, combined CHD, and combined cardiovascular disease. Fatal and nonfatal CHD occurred in 3096 individuals during follow-up. The hazard rates for fatal and nonfatal CHD and the secondary outcomes were similar across antihypertensive treatments. ACE I/D genotype group was not associated with fatal and nonfatal CHD (relative risk of DD versus ID and II, 0.99; 95% CI, 0.91 to 1.07) or any secondary outcome. The 6-year hazard rate for fatal and nonfatal CHD in the DD genotype group was not statistically different from the ID and II genotype group by type of treatment. No secondary outcome measure was statistically different across antihypertensive treatment and ACE I/D genotype strata. CONCLUSIONS: ACE I/D genotype group was not a predictor of CHD, nor did it modify the response to antihypertensive treatment. We conclude that the ACE I/D polymorphism is not a useful marker to predict antihypertensive treatment response. Publication Types: Multicenter Study Randomized Controlled Trial

Clin Adv Hematol Oncol. 2003 Feb;1(2):107-11. Related Articles, Links Using genetic variation to optimize cancer chemotherapy. McLeod HL, Papageorgio C, Watters JW. Washington University School of Medicine, Siteman Cancer Center, St. Louis, MO 63110, USA. hmcleod@im.wustl.edu The high level of interpatient variation in response to chemotherapy and the lack of objective tools to select chemotherapy regimens for a given tumor type have created a clinical problem. A possible solution may be pharmacogenetics: the study of inherited DNA polymorphisms that influence drug disposition and effects in order to individualize drug treatment. Because unpredictable efficacy and high levels of systemic toxicity are common in cancer chemotherapy, pharmacogenetics is particularly appealing to oncologists. Polymorphisms in drug metabolism, drug transport, drug target, and DNA repair genes have been implicated interpatient variability in response to many chemotherapy agents. This review will discuss recent clinically relevant examples of cancer pharmacogenetics and how genetic differences are helping to shape the future of individualized cancer chemotherapy. Publication Types: Review

Clin Adv Hematol Oncol. 2004 Apr;2(4):205-47. Related Articles, Links Current overview of pharmacogenetics. McLeod HL. Washington University, St. Louis 63110, USA.

Clin Adv Hematol Oncol. 2004 Aug;2(8):527-32. Related Articles, Links Dihydropyrimidine dehydrogenase deficiency: impact of pharmacogenetics on 5-Fluorouracil therapy. Lee A, Ezzeldin H, Fourie J, Diasio R. University of Alabama at Birmingham, Birmingham, AL 35294-3300, USA. robert.diasio@ccc.uab.edu. Through the use of pharmacogenetic studies, interindividual variability in response (efficacy and toxicity) to 5-fluorouracil (5-FU) chemotherapy has been linked to the rate-limiting enzyme in the drug's catabolic pathway, known as dihydropyrimidine dehydrogenase (DPD). This pharmacogenetic syndrome, known as "DPD deficiency," results in excessive amounts of 5-FU available to be anabolized to its active metabolites and is relatively undetectable by clinical observation prior to 5-FU administration. Extensive studies have associated both profound and partial deficiency in DPD activity with severe, unanticipated toxicity after 5-FU administration, while research on the molecular basis behind DPD deficiency has been linked to various sequence variants of the DPYD gene. Due to the widespread use of 5-FU, the severity of toxicity associated with DPD deficiency, and the prevalence of DPD deficiency in the population, extensive research is continually being performed to develop quick and accurate phenotypic and genotypic assays suitable for clinical settings that would allow clinicians to identify patients susceptible to adverse 5-FU reactions.

Clin Appl Thromb Hemost. 2004 Apr;10(2):149-54. Related Articles, Links CYP2C9 genetic polymorphisms and warfarin. Redman AR, Dickmann LJ, Kidd RS, Goldstein JA, Ritchie DM, Hon YY. Department of Clinical and Administrative Sciences, Mercer University Southern School of Pharmacy, Atlanta, Georgia 30341-4155, USA. Redman_ar@mercer.edu The objective of this study was to report 2 cases of CYP2C9 genetic polymorphism and elevated warfarin S:R ratios in patients taking low doses of warfarin, and compare the observed characteristics with those in published reports. Two patients of different age groups and races were evaluated for CYP2C9 genotype and warfarin S:R ratios. The patients had been stabilized on weekly warfarin doses of 10.5 mg and 10 mg, respectively. Each patient was found to have at least 1 variant CYP2C9 allele. Elevated warfarin S:R ratios in both patients provided evidence for impaired metabolism of S-warfarin. This report of a CYP2C9*3 heterozygous individual taking a low dose of warfarin is consistent with previous reports in the literature. This summary of a CYP2C9*6 homozygous individual taking a low dose of warfarin is the first such published report. CYP2C9 genotyping in these patients provided a likely explanation for their continued low warfarin dosage requirements. Awareness of a patient's CYP2C9 genotype may provide an explanation for low warfarin dosage requirements in stable patients and may help in determining the optimal dose in patients being initiated on warfarin. Publication Types: Case Reports

Clin Appl Thromb Hemost. 2005 Apr;11(2):113-25. Related Articles, Links Genetics of platelet glycoprotein receptors: risk of thrombotic events and pharmacogenetic implications. Mikkelsson J, Perola M, Karhunen PJ. Tampere University Hospital, Research Unit and Medical School, University of Tampere, Tampere University Hospital, and National Public Health Institute, Helsinki, Finland. jussi.mikkelsson@dnainternet.net Platelet aggregation and coronary thrombosis have a central role in the development of acute coronary syndromes and myocardial infarction (MI). Therapies aimed at inhibiting platelet aggregation have shown great benefit in individuals with coronary disease or with multiple risk factors for coronary disease. Genetic variation in platelet surface receptors mediating thrombus formation has been suggested to be associated with platelet hyperreactivity, with increased risk of MI and possibly with the benefit received from various antithrombotic drug treatments. This review focuses on discrepancies and their likely explanations in studies on platelet glycoprotein genetics. Current knowledge on important issues concerning coronary event phenotypes and pharmacogenetics is analyzed. Possible future applicability of these data to patient treatment is also discussed. Publication Types: Review

Clin Biochem. 2006 Mar;39(3):240-3. Epub 2006 Jan 19. Related Articles, Links Evaluation of an algorithm of tagging SNPs selection by linkage disequilibrium. Tang NL, Pharoah PD, Ma SL, Easton DF. Department of Chemical Pathology, Faculty of Medicine, The Chinese University of Hong Kong, Shatin, Hong Kong. BACKGROUND:: Single nucleotide polymorphisms (SNPs) are the most abundant kind of genetic polymorphism in the human genome. They are important in both genetic research and genetic testing in a clinical setting, such as in the area of pharmacogenetics. In order to improve efficiency, tagging SNPs (tagSNPs) are selected in genes of interest to represent other co-related SNPs in linkage disequilibrium (LD) with the tagSNPs. Various algorithms have been proposed to identify a subset of single nucleotide polymorphisms as tagSNPs. Most algorithms of tagSNPs selection are haplotype-based, in which the spatial relationship between SNPs is considered. Currently, a more efficient cluster-based algorithm is proposed which clusters SNPs solely by a LD parameter, such as r(2). Here, we evaluated the sample distribution of r(2) and its effect on the cluster-based tagSNPs selection. DESIGN AND METHODS:: The genotype data of 198 individual within a 500-kb region on 5q31 was used to evaluate the sample distribution of r(2) and its effect on the cluster-based tagSNPs selection. RESULTS:: It was found that the degree of variation of LD depends on the LD structure of genes. CONCLUSION:: As a cluster-based tagSNPs selection algorithm does not take into account the spatial position of SNPs, a more stringent r(2) threshold is required to achieve more reliable tagSNPs selection.

Clin Breast Cancer. 2004 Aug;5(3):171. Related Articles, Links On not being the "hostess with the mostest". Sledge GW Jr. Publication Types: Editorial

Clin Breast Cancer. 2005 Oct;6(4):283. Related Articles, Links Transforming technologies and breast cancer. Sledge GW Jr. Publication Types: Editorial

Clin Cancer Res. 2004 May 1;10(9):2936-43. Related Articles, Links Synergistic cytotoxicity and pharmacogenetics of gemcitabine and pemetrexed combination in pancreatic cancer cell lines. Giovannetti E, Mey V, Danesi R, Mosca I, Del Tacca M. Division of Pharmacology and Chemotherapy, Department of Oncology, Transplants and Advanced Technologies in Medicine, Pisa, Italy. PURPOSE: Gemcitabine is an inhibitor of ribonucleotide reductase (RR) and DNA synthesis and is an effective agent in the treatment of pancreas cancer. The present study investigates whether the multitargeted antifolate pemetrexed would be synergistic with gemcitabine against MIA PaCa-2, PANC-1, and Capan-1 pancreatic cancer cell lines. EXPERIMENTAL DESIGN: Cells were treated with gemcitabine and pemetrexed, and the type of drug interaction was assessed using the combination index. Cytotoxicity of gemcitabine was examined with inhibitors of (a) deoxycytidine kinase (dCK), which activates gemcitabine by phosphorylation, and (b) 5'-nucleotidase (drug dephosphorylation) and cytidine deaminase (drug deamination), the main inactivating enzymes. The effects of gemcitabine and pemetrexed on cell cycle were analyzed by flow cytometry, and apoptosis was examined by fluorescence microscopy. Finally, quantitative, real-time PCR was used to study the pharmacogenetics of the drug combination. RESULTS: Synergistic cytotoxicity and enhancement of apoptosis was demonstrated, mostly with the sequence pemetrexed-->gemcitabine. Pemetrexed increased cells in S phase, the most sensitive to gemcitabine, and a positive correlation was found between the expression ratio of dCK:RR and gemcitabine sensitivity. Indeed, pemetrexed significantly enhanced dCK gene expression (+227.9, +86.0, and +135.5% in MIA PaCa-2, PANC-1, and Capan-1 cells, respectively), and the crucial role of this enzyme was confirmed by impairment of gemcitabine cytotoxicity after dCK saturation with 2'-deoxycytidine. CONCLUSIONS: These data demonstrate that the gemcitabine and pemetrexed combination displays schedule-dependent synergistic cytotoxic activity, favorably modulates cell cycle, induces apoptosis, and enhances dCK expression in pancreatic cancer cells.

Clin Cancer Res. 2004 Sep 1;10(17):5889-94. Related Articles, Links ABCG2 pharmacogenetics: ethnic differences in allele frequency and assessment of influence on irinotecan disposition. de Jong FA, Marsh S, Mathijssen RH, King C, Verweij J, Sparreboom A, McLeod HL. Department of Medical Oncology, Erasmus University MC-Daniel den Hoed Cancer Center, Rotterdam, The Netherlands. PURPOSE: The ATP-binding cassette transporter ABCG2 (breast cancer resistance protein) is an efflux protein that plays a role in host detoxification of various xenobiotic substrates, including the irinotecan metabolite 7- ethyl-10-hydroxycamptothecin (SN-38). The ABCG2 421C>A polymorphism has been associated with reduced protein expression and altered function in vitro. The aim of this study was to evaluate the ethnic distribution and potential functional consequence of the ABCG2 421C>A genotype in cancer patients treated with irinotecan. EXPERIMENTAL DESIGN: ABCG2 genotyping was performed using Pyrosequencing on DNA from 88 American Caucasians, 94 African Americans, 938 Africans, and 95 Han Chinese, as well as in 84 European Caucasian patients treated with irinotecan undergoing additional blood sampling for pharmacokinetic studies. RESULTS: Significant differences in allele frequencies were observed between the given world populations ($P < 0.001$), the variant allele being most common in the Han Chinese population with a frequency as high as 34%. The mean area under the curve of irinotecan and SN-38 were 19,851 and 639 ng x hour/mL, respectively. The frequency of the variant allele (10.7%) was in line with results in American Caucasians. No significant changes in irinotecan pharmacokinetics were observed in relation to the ABCG2 421C>A genotype, although one of two homozygous variant allele carriers showed extensive accumulation of SN-38 and SN-38 glucuronide. CONCLUSIONS: The ABCG2 421C>A polymorphism appears to play a limited role in the disposition of irinotecan in European Caucasians. It is likely that the contribution of this genetic variant is obscured by a functional role of other polymorphic proteins.

Clin Cancer Res. 2005 Dec 15;11(24 Pt 1):8686-98. Related Articles, Links Comment in: Clin Cancer Res. 2005 Dec 15;11(24 Pt 1):8534-7. Epithelial versus mesenchymal phenotype determines in vitro sensitivity and predicts clinical activity of erlotinib in lung cancer patients. Yauch RL, Januario T, Eberhard DA, Cavet G, Zhu W, Fu L, Pham TQ, Soriano R, Stinson J, Seshagiri S, Modrusan Z, Lin CY, O'Neill V, Amler LC. Department of Molecular Diagnostics, Genentech, Inc., South San Francisco, California 94080, USA. Significant improvements in the outcome of non-small cell lung carcinoma (NSCLC) have been reported in patients treated with the epidermal growth factor receptor (EGFR) inhibitor, erlotinib. To discover biomarkers for the enrichment of patients who might benefit from treatment, a pharmacogenomic approach was used to identify gene signatures that may predict erlotinib activity using in vitro model systems. Erlotinib sensitivity in a panel of 42 NSCLC cell lines was determined by EGFR-mediated proliferative potential, EGFR mutations, and/or EGFR gene amplification, thus supporting an underlying biological mechanism of receptor activation. A strong multigene signature indicative of an epithelial to mesenchymal transition (EMT) was identified as a determinant of insensitivity to erlotinib through both supervised and unsupervised gene expression approaches. This observation was further supported by expression analysis of classic EMT marker proteins, including E-cadherin and vimentin. To investigate the clinical relevance of these findings, we examined expression of the epithelial marker E-cadherin by immunohistochemistry on primary tumor samples from subjects enrolled in a randomized NSCLC clinical trial in which erlotinib in combination with chemotherapy previously failed to show clinical activity. The majority (75%) of the 87 subjects tested showed strong E-cadherin staining and exhibited a significantly longer time to progression (hazard ratio, 0.37; log rank P=0.0028) and a nonsignificant trend toward longer survival with erlotinib plus chemotherapy treatment versus chemotherapy alone. These data support a potential role for

EMT as a determinant of EGFR activity in NSCLC tumor cells and E-cadherin expression as a novel biomarker predicting clinical activity of the EGFR inhibitor erlotinib in NSCLC patients.

Clin Cancer Res. 2005 Jun 1;11(11):4144-50. Related Articles, Links A phase I pharmacologic and pharmacogenetic trial of sequential 24-hour infusion of irinotecan followed by leucovorin and a 48-hour infusion of fluorouracil in adult patients with solid tumors. Wright MA, Morrison G, Lin P, Leonard GD, Nguyen D, Guo X, Szabo E, Hopkins JL, Leguizamo JP, Harold N, Fioravanti S, Schuler B, Monahan BP, Saif MW, Quinn MG, Pang J, Grem JL. Medical Oncology Clinical Research Unit, Center for Cancer Research, National Cancer Institute, Bethesda, Maryland, USA. PURPOSE: In preclinical studies, sequential exposure to irinotecan (CPT-11) then fluorouracil (5-FU) is superior to concurrent exposure or the reverse sequence; a 24-hour infusion of CPT-11 may be better tolerated than shorter infusions. EXPERIMENTAL DESIGN: CPT-11 was first given at four levels (70-140 mg/m(2)/24 hours), followed by leucovorin 500 mg/m(2)/0.5 hours and 5-FU 2,000 mg/m(2)/48 hours on days 1 and 15 of a 4-week cycle. 5-FU was then increased in three cohorts up to 3,900 mg/m(2)/48 hours. RESULTS: Two patients had dose-limiting toxicity during cycle 1 at 140/3,900 of CPT-11/5-FU (2-week delay for neutrophil recovery; grade 3 nausea despite antiemetics); one of six patients at 140/3,120 had dose-limiting toxicity (grade 3 diarrhea, grade 4 neutropenia). Four of 22 patients with colorectal cancer had partial responses, two of which had prior bolus CPT-11/5-FU. The mean 5-FU plasma concentration was 5.1 micromol/L at 3,900 mg/m(2)/48 hours. The end of infusion CPT-11 plasma concentration averaged 519 nmol/L at 140 mg/m(2)/24 hours. Patients with UDP-glucuronosyltransferase (UGT1A1; TA)6/6 promoter genotype had a lower ratio of free to glucuronide form of SN-38 than in patients with >/=1 (TA)7 allele. Thymidylate synthase genotypes for the 28-base promoter repeat were 2/2 (13%), 2/3 (74%), 3/3 (13%); all four responders had a 2/3 genotype. CONCLUSIONS: Doses (mg/m(2)) of CPT-11 140/24 hours, leucovorin 500/0.5 hours and 5-FU 3,120/48 hours were well tolerated. Publication Types: Clinical Trial Clinical Trial, Phase I

Clin Cancer Res. 2005 Nov 15;11(22):8097-104. Related Articles, Links Association of CYP2C8, CYP3A4, CYP3A5, and ABCB1 polymorphisms with the pharmacokinetics of paclitaxel. Henningsson A, Marsh S, Loos WJ, Karlsson MO, Garsa A, Mross K, Mielke S, Vigano L, Locatelli A, Verweij J, Sparreboom A, McLeod HL. Department of Pharmaceutical Biosciences, Faculty of Pharmacy, Uppsala University, Uppsala, Sweden. PURPOSE: To retrospectively evaluate the effects of six known allelic variants in the CYP2C8, CYP3A4, CYP3A5, and ABCB1 genes on the pharmacokinetics of the anticancer agent paclitaxel (Taxol). EXPERIMENTAL DESIGN: A cohort of 97 Caucasian patients with cancer (median age, 57 years) received paclitaxel as an i.v. infusion (dose range, 80-225 mg/m(2)). Genomic DNA was analyzed using PCR RFLP or using Pyrosequencing. Pharmacokinetic variables for unbound paclitaxel were estimated using nonlinear mixed effect modeling. The effects of genotypes on typical value of clearance were evaluated with the likelihood ratio test within NONMEM. In addition, relations between genotype and individual pharmacokinetic variable estimates were evaluated with one-way ANOVA. RESULTS: The allele frequencies for the CYP2C8*2, CYP2C8*3, CYP2C8*4, CYP3A4*3, CYP3A5*3C, and ABCB1 3435C>T variants were 0.7%, 9.2%, 2.1%, 0.5%, 93.2%, and 47.1%, respectively, and all were in Hardy-Weinberg equilibrium. The population typical value of clearance of unbound paclitaxel was 301 L/h (individual clearance range, 83.7-1055 L/h). The CYP2C8 or CYP3A4/5 genotypes were not statistically significantly associated with unbound clearance of paclitaxel. Likewise, no statistically significant association was observed between the ABCB1 3435C>T variant and any of the studied pharmacokinetic variables. CONCLUSIONS: This study indicates that the presently evaluated variant alleles in the CYP2C8, CYP3A4, CYP3A5, and ABCB1 genes do not explain the substantial interindividual variability in paclitaxel pharmacokinetics. Publication Types: Clinical Trial

Clin Chem Lab Med. 2004 Jan;42(1):72-8. Related Articles, Links Association between the CYP2C9 polymorphism and the drug metabolism phenotype. Topic E, Stefanovic M, Samardzija M. Clinical Institute of Chemistry, School of Medicine, Sestre milosrdnice University Hospital, Zagreb, Croatia. elizabeta.topic@zg.htnet.hr CYP2C9, an isoform of the cytochrome P450 enzyme, is involved in the metabolism of most of the drugs of choice for the treatment of thromboembolic disorders. Functional polymorphism is associated with two variant alleles (alleles *2 and *3) encoding CYP2C9 enzymes with a potentially different catalytic activity. The aim of the study was to determine the frequency of the CYP2C9 polymorphism in a representative sample of the Croatian population (n = 177) and to assess the association between the CYP2C9 polymorphism and the warfarin dose in patients with thromboembolism (n = 181). The CYP2C9 genotype was determined by polymerase chain reaction-restriction fragment length poymorphism (PCR-RFLP). According to the CYP2C9 genotype distribution, 31.2% of the healthy subjects were identified with a heterozygous or homozygous CYP2C9 variant genotype. The frequency of 2C9*2 and 2C9*3 alleles was 12.4% and 3.7%, respectively. There was no gender-related genotype or allele difference. In thromboembolism patients, the frequency of CYP2C9 alleles *2 and *3 was 17.4% and 6.6%, respectively, and did not differ significantly from the control group. Almost half (42.5%) of the patients carried at least one variant CYP2C9 genotype. The allele difference between patient subgroups receiving warfarin doses lower and higher than the optimal warfarin dose (4.1 mg/day) was significant (p = 0.027), especially for allele 2C9*3 (p = 0.019; OR 3.250, 95%, CI 1.263-8.413). Comparison of the warfarin dose between patients with different genotypes yielded a significant dose difference between the patients with wild-type genotype and those with variant genotypes (Kruskall-Wallis, chi2 = 9.745, p = 0.008). The results of the association of each of five genotype combinations with the warfarin maintenance dose revealed it to be significantly related to the genotype (Kruskall-Wallis, chi2 = 12.854, p = 0.025). Expressed as percentage of the mean dose in patients with wild-type alleles, the mean warfarin maintenance dose was 92% in 2C9*2 heterozygotes, 74% in 2C*3 heterozygotes, 61% in 2C9*2 homozygotes, 34% in 2C9*3 homozygotes and 63% in compound heterozygotes for 2C9*2 and 2C9*3. Although the mean maintenance dose in homozygous *2/*2 and compound *2/*3 genotype patients was markedly lower (mean 2.66 mg and 2.75 mg, respectively, vs. 4.37 mg), statistical analysis yielded no significance because of the small number of patients carrying these genotypes. A significantly lower maintenance dose was observed in the subgroup of heterozygous *1/*3 genotype patients (p = 0.022). These preliminary results suggest a significant association of the CYP2C9 polymorphism with the warfarin dose and underline the importance of pre-therapeutic genotyping to identify the subjects likely to develop undesirable drug effects.

Clin Chem Lab Med. 2004;42(11):1256-64. Related Articles, Links Pharmacogenomic genotyping methodologies. Jannetto PJ, Laleli-Sahin E, Wong SH. Department of Pathology, Medical College of Wisconsin and Milwaukee County Medical Examiner's Office, Milwaukee, WI, USA. "Personalized medicine" based on an individual's genetic makeup is slowly becoming a reality as pharmacogenomics moves from the research setting to the clinical laboratory. Concordance studies between genotype and phenotype have shown that inherited mutations in several key drug-metabolizing enzymes, such as cytochrome P450 (CYP) 2D6 , 2C9 , and 2C19 , result in several distinct phenotypes that lead to different individual responses following drug administration. One of the major driving forces behind pharmacogenomics and its ability to be used effectively are the technologies that are available. A beneficial genotyping test must identify most or all of the mutations that have a significant impact on the expression or function of drug-metabolizing enzymes, transporter proteins, and/or drug receptors. Selection of the appropriate technology will be based on several issues, including prior knowledge of the mutation/polymorphism, sensitivity/specificity, sample requirements, and cost. Since the future volume of pharmacogenomic testing is anticipated to be large, automation of pharmacogenomics will also become increasingly important. This paper provides an overview of current technologies available for assessing polymorphisms on a small- to large-scale basis. Publication Types: Review

Clin Chem. 2004 Sep;50(9):1498-9. Related Articles, Links Comment on: Clin Chem. 2004 Sep;50(9):1623-33. Fine-tuning pharmacogenetics: paradigm for linking laboratory results to clinical action. Valdes R Jr, Linder MW. Publication Types: Comment Editorial

Clin Chem. 2004 Sep;50(9):1526-7. Related Articles, Links Pharmacogenomics and pharmacogenetics: future role of molecular diagnostics in the clinical diagnostic laboratory. Ito RK, Demers LM. Diagnostic Systems, Protedyne Corporation, Windsor, CT 06095, USA. ralphi@protedyne.com Publication Types: Review

Clin Chem. 2004 Sep;50(9):1528-34. Epub 2004 Jul 9. Related Articles, Links Rapid, long-range molecular haplotyping of thiopurine S-methyltransferase (TPMT) *3A, *3B, and *3C. von Ahsen N, Armstrong VW, Oellerich M. Department of Clinical Chemistry, George-August University, Gottingen, Germany. nahsen@gwdg.de BACKGROUND: Haplotyping is an important technique in molecular diagnostics because haplotypes are often more predictive for individual phenotypes than are the underlying single-nucleotide polymorphisms (SNPs). Until recently, methods for haplotyping SNPs separated by kilobase distances were laborious and not applicable to high-throughput screening. In the case of thiopurine S-methyltransferase (TPMT*), differentiating among TPMT*3A, *3B, and *3C alleles is sometimes necessary for predictive genotyping. METHODS: The genomic region including the two SNPs that define TPMT*3A, *3B, and *3C alleles was amplified by long-range PCR. The resulting PCR product was circularized by ligation and haplotyped by allele-specific amplification PCR followed by product identification with hybridization probes. RESULTS: Critical points were the long-range PCR conditions, including choice of buffer and primers, optimization of the ligation reaction, and selection of primers that allowed for strict allele-specific amplification in the second-round PCR. Different underlying TPMT haplotypes could then be differentiated. Results from the haplotyping method were in full agreement with those from our standard real-time PCR method: TPMT*1/*3A (n = 20); TPMT*1/*3C (n = 4); TPMT*1/*1 (n = 6); and TPMT*3A/*3A (n = 6). One TPMT*1/*3A sample failed to amplify, and no whole blood was available for repeat DNA isolation. CONCLUSIONS: This method for rapid-cycle real-time, allele-specific amplification PCR-assisted long-range haplotyping has general application for the haplotyping of distant SNPs. The procedure is simpler and more rapid than previous methods. With respect to TPMT, haplotyping has the potential to discriminate the genotypes TPMT*1/*3A (intermediate metabolizer) and TPMT*3B/*3C (poor metabolizer).

Clin Chem. 2004 Sep;50(9):1623-33. Epub 2004 Jun 17. Related Articles, Links Comment in: Clin Chem. 2004 Sep;50(9):1498-9. Allele-specific change of concentration and functional gene dose for the prediction of steady-state serum concentrations of amitriptyline and nortriptyline in CYP2C19 and CYP2D6 extensive and intermediate metabolizers. Steimer W, Zopf K, von Amelunxen S, Pfeiffer H, Bachofer J, Popp J, Messner B, Kissling W, Leucht S. Institut fur Klinische Chemie und Pathobiochemie, Technische Universitat Munchen, Munich, Germany. Steimer@KlinChem.med.TU-Muenchen.de BACKGROUND: Recently, new polymorphisms were described in connection with intermediate and ultrarapid CYP2D6 metabolism. These may allow a much desired prediction of metabolic activity within the extensive metabolizer group. The functional consequences are still being discussed with few data available for clinical patients. METHODS: We conducted a prospective, blinded two-center study seeking correlations between CYP2C19 (*2,*3, and *4; conventional PCR) and CYP2D6 genotypes (*1 to *10, *35, and *41; real-time and multiplex PCR) and drug concentrations (Emit and HPLC) in 50 Caucasians receiving amitriptyline (AT; 75 mg twice a day). RESULTS: Eighteen CYP2C19 heterozygotes (*1/*2) had higher AT (P = 0.033) and lower nortriptyline (NT; P = 0.059) concentrations than 30 homozygotes (*1/*1). For CYP2D6, we calculated two new indices, i.e., the allele-specific change of concentration on identical background (ASCOC) and a quantitative functional gene dose. The ASCOC describes the change in NT concentration attributable to a mutant allele compared with the wild type. We found significantly higher concentrations for alleles *4 (95.6%; P <0.0001), *10 (63.3%; P <0.001), and *41 (39.8%; P <0.0001) but not for *2 and *35. Assigning of semiquantitative gene doses of 0, 0.5, or 1 to each allele instead of applying the current classification system (predicted phenotypes: 3 intermediate metabolizers, 46 extensive metabolizers, and 1 ultrarapid metabolizer) produced significant NT concentration differences: gene doses of 0.5 (n =3), 1 (n = 14), 1.5 (n = 11), 2 (n = 21) and 3 (n = 1; P <0.00001). CONCLUSIONS: AT and NT concentrations can be predicted within the group of CYP2D6 extensive metabolizers. The ASCOC provides substantial advantages compared with current methods of analysis. CYP2D6 but not CYP2C19 correlates with the sum of both concentrations used to guide AT therapy. Publication Types: Multicenter Study

Clin Chem. 2005 Feb;51(2):376-85. Epub 2004 Dec 8. Related Articles, Links Amitriptyline or not, that is the question: pharmacogenetic testing of CYP2D6 and CYP2C19 identifies patients with low or high risk for side effects in amitriptyline therapy. Steimer W, Zopf K, von Amelunxen S, Pfeiffer H, Bachofer J, Popp J, Messner B, Kissling W, Leucht S. Institut fur Klinische Chemie und Pathobiochemie, Klinikum rechts der Isar, Technische Universitat Munchen, Munich, Germany. W.Steimer@gmx.de BACKGROUND: Amitriptyline has been replaced in many countries by alternative and more expensive drugs based on claims of improved tolerability and toxicity and despite slightly reduced efficacy. Preliminary studies indicate that adverse effects could be linked to polymorphisms of drug-metabolizing enzymes, but information on their clinical impact remains scanty and includes mainly case reports. We conducted a prospective blinded two-center study seeking correlations between CYP2C19 and CYP2D6 genotypes, drug concentrations, adverse events, and therapy response. METHODS: Fifty Caucasian inpatients with at least medium-grade depressive disorder received amitriptyline at a fixed dose of 75 mg twice a day. Blood samples for concentration monitoring of amitriptyline and nortriptyline were taken weekly until discharge along with evaluations of depression (Hamilton Depression Scale and Clinical Global Impression Scale) and side effect (Dosage Record and Treatment Emergent Symptoms Scale; DOTES) scores. RESULTS: In a ROC analysis, nortriptyline but not amitriptyline concentrations correlated with side effects (DOTES sum score >or=5; area under the curve, 0.733; P = 0.008). Carriers of two functional CYP2D6 alleles had a significantly lower risk of side effects than carriers of only one functional allele (12.1% vs 76.5%; P = 0.00001). The lowest risk was observed for carriers of two functional CYP2D6 alleles combined with only one functional CYP2C19 allele [0 of 13 (0%) vs 9 of 11 (81.8%) for the high-risk group; P = 0.00004]. We found no correlations between drug concentrations or genotypes and therapeutic response. CONCLUSIONS: Combined pharmacogenetic testing for CYP2D6 and CYP2C19 identifies patients with low risk for side effects in amitriptyline therapy and could possibly be used to individualize antidepressive regimens and reduce treatment cost. Identification of genotypes associated with slightly reduced intermediate metabolism may be more important than currently anticipated. It could also be the key to demonstrating cost-effectiveness for CYP2D6 genotyping in critical dose drugs. Publication Types: Clinical Trial

Clin Chem. 2005 Nov;51(11):2074-84. Epub 2005 Sep 15. Related Articles, Links Liquid chromatography-tandem mass spectrometry analysis of erythrocyte thiopurine nucleotides and effect of thiopurine methyltransferase gene variants on these metabolites in patients receiving azathioprine/6-mercaptopurine therapy. Dervieux T, Meyer G, Barham R, Matsutani M, Barry M, Boulieu R, Neri B, Seidman E. Prometheus Laboratories, San Diego, CA 92121, USA. tdervieux@prometheuslabs.com BACKGROUND: Polymorphic thiopurine S-methyltransferase (TPMT) is a major determinant of thiopurine toxicity. METHODS: We extracted 6-thioguanine nucleotides (6-TGNs) and 6-methylmercaptopurine nucleotides (6-MMPNs) from erythrocytes with perchloric acid and converted them to 6-thioguanine (6-TG) and a 6-methylmercaptopurine (6-MMP) derivative during a 60-min acid hydrolysis step. The liquid chromatography system consisted of a C(18) column with an ammonium acetate-formic acid-acetonitrile buffer. 8-Bromoadenine was the internal standard. Analytes were measured with positive ionization and multiple reaction monitoring mode. With PCR-restriction fragment length polymorphism analysis and TaqMan allelic discrimination, common TPMT alleles (*1, *2, *3A, *3B, *3C) were determined in 31 792 individuals. We used perchloric acid extraction, acid hydrolysis, and HPLC with ultraviolet detection to measure erythrocyte 6-TG and 6-MMP nucleotide concentrations in 6189 patients with inflammatory bowel disease receiving azathioprine/6-mercaptopurine therapy. RESULTS: Intra- and interday imprecision were <10% at low and high analyte concentrations. The conversion of 6-TG and 6-MMP nucleoside mono-, di-, and triphosphates was complete after hydrolysis. Allelic frequency for TPMT variant alleles ranged from 0.0063% (*3B) to 3.61% (*3A). Compared with wild types, TPMT heterozygotes had an 8.3-fold higher risk for 6-TGNs >450 pmol/8 x 10(8) erythrocytes (concentration associated with increased risk for leukopenia), but an 8.2-fold lower risk for 6-MMPNs >5700 pmol/8 x 10(8) erythrocytes (concentration associated with increased risk for hepatotoxicity). CONCLUSIONS: The liquid chromatography-tandem mass spectrometry method can be applied to the routine monitoring of thiopurine therapy. The association between TPMT genotype and metabolite concentrations illustrates the utility of pharmacogenetics in the management of patients undergoing treatment with thiopurines.

Clin Chest Med. 2006 Mar;27(1):109-17. Related Articles, Links Pharmacogenetics of asthma: where are we now? Larj MJ, Bleecker ER. Center for Medical Genomics, Wake Forest University Baptist Medical Center, Medical Center Boulevard, Winston Salem, NC 27157, USA. Pharmacogenetics adds value with improved clinical markers and increased ability to predict efficacy with greater clarity. This should lead to individualized and simplified dosing, improved efficacy with specific treatment, and enhanced safety. Improved patient response should lead to enhanced patient compliance. Many challenges remain ahead including ethical issues related to patient confidentiality and banking of DNA. Regulatory issues and guidelines need to be discussed to establish reasonable boundaries. There is also a need for review of diagnosis and treatment combinations and Food and Drug Administration review of the process. Legal issues including patents and commercial issues concerning patient, physician, and managed care acceptance must be addressed.

Clin Chim Acta. 2004 Jun;344(1-2):201-4. Related Articles, Links Metabolic activity of dextromethorphan O-demethylation in healthy Japanese volunteers carrying duplicated CYP2D6 genes: duplicated allele of CYP2D6*10 does not increase CYP2D6 metabolic activity. Ishiguro A, Kubota T, Ishikawa H, Iga T. Department of Pharmacy, Faculty of Medicine, University of Tokyo Hospital, 7-3-1 Hongoh, Bunkyo, Tokyo 113-8655, Japan. BACKGROUND: This study was designed to assess the metabolic activities of dextromethorphan O-demethylation in healthy Japanese subjects carrying duplicated CYP2D6 alleles, CYP2D6*1 x 2, CYP2D6*2 x 2 or CYP2D6*10 x 2. METHODS: Forty-one unrelated healthy Japanese subjects containing carriers who had previously been genotyped as CYP2D6*1 x 2/*2, CYP2D6*1/*2 x 2, and CYP2D6*10/*10 x 2 were phenotyped with dextromethorphan. Results: The metabolic ratios of dextromethorphan/dextrorphan in subjects with CYP2D6*1 x 2/*2 or CYP2D6*1/*2 x 2 were lower than those in subjects with CYP2D6*1/*2, while the metabolic ratios in subjects with CYP2D6*10/*10 x 2, as well as homozygotes for CYP2D6*10, were significantly (P<0.01) higher than those in homozygotes for CYP2D6*1. Conclusions: The results suggested that carriers with three functional CYP2D6 genes, CYP2D6*1 x 2/*2 or CYP2D6*1/*2 x 2, are ultrarapid metabolizer phenotypes in Japanese. The results also suggested that there is no gene-dose effect with the dextromethorphan O-demethylation activities between carriers with two and three CYP2D6*10 mutated genes per genome. Therefore, CYP2D6*10 x 2 may play an important role for the treatment of Japanese patients as well as CYP2D6*10 which is mainly responsible for the intermediate metabolizers in Japanese. Copyright 2004 Elsevier B.V.

Clin Chim Acta. 2005 Dec;362(1-2):147-54. Epub 2005 Jul 15. Related Articles, Links Effects of the CYP3A5 genetic polymorphism on the pharmacokinetics of diltiazem. Yamamoto T, Kubota T, Ozeki T, Sawada M, Yokota S, Yamada Y, Kumagai Y, Iga T. Department of Pharmacy, University of Tokyo Hospital, Hongo, Bunkyo-ku, Japan. BACKGROUND: The cytochrome P450 (CYP) 3A subfamily plays an important role in the metabolism of various endogenous and exogenous compounds. Among CYP3A subfamily members, CYP3A5 is polymorphically expressed and the CYP3A5*3 and CYP3A5*6 alleles are known not to express functional CYP3A5. Thus, these mutant alleles are thought to be responsible for interindividual variability of CYP3A activity. METHODS: Subjects possessing CYP3A5*1/*1, *1/*3 or *3/*3 received oral administration of diltiazem hydrochloride (60 mg), and plasma and urinary concentrations of diltiazem and its metabolite N-desmethyldiltiazem were measured. Before drug intake, cortisol metabolic clearance in each subject was measured to estimate in vivo CYP3A4 activity. RESULTS: The mean values of total oral diltiazem clearance of subjects with *1/*1, *1/*3 and *3/*3 were 183.4 +/- 39.4, 197.9 +/- 49.6 and 293.6 +/- 141.1 (l/h), respectively, and were not significantly different among the 3 genotype groups. The cortisol metabolic clearance was not significantly different among the three genotype groups, indicating that the CYP3A4 activity is not significantly different. CONCLUSION: The results suggest that CYP3A5*3 has only a minor effect on the pharmacokinetics and metabolism of diltiazem. Although our results did not indicate significance of CYP3A5, the effects of CYP3A5*3 on the metabolism of other CYP3A substrates remain to be investigated.

Clin Chim Acta. 2005 Dec;362(1-2):182-8. Epub 2005 Jul 20. Related Articles, Links
Pharmacogenetic study of apolipoprotein E, cholesteryl ester transfer protein and hepatic lipase genes and simvastatin therapy in Brazilian subjects. Fiegenbaum M, da Silveira FR, Van der Sand CR, Van der Sand LC, Ferreira ME, Pires RC, Hutz MH. Departamento de Genetica, Universidade Federal do Rio Grande do Sul, Porto Alegre, Brazil. BACKGROUND: In recent years, one of the focuses of genetic investigation in cardiology has been to identify the genetic factors associated with variable response to statin treatment. Polymorphisms in apolipoprotein E (APOE), cholesteryl ester transfer protein (CETP) and hepatic lipase (LIPC), proteins with major roles in lipid metabolism and homeostasis have been shown associated with lipid-lowering drugs response. METHODS: One hundred forty-six hypercholesterolemic patients of European descent were prospectively enrolled and treated with simvastatin 20 mg per day for over 6 months. Ninety-nine subjects completed the 6-month follow-up. Plasma lipids and lipoproteins were measured before and throughout the study. APOE (E*2, E*3 and E*4), LIPC-250A > G and CETP TaqIB genotypes were determined by PCR and restriction mapping. RESULTS: After a 6-month follow-up, no differences among genotypes in the percentage variation in lipid and lipoprotein concentrations for APOE and LIPC SNPs were observed. After adjustment for covariates, CETP B2B2 homozygotes showed a greater HDL-cholesterol increase compared to B1B2 and B1B1 subjects (14.1% vs. 1.7% and 1.3%, $P < 0.05$, respectively). CONCLUSION: Our study demonstrates that individual plasma HDL-cholesterol response to simvastatin is mediated, in part, by the CETP gene locus, with the B2 homozygotes having more benefit in HDL-C improvement than carriers of B1 allele.

Clin Chim Acta. 2006 Jan;363(1-2):177-86. Epub 2005 Aug 26. Related Articles, Links
Genetic testing for pharmacogenetics and its clinical application in drug therapy. Hiratsuka M, Sasaki T, Mizugaki M. Department of Clinical Pharmaceutics, Tohoku Pharmaceutical University, Aoba-ku, Sendai, Japan. There is wide individual variation in drug responses and adverse effects. As the main causes of the variation in drug responses, attention has focused on the genetic polymorphisms that encode metabolic enzymes regulating pharmacodynamics and receptors modulating the affinity with the responsive sites. Tailor-made drug therapy analyzes genetic polymorphisms involved in drug responses before drug administration and selects drugs and doses suitable for the individual genetic background. Establishment of tailor-made drug therapy is expected to contribute to medical economy by avoiding wasteful drug administration. To promote such medical practice, it is necessary to use simple genetic testing that is clinically convenient. Currently, genetic testing using real-time PCR has been frequently employed at laboratories with its clinical application anticipated. As to the many genes involved in drug responses, to date, the application of patient genetic information to tailor-made drug therapy has been achieved at the practical level. Information on pharmacogenetics will be a critical factor in medical practice in the near future. Publication Types: Review

Clin Colorectal Cancer. 2004 Jun;4 Suppl 1:S43-7. Related Articles, Links

Application of pharmacogenomics in the individualization of chemotherapy for gastrointestinal malignancies. McLeod HL, King CR, Marsh S. Department of Medicine and the Siteman Cancer Center, Washington University School of Medicine, St. Louis, MO 63110-1093, USA. hmcleod@im.wustl.edu The large number of active combination chemotherapy regimens for the treatment of gastrointestinal cancers has led to the need for better information to guide the "standard" treatment for each patient. In an attempt to individualize therapy, pharmacogenomics evaluates the hereditary basis for interindividual differences in drug response. This report will focus on the results of studies assessing the effects of polymorphisms in drug-metabolizing enzymes and drug targets on the toxicity and response to chemotherapy drugs commonly used to treat gastrointestinal malignancies.

Clin Colorectal Cancer. 2005 May;5(1):61-4. Related Articles, Links Severe irinotecan-induced toxicities in a patient with uridine diphosphate glucuronosyltransferase 1A1 polymorphism. Mehra R, Murren J, Chung G, Smith B, Psyrri A. Department of Medical Oncology, Yale University Cancer Center, New Haven, CT 06520, USA. Irinotecan is an analogue of camptothecin, a topoisomerase I inhibitor, that has an important role in the management of advanced colorectal cancer. It is approved as first-line therapy in combination with 5-fluorouracil and leucovorin or as monotherapy in the second-line setting. Its clinical use has been associated with variability in terms of pharmacokinetic behavior and toxicities, especially myelosuppression and diarrhea. Irinotecan is metabolized to the active compound SN-38; it is now known that the metabolism of irinotecan and the inactivation of SN-38 by glucuronidation are mediated by genetic differences, which contributes to the variability. In this article, a case is presented that illustrates this, and there is a brief discussion of the clinical pharmacology of irinotecan and some of the genetic variations that affect its cellular metabolism. Publication Types: Case Reports

Clin Exp Allergy. 2005 Sep;35(9):1162-7. Related Articles, Links Association between bronchodilating response to short-acting beta-agonist and non-synonymous single-nucleotide polymorphisms of beta-adrenoceptor gene. Cho SH, Oh SY, Bahn JW, Choi JY, Chang YS, Kim YK, Min KU, Kim YY. Department of Internal Medicine, Seoul National University College of Medicine, 28 Yongon-dong, Chongno-gu, Seoul 110-744, Korea. BACKGROUND: With beta-agonists being the most widely used agents in the treatment of asthma, in vitro studies reported that beta(2)-adrenergic receptor (ADRB2) polymorphisms are associated with agonist-promoted down-regulation. OBJECTIVE: The present population-based study aimed to evaluate the association between bronchodilating response to inhaled short-acting beta-agonist and two non-synonymous single-nucleotide polymorphisms (SNPs) of ADRB2 (ADRB2-16 and ADRB2-27). METHODS: Two hundred and nine children with reduction in forced expiratory volume in 1 s of more than 20% on methacholine bronchial challenge underwent bronchodilating response testing 5 min after the inhalation of 200 mug of albuterol. Of these 209, 195 gave peripheral blood for genotyping of ADRB2 polymorphisms. RESULTS: The bronchodilating response was significantly higher in subjects with the homozygous Arg16 than in those with the homozygous

Gly16. It was further demonstrated that haplotype pairs of the homozygous Arg16Gln27 and of the heterozygous Arg16Gln27/Gly16Glu27 showed the highest bronchodilating responses, and the haplotype pairs of the homozygous Gly16Gln27 the lowest response. As a whole, the bronchodilating response was more positively associated with the combined quantity of Arg16 and Glu27 polymorphisms than with that of Arg16 alone. CONCLUSION: Non-synonymous SNPs of ADRB2 at codons 16 and 27 is significantly associated with bronchodilating response to inhaled short acting beta-agonists.

Clin Exp Pharmacol Physiol. 2005 Nov;32(11):975-8. Related Articles, Links Individualized drug and dose: the clinical pharmacologist's calling or curse? Begg EJ. Department of Medicine, Christchurch School of Medicine, Christchurch, New Zealand. evan.begg@chmeds.ac.nz 1. The role of the clinical pharmacologist is to promote the rational, safe and effective use of medicines. This revolves around the notion of variability, between and within patients and between and within drugs, in terms of both pharmacokinetics and pharmacodynamics. Ideal therapeutics involves tailoring the drug and its dosing to the individual patient, taking into account this variability. 2. In the 25 years of my membership of the Australasian Society of Clinical and Experimental Pharmacologists and Toxicologists, three themes have dominated my research: (i) drugs and breast feeding; (ii) aminoglycoside dosing; and (iii) pharmacogenetics. In all these, the research has been orientated towards identifying factors involved in variability and working towards dose individualization based on the understanding of these factors. 3. Our model for predicting drug concentrations in milk has assisted not only in estimating the safety of drug ingestion via breast milk, but also in the understanding of the processes involved in drug transfer. 4. The aminoglycoside studies have assisted in the understanding of the basis behind extended interval dosing, leading to a model for dose prediction that is widely used, especially in Australasia. 5. Pharmacogenetics is a field widely acclaimed as having a huge future in terms of individualization of drug therapy. Our early studies in this area lend only cautious support to this optimism.

Clin Experiment Ophthalmol. 2004 Jun;32(3):236-7. Related Articles, Links Comment on: Clin Experiment Ophthalmol. 2004 Jun;32(3):305-24. The promise and challenges of personalized medicine for eye diseases. McCarty CA. Publication Types: Comment Editorial

Clin Gastroenterol Hepatol. 2006 Jan;4(1):21-8. Related Articles, Links Pharmacogenomics in inflammatory bowel disease. Egan LJ, Derijks LJ, Hommes DW. Department of Pharmacology, National University of Ireland, Galway, Ireland. laurence.egan@nuigalway.ie Inherited variations in the nucleotide sequence of genes influence how individual patients respond to drugs. Most commonly, clinically significant genetic variations consist of single nucleotide polymorphisms (SNPs) within genes that affect drug disposition or drug targets. Up to now, relatively few clinically important examples of inherited traits that affect drug responses have been studied in detail. However, one of the well-characterized examples is highly relevant to inflammatory bowel disease therapeutics, that of thiopurine methyltransferase pharmacogenetics. Individuals with 2 normal alleles of the gene encoding thiopurine methyltransferase metabolize and clear thiopurines such as azathioprine and 6-mercaptopurine rapidly. Individuals with 1 normal and 1 variant allele are intermediate, whereas those with 2 variant alleles clear thiopurines very slowly. Intermediate and slow metabolizers are predisposed to have high active thiopurine drug levels and develop bone marrow suppression. Genomic era technology permits determination of large numbers of SNPs in large numbers of individuals. This capability is allowing the field of pharmacogenomics to become one of the most productive interfaces in translational biomedical research at present. By using high-throughput SNP genotyping, combined with careful phenotypic characterization of disease, pharmacogenomic research carries the potential of identifying individual biomarkers that predict the relative likelihood of benefit or risk from a therapeutic intervention. If this promise can be realized, pharmacogenomics will deliver the opportunity for personalized medicine.

Clin Infect Dis. 2004 Jul 1;39(1):98-106. Epub 2004 Jun 1. Related Articles, Links The pharmacogenetics of antiretroviral therapy: a review of studies to date. Quirk E, McLeod H, Powderly W. Department of Medicine, Washington University School of Medicine, St. Louis, Missouri 63110, USA. equirk@im.wustl.edu Although the ever-expanding armamentarium of antiretroviral drugs has significantly decreased the morbidity and mortality due to human immunodeficiency virus infection, patients and clinicians are increasingly faced with the problems of inadequate or toxic response to therapy that may be genetically mediated. Significant evidence now exists that interindividual differences, such as efficacy of therapy, hypersensitivity reactions, and metabolic complications as a result of antiretroviral therapy, are in part genetically determined. This article reviews the significant studies published to date in the area of the pharmacogenetics of antiretroviral therapy and summarizes current trends, as well as areas where further research is needed.

Clin Infect Dis. 2005 Nov 15;41 Suppl 7:S449-52. Related Articles, Links Pharmacogenetic analysis of clinically relevant genetic polymorphisms. McLeod HL. Department of Medicine, The Alvin J. Siteman Cancer Center, Washington University School of Medicine, St. Louis, MO 63110, USA. hmcleod@im.wustl.edu The ascertainment of the human genome sequence has generated great enthusiasm for the use of gene-based approaches to improve virtually all aspects of medical care. Particular interest has focused on the field of pharmacogenetics--for example, the use of an individual's genetic profile to optimize drug prescription. This approach takes advantage of the presence of single-nucleotide polymorphisms (SNPs) or other genetic variants in every gene in the human genome. There are currently > 9 million SNPs in the human SNP database dbSNP, with an estimated 11 million variants ultimately to be found in the human population. To date, the preponderance of interest in this field has centered on the potential of applying this approach to subacute or chronic illnesses, such as cancer, cardiovascular disease, human immunodeficiency virus infection, or rheumatologic disorders. In contrast, little attention has been devoted to the potential utility of implementing the pharmacogenomic methodology for guiding drug selection for acutely ill patients in the critical care environment. Although such an approach has theoretical appeal as a means of enhancing quality and improving outcomes in this setting, several obstacles currently exist and slow the progress toward clinical application.

Clin Infect Dis. 2006 Feb 1;42(3):401-7. Epub 2005 Dec 27. Related Articles, Links Pharmacogenetics of plasma efavirenz exposure after treatment discontinuation: an Adult AIDS Clinical Trials Group Study. Ribaudo HJ, Haas DW, Tierney C, Kim RB, Wilkinson GR, Gulick RM, Clifford DB, Marzolini C, Fletcher CV, Tashima KT, Kuritzkes DR, Acosta EP; Adult AIDS Clinical Trials Group Study. Statistical Data Analysis Center, Harvard School of Public Health, Harvard Medical School, Boston, MA, USA. BACKGROUND: Efavirenz has a long plasma half-life and a low genetic barrier to resistance. Simultaneously stopping treatment with all agents in efavirenz-containing regimens may result in functional efavirenz monotherapy that selects for drug-resistant human immunodeficiency virus type 1. Lower plasma efavirenz clearance is associated with a cytochrome P450 2B6 gene (CYP2B6) polymorphism (516G-->T) that is more frequent among African American individuals than among European American individuals. METHODS: We characterized relationships between this polymorphism and predicted plasma efavirenz concentration-time profiles after discontinuation of therapy with use of data obtained from subjects receiving therapy. Pharmacokinetic parameters were estimated using population-based methods. Concentrations after discontinuation of therapy were predicted from subject-specific estimates. RESULTS. Median estimated efavirenz half-lives were 23, 27, and 48 h for patients with CYP2B6 position 516 GG (78 patients), GT (60), and TT (14) genotypes, respectively (P<.001). After therapy was stopped, plasma efavirenz concentrations in patients with GG, GT, and TT genotypes were predicted to exceed 46.7 ng/mL (the estimated protein-adjusted 95% inhibitory concentration for wild-type virus) for a median of 5.8 days (interquartile range [IQR], 4.4-8.3 days), 7.0 days (IQR, 5.0-8.0 days), and 14 days (IQR, 11.1-21.2 days), respectively (P<.001). Plasma efavirenz levels were predicted to exceed 46.7 ng/mL for >21 days in 5% of subjects with GG genotype, 5% of subjects with GT genotype, and 29% of subjects with TT genotype. CONCLUSIONS: The CYP2B6 position 516 TT genotype or a prolonged measured elimination half-life may predict increased risk of developing drug resistance among patients who discontinue efavirenz-containing regimens. This has implications for strategies to safely discontinue antiretroviral regimens while avoiding the emergence of drug resistance.

Clin Invest Med. 2004 Feb;27(1):14-5. Related Articles, Links Genetic medicine: ethical and practical issues of application of the new technology. Kotalik J, Silverman M. Department of Medicine, McMaster University.

Clin Invest Med. 2004 Feb;27(1):5-6. Related Articles, Links Genes, race and drugs. Bevan D. Publication Types: Editorial

Clin Lab. 2004;50(3-4):141-8. Related Articles, Links Development and evaluation of a rapid and reliable method for cytochrome P450 2C8 genotyping. Weise A, Grundler S, Zaumsegel D, Klotzek M, Grondahl B, Forst T, Pfutzner A. Institute for Clinical Research and Development, IKFE GmhH, Mainz, Germany. The analysis of gene polymorphisms has started to become an interesting field of new services to be provided by clinical laboratories for both, clinical research and routine determinations. To expand the use of these methods and to increase the benefit for patients and the society, cheap and reliable methods for genotyping also allowing for high-turnover analysis need to be established in clinical laboratories. The presented investigation was performed to develop and evaluate a fast real-time PCR method for the detection of three different allele mutations of Cytochrome P450 isoenzyme 2C8 (CYP2C8*2, *3, and *4), which have been demonstrated to influence drug metabolism (and thus the efficacy) of a variety of drugs. The DNA of 122 Caucasian subjects (56 male, 66 female, age (mean +/- STD): 50 +/- 16 years) was analyzed for these mutations by means of classical RFLP-PCR and a new protocol developed for the LightCycler real-time PCR method. The polymorphisms within the CYP2C8 gene were detected by use of two primer pairs and three different pairs of hybridization probes. The results of both methods were perfectly concordant and comparable to results published in the literature (allele frequencies: CYP2C8*2: 0.016, *3: 0.140, *4: 0.074). A subsequent analysis of the related costs revealed comparable resource requirements but substantially longer time needs for RFLP-PCR, resulting in higher overall analysis costs for the older method. In conclusion, the elaborated protocol for real-time PCR analysis of gene mutations CYP2C8*2, *3, and *4 is reliable and cost effective, and thus, suitable for routine laboratory use. Publication Types: Evaluation Studies

Clin Lung Cancer. 2004 Dec;6 Suppl 1:S30-4. Related Articles, Links Predictors of sensitivity and resistance to epidermal growth factor receptor inhibitors. Perea S, Hidalgo M. The Sidney Kimmel Comprehensive Cancer Center, Johns Hopkins University School of Medicine, Baltimore, MD 21231, USA. Lung cancer is one of the leading types of cancer with an associated high mortality. Currently, treatment with conventional cytotoxic agents remains suboptimal. Inhibition of the epidermal growth factor receptor (EGFR) with monoclonal antibodies or small-molecule inhibitors of the tyrosine kinase (TK) domain of the receptor have demonstrated modest, albeit significant, antitumor activities in patients with non-small-cell lung cancer (NSCLC). The goal of any targeted therapy is to direct treatment to those patients who are more likely to derive benefit from such a treatment. Two interventions may improve the predicted sensitivity to these agents: (1) the use of a real predictor before treatment, represented by pharmacodiagnostic tests, and (2) studying the relationship between an early event after treatment and outcome, represented by pharmacodynamic tests. Pharmacodiagnostic factors that have been studied include the clinical features and histologic subtype of the tumor, the presence of somatic mutations in the TK domain of the EGFR, the expression of the receptor itself, and the activation of the receptor signaling pathway. Pharmacodynamic events associated with improved outcome include drug-induced rash and regulation of the receptor expression. Currently, the best established determinant of response to small-molecule inhibitors of the EGFR is the presence of activating mutations in the receptor TK domain. However, it is not known whether these functional mutations are involved in the response of NSCLC to monoclonal antibodies. Further investigation is needed to better predict patients who are more likely to benefit from these drugs. Publication Types: Review

Clin Lung Cancer. 2004 Sep;6(2):79-82. Related Articles, Links Impact of genetic polymorphisms in DNA repair enzymes on drug resistance in lung cancer. [No authors listed] Publication Types: Review

Clin Med. 2005 Sep-Oct;5(5):476-81. Related Articles, Links Molecular genetics goes to the diabetes clinic. Hattersley AT. Peninsu Medical School, Exeter. A.T.Hattersley@exeter.ac.uk Diabetes has historically been thought of as a medical specialty which primarily deals with treatment rather than diagnosis. Molecular genetic testing can now be used to make a diagnosis of the 1-2% of all diabetic patients with monogenic diabetes. Making a diagnosis of monogenic diabetes is important as it can have a dramatic effect on the treatment a patient should receive: glucokinase MODY patients need no treatment; HNF1alpha MODY patients are very sensitive to low dose sulphonylureas; and patients with neonatal diabetes due to Kir6.2 mutations, despite being insulin dependent, can discontinue insulin and be well controlled on high dose sulphonylurea tablets. The challenge for diabetologists is to use clinical skills to detect these monogenic patients whose care will be greatly helped by the treatment changes that follow molecular genetic testing.

Clin Nurse Spec. 2004 May-Jun;18(3):126-32; quiz 133-4. Related Articles, Links Genetic practice, education, and research: an overview for advanced practice nurses. Beery TA, Hern MJ. Adult Health Nursing, College of Nursing, University of Cincinnati, Cincinnati, Ohio, USA. PURPOSE/OBJECTIVES: The purpose of this article is to describe how the new genomic era will affect advanced practice registered nurses (APRNs) patient care, education, and research. BACKGROUND/RATIONALE: Given the exponential growth of genetic information and that 9 of the top 10 leading causes of mortality have genetic components (www.cdc.gov), it is imperative to educate advanced practice nurses about this salient topic. DESCRIPTION OF THE PROCESS: Because few APRNs in practice or academia have had formal education on genetics, the first step of nursings' own gene discovery is recognizing that there is an ongoing need to understand state of the science genetic information to gain clinical and educational utility. OUTCOMES: By recognizing APRNs need to know genetics, APRNs will clamor within their workplace for continuing education about this dynamic information. It is critical knowledge for APRNs to classify risk based on family history, target individualized patient prevention and education, modify pharmacologic interventions, and refer when genetic testing is necessary. INTERPRETATION/CONCLUSION: This article stresses the timely relevance of applying genetics and genomics to practice, teaching, and research. IMPLICATIONS FOR NURSING PRACTICE: APRNs need to maintain a place at the genetic table with all healthcare providers by developing strategies to expand this nursing knowledge to their practice, teaching, and research. Nurses need to be cognizant of the keen genetic value of family histories, how risk classification will individualize prevention recommendations, and the exciting role of pharmacogenetics, given many APRNs' prescriptive authority. Our core professional belief that each human is highly unique has probably never been more accurate than with the future in genetic and genomic nursing. Publication Types: Review

Clin Obstet Gynecol. 2005 Sep;48(3):737-42. Related Articles, Links Future considerations in pelvic reconstructive surgery. Cornella JL. Department of Obstetrics and Gynecology, Mayo Clinic College of Medicine, Mayo Clinic Scottsdale, Scottsdale, Arizona, USA. Cornella.Jeffrey@mayo.edu Publication Types: Review

Clin Perinatol. 2004 Mar;31(1):53-67. Related Articles, Links The role of molecular genetics in the pathogenesis and diagnosis of neonatal sepsis. Del Vecchio A, Laforgia N, Capasso M, Iolascon A, Latini G. Neonatal Intensive Care Unit, Azienda U.S.L. BR/1, Ospedale A. Perrino, Brindisi 72100, Italy. delveccant@libero.it Polymorphisms within genes encoding endogenous mediators of inflammation are good candidates for the individual differences in systemic inflammatory responses of neonates to infection. Ina similar manner, polymorphisms in the genes encoding drug metabolizing enzymes, drug transporters, and drug receptors can influence a neonate's risk of an adverse drug reaction or can alter the efficacy of drug treatment. Additionally, molecular tools are proving valuable in the diagnosis of neonatal infection. This article gives an overview of the genetic susceptibility to sepsis, discusses the use of molecular genetics in diagnostic tests for infection, and reviews the potential for more effective and specific therapies for sepsis based on genetic variability. Publication Types: Review

Clin Pharmacokinet. 2004;43(14):983-1013. Related Articles, Links Genetic predictors of the clinical response to opioid analgesics: clinical utility and future perspectives. Lotsch J, Skarke C, Liefhold J, Geisslinger G. Pharmazentrum Frankfurt/ZAFES, Institute of Clinical Pharmacology, Johann Wolfgang Goethe-University, Theodor-Stern-Kai 7, D-60590 Frankfurt, Germany. j.loetsch@em.uni-frankfurt.de This review uses a candidate gene approach to identify possible pharmacogenetic modulators of opioid therapy, and discusses these modulators together with demonstrated genetic causes for the variability in clinical effects of opioids.Genetically caused inactivity of cytochrome P450 (CYP) 2D6 renders codeine ineffective (lack of morphine formation), slightly decreases the efficacy of tramadol (lack of formation of the active O-desmethyl-tramadol) and slightly decreases the clearance of methadone. MDR1 mutations often demonstrate pharmacogenetic consequences, and since opioids are among the P-glycoprotein substrates, opioid pharmacology may be affected by MDR1 mutations. The single nucleotide polymorphism A118G of the mu opioid receptor gene has been associated with decreased potency of morphine and morphine-6-glucuronide, and with decreased analgesic effects and higher alfentanil dose demands in carriers of the mutated G118 allele. Genetic causes may also trigger or modify drug interactions, which in turn can alter the clinical response to opioid therapy. For example, by inhibiting CYP2D6, paroxetine increases the steady-state plasma concentrations of (R)-methadone in extensive but not in poor metabolisers of debrisoquine/sparteine.So far, the clinical consequences of the pharmacogenetics of opioids are limited to codeine, which should not be administered to poor metabolisers of debrisoquine/sparteine. Genetically precipitated drug interactions might render a standard opioid dose toxic and should, therefore, be taken into consideration. Mutations affecting opioid receptors and pain perception/processing are of interest for the study of opioid actions, but with modern practice of on-demand administration of opioids their utility may be limited to explaining why some patients need higher opioid doses; however, the adverse effects profile may be modified by these mutations. Nonetheless, at a limited level, pharmacogenetics can be expected to facilitate individualised opioid therapy. Publication Types: Review

Clin Pharmacokinet. 2006;45(3):253-85. Related Articles, Links Genetic polymorphisms of drug-metabolising enzymes and drug transporters in the chemotherapeutic treatment of cancer. Bosch TM, Meijerman I, Beijnen JH, Schellens JH. Department of Pharmacy and Pharmacology, The Netherlands Cancer Institute/Slotervaart Hospital, Amsterdam, The Netherlands. There is wide variability in the response of individuals to standard doses of drug therapy. This is an important problem in clinical practice, where it can lead to therapeutic failures or adverse drug reactions. Polymorphisms in genes coding for metabolising enzymes and drug transporters can affect drug efficacy and toxicity. Pharmacogenetics aims to identify individuals predisposed to a high risk of toxicity and low response from standard doses of anti-cancer drugs. This review focuses on the clinical significance of polymorphisms in drug-metabolising enzymes (cytochrome P450 [CYP] 2C8, CYP2C9, CYP2C19, CYP2D6, CYP3A4, CYP3A5, dihydropyrimidine dehydrogenase, uridine diphosphate glucuronosyltransferase [UGT] 1A1, glutathione S-transferase, sulfotransferase [SULT] 1A1, N-acetyltransferase [NAT], thiopurine methyltransferase [TPMT]) and drug transporters (P-glycoprotein [multidrug resistance 1], multidrug resistance protein 2 [MRP2], breast cancer resistance protein [BCRP]) in influencing efficacy and toxicity of chemotherapy.The most important example to demonstrate the influence of pharmacogenetics on anti-cancer therapy is TPMT. A decreased activity of TPMT, caused by genetic polymorphisms in the TPMT gene, causes severe toxicity with mercaptopurine. Dosage reduction is necessary for patients with heterozygous or homozygous mutation in this gene.Other polymorphisms showing the influence of pharmacogenetics in the chemotherapeutic treatment of cancer are discussed, such as UGT1A1*28. This polymorphism is associated with an increase in toxicity with irinotecan. Also, polymorphisms in the DPYD gene show a relation with fluorouracil-related toxicity; however, in most cases no clear association has been found for polymorphisms in drug-metabolising enzymes and drug transporters, and pharmacokinetics or pharmacodynamics of anti-cancer drugs. The studies discussed evaluate different regimens and tumour types and show that polymorphisms can have different, sometimes even contradictory, pharmacokinetic and pharmacodynamic effects in different tumours in response to different drugs.The clinical application of pharmacogenetics in cancer treatment will therefore require more detailed information of the different polymorphisms in drug-metabolising enzymes and drug transporters. Larger studies, in different ethnic populations, and extended with haplotype and linkage disequilibrium analysis, will be necessary for each anti-cancer drug separately.

Clin Pharmacol Ther. 2004 Apr;75(4):253-8. Related Articles, Links Pharmacogenetics: inherited variation in amino acid sequence and altered protein quantity. Weinshilboum R, Wang L. Department of Molecular Pharmacology and Experimental Therapeutics and Medicine, Mayo Medical School-Mayo Clinic-Mayo Foundation, Rochester, MN 55905, USA.

weinshilboum.richard@mayo.edu
Publication Types: Review

Clin Pharmacol Ther. 2004 Aug;76(2):104-12. Related Articles, Links Effect of the CYP3A5 genotype on the pharmacokinetics of intravenous midazolam during inhibited and induced metabolic states. Yu KS, Cho JY, Jang IJ, Hong KS, Chung JY, Kim JR, Lim HS, Oh DS, Yi SY, Liu KH, Shin JG, Shin SG. Department of Pharmacology and Clinical Pharmacology Unit, Seoul National University College of Medicine and Hospital, Seoul, South Korea. OBJECTIVE: Our objective was to investigate the effect of the CYP3A5 genotype on the systemic clearance of midazolam in constitutive, inhibited, and induced metabolic conditions. METHODS: Nineteen healthy volunteers were grouped with regard to the CYP3A5*3 allele, into homozygous wild-type (CYP3A5*1/*1, n = 6), heterozygous (CYP3A5*1/*3, n = 6), and homozygous variant-type (CYP3A5*3/*3, n = 7) subject groups. The pharmacokinetic profile of intravenous midazolam was characterized before and after itraconazole administration (200 mg once daily for 4 days) and also after rifampin (INN, rifampicin) pretreatment (600 mg once daily for 10 days), with a washout period of 2 weeks in between. RESULTS: The pharmacokinetic profiles of midazolam and of its hydroxy metabolites did not show differences between the genotype groups under basal and induced metabolic conditions. However, during the inhibited metabolic state, the CYP3A5*3/*3 group showed a greater decrease in systemic clearance than was seen in the CYP3A5*1/*1 group (8.5 +/- 3.8 L. h(-1). 70 kg(-1) versus 13.5 +/- 2.7 L. h(-1). 70 kg(-1), P =.027). The 1'-hydroxymidazolam-to-midazolam area under the plasma concentration-time curve ratio was also significantly lower in the CYP3A5*3/*3 group (0.58 +/- 0.35 versus 1.09 +/- 0.37 for the homozygous wild-type group, P =.026). CONCLUSIONS: The CYP3A5 genotype did not affect the pharmacokinetics of intravenous midazolam in the basal or induced states. However, during cytochrome P450 (CYP) 3A inhibition by itraconazole, individuals carrying the CYP3A5*1 allele were found to be less susceptible to changes in systemic clearance and showed higher 1'-hydroxymidazolam-to-midazolam area under the plasma concentration-time curve ratios, probably resulting from the relatively CYP3A4-specific inhibition caused by itraconazole.

Clin Pharmacol Ther. 2004 Aug;76(2):113-8. Related Articles, Links Functional impact of CYP2C95, CYP2C96, CYP2C98, and CYP2C911 in vivo among black Africans. Allabi AC, Gala JL, Horsmans Y, Babaoglu MO, Bozkurt A, Heusterspreute M, Yasar U. Centre d'Investigations Cliniques et de Recherches Therapeutiques, Cove, Republique du Benin. Background and aim Previous data indicate that the urinary losartan/E-3174 ratio is a marker for cytochrome P450 (CYP) 2C9 activity in vivo. The functional impact of CYP2C9*5, *6, *8, and *11 polymorphisms in vivo has not been investigated previously in humans. METHODS: A single oral dose of losartan (25 mg) was given to 19 Beninese subjects with CYP2C9*1/*1 (n = 9), *1/*5 (n = 1), *1/*6 (n = 1), *1/*8 (n = 2), *1/*11 (n = 3), *5/*6 (n = 1), *5/*8 (n = 1), and *8/*11 (n = 1) genotypes. Concentrations of losartan and its active metabolite E-3174 were determined in urine from 0 to 8 hours by HPLC. The losartan/E-3174 metabolic ratio was used as a measure of losartan oxidation in vivo. RESULTS: The urinary losartan/E-3174 ratio in the various genotypes was as follows: 1.85 +/- 2.4 (mean +/- SD) for CYP2C9*1/*1, 14.6 for CYP2C9*1/*5, 4.2 for CYP2C9*1/*6, 188 for CYP2C9*5/*6, 11.6 for CYP2C9*5/*8, 0.44 +/- 0.13 (mean +/- SD) for CYP2C9*1/*8, 2.2 for CYP2C9*8/*11, and 5.72 +/- 4.5 (mean +/- SD) for CYP2C9*1/*11. Compared with the CYP2C9*1/*1 genotypes, the losartan/E-3174 ratio was significantly different in the CYP2C9*5 allele carriers (CYP2C9*1/*5, CYP2C9*5/*8, and CYP2C9*5/*6 genotypes) (P =.01, Mann-Whitney) but was not different in CYP2C9*1/*8 (P =.16) and CYP2C9*1/*11 (P =.11) carriers. The urinary losartan/E-3174 ratio of the single CYP2C9*1/*6 subject was higher than the 95% confidence interval of the mean of the CYP2C9*1/*1 group (0.0-3.7), whereas the metabolic ratio of the CYP2C9*8/*11 carrier was inside the 95% confidence interval of the means of the CYP2C9*1/*1 and CYP2C9*1/*11 groups (0.0-18). CONCLUSIONS: The CYP2C9*5 and *6 alleles are associated with decreased enzyme activity in vivo compared with the wild-type variant, whereas the CYP2C9*8 and *11 variants did not appear to have large in vivo effects.

Clin Pharmacol Ther. 2004 Aug;76(2):185-6; author reply 186. Related Articles, Links Caution with beta1-adrenergic receptor genotyping. Lanfear DE, Marsh S, McLeod HL. Publication Types: Letter

Clin Pharmacol Ther. 2004 Aug;76(2):99-103. Related Articles, Links Genetic variability in cytochrome P450 3A5 and in vivo cytochrome P450 3A activity: some answers but still questions. Wilkinson GR. Department of Pharmacology, Vanderbilt University School of Medicine, Nashville, Tenn 37232-6602, USA . grant.wilkinson@vanderbilt.edu Publication Types: Editorial

Clin Pharmacol Ther. 2004 Dec;76(6):528-35. Related Articles, Links Pharmacogenetics of human carboxylesterase 2, an enzyme involved in the activation of irinotecan into SN-38. Charasson V, Bellott R, Meynard D, Longy M, Gorry P, Robert J. Laboratory of Pharmacology of Anticancer Agents, Institut Bergonie and Universite Victor Segalen Bordeaux 2, 33076 Bordeaux Cedex, France. PURPOSE: Irinotecan, a drug widely used in the treatment of advanced colorectal cancers, is a prodrug requiring activation to 7-ethyl-10-hydroxycamptothecin (SN-38) by carboxylesterase 2 (hCE2). The existence of functional polymorphisms in the gene encoding this enzyme could explain the individual variability in drug efficacy and toxicity. We have explored this possibility in looking for single nucleotide polymorphisms and their functional consequence. METHODS: In a series of 115 human deoxyribonucleic acid samples, we have explored the 12 exons of the hCE2 gene, the intron-exon junctions, and the 5'- and 3'-untranslated regions, by denaturing HPLC and sequencing of polymerase chain reaction products. The functionality of the variations identified was studied in 60 human liver samples by measuring hCE2 gene expression by real-time reverse transcriptase-polymerase chain reaction of messenger ribonucleic acid extracts and carboxylesterase activity by use of irinotecan as a substrate. RESULTS: We have identified a total of 11 single nucleotide polymorphisms, none of them able to alter the amino acid sequence of the protein. They are distributed in 10 distinct genotypes in addition to the wild type. The most frequent variation (localized in IVS10) has an allele frequency of 0.17 and has been identified at the homozygous state in 1 sample. hCE2 gene expression and carboxylesterase activity in the variants identified were not significantly different from those measured in wild-type samples. CONCLUSION: The hCE2 gene presents several polymorphisms, none of which seems to be involved in significant variations in protein activity and, therefore, in irinotecan activation.

Clin Pharmacol Ther. 2004 Jul;76(1):1-17. Related Articles, Links Comment in: Clin Pharmacol Ther. 2005 Jul;78(1):92-3. Clin Pharmacol Ther. 2005 May;77(5):451. Health risks of herbal remedies: an update. De Smet PA. Scientific Institute Dutch Pharmacists, The Hague, The Netherlands. pdesmet@winap.nl Publication Types: Review

Clin Pharmacol Ther. 2004 Jul;76(1):97-8; author reply 98. Related Articles, Links Comment on: Clin Pharmacol Ther. 2003 Sep;74(3):197-202. Optimizing drug therapy. Spector R. Publication Types: Comment Letter

Clin Pharmacol Ther. 2004 May;75(5):376-80. Related Articles, Links CYP2C9 and oral anticoagulation therapy with acenocoumarol and warfarin: similarities yet differences. Takahashi H, Wilkinson GR, Padrini R, Echizen H. Department of Pharmacotherapy, Meiji Pharmaceutical University, Tokyo, Japan. harumit@my-pharm.ac.jp Publication Types: Review

Clin Pharmacol Ther. 2004 May;75(5):403-14. Related Articles, Links Pharmacogenetics of acenocoumarol pharmacodynamics. Morin S, Bodin L, Loriot MA, Thijssen HH, Robert A, Strabach S, Verstuyft C, Tregouet DA, Dubert L, Laurent-Puig P, Funck-Brentano C, Jaillon P, Beaune PH, Becquemont L. Pharmacology Department, Saint-Antoine University Hospital, Paris, France. OBJECTIVE: The aim of this study was to investigate the respective contribution of the different cytochrome P450 (CYP) 2C9 genetic polymorphisms to the interindividual variability of acenocoumarol pharmacodynamic response. METHODS: A total of 263 healthy volunteers were genotyped for CYP2C9*2, CYP2C9*3, CYP2C9*4, and CYP2C9*5 alleles, as well as for the nicotinamide adenine dinucleotide phosphate, reduced, quinone oxidoreductase 1 genetic polymorphism (NQO1*2). Moreover, the 5'-flanking region of the CYP2C9 gene was investigated for new polymorphisms, and haplotype analysis was then performed. Finally, CYP2C9 phenotype was evaluated after a single oral dose of 4 mg of acenocoumarol. Factor VII coagulant activity was measured before and 24 hours after acenocoumarol intake. RESULTS: The CYP2C9*3 allele was the only nonsynonymous single nucleotide polymorphism (SNP) influencing acenocoumarol pharmacodynamics; the percentages of remaining factor VII were 60% +/- 19%, 39% +/- 17%, and 17% for CYP2C9*1/CYP2C9*1, CYP2C9*1/CYP2C9*3, and CYP2C9*3/CYP2C9*3 subjects, respectively (P =.001). Among the white subjects, the CYP2C9 promoter showed the existence of 6 SNPs at positions G-1538A, T-1189C, G-1097A, G-982A, T-640 del, and G-620T with allelic frequencies of 0.085, 0.0398, 0.136, 0.086, 0.005, and 0.0138, respectively. Four major haplotypes could be inferred among white subjects. The haplotype that contains the CYP2C9*3 allele was the only one influencing acenocoumarol pharmacodynamics, explaining 14.3% of its interindividual variability. Body weight explained 5% of acenocoumarol pharmacodynamic variability, whereas the NQO1*2 allele had no significant effect. CONCLUSION: Overall, CYP2C9-related genetic variability accounts for 14% of the interindividual variability in acenocoumarol pharmacodynamic response. The information found by haplotype analysis is mainly related to the CYP2C9*3 SNP.

Clin Pharmacol Ther. 2004 May;75(5):415-21. Related Articles, Links Evidence for inverse effects of OATP-C (SLC21A6) 5 and 1b haplotypes on pravastatin kinetics. Mwinyi J, Johne A, Bauer S, Roots I, Gerloff T. Institute of Clinical Pharmacology, Humboldt University, Berlin, Germany. OBJECTIVE: We compared the pharmacogenetic effects of OATP-C (organic anion transporting polypeptide C) *1a, *1b (A388G), and *5 (T521C) haplotypes on single-dose pharmacokinetics of pravastatin in white subjects. METHODS: Thirty healthy white male subjects were grouped according to their OATP-C haplotype. Each group contained 10 individuals who were either homozygous or heterozygous carriers of the *1a, *1b, or *5 haplotype. After a single oral dose of 40 mg pravastatin, we analyzed kinetic parameters of pravastatin disposition. RESULTS: Values for the area under the plasma concentration-time curve from time 0 to 6 hours [AUC(0-6)] in *1a/*1a, *1a/*1b or *1b/*1b, and *1a/*5 individuals were 114.5 +/- 68.6 microg. L(-1). h, 74.8 +/- 35.6 microg. L(-1). h, and 163.0 +/- 64.6 microg. L(-1). h, respectively, with highly significant differences across all 3 study groups (P =.006) and between subjects carrying the *1b and *5 haplotype (P =.002). Strikingly, values of AUC(0-6) from the OATP-C *1b group were more than 60% lower than those derived from carriers of the wild-type OATP-C *1a haplotype, although this difference failed to reach statistical significance. However, the amount of pravastatin excreted into the urine from time 0 to 12 hours [Ae(0-12)] was significantly diminished in the OATP-C *1b haplotype group (1729 +/- 907 microg) compared with *1a wild-type control subjects (2974 +/- 1590 microg) (P =.049). CONCLUSION: There was a significant effect of tested OATP-C variant haplotypes on pravastatin disposition. Whereas *5 expression delayed the hepatocellular uptake of pravastatin, *1b expression seemed to accelerate OATP-C-dependent uptake of the drug.

Clin Pharmacol Ther. 2005 Dec;78(6):656-63. Related Articles, Links Arg16 homozygosity of the beta2-adrenergic receptor improves the outcome after beta2-agonist tocolysis for preterm labor. Landau R, Morales MA, Antonarakis SE, Blouin JL, Smiley RM. Division of Anesthesiology and Department of Obstetrics and Gynecology, University Hospital of Geneva, University of Geneva Medical School, Geneva, Switzerland. ruth.landau@hcuge.ch BACKGROUND: Beta(2)-adrenergic receptor (beta(2)AR) agonists are not consistently successful when administered as tocolytic therapy. The beta(2)AR displays genetic variability; an arginine-to-glycine substitution at codon 16 (Arg16Gly) has been shown to increase receptor desensitization in response to agonist exposure, whereas a substitution of glutamate for glutamine at codon 27 (Gln27Glu) decreases down-regulation. We have demonstrated that homozygosity for Arg16 protects against preterm delivery. Our goal was to determine whether beta(2)-agonists are more effective in women with the Arg16 genotype and preterm labor. METHODS: Sixty white women with preterm labor between 24 and 34 weeks' gestation were treated for 48 hours with intravenous hexoprenaline. The effect of tocolysis and outcome of pregnancy were recorded. The beta(2)AR genotypes at codons 16 and 27 of ADRB2 were determined. A control group of 116 women delivered at term was also genotyped. RESULTS: Preterm labor was not associated with beta(2)AR genotype at codon 16 (17% of patients with preterm labor were Arg16 homozygotes versus 19% of control subjects) or codon 27. Gestation was significantly prolonged in Arg16 homozygotes (median, 69 days; interquartile range, 63-79 days) compared with the other 2 genotypes (median, 58 days; interquartile range, 2-72 days) (P = .04). Tocolysis was 100% successful in delaying delivery for 48 hours in Arg16 homozygotes (n = 10), just failing to achieve statistical significance (P = .069). In contrast, only 37 of 50 women carrying 1 or 2 glycine alleles (74%) had delivery delayed by more than 48 hours with tocolysis. Neonatal outcomes were significantly better in babies born to mothers homozygous for arginine than in women with 1 or 2 Gly16 alleles. CONCLUSIONS: This is the first study examining the pharmacogenetics of beta(2)AR agonist therapy for preterm labor. It appears that Arg16 homozygosity improves pregnancy outcome after beta(2)-agonist tocolysis. The relatively low frequency of Arg16 homozygotes in our population limited the power of this investigation. Future assessments of tocolytic therapy may need to assess beta(2)AR genotype.

Clin Pharmacol Ther. 2005 Jan;77(1):1-16. Related Articles, Links Clinical consequences of cytochrome P450 2C9 polymorphisms. Kirchheiner J, Brockmoller J. Department of Pharmacology, University of Cologne, 50931 Koln, Germany. julia.kirchheiner@uk-koelen.de The gene coding for the cytochrome P450 (CYP) enzyme 2C9 (CYP2C9) carries numerous inherited polymorphisms. Those coding for R144C (*2) and I359L (*3) amino acid substitutions have both significant functional effects and appreciable high population frequencies, and their in vivo consequences have been studied in humans with regard to drug metabolism. This review summarizes present knowledge about the pharmacokinetics, drug responses, and outcomes of clinical studies in individuals with different CYP2C9 genotypes. Tentative estimates of how CYP2C9 genotyping might be applied to dose adjustments in clinical therapy were based on dose-related pharmacokinetic parameters such as clearance or trough drug concentrations. Mean clearances in homozygous carriers of the *3 allele were below 25% of that of the wild type for S - warfarin, tolbutamide, glipizide, celecoxib, and fluvastatin. In the more frequent heterozygous carriers (genotype *1/*3), the clearances were between 40% and 75%. In these cases in which individual dosages are derived from clinical drug effects, such as for the oral anticoagulants, the pharmacogenetics-based dose adjustments showed a good correlation with the genotype-specific empirically derived doses. In addition to its role in pharmacokinetics, CYP2C9 contributes to the metabolism of fatty acids, prostanoids, and steroid hormones, and it may catalyze potentially toxic bioactivation reactions. However, our current understanding of the role of CYP2C9 in biotransformation of endogenous signaling molecules and in drug toxicity is relatively meager. Publication Types: Review

Clin Pharmacol Ther. 2005 Jan;77(1):76-89. Related Articles, Links Population pharmacokinetics of CCI-779: correlations to safety and pharmacogenomic responses in patients with advanced renal cancer. Boni JP, Leister C, Bender G, Fitzpatrick

V, Twine N, Stover J, Dorner A, Immermann F, Burczynski ME. Department of Clinical Pharmacology, Wyeth Research, Collegeville, PA 19426, USA. bonij@wyeth.com OBJECTIVE: Our objective was to estimate the pharmacokinetic parameters of CCI-779 and its metabolite, sirolimus, and evaluate associations of exposure parameters with safety and clinical activity. Exposure parameters were also correlated with pharmacogenomic responses in peripheral blood mononuclear cells (PBMCs). METHODS: In this randomized, double-blind, multicenter trial, once-weekly intravenous doses of 25, 75, or 250 mg CCI-779 were administered to patients with advanced renal cancer. Whole blood for CCI-779 and sirolimus concentrations was drawn. Population pharmacokinetic analyses yielded Bayesian-predicted exposure metrics that were correlated with severity and duration of adverse events and survival. PBMC samples taken before and after treatment were examined for pharmacogenomic responses. Ribonucleic acid samples were converted to labeled probes and hybridized to oligonucleotide arrays containing more than 12,600 human sequences. RESULTS: The final population pharmacokinetic models of CCI-779 and sirolimus included 235 and 305 observations, respectively, from 50 patients. For CCI-779, dose, single versus multiple dose, and body surface area were significant pharmacokinetic covariates. For sirolimus, dose and hematocrit were significant covariates. Age, sex, or race did not influence drug disposition. CCI-779 area under the curve correlated with adverse event severity for thrombocytopenia (P = .007), pruritus (P = .011), and hyperlipemia (P = .040). Exposure (CCI-779 cumulative area under the curve) correlated with a specific subset of gene transcripts in PBMCs following 16 weeks after therapy (P < .001, Spearman correlation). CONCLUSIONS: Concentrations of CCI-779 and sirolimus were adequately described with a population model incorporating factors for dose, attenuated exposure of multiple doses, body surface area, and hematocrit. Correlations with adverse event severity and duration profiles were provided to aid in the detection of treatment-emergent effects. Pharmacogenomic profiling of PBMCs identified altered ribonucleic acid transcript expression levels that correlate with exposure. These transcripts represent potential biomarkers of CCI-779 exposure in peripheral blood. Publication Types: Clinical Trial Multicenter Study Randomized Controlled Trial

Clin Pharmacol Ther. 2005 Jun;77(6):458-67. Related Articles, Links Tramadol as a new probe for cytochrome P450 2D6 phenotyping: a population study. Pedersen RS, Damkier P, Brosen K. Institute of Public Health, Fuculty of Health Sciences, Clinical Pharmacology, University of Southern Denmark, Winslowparken 19, DK-5000 Odense C, Denmark. rpedersen@health.sdu.dk BACKGROUND AND OBJECTIVE: Polymorphic cytochrome P450 (CYP) 2D6 activity has been shown to be a determinant of the pharmacokinetics and pharmacodynamics of tramadol via hepatic phase I O -demethylation of (+)-tramadol to (+)-O-desmethyltramadol. Our objective was to investigate whether tramadol can be used as a probe for CYP2D6 phenotyping by determining the concordance between the 8-hour tramadol and 12-hour sparteine metabolic urinary ratios. METHODS: Sparteine phenotyping test was carried out in 278 healthy, white subjects. At a minimum of 2 weeks later, each subject took 50 mg tramadol hydrochloride followed by 8-hour urine collection, and a venous blood sample was drawn from 276 subjects. Urine and plasma concentrations of (+/-)-tramadol and (+/-)-O-desmethyltramadol were determined. CYP2D6 genotyping was performed with regard to *3, *4, *6, and *9 alleles. RESULTS: There were 28 poor metabolizers of sparteine (10.1% [confidence interval, 6.8%-14.2%]). Very low recoveries of (+)-M1 were found in poor metabolizers (0.53% [range, 0.1%-1.1%]) compared with extensive metabolizers (8.7% [range, 1.7%-23.2%]). A bimodal distribution of the metabolic ratio of (-)-M1/(+)-M1 was found. The visual antimode was 2.0. This new phenotype test had only 1 misclassified subject compared with sparteine phenotyping (sensitivity and negative predictive value, 100%; specificity, 99.6%; positive predictive value, 96.6%). Of the 28 sparteine poor metabolizers, 26 were found to be genotypically poor metabolizers with regard to the inactivating mutations *3, *4, and *6. CONCLUSION: Fifty milligrams of tramadol is an alternative CYP2D6 phenotype probe by use of the 8-hour urinary ratio of (-)-M1/(+)-M1. The poor metabolizers have a metabolic ratio of 2.0 or higher.

Clin Pharmacol Ther. 2005 Mar;77(3):123-6. Related Articles, Links Comment on: Clin Pharmacol Ther. 2005 Mar;77(3):127-37. Pharmacogenetics and response to beta-adrenergic receptor antagonists in heart failure. Muszkat M, Stein CM. Unit of Clinical Pharmacology, Department of Medicine, Hadassah University Hospital, Jerusalem, Israel. muszhatm@hadassah.org.it Publication Types: Comment Review

Clin Pharmacol Ther. 2005 Mar;77(3):127-37. Related Articles, Links Comment in: Clin Pharmacol Ther. 2005 Mar;77(3):123-6. beta-Adrenergic receptor polymorphisms and responses during titration of metoprolol controlled release/extended release in heart failure. Terra SG, Pauly DF, Lee CR, Patterson JH, Adams KF, Schofield RS, Belgado BS, Hamilton KK, Aranda JM, Hill JA, Yarandi HN, Walker JR, Phillips MS, Gelfand CA, Johnson JA. Department of Pharmacy Practice, University of Florida, Gainsville, FL 32610, USA. OBJECTIVE: beta-Blockers require careful initiation and titration when used in patients with heart failure. Some patients tolerate beta-blocker therapy initiation without difficulty, whereas in other patients this period presents clinical challenges. We tested the hypothesis that polymorphisms at codons 389 (Arg389Gly) and 49 (Ser49Gly) of the beta(1)-adrenergic receptor would be associated with differences in initial tolerability of beta-blocker therapy in patients with heart failure. We also tested whether polymorphisms in the beta(2)-adrenergic receptor, G-protein alpha s subunit (G(s)alpha), and cytochrome P450 (CYP) 2D6 genes or S-metoprolol plasma concentrations were associated with beta-blocker tolerability. METHODS: Sixty-one beta-blocker-naive patients with systolic heart failure were prospectively enrolled. Patients began taking 12.5 to 25 mg metoprolol controlled release/extended release with titration every 2 weeks (as tolerated) to 200 mg/d or the maximum tolerated dose over a period of 8 to 10 weeks. Decompensation was the composite of death, heart failure hospitalization, increase in other heart failure medications, or need to discontinue metoprolol. End points were assessed during the titration period. RESULTS: The overall rate of decompensation was not different between the codon 49 or 389 genotypes. However, a significantly greater percentage of patients with the Gly389 variant required increases in heart failure medications as compared with Arg389 homozygotes (48% versus 14%, respectively; P = .006). Similarly, patients with the Ser49 homozygous genotype were significantly more likely to require increases in concomitant heart failure therapy as compared with Gly49 carriers (41% versus 11%, respectively; P = .03). Neither CYP2D6 genotypes nor metoprolol pharmacokinetics differed between patients with and those without a decompensation event. There was no association between the beta(2)-adrenergic receptor or G(s)alpha polymorphisms with decompensated heart failure. CONCLUSIONS: Patients with the Gly389 variant and Ser49Ser genotype were significantly more likely to require increases in heart failure medications during beta-blocker titration and thus may require more frequent follow-up during titration. Publication Types: Clinical Trial Multicenter Study

Clin Pharmacol Ther. 2005 May;77(5):341-52. Related Articles, Links Erratum in: Clin Pharmacol Ther. 2005 Aug;78(2):153. Cytochrome P450 2C8: substrates, inhibitors, pharmacogenetics, and clinical relevance. Totah RA, Rettie AE. Department of Medicinal Chemistry, University of Washington, Seattle, WA 98195, USA. Cytochrome P450 (CYP) 2C8 [corrected] has been a relatively neglected member of the human CYP2C family. Over the period from 2000 through 2003, PubMed searches with the key word CYP2C8 returned only 10% to 15% of the citations obtained for all of the CYP2C enzymes combined. However, in the past year a crystal structure for CYP2C8 has been described, new inhibitors and probe substrates for the enzyme have been in development, the first case study was published linking CYP2C8 genetic polymorphisms to a disease state, and there has been an increasing awareness of the role that CYP2C8 plays in the disposition of therapeutic agents, especially from the pharmacogenetic and drug-drug interaction perspectives. This report discusses baseline characteristics of the enzyme and summarizes recent developments in these areas and their clinical relevance. Publication Types: Review

Clin Pharmacol Ther. 2005 May;77(5):373-87. Related Articles, Links Genotype-phenotype associations of cytochrome P450 3A4 and 3A5 polymorphism with midazolam clearance in vivo. He P, Court MH, Greenblatt DJ, Von Moltke LL. Department of Pharmacology and Experimental Therapeutics, Tufts University School of Medicine, 136 Harrison Ave, Boston, MA 02111, USA. The molecular basis for the wide interindividual variability of cytochrome P450 (CYP) 3A metabolic activity was studied in vivo at a genetic level. A single oral dose of midazolam was administered to 26 healthy subjects. The variability in midazolam oral clearance was 11-fold. No differences in midazolam oral clearance related to gender or ethnicity were observed. Selective sequencing of CYP3A4 and CYP3A5 genes revealed 18 single nucleotide polymorphisms (SNPs), including 8 novel CYP3A4 SNPs. Thirteen novel CYP3A4 haplotypes, 2 novel CYP3A5 haplotypes, and 1 major novel multigene haplotype (CYP3A4*VI - CYP3A5*3A) were also identified. No significant genotype-phenotype or haplotype-phenotype associations were found for any of the SNPs or haplotypes studied, including CYP3A4*1B , CYP3A5*3 , and CYP3A5*6 , even when ethnicity was considered. The only exceptions were the haplotype CYP3A4*VI and the multigene haplotype

CYP3A4*VI - CYP3A5*3A . The carriers of the haplotype CYP3A4*VI had a 1.8-fold higher clearance of midazolam in black subjects (ANOVA on ranks, P = .028) compared with other individuals, and the carriers of the multigene haplotype CYP3A4*VI - CYP3A5*3A had a 1.7-fold higher clearance in the entire population (ANOVA on ranks, P = .012). In conclusion, these results indicate that the genetic variants identified so far in the CYP3A4 and CYP3A5 genes have only a limited impact on CYP3A-mediated drug metabolism in vivo.

Clin Pharmacol Ther. 2005 May;77(5):388-403. Related Articles, Links Human response to alpha2-adrenergic agonist stimulation studied in an isolated vascular bed in vivo: Biphasic influence of dose, age, gender, and receptor genotype. King D, Etzel JP, Chopra S, Smith J, Cadman PE, Rao F, Funk SD, Rana BK, Schork NJ, Insel PA, O'Connor DT. Department of Medicine and Center for Molecular Genetics (0838), University of California at San Diego, and VA San Diego Healthcare System, 9500 Gilman Dr, La Jolla, CA 92093-0838, USA. BACKGROUND AND OBJECTIVES: Activation of alpha 2 -adrenergic receptors regulates a broad spectrum of physiologic responses, including blood pressure (centrally and peripherally), sedation, analgesia, insulin release, renal function, cognition, and behavior. The purpose of this study was to explore systematically the local vascular responses in humans triggered by a highly selective alpha 2 -adrenergic agonist (azepexole [B-HT 933]) and whether such responses are dose-dependent or influenced by age, gender, or allelic variation at the drug's receptor. METHODS: We evaluated dorsal hand vein vascular responses to the infusion of a wide spectrum of doses of azepexole, assessing any venodilation, as well as the maximal extent of venoconstriction (B max) and the dose that produced a half-maximal effect (K d), in 50 healthy normotensive adults of both genders and 4 ethnicities. Genomic deoxyribonucleic acid from the study subjects was evaluated at polymorphisms of the alpha 2B -adrenergic receptor gene (ADRA2B). RESULTS: We found previously unreported initial venodilation to low doses (10-100 ng/min) of azepexole, followed by progressive, intense venoconstriction to higher doses (200-100,000 ng/min) of the drug. Younger individuals (aged <30 years) had less venodilation than older individuals (aged >30 years) with low doses of azepexole but had a greater extent of venoconstriction at higher doses of azepexole (ANOVA, P = .001). Men had less venodilation than women with low doses of azepexole but greater venoconstriction with higher doses (ANOVA, P = .036). Several common polymorphisms (>10% minor allele frequency) at ADRA2B (insertion/deletion polymorphism [Glu 322-325], G-98C, C1182A, and C1776A) did not show an association with either B max or K d for the drug response. The A36G (Thr12Thr) synonymous single nucleotide polymorphism displayed a nonsignificant trend (P = .073) toward higher K d in A/G heterozygotes compared with A/A homozygotes. CONCLUSIONS: Local infusion into the human dorsal hand vein of a highly selective alpha 2 -adrenergic agonist, azepexole, produces biphasic responses, with venodilation at a low dose and intense venoconstriction at a higher concentration. These responses to azepexole show prominent differences as a function of age and gender but appear not to depend on common allelic variations at the ADRA2B receptor.

Clin Pharmacol Ther. 2005 Oct;78(4):330-41. Related Articles, Links Comment in: Clin Pharmacol Ther. 2005 Oct;78(4):311-6. Rosuvastatin pharmacokinetics and pharmacogenetics in white and Asian subjects residing in the same environment. Lee E, Ryan S, Birmingham B, Zalikowski J, March R, Ambrose H, Moore R, Lee C, Chen Y, Schneck D. National University Hospital and Changi General Hospital, Singapore. BACKGROUND: Systemic exposure to rosuvastatin had been observed to be approximately 2-fold higher in Japanese subjects living in Japan compared with white subjects in Western Europe or the United States. The organic anion transporting polypeptide 1B1 contributes to the hepatic uptake of rosuvastatin. Polymorphisms in the SLCO1B1 gene can lead to reduced transport function in vitro (T 521>C). This study was conducted to determine whether the pharmacokinetic differences between Japanese and white subjects extended to other Asian ethnic groups and to determine whether polymorphisms in the SLCO1B1 gene contribute to any pharmacokinetic differences observed. METHODS: Rosuvastatin pharmacokinetics was studied in an open-label, parallel-group, single-oral dose (40 mg) study in 36 white, 36 Chinese, 35 Malay, and 35 Asian-Indian subjects living in Singapore, Singapore. Plasma concentrations of rosuvastatin and metabolites were determined by HPLC-mass spectrophotometry. Two SLCO1B1 polymorphisms (A 388>G and T 521>C) were genotyped. RESULTS: Ratios for rosuvastatin area under the plasma concentration-time curve from time 0 to the time of the last quantifiable concentration were 2.31, 1.91, and 1.63 and ratios for maximum plasma concentration were 2.36, 2.00, and 1.68 in Chinese, Malay, and Asian-Indian subjects, respectively, compared with white subjects. Similar increases in exposure to N-desmethyl rosuvastatin and rosuvastatin-lactone were observed. SLCO1B1 genotypes did not account for the observed pharmacokinetic differences between Asians and white subjects. CONCLUSIONS: Plasma exposure to rosuvastatin and its metabolites was significantly higher in Chinese, Malay, and Asian-Indian subjects compared with white subjects living in the same environment. Publication Types: Clinical Trial Multicenter Study

Clin Rev Allergy Immunol. 2004 Dec;27(3):197-205. Related Articles, Links Asthma treatment in the 21st century: what's next? Peters SP. Center for Human Genomics and Department of Medicine, Section on Pulmonary and Critical Care Medicine, Wake Forest University School of Medicine, Winston-Salem, North Carolina, USA. sppeters@wfubmc.edu Asthma treatment is evolving as we enter the 21st century. This review focuses on several different areas of asthma treatment now in evolution. These include: (1) the proper role of various asthma controllers--either already approved or under investigation--besides inhaled corticosteriods in asthma therapy; (2) the potential role for immune and cytokine modulation for asthma therapy; (3) the potential role for pharmacogenetics in asthma therapy; and (4) whether single-inhaler therapy with a combination of an inhaled corticosteriod and a long-acted beta-agonist could be used for both maintenance and rescue in patients with asthma. Publication Types: Review

Clin Toxicol (Phila). 2005;43(2):121-6. Related Articles, Links The use of toxicogenomic data in risk assessment: a regulatory perspective. Chan VS, Theilade MD.

Innovative Therapeutics Group, Centre for Drug Administration, Health Sciences Authority, Singapore. Vivian_CHAN@hsa.gov.sg Recent advances in genomic research have provided new insights into mechanisms of toxicity evoked by drugs or xenobiotics. Several governmental and commercial organizations are at present actively building up databases containing large amounts of toxicogenomics information. With promises to improve our ability to characterize hazard, scientists are facing the challenge as to how to link patterns of gene expression and gene clustering to specific adverse effects of toxicants or classes of toxicants. The future of toxicogenomics lies in the robustness of the databases generated. Regulators are working together with institutes and industry in exploring the potential use of these databases in regulatory purposes. It is, however, anticipated that regulatory use of the toxicogenomic databases as supportive information in the assessment procedure of new drug applications will be on a case-by-case basis until the predictive value of the databases is firmly established. Publication Types: Review

Comb Chem High Throughput Screen. 2004 May;7(3):207-11. Related Articles, Links DNA microarrays as a tool in toxicogenomics. de Longueville F, Bertholet V, Remacle J. Eppendorf Array Technologies, 20 rue du seminaire, 5000 Namur, Belgium. delongueville.f@eppendorf.be Toxicogenomics is an emerging technology that defines the use of novel genomic techniques to investigate the adverse effects of xenobiotic on gene expression. Toxicogenomics is based on the fact that most of relevant toxicological effects of a compound affect directly or indirectly the gene expression. The most common methods to profile gene expression at the transcript level are Northern Blotting and the real-time PCR. While commonly used and well accepted, these techniques are now superseded by new technologies allowing the analysis of the expression for multiple genes simultaneously. DNA microarrays are now developed for simultaneous gene analysis but inherent to such multiple assays, their quantitative aspect and their relevance for toxicogenomics have been questioned. We will review here recent studies on their use for toxicogenomics and examine the possible future of such technology in complementation with the other toxicology methods. Publication Types: Review

Community Genet. 2006;9(1):50-4. Related Articles, Links Pharmacogenetics, adverse drug reactions and public health. Kollek R, van Aken J, Feuerstein G, Schmedders M. Forschungsschwerpunkt Biotechnik, Gesellschaft und Umwelt, Universitat Hamburg, Hamburg, Germany. kollek@uni-hamburg.de Adverse drug reactions (ADRs) are a major public health problem. Pharmacogenetic testing prior to drug treatment is supposed to considerably alleviate this problem. The state of pharmacogenetic development was assessed by a systematic literature review, supplemented by expert interviews. Analysis of three case examples revealed that - with the exception of thiopurine methyltransferase (TPMT) - studies are lacking which unambiguously prove the clinical value of pharmacogenetic testing. Testing can prevent some, but by far not all ADRs. Since it does not compensate for clinical monitoring, pharmacogenetics can be regarded as add-on technology, applied in addition to established methods. A non-representative, explorative survey conducted amongst members of the German Society of Laboratory Medicine revealed that the demand for testing is limited and has not increased much, although a certain increase is expected in the future. Copyright (c) 2006 S. Karger AG, Basel.

Congest Heart Fail. 2004 Nov-Dec;10(6):273, 288. Related Articles, Links Comment on: Congest Heart Fail. 2004 Nov-Dec;10(6):274-78; quiz 279-80. Pharmacogenomics and heart failure: tailor-made therapy? Iyengar S, Abraham WT. The OSU Heart Center, Division of Cardiovascular Medicine, 473 West 12th Avenue, Room 110P DHLRI, Columbus, OH 43210-1252, USA. Publication Types: Comment

Congest Heart Fail. 2004 Nov-Dec;10(6):281-8. Related Articles, Links The emerging pharmacogenomics of the beta-adrenergic receptors. Taylor MR, Bristow MR. CU-Cardiovascular Institute, Division of Cardiology, Adult Medical Genetics Program, University of Colorado Health Sciences Center, Aurora, CO, USA. matthew.taylor@uchsc.edu Beta-adrenergic signaling mechanisms are of central importance to cardiovascular health and disease. Modulation of these pathways represents an important pharmacologic approach to the treatment of heart failure and hypertension. Advances in molecular genetics have identified genetic polymorphisms in the human beta-adrenergic receptor genes; some of this variation predicts changes in protein sequence/structure, and potentially changes in function, of the b-adrenergic receptors. This article reviews the current state of knowledge and understanding of the genetic variation present in the three human beta-adrenergic receptor genes. Already, variation in these genes has been associated with observed differences in several cardiovascular phenotypes. This work has led to the demonstration of functional differences in activity between receptors with certain known polymorphisms and "wild-type" receptors. An understanding of these polymorphisms is key to the development of studies of how differences in drug response/effects may be mediated by these polymorphisms. Such studies are anticipated to provide a foundation for the development of novel pharmacologic approaches where selection of and dosing of cardiovascular therapy is tailored to individuals on the basis of each patient's specific genetic makeup. Publication Types: Review

Congest Heart Fail. 2004 Nov-Dec;10(6):289-92. Related Articles, Links Tumor necrosis factor alpha polymorphism in heart failure/cardiomyopathy. Vadlamani L, Iyengar S. Department of Cardiovascular Medicine, Ohio State University, Suite 200, Davis Heart and Lung Research Institute, 473 West 12th Avenue, Columbus, OH 43210-1252, USA. vadlamani-1@medctr.osu.edu Tumor necrosis factor a (TNF-alpha) is a proinflammatory cytokine that is produced by activated macrophages. It has been shown to stimulate the release of endothelial cytokines and NO, increase vascular permeability, decrease contractility, and induce a prothrombotic state. The most studied TNF-a gene mutation in heart disease is a gamma to alpha substitution, which occurs when 308 nucleotides move upstream from the transcription initiation site in the TNF promoter and has been associated with elevated levels of TNF-alpha. The TNF1 allele (wild type) contains gamma at this site, while the TNF2 allele has an alpha substitution at the site. The TNF2 allele is a more powerful transcriptional activator, therefore leading to higher TNF-alpha levels. Most of the studies to date have failed to conclusively show any link between the polymorphism and heart disease, both coronary artery disease and cardiomyopathy/heart failure. Publication Types: Review

Congest Heart Fail. 2004 Nov-Dec;10(6):302-8. Related Articles, Links Pharmacogenetics in heart failure: genomic markers of endothelial and neurohumoral function. McNamara DM. Heart Failure/Transplantation Program, Genetics Core Laboratory, University of Pittsburgh Medical Center, S-558 Lothrop Street, Pittsburgh, PA 15213, USA. mcnamaradm@msx.upmc.edu There is a high potential for pharmacogenetic interaction in the management of many diseases including heart failure. Although genetic tailoring of therapy is not yet a common medical practice, it is foreseeable that some forms of genetic targeting will become standard care by the end of the current decade. This review will summary how genetic variation in two genes involved in both endothelial function and heart failure pathogenesis, angiotensin-converting enzyme and endothelial nitric oxide synthase, influence both heart failure outcomes and the effects of standard therapies. Publication Types: Review

Crit Rev Clin Lab Sci. 2005;42(4):311-92. Related Articles, Links The G protein-coupled receptors: pharmacogenetics and disease. Thompson MD, Burnham WM, Cole DE. Department of Laboratory Medicine and Pathobiology, Banting Institute, University of Toronto, ON, Canada. miles.thompson@utoronto.ca Genetic variation in G-protein coupled receptors (GPCRs) is associated with a wide spectrum of disease phenotypes and predispositions that are of special significance because they are the targets of therapeutic agents. Each variant provides an opportunity to understand receptor function that complements a plethora of available in vitro data elucidating the pharmacology of the GPCRs. For example, discrete portions of the proximal tail of the dopamine D1 receptor have been discovered, in vitro, that may be involved in desensitization, recycling and trafficking. Similar in vitro strategies have been used to elucidate naturally occurring GPCR mutations. Inactive, over-active or constitutively active receptors have been identified by changes in ligand binding, G-protein coupling, receptor desensitization and receptor recycling. Selected examples reviewed include those disorders resulting from mutations in rhodopsin, thyrotropin, luteinizing hormone, vasopressin and angiotensin receptors. By comparison, the recurrent pharmacogenetic variants are more likely to result in an altered predisposition to complex disease in the population. These common variants may affect receptor sequence without intrinsic phenotype change or spontaneous induction of disease and yet result in significant alteration in drug efficacy. These pharmacogenetic phenomena will be reviewed with respect to a limited sampling of GPCR systems including the orexin/hypocretin system, the beta2 adrenergic receptors, the cysteinyl leukotriene receptors and the calcium-sensing receptor. These developments will be discussed with respect to strategies for drug discovery that take into account the potential for the development of drugs targeted at mutated and wild-type proteins. Publication Types: Review

Curr Allergy Asthma Rep. 2005 Mar;5(2):101-8. Related Articles, Links Pharmacogenetic approaches in the treatment of asthma. Sayers I, Hall IP. Division of Therapeutics and Molecular Medicine, University Hospital of Nottingham, D Floor, South

Block, Nottingham, NG7 2UH, UK. A patient's response to asthma therapy is determined by both genetic and environmental factors. In the past 10 years, we have witnessed significant progress in the field of asthma pharmacogenetics--the study of how a patient's genetic background determines the efficacy and potential for adverse effects to current asthma medication. There are now clear examples of gene polymorphisms that can influence responses to beta(2)-agonists, glucocorticosteroids, and leukotriene modifier drugs, the three main classes of medication used clinically to treat asthma. Identification of genetic polymorphism that predicts drug responses has the potential to lead to the development of new therapeutics, improve asthma management, and reduce serious episodes and hospitalizations. In this review, we discuss the current understanding of asthma pharmacogenetics, focusing on the main three classes of drugs currently used clinically. Publication Types: Review

Curr Atheroscler Rep. 2005 May;7(3):177-8. Related Articles, Links Pharmacogenetic study of statin therapy and cholesterol reduction. Marian AJ.

Curr Atheroscler Rep. 2005 May;7(3):204-8. Related Articles, Links Pharmacogenetics of response to statins: where do we stand? Maitland-van der Zee AH, Boerwinkle E. Human Genetics Center, Health Science Center at Houston, University of Texas, 1200 Hermann Pressler, Houston, TX 77030, USA. Cardiovascular disease is one of the leading causes of death, especially in developed countries. Blood cholesterol lowering by way of statin therapy is a common risk-lowering therapy. The risk reduction for coronary artery disease for patients using statins is 27%. These reductions, however, are average effects for all patients included in the trials. There is notable interindividual variation in response to statins, and the origins of this variation are poorly understood. Pharmacogenetics seeks to determine the role of genetic factors in variation of drug response. In patients with primary hypercholesterolemia, 23 studies have examined the effects of genetic polymorphisms at 20 different loci on the lipid response to statin treatment, and 18 studies examined genetic polymorphisms involved in the benefits of statin therapy in the prevention of cardiovascular disease. Even though many studies have been performed, few results have been replicated. It is our contention that larger sample sizes and consideration of multiple genes are needed in the field of pharmacogenetics of statin response. Publication Types: Review

Curr Biol. 2005 Jan 26;15(2):R36-7. Related Articles, Links New support to tackle pathogen secrets. Tebb G. The European Commission recently announced the launch of PathoGenoMics, to coordinate funding for research on disease-causing microbes. Graham Tebb reports.

Curr Drug Deliv. 2004 Jan;1(1):73-80. Related Articles, Links Challenges in current drug delivery from the potential application of pharmacogenomics and personalized medicine in clinical practice. Vizirianakis IS. Laboratory of Pharmacology, Department of Pharmaceutical Sciences, Aristotle University of Thessaloniki, GR-54124 Thessaloniki, Greece. ivizir@pharm.auth.gr The recent technological achievements in biotechnology and recombinant DNA technology have provided multiple new methods, molecular targets, and DNA-based diagnostics to pharmaceutical research that can be utilized in assays for screening and developing potential biotechnology-based drugs, as well as in biomedicine, health and pharmaceutical care. Furthermore, such advances opened up new opportunities by applying genetic information data in pharmacotherapy and drug delivery, thus ensuring better drug efficacy and safety in clinical practice. Now the concepts of personalized medicine and pharmacogenomics are likely improving the area of pharmacodynamics and pharmacokinetics, since they favor differentiation of the conventional clinical diagnosis and drug selection into separate molecular subtypes of individuals belonging within a group of patients suffering from the same disease. Genetic polymorphisms have already been detected and analyzed in genes encoding drug-metabolizing enzymes, transporters as well as targets (e.g. receptors). The potential of applying genotyping and haplotyping analysis in future pharmaceutical care could eventually lead to pharmacotyping, i.e. individualized drug delivery profiling based on genetic-bioinformatic data in routine patient care. However, the steps towards this direction of drug delivery in clinical practice still have a long way to go to be fully achieved; until then, the critical evaluation of all available clinical data including pharmacodynamic, pharmacokinetic and genomic must be assessed for ensuring drug efficacy and safety. In this way, there has been great progress in elucidating genetic determinants contributing to the observed interindividual differences in drug disposition and effects, thus implementing current drug delivery with molecular genetics and diagnostics. Publication Types: Review

Curr Drug Deliv. 2005 Oct;2(4):429-41.
Related Articles, Links Toxicogenomics of cationic lipid-based vectors for gene therapy: impact of microarray technology. Omidi Y, Barar J, Akhtar S. Department of Pharmaceutics, Faculty of Pharmacy, Tabriz University of Medical Sciences, Tabriz, Iran. yomidi@yahoo.com
Implementation of the high-throughput microarray gene expression profiling technology towards "toxicogenomics" has advanced identification process for safer drugs in the century of 'omics' technology. Applying such technology, in fact, to identify mechanisms for cellular toxicity can provide a means to clarify safety liabilities early in the drug discovery and developments process. The underlying principle in gene therapy is primarily targeting a specific gene (e.g., for silencing). Hence, massive efforts have been devoted to validate the gene-based therapeutics, regardless of toxicogenomics potential of delivery systems. Of the gene delivery systems, viral and non-viral vectors, as two main paradigms, have so far been widely used for delivering of the genome-based therapeutics such as oligonucleotide, small interfering RNA and DNA. However, the use of viral vectors was narrowed due to the safety concerns. Non-viral vectors were utilized as safer alternatives for gene delivery in vitro and ex-vivo; though their success for in vivo gene therapy has been limited due to low efficiency and safety issues. Fundamental principle for gene therapy is to deliver gene-based therapeutics into target cells for specific gene targeting ideally with minimal cellular toxicity. Until now, few works have been conducted about geno-compatibility of delivery systems itself, including cationic lipid-based nanosystems. Inadvertent toxicogenomic impact of gene delivery systems (e.g., cationic lipids) may intrinsically affect the outcome of gene therapy, where often only a single desired genetic change is sought. Further, there exists a possibility that gene

changes induced by the lipid delivery system itself could exacerbate, attenuate or even mask the desired effects of the gene-based therapeutics. This review will focus on toxicogenomics impact of the cationic lipid-based formulations for gene therapy. Publication Types: Review

Curr Drug Metab. 2005 Aug;6(4):369-83. Related Articles, Links Genetic variants of PXR (NR1I2) and CAR (NR1I3) and their implications in drug metabolism and pharmacogenetics. Lamba J, Lamba V, Schuetz E. Department of Pharmaceutical Sciences, Mail Stop 313, St. Jude Children's Research Hospital, 332 N. Lauderdale Street, Memphis, TN 38105, USA. The defense mechanisms responsible for protecting the body from endogenous toxins are also involved in the metabolism of drugs and are composed of phase I and phase II drug metabolizing enzymes, as well as drug transporters. Numerous drugs and chemicals have been shown to modulate the expression of the genes involved in these three drug-detoxifying processes. Induction of these genes contributes to both auto-induction of drug clearance and to drug-drug interactions in combination therapies. The orphan nuclear receptors PXR (pregnane X receptor) and CAR (Constitutive androstane receptor) are xenosensors that mediate drug-induced changes by increasing transcription of genes that are involved in drug clearance and disposition. Co-administration of drugs, one of which is a nuclear receptor agonist or antagonist, can either lead to altered clearance of the second drug and severe toxicity, or a loss of therapeutic efficacy or an imbalance in physiological substrate concentrations, providing a novel molecular mechanism for drug-drug interactions. Thus, genetic variability in these nuclear receptors will contribute to human variation in the magnitude of clinically significant drug-drug interactions. This review describes common PXR and CAR genetic variants that have been identified to date in the human population and the functional consequence of these variant alleles. In addition, alternatively spliced variants of PXR and CAR that may also contribute to individual variability as well as tissue specific expression of these receptors are also described. Identification of PXR and CAR genetic variants and alternatively spliced mRNAs may ultimately allow predictions of interindividual differences in target gene induction and drug-drug interactions. Publication Types: Review

Curr Drug Targets Immune Endocr Metabol Disord. 2005 Dec;5(4):439-48. Related Articles, Links Hormonal effects on drug metabolism through the CYP system: perspectives on their potential significance in the era of pharmacogenomics. Sarlis NJ, Gourgiotis L. Department of Endocrine Neoplasia and Hormonal Disorders, The University of Texas M. D. Anderson Cancer Center, 1515 Holcombe Blvd., Unit 435, Houston, TX 77030-4009, USA. njsarlis@mdanderson.org Cytochrome P450 (CYP) is a group of enzymes that metabolize drugs to a more water-soluble form, rendering them available for renal excretion. The major site of CYP expression is the liver. Nearly 50% of all medications currently on the market are metabolized by the enzyme CYP3A4, while metabolism of another 35-40% occurs through enzymes CYP1A2, CYP2C19, CYP2D6, CYP3A5 CYP3A6, and CYP3A7. Here, we summarize the current knowledge of the effects of hormones on the CYP family. The term "hormone" is used in its broad sense and includes products of the major endocrine glands (i.e., thyroid, adrenals, gonads, pancreas) and compounds that are not classically considered hormones, such as neurogenic amines, cytokines, interleukins, and eicosanoids. In addition, we comment on the effects on CYP expression of states associated with profound hormonal changes, such as pregnancy, malnutrition, obesity, diabetes mellitus, systemic inflammation, and conditions of altered extracellular fluid volume or osmolality. Available data are limited and are derived primarily from in vitro and animal studies. Moreover, the picture is obscured by conflicting results among studies and the complexity of the regulation of the expression and activity of elements of the CYP system. While the clinical significance of hormonal effects on the CYP system remains to be determined, we anticipate that such effects will be most pertinent to drugs with a narrow therapeutic range. Further research is needed to determine the scope and significance of these effects in view of rapid advances in the field of pharmacogenomics and the ever-increasing number of drugs available for therapeutic use. Publication Types: Review

Curr HIV/AIDS Rep. 2004 Jun;1(2):89-96. Related Articles, Links Drug interactions with antiretrovirals. Catanzaro LM, Slish JC, DiCenzo R, Morse GD. Department of Pharmacy Practice, School of Pharmacy and Pharmaceutical Sciences, University at Buffalo, Amherst, NY 14260, USA. The recent development of new antiretroviral drugs, along with the evolution in clinical practice guidelines that include the recommendation of the use of three- to four-drug combination regimens for achieving optimal suppression of viral replication, has focused clinicians on the relevance of drug-drug interactions in the chronic care of HIV-infected individuals. However, the routine clinical management of drug interactions is complicated by our expanding knowledge of the physiologic mechanisms underlying pharmacokinetic interactions, particularly as they relate to drug transport and tissue distribution (eg, P-glycoprotein) and biotransformation (hepatic cytochrome p450 mono-oxygenase induction and inhibition). This review provides an updated summary of key drug interactions that have been reported since its initial publication. Publication Types: Review

Curr Hypertens Rep. 2005 Feb;7(1):21-30. Related Articles, Links Gene markers and antihypertensive therapy. Turner ST, Schwartz GL. Division of Nephrology and Hypertension, Department of Internal Medicine, Mayo Clinic College of Medicine, 200 First Street SW, Rochester, MN 55905, USA. turner.stephen@mayo.edu Increasingly, detailed characterization of human molecular genetic variation will facilitate the use of genetic information in preventing, diagnosing, and treating common diseases. One promising application is the identification of genetic variants influencing responses to drugs used to lower blood pressure (BP) and prevent target-organ complications of hypertension. This update on gene markers to guide antihypertensive therapy highlights polymorphisms recently reported to predict interindividual differences in response to antihypertensive medications. However, single-site variation in most genes makes only a small contribution to differences in BP response, and, after all known genetic and environmental predictors have been considered, most variation in responses still remains unexplained. Advancing beyond our current "trial-and-error" approach to selecting drug therapy in individual patients will undoubtedly require whole-genome approaches to discover additional, novel genetic pathways influencing drug response. In addition, larger samples will be required to more fully characterize genetic variation within candidate genes and to consider the joint effects of gene-gene and gene-environment interactions. Eventually, knowledge of genetic variants that influence BP responses may allow more individualized tailoring of therapy to optimally reduce BP and target-organ damage. Publication Types: Review

Curr Med Chem Cardiovasc Hematol Agents. 2005 Oct;3(4):357-64. Related Articles, Links Pharmacogenetics in cardiovascular antithrombotic therapy. Marin F, Roldan V, Gonzalez-Conejero R, Corral J. Cardiology Department, Hospital General Universitario, C/ Pintor Baeza s/n, Alicante, Spain. fcomarino@hotmail.com Thrombosis is the most important underlying mechanism of coronary heart disease and embolic stroke. Therefore, antithrombotic therapy is commonly used in cardiovascular diseases. Unfortunately, the benefits are limited, and an important proportion of treated patients will suffer a new thrombotic event. Lack of clinical benefits may be related to heterogeneous response to antithrombotic treatment among individuals (inter-individual heterogeneity). Few factors have been identified to be involved in this inter-individual heterogeneity. Recently, pharmacogenetic has emerged as a new field in medicine that tries to identify gene variants able to explain the heterogeneity in patient's response to a drug. Polymorphisms affecting disposition, metabolism, transporters or targets of the drug could modify the individual response to one therapy, and probably its side effects. The present review article explores the genetic influence on antithrombotic drug efficacy, analysing the modulating role of different polymorphisms on individuals' response to drugs commonly used in current day practice. Publication Types: Review

Curr Med Res Opin. 2005 Jul;21(7):1041-7. Related Articles, Links Pharmacogenomics: questions and concerns. Mahlknecht U, Voelter-Mahlknecht S. University of Heidelberg Medical Center, Department of Hematology/Oncology, Im Neuenheimer Feld 410, 69120 Heidelberg, Germany. Ulrich.Mahlknecht@med.uni-heidelberg.de The progressively aging population in the western world, rising socioeconomic expenditure and increasing costs for the treatment of adverse drug reactions, lead to increasing pressure on public spending. The public acceptance of pharmacogenomics is high, therefore, because it promises individualized safe and effective treatment at lower cost. Pharmacogenomics studies the genetic polymorphisms that underlie the variability in drug response between individuals. Despite the great benefits being awaited from this new field, a number of ethical, social and legal concerns arise, which demand rapid strict international regulations in order to prevent discrimination or harm of any kind from society, industry, groups or individuals. Publication Types: Review

Curr Mol Med. 2005 Feb;5(1):103-10. Related Articles, Links Development of oncology drug response markers using transcription profiling. Dracopoli NC. Bristol-Myers Squibb, Princeton, NJ 08540, USA. Nicholas.Dracopoli@bms.com Transcriptional profiling of a tumor's entire genomic complement has become a key tool in the analysis of human cancers and identification of novel markers to predict disease state, outcome, and response to therapy. At present, this technology provides the most comprehensive approach for the analysis of somatic changes altering critical pathways during transformation of stable diploid cells into unstable tumor cells. Such analyses are impacting the development of novel anti-cancer drugs through the early detection of cancer, development of targeted therapies, identification of optimal dose and regimens for new drugs, and segmentation of patients to enrich response rates and reduce risk of adverse events. Publication Types: Review

Curr Mol Med. 2005 Feb;5(1):111-20. Related Articles, Links DNA microarrays in clinical cancer research. Wadlow R, Ramaswamy S. Massachusetts General Hospital Cancer Center and Harvard Medical School, MA, USA. The recent sequencing of the human genome, coupled with advances in biotechnology, is enabling the comprehensive molecular "profiling" of human tissues. In particular, DNA microarrays are powerful tools for obtaining global views of human tumor gene expression. Complex information from tumor "expression profiling" studies can, in turn, be used to create novel molecular cancer diagnostics. We discuss the utility of DNA microarray-based tumor profiling in clinical cancer research, highlight some important recent studies, and identify future avenues of research in this evolving field. Publication Types: Review

Curr Mol Med. 2005 Feb;5(1):53-64. Related Articles, Links The role of transcriptome analysis in pre-clinical toxicology. Searfoss GH, Ryan TP, Jolly RA. Lilly Research Laboratories, Department of Investigative Toxicology, Eli Lilly and Company, Greenfield, IN 46140, USA. searfgh@lilly.com A major benefit of the genomics revolution in biomedical research has been the establishment of transcriptome analysis as an enabling technology in the drug development process. Nowhere in the realm of drug development has the expectation of the impact of transcriptome analysis been greater than in the area of pre-clinical toxicology. Transcriptome analysis, along with other new high-content data generating technologies, has the potential to radically improve the drug safety assessment process by allowing drug development teams to identify potential toxicity liabilities earlier, and thus proceed only with those molecules that have both efficacy at the target and a low potential for toxicity in the human population. In this review we will briefly describe the major ways in which transcriptome analysis is being applied in the pre-clinical safety assessment process, focusing primarily on four areas where transcriptome analysis has already begun to have impact. These include using transcriptome analysis to: 1) understand mechanisms of toxicity: 2) predict toxicity: 3) develop in vivo and in vitro surrogate models and screens; and, 4) develop toxicity biomarkers. We will close by briefly addressing future trends and needs in the application of transcriptome analysis to drug safety assessment. Publication Types: Review

Curr Mol Med. 2005 Feb;5(1):83-102. Related Articles, Links Clinical pharmacogenomics and transcriptional profiling in early phase oncology clinical trials. Burczynski ME, Oestreicher JL, Cahilly MJ, Mounts DP, Whitley MZ, Speicher LA, Trepicchio WL. Discovery Medicine, Wyeth Research, Cambridge, MA 01810, USA. mburczynski@wyeth.com Microarray-based expression profiling studies in the field of oncology have demonstrated encouraging correlations between tumor transcriptional profiles and eventual patient outcomes. These findings have fueled great interest in the application of transcriptional profiling to samples available from real-time clinical trials, and clinical pharmacogenomic objectives utilizing transcriptional profiling strategies are becoming increasingly incorporated into clinical trial study designs. Over the last few years several retrospective studies based on the profiling of archival tumor tissues suggest that transcriptional analysis of oncology samples may provide general prognosis measures, and in some cases may even predict response to specific therapies. Recently the FDA released a voluntary genomic data guidance meant to assist both regulatory agencies and pharmaceutical companies alike in evaluating the potential benefit of implementing expression profiling studies during the preclinical and clinical phases of drug development. Despite the great promise afforded by this technology, the ultimate benefit of applying transcriptional profiling in prospective clinical trials has yet to be realized because a number of practical impediments to this process exist. The multi-fold purpose of the current review is to highlight the increasing evidence from studies that have identified transcriptional signatures in archived tumors prognostic of patient outcome, to describe some of the drivers for the implementation of transcriptional profiling strategies in real-time drug development, to discuss the use of transcriptional profiling in the context of increasingly complex translational medicine strategies, and to highlight the practical issues and potential approaches involved in the successful application of clinical pharmacogenomic objectives during real-time clinical trials. Strategic implementation of transcriptional profiling in early oncology clinical trials can provide an opportunity to identify predictive markers of clinical response and eventually provide a substantial step forward towards the era of personalized medicine. Publication Types: Review

Curr Oncol Rep. 2005 May;7(3):181-5. Related Articles, Links Adjuvant therapy for colon cancer. Sun W, Haller DG. Abramson Cancer Center, University of Pennsylvania, 16 Penn Tower, 3400 Spruce Street, Philadelphia, PA 19104-4283, USA. weijing.sun@uphs.upenn.edu As there have been advances in the treatment of metastatic colorectal cancer, exciting developments have also been achieved in the adjuvant treatment of colon cancer. At the same time, more questions have been raised, and some controversies remain. The results of the MOSAIC trial demonstrated the benefit of adding oxaliplatin to 5-fluorouracil (5-FU) and leucovorin (FOLFOX) in adjuvant therapy for stage II and III disease, but the optimal duration of therapy and the management of toxicities remain to be resolved. Capecitabine is at least equivalent to the Mayo Clinic bolus 5-FU and leucovorin regimen in the adjuvant treatment of stage III colon cancer with a lower incidence profile of adverse events, allowing additional options for patients and physicians. Routine adjuvant systemic therapy in all patients with stage II colon cancer is still debatable. Although a statistically significant advantage for adjuvant treatment in stage II disease was shown for the first time from a large randomized study (QUASAR), the subsets of patients who truly benefit from therapy need to be identified. The application of pharmacogenetics and pharmacogenomics in adjuvant therapy for colorectal cancer will help to distinguish those patients with risk factors and to guide individualized therapy. Publication Types: Review

Curr Oncol Rep. 2005 Nov;7(6):475-9. Related Articles, Links What are SNPs and haplotypes and how will they help us manage the prevention of adult cancer? Velasquez JL, Lipkin SM. Department of Medicine, Division of Hematology-Oncology, University of California, Irvine, 839 Medical Sciences Court, 2nd Floor, Sprague Hall--Lab 250, Irvine, CA 92697, USA. Human genetic variation data are now publicly available on a large scale, from public and private discovery efforts. Datasets from the International Haplotype Map Consortium and Perlegen Sciences provide a level of knowledge about human genetic variation that is unprecedented. In combination with novel high-throughput genotyping technologies, these new resources will allow cancer prevention investigators to identify in a more precise way which genetic subsets of patients are likely to benefit most from chemoprevention and screening interventions. Publication Types: Review

Curr Oncol Rep. 2005 Sep;7(5):323-32. Related Articles, Links Advances in the molecular genetics of acute leukemia. Scandura JM. Memorial Sloan-Kettering Cancer Center, New York, NY 10021, USA. scandurj@mskcc.org Acute leukemias are characterized by the unrestrained clonal proliferation of hematopoietic precursor cells coupled with aberrant or arrested differentiation. The molecular basis of hematopoiesis and leukemogenesis is still being defined, yet it is increasingly evident that acute leukemias have recurrent molecular features that can be exploited for diagnostic, prognostic, and therapeutic purposes. Modern molecular technologies already influence treatment strategies for these diseases, and it is likely that as such technology matures it will have an increasing impact on all aspects of acute leukemia management. This article reviews recent developments in the molecular classification, prognostication, and treatment of the acute leukemias. Publication Types: Review

Curr Opin Allergy Clin Immunol. 2004 Feb;4(1):37-8. Related Articles, Links Pharmacogenetics: the new science of personalizing treatment. Holgate ST. Publication Types: Editorial

Curr Opin Allergy Clin Immunol. 2005 Aug;5(4):309-16. Related Articles, Links Epidemiology of hypersensitivity drug reactions. Gomes ER, Demoly P. Allergy Department, INSERM U454 - IFR3, Arnaud de Villeneuve Hospital, University Hospital of Montpellier, Montpellier, France. PURPOSE OF REVIEW: Hypersensitivity drug reactions are but one of the many different types of adverse drug reactions. They may be potentially life-threatening, prolong hospitalization, affect drug prescribing patterns of physicians and result in socioeconomic costs. This review summarizes current knowledge on the incidence, prevalence, mortality and risk factors for these reactions in different populations. RECENT FINDINGS: Hypersensitivity reactions represent about one third of all adverse drug reactions. Adverse drug reactions affect 10-20% of hospitalized patients and more than 7% of the general population. Severe reactions including anaphylaxis, drug hypersensitivity syndromes, Stevens Johnson syndrome and toxic epidermal necrolysis are also associated with significant morbidity and mortality. Although several risk factors have been identified, their clinical importance has not been fully understood. Future progress in immunogenetics and pharmacogenetics may help identify populations at risk for specific types of reactions. SUMMARY: Well designed epidemiological studies on hypersensitivity drug reactions are lacking as most studies have been on adverse drug reactions. Such studies will be helpful in identifying patients at risk of developing such reactions, in particular severe reactions, and implementing early preventive measures. Publication Types: Review

Curr Opin Chem Biol. 2005 Aug;9(4):381-6. Related Articles, Links Genomic medicine: bringing biomarkers to clinical medicine. Seo D, Ginsburg GS. Center for Genomic Medicine, Institute for Genome Sciences and Policy, Duke University Medical Center, Durham, NC 27710, USA. An important by-product of sequencing the human genome has been the development of a novel 'toolbox' for biomarker discovery and development. Genomic medicine is an emerging discipline in the genome sciences that integrates these tools to interrogate genomic variation in well-defined populations in order to develop predictors of disease susceptibility, progression and drug response. Several important classes of biomarkers result from these analyses which, when translated to clinical medicine and drug development, will have an important impact on human health and disease. This review highlights both the opportunities and challenges in bringing biomarkers into clinical medicine. Publication Types: Review

Curr Opin Drug Discov Devel. 2005 Jan;8(1):100-6. Related Articles, Links In vivo zebrafish assays for toxicity testing. Parng C. Phylonix Pharmaceuticals Inc, Cambridge, MA 02139, USA. Chuenlei@phylonix.com Toxicity, due to complications of in vivo adsorption, distribution, metabolism and excretion (ADME), is a major cause of failure during drug development; many drugs shown to be safe in cell culture prove toxic in animal studies. Effective in vivo toxicity screening early in the development process can reduce the number of compounds that progress to laborious and costly late-stage animal testing. The transparent zebrafish provides accessibility to internal organs, tissues and even cells, and has emerged as an invaluable model organism for toxicity testing and drug discovery. Straightforward in vivo zebrafish assays can serve as an intermediate step between cell-based and mammalian testing, thus streamlining the drug development time-line. Publication Types: Review

Curr Opin Drug Discov Devel. 2005 Jan;8(1):78-88. Related Articles, Links In vitro ADME phenotyping in drug discovery: current challenges and future solutions. Williams JA, Bauman J, Cai H, Conlon K, Hansel S, Hurst S, Sadagopan N, Tugnait M, Zhang L, Sahi J. Pfizer Global Research and Development, Pharmacokinetics, Dynamics and Metabolism, Ann Arbor, MI 48103, USA. james.williams2@pfizer.com Drug-metabolizing enzymes and drug transporters are key regulators of drug disposition and pharmacodynamics, which are closely linked to drug efficacy and safety. In this article, current challenges and future solutions to predicting their influence on pharmacokinetics and inter-organ distribution in humans, from data generated during the drug discovery decision-making process, are presented. In vitro phenotyping strategies for drug metabolizing enzymes (eg, CYP3A4, UGT1A1) and transporters (eg, OATP1B1) are offered, including perspectives on a selection of in vitro systems, novel in vitro phenotyping reagents and remaining technology gaps, challenges in extrapolating in vitro data to the in vivo situation, in silico models for the prediction of whether compounds are enzyme or transporter substrates, and the impact of pharmacogenomics. Publication Types: Review

Curr Opin Genet Dev. 2004 Jun;14(3):287-91. Related Articles, Links Society and ethics - the genetics of disease. Thomas SM. Nuffield Council on Bioethics, 28 Bedford Square, London WC1B 3JS, UK. sthomas@nuffieldfoundation.org Established guidance for the protection of human subjects in research has provided the framework for research and clinical practice in genetics. Three key principles to emerge are the requirements for consent, privacy and confidentiality. However, recent research on genetic susceptibility to common diseases indicates that it may be more difficult to decide if and when genetic testing will be appropriate. Risks of disease may be low and interventions may not be available. Today, debate is primarily focussed on ethical issues raised by the use and storage of genetic information. One of the earliest experiences of genetic testing for some people is likely to be in the area of pharmacogenetics. Debate about ethical issues has been focused on the implications of patient stratification, particularly with regard to the availability of medicines for small groups and the significance of racial variation in response to medicines. The possible use of personal genetic information by insurance companies and employers has also been an issue that legislators have taken seriously. Publication Types: Review

Curr Opin Hematol. 2004 Nov;11(6):434-8. Related Articles, Links Pharmacogenetics of acute lymphoblastic leukemia. Mehta PA, Davies SM. Cincinnati Children's Hospital Medical Center, Cincinnati, Ohio 45229, USA. Parinda.Mehta@cchmc.org PURPOSE OF REVIEW: The outcome in children with acute lymphoblastic leukemia has improved significantly over the past four decades. Current therapy results in event-free survival exceeding 80% for most patients. The development of risk-adapted therapy based on characteristics of the child (age), leukemia (leukocyte count, acquired genetic characteristics) and early response to therapy allows dose intensification for children with higher-risk disease. Much less attention has been given to the role of host variability (pharmacogenetic polymorphism) in determining outcome. This review discusses literature reports in this area and describes some of the challenges facing the field as it moves forward. RECENT FINDINGS: Polymorphisms in many different metabolic pathways have been demonstrated in single gene studies to influence the outcome of acute lymphoblastic leukemia. Challenges arise in establishing the generalizability of observations and interpreting complex gene-gene interactions in multigene pathways. Recent studies also illustrate the importance of correlation of clinical associations with biological mechanisms. SUMMARY: Despite significant progress in the treatment of childhood acute lymphoblastic leukemia, therapy is still unsuccessful in 20% of patients. Further knowledge of and insight into the role of host genetic polymorphisms will improve the results by integrating pharmacodynamic and pharmacogenomic studies in individualizing therapy for children with acute lymphoblastic leukemia. Publication Types: Review

Curr Opin Infect Dis. 2005 Dec;18(6):543-9. Related Articles, Links Host determinants

of antiretroviral drug activity. Boffito M, Winston A, Owen A. St. Stephen's Centre-Chelsea and Westminster Hospital, 369 Fulham Road, London SW10 9NH, UK. marta.boffito@chelwest.nhs.uk PURPOSE OF REVIEW: As physicians are confronted with a diversity of adverse events and variability in response to medication among patients, this review will focus on the available evidence regarding the impact of genetic variation on drug response. Specifically, variation in drug metabolizing enzymes such as the cytochrome P450s, drug transporters and human leucocyte antigen (for idiosyncratic drug reactions). The potential role of pharmacogenetics in the management of HIV-1 infected individuals and drug discovery will be discussed. RECENT FINDINGS: Wide inter-individual variability of antiretroviral therapy efficacy and toxicity in HIV-infected patients has been extensively reported in the literature. Since treatment involves multiple drugs and drug classes with the potential for significant variability in drug-host as well as drug-drug interactions, antiretroviral drug therapy represents a significant challenge. Despite this inherent complexity, considerable recent advances have led to a greater understanding of interactions between genetic and host factors that influence the efficacy and toxicity of these agents. SUMMARY: The goal of pharmacogenetics in antiretroviral therapy is to outline differences within a given population that influence drug efficacy and toxicity. Although to date, despite the numerous studies available in the literature, conclusions on how the analysis of the relationship between single nucleotide polymorphisms and drug efficacy may not always be clinically useful. Further studies are warranted to clarify the role of pharmacogenetics and antiretroviral drug management.
Publication Types: Review

Curr Opin Mol Ther. 2004 Dec;6(6):600-7. Related Articles, Links Genomic and proteomic profiling for biomarkers and signature profiles of toxicity. Merrick BA, Bruno ME. National Center for Toxicogenomics, National Institute of Environmental Health Sciences, PO Box 12233, Research Triangle Park, NC 27709, USA. merrick@niehs.nih.gov Toxicity profiling measures and compares all gene expression changes among biological samples after toxicant exposure. Toxicity profiling with DNA microarrays to measure all mRNA transcripts (transcriptomics), or by global separation and identification of proteins (proteomics), has led to the discovery of better descriptors of toxicity, toxicant classification and exposure monitoring than current indicators. A shared goal in transcript and proteomic profiling is the development of biomarkers and signatures of chemical toxicity. In this review, biomarkers and signature profiles are described for specific chemical toxicants that affect target organs such as liver, kidney, neural tissues, gastrointestinal tract and skeletal muscle, for specific disease models such as cancer and inflammation, and for unique chemical-protein adducts underlying cell injury. The recent introduction of toxicogenomics databases support researchers in sharing, analyzing, visualizing and mining expression data, assist the integration of transcriptomics, proteomics and toxicology datasets, and eventually will permit in silico biomarker and signature pattern discovery.
Publication Types: Review

Curr Opin Mol Ther. 2004 Dec;6(6):608-15. Related Articles, Links Gels and more gels: probing toxicity. Witzmann FA, Bai

F, Hong SM, Liu S, Pedrick N, Ringham H, Tan J. Indiana University School of Medicine, Department of Cellular and Integrative Physiology, Biotechnology and Research Training Center, 1345 West 16th Street, Indianapolis, IN 46202, USA. fwitzman@iupui.edu Two-dimensional electrophoresis (2-DE) remains an important technology in the study of protein expression. In many applications, 2-DE has been supplanted by liquid chromatographic and mass spectrometric approaches that overcome some of its limitations and labor intensiveness. Nevertheless, 2-DE has exceptional relevance in toxicology and, despite the challenges, its implementation continues to support toxicologists in understanding the biological effects of chemical exposures in living systems. This review will address the use of 2-DE-based proteomics in toxicology and recent developments in this strategy, considering the unique nature of toxicity testing and the issues of dynamic range and reproducibility that have previously limited the overall utility of 2-DE in this field. Publication Types: Review

Curr Opin Mol Ther. 2004 Jun;6(3):296-301. Related Articles, Links Pharmacogenomics in breast cancer: current trends and future directions. Wajapeyee N, Somasundaram K. Indian Institute of Science, Department of Microbiology and Cell Biology, Bangalore 560 012, India. Pharmacogenomics is the study of genetic variations between individuals to predict the risk of toxic side effects and the probability that a patient will respond to single- or multidrug chemotherapy. Breast cancer remains one of the most common cancers among women worldwide and is second only to lung cancer in cancer-related death. A better understanding of the mechanisms of initiation and progression of breast cancer is needed for early diagnosis and development of better therapeutic methodologies. Differences in cancer patients' responses to chemotherapy have often been attributed to pathogenesis and severity of the disease, drug interactions, patient's age, gender, nutritional status, organ functions and tumor biology. It is now well recognized that genetic variations in drug target genes, disease pathway genes and drug metabolizing enzymes can have greater influence on drug efficacy and toxicity. In addition, germline variants can be used to study breast cancer susceptibility, as well as the variable response to both drug and radiation therapy used in the treatment of breast cancer. This review discusses clinically relevant individual gene variations that influence breast cancer susceptibility and cancer therapy, as well as the microarray-based expression profiling studies that have great potential in cancer pharmacogenomics in terms of tumor classification, drug and biomarker discovery and drug efficacy testing. Publication Types: Review

Curr Opin Mol Ther. 2004 Jun;6(3):302-7. Related Articles, Links Pharmacogenomics of HIV. Ast O, Luke W. Berlex Biosciences, 2600 Hilltop Drive, PO Box 4099, CA 94804-0099, USA. Oliver_Ast@berlex.com The antiretroviral treatment of HIV infection has expanded tremendously in the last few years. This trend is mainly a result of new assays, genetic advances and recombinant DNA technologies providing new insights into HIV virology, pathology and resistance mechanisms. Since 1995, the use of highly active antiretroviral therapy (HAART) as a combination of substances directed against various steps in the viral life cycle, has led to significant decreases in the morbidity and mortality associated with HIV infections. The ability to quantify viral load and to perform sequence analyses represent valuable tools both for understanding the pathogenic actions of the virus and for clinical drug monitoring of HIV-infected patients. Laboratory tests have been developed and validated to help predict which antiviral substances may be more effective to control viral replication in a given patient. Genotypic and phenotypic assays have been developed to assess HIV antiviral resistance. The ability to predict drug response from a certain genotypic or phenotypic setting with respect to drug absorption, drug metabolism and drug elimination is continually evolving. This may lead to significant changes in drug plasma concentrations and may affect the efficacy and toxicity of antivirals. More recently, drug/drug interactions and mutation/drug correlations have been discovered. However, the optimal usage of pharmacogenetic and pharmacogenomic tools in the clinic still remains to be defined. This review summarizes mechanisms of drug bioavailability with respect to pharmacogenomics and discusses the impact and clinical benefit of 'personalized' HIV therapy. Publication Types: Review

Curr Opin Mol Ther. 2005 Dec;7(6):551-6. Related Articles, Links Stem cell pharmacogenomics: a reality check on stem cell therapy. Bapat SA, Mishra GC. National Centre for Cell Science, Ganeshkhind, Pune 411007, India. sabapat@nccs.res.in Widespread applications of stem cell-based therapies in the clinic are being reported, yet there is a surprising lack of resolution of the factors that lead to failure of such therapies on a long-term basis. While classical pharmacogenomics aids the prediction of drug responses in an individual based on genetic variation and pharmacological responses, stem cell therapy involves an additional dimension of host-donor cell interactions and adaptability. We propose the development of concise guidelines based on pharmacogenetic and donor/host-related cellular factors studied more extensively in larger data sets, and used in prospective studies to individualize stem cell therapy. Publication Types: Review

Curr Opin Mol Ther. 2005 Jun;7(3):202-8. Related Articles, Links Smoking cessation treatment: pharmacogenetic assessment. Munafo MR, Lerman C, Niaura R, Shields AE, Swan GE. University of Bristol, Department of Experimental Psychology Bristol, UK. marcus.munafo@bristol.ac.uk This review focuses on the current status and future directions of pharmacogenetics research into responses to treatments for nicotine dependence and smoking cessation. Research remains in its infancy and, although the potential for individualized treatment tailored to genotype is promising, there are practical, ethical and social considerations that must be addressed before such research is translated into clinical practice. In particular, future studies that need to be conducted before such research is translated into clinical practice and potential limitations and barriers to this translation are described. Publication Types: Review

Curr Opin Mol Ther. 2005 Jun;7(3):209-17. Related Articles, Links The pharmacogenetics of asthma: an update. Tantisira KG, Weiss ST. Brigham and Women's Hospital and Harvard Medical School, Channing Laboratory, 181 Longwood Avenue, Boston, MA 02115, USA. kelan.tantisira@channing.harvard.edu Responses to the three major classes of asthma therapy, beta-agonists, leukotriene antagonists and inhaled corticosteroids, demonstrate wide inter-individual variability. Moreover, both asthma and the traits measured in response to asthma therapy, including forced expiratory volume at 1 s, are highly heritable. This indicates that genetics may play a prominent role in the determination of the therapeutic response to asthma. The human genetic association trials that investigate responses to each of the three major classes of asthma therapy will be summarized, and recent findings in the literature highlighted. Altogether, the available data indicate that genetics influences the likelihood of an individual responding to a given therapy, indicating that, in the future, optimal care for individuals with asthma may include genetic testing. Publication Types: Review

Curr Opin Mol Ther. 2005 Jun;7(3):218-25. Related Articles, Links Hypertension pharmacogenomics: current status and future directions. Johnson JA, Turner ST. University of Florida, Departments of Pharmacy Practice and Medicine (Cardiology) and Center for Pharmacogenomics, Box 100486, Gainesville, FL 32610-0486, USA. johnson@cop.ufl.edu Hypertension is the most common chronic disease in the Western world, and while there are many drug classes from which to choose therapy, only 34% of North Americans currently have their blood pressure controlled. The potential clinical utility of pharmacogenomics in helping to guide antihypertensive drug therapy selection is described. The hypertension pharmacogenetics literature is reviewed, which highlights that only a small fraction of the genes that likely contribute to antihypertensive response have been studied to date. The genes for alpha-adducin (diuretic response), the beta1-adrenergic receptor (beta-blocker response) and angiotensinogen (response to multiple drug classes) are among the genes with the most compelling data (based on replication) as pharmacogenetic candidates. Potential limitations of current studies are also discussed. These include reliance on clinic blood pressure, which is probably a suboptimal response phenotype, and the relatively small sample sizes of most studies to date. Also discussed is the relatively simplistic genetic approach that has been taken, which has focused largely on a single gene or single nucleotide polymorphism within a gene. Multiple ways to overcome these potential limitations are described. Hypertension pharmacogenomics holds tremendous potential for providing a mechanism by which management of hypertensive patients might be improved, and future studies should help move this field towards its clinical potential. Publication Types: Review

Curr Opin Mol Ther. 2005 Jun;7(3):246-50. Related Articles, Links Gene expression-driven diagnostics and pharmacogenomics in cancer. Wang Y. Veridex LLC, a Johnson and Johnson Company, 3210 Merryfield Row, San Diego, CA 92121, USA. ywang44@vrxus.jnj.com The advancement of microarray technologies for characterizing tumors at the gene expression level has made a significant impact on the field of oncology. Profiling gene expression of various human tumors has led to the identification of gene expression patterns or signatures related to tumor classification, disease outcome and response to therapy. This technology can also be used to study the mechanism of action of specific therapeutics. Routine application of microarrays in clinical practice will require significant efforts to standardize the array manufacturing techniques, assay protocols and analytical methods used to interpret the data. Extensive, independent validation using large, statistically sound datasets will also be necessary. Studies on gene expression profiling of clinically relevant tissue samples with the aim of finding gene markers to support disease prognosis and therapy decisions are reviewed. Publication Types: Review

Curr Opin Nephrol Hypertens. 2005 Sep;14(5):428-34. Related Articles, Links New directions in the assessment and treatment of hypertensive heart disease. Gonzalez A, Lopez B, Diez J. Division of Cardiovascular Pathophysiology, Centre for Applied Medical Research, University Clinic, School of Medicine, University of Navarra, C/Pio XII 55, 31008 Pamplona, Spain. PURPOSE OF REVIEW: This article will review briefly the emerging new concepts in the diagnosis and treatment of myocardial fibrosis in patients with hypertensive heart disease. RECENT FINDINGS: Although hypertensive heart disease is characterized clinically by development of left-ventricular hypertrophy in the absence of a cause other than arterial hypertension, changes in the composition of myocardial tissue also develop in arterial hypertension leading to structural remodeling of the myocardium (e.g. fibrosis). Recent available data on the determination of serum concentrations of collagen-derived serum peptides and quantitative analysis of echoreflectivity to address the presence of fibrosis in the myocardium of hypertensive patients are promising. In addition, preliminary data suggest that the goal of reducing myocardial fibrosis is achievable in patients with hypertensive heart disease using specific antihypertensive agents (e.g. those interfering with angiotensin II). SUMMARY: The time has come to revisit the current management of hypertensive heart disease simply focused on detecting left-ventricular hypertrophy and controlling blood pressure to reduce left-ventricular mass. It is necessary to develop new approaches aimed at assessing and repairing alterations of myocardial structure and protect myocardial function and, in so doing, to reduce in a more-effective manner adverse risk associated with hypertensive heart disease. Publication Types: Review

Curr Opin Pharmacol. 2005 Dec;5(6):604-9. Epub 2005 Sep 30. Related Articles, Links Pediatric gastrointestinal diseases: are drugs the answer? Jones NL, Wine E. Department of Paediatrics, Hospital for Sick Children, University of Toronto, Toronto, Canada. nicola.jones@sickkids.ca Owing to the lack of large randomized controlled studies, which would produce level 1 evidence, to guide management of gastrointestinal disorders in children, data are often extrapolated from adult studies to aid in treatment strategies. However, there are unique aspects to the management of children and adolescents with these chronic diseases, including issues of growth, side effects, long-term outcomes and psychosocial factors that might not be considered in adult trials. There is a major need for increased research in this population. In the future, a better understanding of the pathophysiologic mechanisms of these diseases should guide the development of rational novel therapies with better safety profiles for children with gastrointestinal disorders. Publication Types: Review

Curr Pharm Des. 2006;12(3):273-86. Related Articles, Links An update on overcoming MDR1-mediated multidrug resistance in cancer chemotherapy. Takara K, Sakaeda

T, Okumura K. Department of Hospital Pharmacy, School of Medicine, Kobe University, 7-5-2 Kusunoki-cho, Chuo-ku, Kobe 650-0017, Japan. The intrinsic or acquired resistance to anticancer drugs remains one of the most significant factors impeding the progress of cancer chemotherapy. This phenomenon often involves simultaneous resistance to other anticancer drugs that differ in their chemical structure and mode of action and are not even used in chemotherapy. This phenotype has been called multidrug resistance (MDR). Although the cellular basis underlying MDR is not fully understood, several factors mediating therapy resistance in tumors have been proposed. One of the mechanisms leading to chemoresistance of tumor cells is the increased activity of transporter proteins. The best-characterized transporter protein is MDR1/P-glycoprotein, and a number of clinical investigations have suggested that its intrinsic or acquired overexpression resulted in a poor clinical outcome of chemotherapy. Various types of compounds and techniques for the reversal of MDR1/P-glycoprotein-mediated MDR have been developed, and efforts have concentrated on the inhibition of function and suppression of expression. This review summarizes the current state of knowledge of MDR1/P-glycoprotein and the modulation of MDR by targeting MDR1/P-glycoprotein. Publication Types: Review

Curr Top Med Chem. 2004;4(13):1329-45. Related Articles, Links The use of DNA microarrays to investigate the pharmacogenomics of drug response in living systems. Villeneuve DJ, Parissenti AM. Northeastern Ontario Regional Cancer Centre, Research Department, 41 Ramsey Lake Road, Sudbury, ON, Canada P3E 5J1. aparissenti@hrsch.on.ca With the advent of DNA microarray analysis, it is now possible to examine the response of virtually the entire human genome to cellular drug exposure and to uncover a wide variety of genes correlating with the establishment of drug resistance. This relatively new field of "pharmacogenomics" is likely to vastly increase our understanding of the mechanisms of drug action and how cells respond and adapt to drug exposure. However, DNA microarray studies typically result in the identification of hundreds of genes that may or may not be of relevance in vivo-particularly when large, genetically diverse study populations are used. The challenge to the researcher is to design experimental systems and approaches which minimize variability in the data, increase the reproducibility amongst experiments, allow array data from multiple experiments to be assessed by a variety of statistical, supervised learning, and data clustering approaches, and provide a clear link between drug response and the expression of specific genes. This review provides a description and critical analysis of recent studies on the pharmacogenomics of drug response and discusses current guidelines and approaches for the performance and analysis of DNA microarray experiments in this area. Publication Types: Review

Curr Top Med Chem. 2004;4(13):1347-56. Related Articles, Links Growth factor signaling and resistance to cancer chemotherapy. Dai Z, Huang Y, Sadee W. Program of Pharmacogenomics, Department of Pharmacology, College of Medicine and Public Health, The Ohio State University, 5168 Graves Hall, 333 West 10th Avenue, Columbus, OH 43210, USA. dai.15@osu.edu Multiple mechanisms contribute to chemoresistance, eventually leading to failure of cancer chemotherapy. Deregulated growth factor signaling pathways promote cell proliferation and render cancer cells resistant to apoptosis, a common mechanism of chemoresistance. Therefore, inhibitors of growth factor signaling, including antibodies and small molecules, are promising drug candidates for chemotherapy, either given alone or as adjuvants to overcome general drug resistance. While dramatic responses have been attained in some cases, innate or acquired resistance to these novel anticancer drugs is common and limits broad applicability. Treatment failure may arise from complexity of growth factor signaling, with numerous parallel pathways and diverse downstream events. This review discusses the use of pharmacogenomics, assessing multiple growth factor signaling pathways and complex chemoresistance mechanisms. Monitoring expression profiles and activating mutations in growth factor receptors holds promise for the design of individualized therapy with a combination of drugs. Publication Types: Review

Curr Top Med Chem. 2004;4(13):1357-70. Related Articles, Links Analysis of DNA microarray data. Hackl H, Sanchez Cabo F, Sturn A, Wolkenhauer O, Trajanoski Z. Institute for Genomics and Bioinformatics and Christian Doppler Laboratory for Genomics and Bioinformatics, Graz University of Technology, Petersgasse 14, A-8010 Graz, Austria. Recent advances in DNA microarray technology have great impact on many areas of biomedical research and pharmacogenomics: discovering novel targets and genes, elucidating signatures of complex diseases, transcriptional profiling of models for diseases, and the development of individually optimized drugs based on differential gene expression patterns. Consequently, there is demand for robust methods for data analysis and the choice of adequate statistical tests. This review guides through all steps in the cDNA microarray data analysis pipeline and gives a basic understanding of the challenges in interpreting large microarray datasets. Publication Types: Review

Curr Top Med Chem. 2004;4(13):1371-83. Related Articles, Links Stem cell pharmacogenomics. Bapat SA, Mishra GC. National Centre for Cell Science, NCCS Complex, Ganeshkhind, Pune 411 007, Maharashtra, India. sabapat@nccs.res.in Therapeutic stem cell applications represent a newly evolving approach for the treatment of several genetic and degenerative diseases. The advent of pharmacogenomics too, holds promise for an individualized, optimal treatment regime for a large variety of medical conditions. A combination of the benefits of these two technologies creates a new niche in therapeutic medicine research viz. that of stem cell pharmacogenomics (SCP). The development of this approach requires the application of existing technologies in genomics, proteomics and bioinformatics to resolve the various issues involved in advancing the therapeutic applications of stem cell medicine. In this brief overview of the subject, we attempt to provide fresh insights into the exclusive niche of stem cell pharmacogenomics and discuss some of the priority issues that need to be targeted, based on the existing principles of pharmacogenomics, stem cell characteristics and transplantation medicine. Advances in these areas are imperative in realizing the dream of stem cell therapies contributing towards the improvisation of the quality of human life. Publication Types: Review

Curr Top Med Chem. 2004;4(13):1385-98. Related Articles, Links Pharmacogenetics of drug transporters and its impact on the pharmacotherapy. Sakaeda T, Nakamura T, Okumura K. Department of Hospital Pharmacy, School of Medicine, Kobe University, 7-5-2 Kusunoki-cho, Chuo-ku, Kobe 650-0017, Japan. Most drug responses are determined by the interplay of several gene products that influence pharmacokinetics and pharmacodynamics, i.e., drug metabolizing enzymes, drug transporters, and drug targets. With the sequencing of the human genome, it has been estimated that approximately 500-1200 genes code for drug transporters. Concerning the effects of genetic polymorphisms on pharmacotherapy, the best characterized drug transporter is the multidrug resistant transporter P-glycoprotein/MDR1, the gene product of MDR1. Little such information is available on other drug transporters. MDR1 is a glycosylated membrane protein of 170 kDa, belonging to the ATP-binding cassette superfamily, and is expressed mainly in intestines, liver, kidneys and brain. A number of various types of structurally unrelated drugs are substrates for MDR1, and their intestinal absorption, hepatobiliary secretion, renal secretion and brain transport are regulated by MDR1. The first investigation on the effects of MDR1 genotypes on pharmacotherapy was reported in 2000: a silent single nucleotide polymorphism (SNP), C3435T in exon 26, was found to be associated with the duodenal expression of MDR1, and thereby the plasma concentration of digoxin after oral administration. At present, a total of 28 SNPs have been found at 27 positions on the MDR1 gene. Clinical investigations on the association of MDR1 genotypes with the expression and function of MDR1 in tissues, and with pharmacokinetics and pharmacodynamics have mainly focused on C3435T; however, there are still discrepancies in the results, suggesting that the haplotype of the gene should be analyzed instead of a SNP. C3435T is also reported to be a risk factor for a certain class of diseases including the inflammatory bowel diseases, Parkinson's disease and renal epithelial tumor, and this also might be explained by the effects on MDR1 expression and function. In this review, the latest reports on the effects of genetic polymorphisms of MDR1 on pharmacotherapy are summarized, and the pharmacogenetics of other transporters is briefly introduced. Publication Types: Review

Curr Top Med Chem. 2004;4(13):1399-409. Related Articles, Links Pharmacogenomics: the influence of genomic variation on drug response. Thomas FJ, McLeod HL, Watters JW. Washington University School of Medicine, Department of Medicine, Campus Box 8069, St. Louis, MO 63110, USA. jwatters@im.wustl.edu Unpredictable efficacy and toxicity are major hurdles in the administration of many medications. By identifying inherited DNA polymorphisms that influence drug disposition and effects, pharmacogenomics is an exciting tool for the individualization of drug therapies. Single nucleotide polymorphisms (SNP) in genes encoding drug metabolizing enzymes, drug transporters, and DNA repair genes have recently been shown to influence drug toxicity and efficacy. This review will discuss clinically relevant examples of genetic polymorphisms that influence the outcome of drug therapy, and possibilities for future applications of pharmacogenomics. Publication Types: Review

Curr Top Med Chem. 2004;4(13):1411-21. Related Articles, Links Genotyping as a tool to predict adverse drug reactions.

Guzey C, Spigset O. Department of Clinical Pharmacology, St. Olav's University Hospital, 7006 Trondheim, Norway. During the last decades, the rapid development in molecular biology has contributed to the understanding of genetic factors underlying many adverse drug reactions. Until recently, most research in this area has focused on genes coding for drug-metabolizing enzymes. Inactivating mutations have been found in genes coding for enzymes belonging to the cytochrome P-450 system, which is the major system for drug metabolism in humans, but also in genes coding for other enzymes. Subjects with a lack of functional activity in these enzymes should be treated with very low doses of drugs metabolized by the same enzyme in order to avoid excessive drug levels and thereby toxic effects. In the last years, increasing attention has been directed towards genes coding for drug targets. Hitherto, most studies have been carried out on single genes known to be or assumed to be functionally related to a given adverse drug reaction. Another approach, which may become more common in the future, is testing for complex single nucleotide polymorphism patterns that may be associated with adverse drug reactions, although the functional relationship between them may be completely unknown. Due to the influence of non-genetic factors in the development of adverse drug reactions, the association between a specific genotype and an adverse drug reaction will always be lower than 100%. Therefore, there is a need for prospective large-scale studies in order to elucidate the extent of environmental influences on the adverse drug reactions for which a genetic basis has been suggested. Despite these obstacles, pharmacogenetic testing will hopefully in the future identify at least some clear-cut situations where a drug should be avoided in certain individuals in order to reduce the risk of adverse drug reactions. Publication Types: Review

Curr Top Med Chem. 2004;4(13):1423-31. Related Articles, Links SNP discovery and typing technologies for pharmacogenomics. Twyman RM. Department of Biology, University of York, Heslington, York YO10 5DD, UK. richard@writescience.com Genetic variation in the human genome occurs predominantly as single nucleotide polymorphisms (SNPs). Our DNA may contain as many as ten million SNPs, of which three million or more are likely to differ between any two unrelated individuals. These three million genetic differences make a significant contribution to the observed variation in complex human phenotypes, such as disease susceptibility and our responses to drugs or environmental chemicals. Large-scale association studies taking place throughout the drug development process can help to identify such differences and tailor drugs and dose regimens to particular genotype classes. The need for such large-scale studies has driven the development of high-throughout SNP discovery and typing technologies, which are the subject of this review. Publication Types: Review

Curr Top Med Chem. 2004;4(13):1455-60. Related Articles, Links The regulation of pharmacogenomics-based drugs and policy making. Issa AM. UCLA School of Public Health, CHS Room 31-245A, Box 951772, Los Angeles, CA 90095-1772, USA. aissa1@ucla.edu In addition to potential future clinical benefits such as reducing adverse drug reactions and optimizing therapeutic efficacy, pharmacogenomic applications promise numerous benefits for the pharmaceutical and biotechnology industries, including decreasing the size and expense of clinical trials and streamlining the drug development process. The application of pharmacogenomics and related technological advances to drug development has prompted various regulatory agencies such as the United States Food and Drug Administration to issue guidance documents and other advisory statements. This article delineates the impact of pharmacogenomic-guided drug development on the regulatory process in the United States including relevant highlights of industry guidance documents and policy statements. Hypothetical vignettes are used to illustrate a number of issues that are challenging to policy makers and the potential impact of pharmacogenomic based drug research and development on the regulatory environment.

Curr Top Med Chem. 2004;4(16):1733-44. Related Articles, Links Pharmacogenetics of the cytochromes P450. Daly AK. Pharmacogenetics Group, School of Clinical and Laboratory Sciences, University of Newcastle upon Tyne, Medical School, Framlington Place, Newcastle upon Tyne NE2 4HH, UK. A.K.Daly@ncl.ac.uk The cytochromes P450 are a family of heme-containing proteins with a major role in the oxidation of both xenobiotics (including prescribed drugs) and endogenous compounds. There are at least 57 human P450s (termed isoforms) which are all encoded by separate genes but only 10 of these contribute to drug metabolism, with the major contribution coming from only 3 isoforms, CYP3A4, CYP2D6 and CYP2C9. It is now well recognised that most cytochrome P450 genes are subject to genetic polymorphism and that therefore some individuals have sequence changes present that result in the production of an enzyme with altered catalytic activity or give rise to abnormal gene expression. This article describes the range of genetic polymorphisms now known to occur in the drug metabolizing cytochromes P450 with particular reference to their functional effects and the influence of ethnic origin on the frequency of variant alleles. The relevance of the various polymorphisms to drug response and toxicity is considered as well as the possibility that genotype for these polymorphisms may be a determinant for "personalized prescribing" in the future. Publication Types: Review

Curr Top Med Chem. 2005;5(11):1039-46. Related Articles, Links Pharmacogenomics: integration into drug discovery and development. Johnson K, Thompson J, Power A. Clinical Pharmacogenomics, Pfizer Global Research and Development, Ann Arbor, Michigan, USA. To deliver on the promise of personalized medicine requires the integration of pharmacogenomics into the discovery and development of medicines. Over the last few years the pharmaceutical industry has been building considerable resources to achieve that. However, this requires new skill sets, capabilities and infrastructures which have not been a traditional part of the industry's efforts. In this article we describe how the integration of genetics and pharmacogenomics data has begun to deliver success and illustrate the challenges that the new science and technologies bring and how these challenges can be addressed in order to deliver on the promise. Publication Types: Review

Cytokine. 2006 Mar 7; [Epub ahead of print] Related Articles, Links Cytokine pharmacogenetics. Maxwell JR, Wilson AG. Academic Rheumatology Group, Royal Hallamshire Hospital, Sheffield,

UK; Division of Genomic Medicine, Sheffield Medical School, University of Sheffield, Sheffield, UK. Genetic variation plays a significant role in the normal functioning of the immune system, and also in the interaction between many common drugs and cellular pathways. With a growing number of cytokine-based therapies now in mainstream clinical use, the prospect of targeting these agents to the individuals likely to benefit from them most is an appealing one. This review outlines the potential clinical impact of cytokine pharmacogenetics in targeting these therapies to individuals with favourable genetic profiles. The use of such approaches may have important pharmacoeconomic benefits and lead to improved therapeutic profiles for these treatments. y publisher]

De Paul Law Rev. 2004 Spring;53(3):1111-26. Related Articles, Links Race as a proxy for drug response: the dangers and challenges of ethnic drugs. Bowser R. University of Illinois College of Law, USA.

Del Med J. 2002 Dec;74(12):469-73. Related Articles, Links Epstein-Barr virus-associated lymphoproliferative disorder in a patient with rheumatoid arthritis on methotrexate and rofecoxib: idiosyncratic reaction or pharmacogenetics? Vincent S, Slease RB, Rocca PV. Clinical Pharmacology/MSCI fellow at Vanderbilt University School of Medicine in Nashville, Tennessee, USA. Rheumatoid arthritis (RA) is an autoimmune disease associated with altered immunoregulation and resulting in a deforming polyarthritis. Methotrexate (MTX) is a commonly used second line agent for RA, and there have been several recent reports of Epstein-Barr virus (EBV)-associated polyclonal B cell lymphoproliferative disorder in MTX-treated RA patients. The patient in this report had long standing RA treated with MTX and had recently begun taking a cyclooxygenase-2 (COX-2) inhibitor. She developed a febrile illness associated with severe pancytopenia and leukocytoclastic vasculitic rash followed by diffuse adenopathy, with serologic and pathologic evidence of EBV infection. Previous studies have demonstrated the interaction of MTX and a variety of non-steroidal, anti-inflammatory drugs (NSAIDs) with various clinical manifestations including acute renal failure, pancytopenia, vomiting, diarrhea, elevated liver transaminases, jaundice, mucosal ulcerations, and pyrexia. However, we have not identified previous reports suggesting interaction between MTX and COX-2 inhibitors. We hypothesize that decreased renal elimination of MTX induced by the COX-2 inhibitor resulted in enhanced hematopoietic toxicity and immunosuppression causing the EBV-associated lymphoproliferative disease. Publication Types: Case Reports

Diabetes Care. 2004 Jun;27(6):1394-8. Related Articles, Links The Arg972 variant in insulin receptor substrate-1 is associated with an increased risk of secondary failure to sulfonylurea in patients with type 2 diabetes. Sesti G, Marini MA, Cardellini M, Sciacqua A, Frontoni S, Andreozzi F, Irace C, Lauro D, Gnasso A, Federici M, Perticone F, Lauro R. Dipartimento di Medicina Sperimentale e Clinica, Universita Magna Graecia di Catanzaro-Via Tommaso Campanella, 115 88100 Catanzaro, Italy. sesti@unicz.it OBJECTIVE: The aim of this study was to investigate whether diabetic patients carrying the Arg(972) insulin receptor substrate-1 (IRS-1) variant are at increased risk for secondary failure to sulfonylurea. RESEARCH DESIGN AND METHODS: A total of 477 unrelated Caucasian type 2 diabetic patients were recruited according to the following criteria: onset of diabetes after age 35 years, absence of ketonuria at diagnosis, and anti-GAD(-) antibody. Type 2 diabetes was diagnosed according to the American Diabetes Association criteria. Patients with secondary sulfonylurea failure were defined as those requiring insulin due to uncontrolled hyperglycemia (fasting plasma glucose >300 mg/dl) despite sulfonylurea-metformin combined therapy, appropriate diet, and absence of any conditions causing hyperglycemia. RESULTS: Of the total patients, 53 (11.1%) were heterozygous for the Arg(972) IRS-1 variant, 1 (0.2%) was homozygous, and the remainder (88.7%) were homozygous for the wild-type allele. The genotype frequency of the Arg(972) IRS-1 variant was 8.7% among diabetic patients well controlled with oral therapy and 16.7% among patients with secondary failure to sulfonylurea (odds ratio 2.1 [95% CI 1.18-3.70], P = 0.01). Adjustment for age, sex, BMI, metabolic control, age at diagnosis, duration of diabetes, and Pro12Ala polymorphism of peroxisome proliferator-activated receptor-gamma2 gene in a logistic regression analysis with secondary failure to sulfonylurea as a dependent variable did not change this association (2.0 [1.38-3.86], P = 0.038). CONCLUSIONS: These data demonstrate that the Arg(972) IRS-1 variant is associated with increased risk for secondary failure to sulfonylurea, thus representing a potential example of pharmacogenetics in type 2 diabetes.

Diabetes. 2004 Oct;53(10):2713-8. Related Articles, Links Permanent neonatal diabetes due to mutations in KCNJ11 encoding Kir6.2: patient characteristics and initial response to sulfonylurea therapy. Sagen JV, Raeder H, Hathout E, Shehadeh N, Gudmundsson K, Baevre H, Abuelo D, Phornphutkul C, Molnes J, Bell GI, Gloyn AL, Hattersley AT, Molven A, Sovik O, Njolstad PR. Section of Pediatrics, Department of Clinical Medicine, University of Bergen, N-5021 Bergen, Norway. Permanent neonatal diabetes (PND) can be caused by mutations in the transcription factors insulin promoter factor (IPF)-1, eukaryotic translation initiation factor-2alpha kinase 3 (EIF2AK3), and forkhead box-P3 and in key components of insulin secretion: glucokinase (GCK) and the ATP-sensitive K(+) channel subunit Kir6.2. We sequenced the gene encoding Kir6.2 (KCNJ11) in 11 probands with GCK-negative PND. Heterozygous mutations were identified in seven probands, causing three novel (F35V, Y330C, and F333I) and two known (V59M and R201H) Kir6.2 amino acid substitutions. Only two probands had a family history of diabetes. Subjects with the V59M mutation had neurological features including motor delay. Three mutation carriers tested had an insulin secretory response to tolbutamide, but not to glucose or glucagon. Glibenclamide was introduced in increasing doses to investigate whether sulfonylurea could replace insulin. At a glibenclamide dose of 0.3-0.4 mg. kg(-1). day(-1), insulin was discontinued. Blood glucose did not deteriorate, and HbA(1c) was stable or fell during 2-6 months of follow-up. An oral glucose tolerance test performed in one subject revealed that glucose-stimulated insulin release was restored. Mutations in Kir6.2 were the most frequent cause of PND in our cohort. Apparently insulin-dependent patients with mutations in Kir6.2 may be managed on an oral sulfonylurea with sustained metabolic control rather than insulin injections, illustrating the principle of pharmacogenetics applied in diabetes treatment.

Diabetes. 2005 Jun;54(6):1854-62. Related Articles, Links Pharmacogenetic analysis of rosiglitazone-induced hepatosteatosis in new mouse models of type 2 diabetes. Pan HJ, Reifsnyder P, Vance DE, Xiao Q, Leiter EH. The Jackson Laboratory, 600 Main St., Bar Harbor, ME 04609, USA. Although thiazolidinediones suppress hyperglycemia in diabetic (NON x NZO)F1 males, these mice exhibit unusual sensitivity to drug-induced exacerbation of an underlying hepatosteatosis only rarely experienced in human patients. To establish the pharmacogenetic basis for this sensitivity, a panel of recombinant congenic strains (RCSs) with varying degrees of obesity and diabetes was generated by fixing selected NZO HlLt alleles on the diabetes- and hepatosteatosis-resistant NON/Lt background. Four new strains in this panel were exposed to chronic rosiglitazone treatment. Only one, NONcNZO8 (designated RCS8), exhibited an F1-like hepatosteatotic response. In both the F1 and RCS8 males, this adverse effect correlated with rosiglitazone suppression of already impaired hepatic phosphatidylcholine biosynthetic enzymes in both arms of the biosynthetic pathway, the phosphatidylethanolamine methyl-transferase pathway, and the CDP-choline pathway, including choline kinase and CTP-cholinephosphate cytidylyltransferase. This adverse response was not reproduced by CL316,243, a beta3-adrenergic receptor agonist with potent antihyperlipemic effects. Genome comparison showed that RCS8 differed from the other strains in carrying NZO-derived genome on virtually all of chromosome 16 and in smaller segments on chromosomes 6, 14, and 17. Thus, these RCSs present a panel of new mouse models exhibiting differential levels of obesity and diabetes as well as different drug responses. This panel can be used to screen for treatments for type 2 diabetes and its complications.

Diabetes. 2005 Nov;54(11):3319-25. Related Articles, Links Sequence variation in PPARG may underlie differential response to troglitazone. Wolford JK, Yeatts KA, Dhanjal SK, Black MH, Xiang AH, Buchanan TA, Watanabe RM. Genetic Basis of Human Disease Division, Translational Genomics Research Institute, Phoenix, Arizona, USA. Thiazolidinediones (TZDs) are peroxisome proliferator-activated receptor-gamma (PPARG) agonists used to treat type 2 diabetes. TZDs can also be used to reduce rates of type 2 diabetes in at-risk individuals. However, a large fraction of TZD-treated patients (30-40%) do not respond to TZD treatment with an improvement in insulin sensitivity (Si). We hypothesized that variation within the gene encoding PPARG may underlie this differential response to TZD therapy. We screened approximately 40 kb of PPARG in 93 nondiabetic Hispanic women (63 responders and 30 nonresponders) with previous gestational diabetes who had participated in the Troglitazone In the Prevention Of Diabetes study. TZD nonresponse was defined as the lower tertile in change in Si after 3 months of treatment. Baseline demographic and clinical measures were not different between responders and nonresponders. We identified and genotyped 131 variants including 126 single nucleotide polymorphisms and 5 insertion-deletion polymorphisms. Linkage disequilibrium analysis identified five haplotype blocks. Eight variants were associated with TZD response ($P < 0.05$). Three variants were also associated with changes in Si as a continuous variable. Our results suggest that PPARG variation may underlie response to TZD therapy in women at risk for type 2 diabetes. Publication Types: Randomized Controlled Trial

Diabetes. 2005 Sep;54(9):2645-54. Related Articles, Links ATP and sulfonylurea sensitivity of mutant ATP-sensitive K+ channels in neonatal diabetes: implications for pharmacogenomic therapy. Koster JC, Remedi MS, Dao C, Nichols CG. Department of Cell Biology and Physiology, Washington University School of Medicine, St. Louis, MO 63110, USA. cnichols@cellbio.wustl.edu The prediction that overactivity of the pancreatic ATP-sensitive K(+) channel (K(ATP) channel) underlies reduced insulin secretion and causes a diabetic phenotype in humans has recently been borne out by genetic studies implicating "activating" mutations in the Kir6.2 subunit of K(ATP) as causal in both permanent and transient neonatal diabetes. Here we characterize the channel properties of Kir6.2 mutations that underlie transient neonatal diabetes (I182V) or more severe forms of permanent neonatal diabetes (V59M, Q52R, and I296L). In all cases, the mutations result in a significant decrease in sensitivity to inhibitory ATP, which correlates with channel "overactivity" in intact cells. Mutations can be separated into those that directly affect ATP affinity (I182V) and those that stabilize the open conformation of the channel and indirectly reduce ATP sensitivity (V59M, Q52R, and I296L). With respect to the latter group, alterations in channel gating are also reflected in a functional "uncoupling" of sulfonylurea (SU) block: SU sensitivity of I182V is similar to that of wild-type mutants, but the SU sensitivity of all gating mutants is reduced, with the I296L mutant being resistant to block by tolbutamide (</=10 mmol/l). These results have important implications for the use of insulinotropic SU drugs as an alternative therapy to insulin injections.

Diagn Microbiol Infect Dis. 2004 Jun;49(2):89-97. Related Articles, Links Accurate mapping of mutations of pyrazinamide-resistant Mycobacterium tuberculosis strains with a scanning-frame oligonucleotide microarray. Wade MM, Volokhov D, Peredelchuk M, Chizhikov V, Zhang Y. Department of Molecular Microbiology and Immunology, Bloomberg School of Public Health, Johns Hopkins University, Baltimore, MD, USA. The increasing emergence of drug-resistant Mycobacterium tuberculosis poses significant threat to the treatment of tuberculosis. Conventional susceptibility testing for the front-line tuberculosis drug pyrazinamide (PZA) is difficult, because of the requirement for acid pH for the drug to show activity. Resistance to PZA in M. tuberculosis is caused by mutations in the pncA gene, and detection of pncA mutations can be an indicator of PZA resistance. In this study, we examined the feasibility of a microarray-based approach exploiting short overlapping oligonucleotides (sliding-frame array) to rapidly detect pncA mutations (substitutions, deletions, and insertions) in multiple strains of PZA-resistant M. tuberculosis. The genetic mapping of these mutations is necessary to link the gene sequence to the protein function defined by mutant phenotype. Microarray analysis was performed in a blind manner using 57 isolates of M. tuberculosis for which the sequence of the pncA gene was previously determined. Our results showed that all mutations could be unambiguously detected, suggesting that microarray can be a routine and valuable tool for rapid identification of drug-resistant M. tuberculosis isolates. We expect that mutation mapping with a sliding-frame microarray will accelerate the molecular analysis of drug-resistant M. tuberculosis bacteria and the microorganism populations. Copyright 2004 Elsevier Inc.

Diagn Microbiol Infect Dis. 2004 Sep;50(1):25-32. Related Articles, Links Evaluation of fluconazole resistance mechanisms in candida albicans clinical isolates from HIV-infected patients in Brazil. Goldman GH, da Silva Ferreira ME, dos Reis Marques E, Savoldi M, Perlin D, Park S, Godoy Martinez PC, Goldman MH, Colombo AL. Faculdade de Ciencias Farmaceuticas de Ribeirao Preto, Universidade de Sao Paulo, Sao Paulo, Brazil. ggoldman@usp.br In this study, we describe resistance mechanisms in fluconazole-resistant isolates of C. albicans isolated from AIDS patients from nine Brazilian hospitals. These mechanisms include the presence of point mutations in the ERG11 gene and overexpression of ERG11, and several genes encoding efflux pumps, as measured by quantitative real-time reverse transcriptase polymerase chain reaction. Several fluconazole-resistant strains had multiple mechanisms of resistance. Four mutations previously described, Y132F, K143R, E266D, and V437I, were identified among the strains, whereas some isolates contained more than one mutation. Fourteen novel mutations were identified. Interestingly, all Brazilian fluconazole-resistant isolates showed homozygosity at mating-type loci (MTL) associated with fluconazole resistance. This is the first comprehensive assessment at molecular level of mechanisms of fluconazole resistance in C. albicans isolates from South America.

Dialogues Clin Neurosci. 2005;7(3):223-30. Related Articles, Links Pharmacogenomics in depression and antidepressants. Bondy B. Psychiatric Clinic of University Munich, Department of Neurochemistry, Munich, Germany. Genetic factors are believed to play a major role in the variation of treatment response and the incidence of adverse effects to medication. The aim of pharmacogenetics is to elucidate this variability according to hereditary differences. Considering current hypotheses for the mechanisms of action of antidepressants, most investigations to date have concentrated on mutations in genes coding either for the pathways in the serotonergic and noradrenergic systems or for drug-metabolizing enzymes. Recent studies shifted the emphasis on the main mechanism of drug action from changes in neurotransmitter concentration or receptor function toward long-lasting adaptive processes within the neurons. Although the results are controversial, many studies support the hypothesis that psychopharmacogenetics will help predict an individual's drug response, while minimizing the side effects. The inclusion of functional genomics, which investigates the complex gene and/or protein expression in response to a given drug, may lead to the development of novel and safer drugs. Publication Types: Review

Dig Liver Dis. 2005 Apr;37(4):282-97. Related Articles, Links Thiopurines in inflammatory bowel disease: pharmacogenetics, therapeutic drug monitoring and clinical recommendations. Al Hadithy AF, de Boer NK, Derijks LJ, Escher JC, Mulder CJ, Brouwers JR. Department of Pharmacotherapy and Pharmaceutical Care, Groningen University Institute of Drug Exploration, University of Groningen, Bloemsingel 1, 9713 BZ Groningen, The Netherlands. There is a growing interest in the use of thiopurines (azathioprine, 6-mercaptopurine and 6-thioguanine) for the management of inflammatory bowel disease. The genetically controlled thiopurine (S)-methyltransferase enzyme is involved in the metabolism of these agents and is hypothesised to determine the clinical response to thiopurines. Diminished activity of this enzyme decreases the methylation of thiopurines, theoretically resulting in potential overdosing, while high thiopurine (S)-methyltransferase status leads to overproduction of toxic metabolites and ineffectiveness of azathioprine and 6-mercaptopurine. In practice, controversies exist regarding the utility of standard thiopurine (S)-methyltransferase pheno- and genotyping. Current pharmacogenetic insights suggest that another enzyme system may participate in the efficacy and toxicity of thiopurines; inosine triphosphate pyrophosphatase. Other topics discussed in this review are the utilisation of therapeutic drug monitoring and the experimental use of 6-thioguanine in the treatment of inflammatory bowel disease. 6-Thioguanine has a less genetically controlled metabolism and skips genetically determined metabolic steps. On theoretical basis, 6-thioguanine might therefore have a more predictable profile than azathioprine and 6-mercaptopurine. However, the use of 6-thioguanine has been associated with an increased risk of nodular regenerative hyperplasia of the liver and veno-occlusive disease. Further research is warranted before 6-thioguanine can be considered as a treatment option for inflammatory bowel disease. Publication Types: Review

Dis Manag. 2004;7 Suppl 2:S17-9. Related Articles, Links "Personalized" medicine: changing the practice and economics of healthcare. Wallner C. Synvisc, USA.

Drug Discov Today. 2004 Jul 1;9(13):567-73. Related Articles, Links Translating pharmacogenetics and pharmacogenomics into drug development for clinical pediatrics and beyond. Leeder JS. Section of Developmental Pharmacology and Experimental Therapeutics, Children's Mercy Hospital, 2401 Gillham Road, Kansas City, MO 64108, USA. sleeder@cmh.edu Pharmacogenetic and pharmacogenomic investigations conducted in children must consider that human development from conception through to adolescence is a rapidly changing, dynamic process. An improved understanding of the gene networks that are involved in growth and development and of the unintended consequences of modulating those systems could provide insights into the susceptibility of an individual to drug-induced birth defects and to pediatric adverse drug reactions. Furthermore, these technologies potentially present the opportunity to develop novel, effective treatments for childhood diseases and for adult diseases that manifest primarily during childhood. The lack of pharmacogenetic and pharmacogenomic investigations in children and the potential to impact on all age groups provides a considerable incentive to invest in this area of research. Publication Types: Review

Drug Discov Today. 2004 Oct 1;9(19):838-45. Related Articles, Links Combining genome-wide and targeted gene expression profiling in drug discovery: microarrays and real-time PCR. Brazeau DA. Pharmaceutical Genetics Laboratory, Department of Pharmaceutical Sciences, University at Buffalo State, University of New York, Buffalo, NY, USA. dbrazeau@acsu.buffalo.edu Publication Types: Review

Drug Discov Today. 2005 Aug 15;10(16):1076-7. Related Articles, Links

Drugs tailored to race move a step closer to reality. Senior K. Publication Types: News

Drug Discov Today. 2005 Nov 15;10(22):1485-7. Related Articles, Links Overcoming challenges of using blood samples with gene expression microarrays to advance patient stratification in clinical trials. McPhail S, Goralski TJ. The advances in blood protocols enable improved identification of biomarkers based on RNA expression profiles and might assist us in realizing the promise of pharmacogenomics. Publication Types: Editorial

Drug Discov Today. 2005 Oct 15;10(20):1369-75. Related Articles, Links Automation and validation of DNA-banking systems. Thornton M, Gladwin A, Payne R, Moore R, Cresswell C, McKechnie D, Kelly S, March R. RandD Genetics, AstraZeneca Pharmaceuticals, Mereside, Alderley Park, Macclesfield, Cheshire SK10 4TG, UK. melissa.thornton@astrazeneca.com DNA banking is one of the central capabilities on which modern genetic research rests. The DNA-banking system plays an essential role in the flow of genetic data from patients and genetics researchers to the application of genetic research in the clinic. Until relatively recently, large collections of DNA samples were not common in human genetics. Now, collections of hundreds of thousands of samples are common in academic institutions and private companies. Automation of DNA banking can dramatically increase throughput, eliminate manual errors and improve the productivity of genetics research. An increased emphasis on pharmacogenetics and personalized medicine has highlighted the need for genetics laboratories to operate within the principles of a recognized quality system such as good laboratory practice (GLP). Automated systems are suitable for such laboratories but require a level of validation that might be unfamiliar to many genetics researchers. In this article, we use the AstraZeneca automated DNA archive and reformatting system (DART) as a case study of how such a system can be successfully developed and validated within the principles of GLP. Publication Types: Review

Drug Discov Today. 2005 Sep 15;10(18):1216-8. Related Articles, Links Evolution of biomarkers: drug discovery to personalized medicine. Mukhtar M. Neurovirology Section, Thomas Jefferson University, 1020 Locust Street, Philadelphia, PA 19107, USA. mukhtar.muhammad@gmail.com

Drug Discov Today. 2006 Jan;11(1-2):1-3. Related Articles, Links Pharmacogenomics: an in-house advantage? Borchardt PE. Publication Types: Editorial

Drug Metab Dispos. 2005 Jun;33(6):749-53. Epub 2005 Mar 11. Related Articles, Links Role of CYP2C9 and its variants (CYP2C9*3 and CYP2C9*13) in the metabolism of lornoxicam in humans. Guo Y, Zhang Y, Wang Y, Chen X, Si D, Zhong D, Fawcett JP, Zhou H. College of Life Science, Jilin University, No.115 Jiefang Road, Changchun, 130023, China. CYP2C9 is an important member of the cytochrome P450 enzyme superfamily with some 12 CYP2C9 alleles (*1-*12) being previously reported. Recently, we identified a new CYP2C9 allele with a Leu90Pro mutation in a Chinese poor metabolizer of lornoxicam [Si D, Guo Y, Zhang Y, Yang L, Zhou H, and Zhong D (2004) Pharmacogenetics 14:465-469]. The new allele, designated CYP2C9*13, was found to occur in approximately 2% of the Chinese population. To examine enzymatic activity of the CYP2C9*13 allele, kinetic parameters for lornoxicam 5'-hydroxylation were determined in COS-7 cells transiently transfected with pcDNA3.1 plasmids carrying wild-type CYP2C9*1, variant CYP2C9*3, and CYP2C9*13 cDNA. The protein levels of cDNA-expressed CYP2C9*3 and *13 in postmitochondrial supernatant (S9) from transfected cells were lower than those from wild-type CYP2C9*1. Mean values of Km and Vmax for CYP2C9*1, *3, and *13 were 1.24, 1.61, and 2.79 microM and 0.83, 0.28, and 0.22 pmol/min/pmol, respectively. Intrinsic clearance values (Vmax/Km) for variant CYP2C9*3 and CYP2C9*13 on the basis of CYP2C9 protein levels were separately decreased to 28% and 12% compared with wild type. In a subsequent clinical study, the AUC of lornoxicam was increased by 1.9-fold and its oral clearance (CL/F) decreased by 44% in three CYP2C9*1/*13 subjects, compared with CYP2C9*1/*1 individuals. This suggests that the CYP2C9*13 allele is associated with decreased enzymatic activity both in vitro and in vivo.

Drug Metab Rev. 2004 May;36(2):159-97. Related Articles, Links Cytochrome P450: what have we learned and what are the future issues? Guengerich FP. Department of Biochemistry, Center in Molecular Toxicology, Vanderbilt University School of Medicine, Nashville, Tennessee 37232-0146, USA. f.guengerich@vanderbilt.edu The cytochrome P450 (P450) field came out of interest in the metabolism of drugs, carcinogens, and steroids, which remain major focal points. Over the years we have come to understand the P450 system components, the multiplicity of P450s, and many aspects of the regulation of the genes and also the catalytic mechanism. Many crystal structures are now becoming available. The significance of P450 in in vivo metabolism is appreciated, particularly in the context of pharmacogenetics. Current scientific issues involve posttranslational modification, gene regulation, component interactions, structures of P450 complexed with ligands, details of high-valent oxygen chemistry, the nature and influence of rate-limiting steps, greater details about some reaction steps, cooperativity, and the relevance of P450 variations to cancer risk. Some emerging research areas involve new methods of analysis of ligand interactions, roles of conformational changes linked to individual reaction steps, functions of orphan P450s, "molecular breeding" of new P450 functions and enhanced activity, and the utilization of P450s in chemical synthesis. Publication Types: Review

Drug Metab Rev. 2004 Oct;36(3-4):475-86. Related Articles, Links Where is toxicology headed in the future? Guengerich FP. Department of Biochemistry and Center in Molecular Toxicology, Vanderbilt University School of Medicine, Nashville, Tennessee 37232-0146, USA. f.guengerich@vanderbilt.edu Herbert Remmer was a pioneer in the study of the phenomenon of enzyme induction. He was also a leading figure, if not the foremost, in the development of the discipline of toxicology in Germany during his tenure as Professor of Toxicology at the University of Tubingen. Included here are some brief thoughts about where toxicology came from, where it is today, and what the future is. Toxicology is at a crossroads today, at an interface between basic science and applied projects. From its past as a descriptive discipline, it has incorporated a medley of concepts and technology from basic science. The usefulness of many approaches is now being evaluated. The hope is that toxicology will be able to be much more predictive in the future; a great need exists in the pharmaceutical industry. The shape of academic toxicology is also changing. Publication Types: Biography Historical Article Personal Name as Subject: Remmer H

Drug Metab Rev. 2004 Oct;36(3-4):617-38. Related Articles, Links Pharmacogenetics-based new therapeutic concepts. Roots I, Gerloff T, Meisel C, Kirchheiner J, Goldammer M, Kaiser R, Laschinski G, Brockmoller J, Cascorbi I, Kleeberg U, Hildebrandt AG. Institut fur Klinische Pharmakologie, Charite-Universitatsmedizin Berlin, Campus Charite Mitte, Humboldt-Universitat zu Berlin, Berlin, Germany. ivar.roots@charite.de Pharmacogenetics, one of the fields of clinical pharmacology, studies how genetic factors influence drug response. If hereditary traits are taken into account appropriately before starting drug treatment, the type of drug and its dosage can be tailored to the individual patient's needs. Pharmacogenetics adds a considerable amount of stringency to the doctor's therapeutic approach. Today, it is the relationship between dosage requirements and genetic variations in drug metabolizing enzymes like cytochrome P450 (CYP) 2D6 and CYP2C19, or in drug transporters like p-glycoprotein, that is substantiated best. A standard dose will bring about more adverse effects than usual if enzymatic activity is lacking or feeble. Sometimes, however, therapeutic response might be better due to higher concentrations: proton pump inhibitors for eradication of Helicobacter pylori are more efficacious in carriers of a deficient CYP2C19 variant. The drug's interaction with its target (e.g. receptor) also depends on genetic factors. In some cases genetic tests can help distinguish between responders and non-responders of a specific drug treatment. The first pharmacogenetic tests are already on the market. Publication Types: Review

Drug Metab Rev. 2004 Oct;36(3-4):845-52. Related Articles, Links Pharmacology, drug efficacy, and the individual. Hildebrandt AG. alfred.hildebrandt@charite.de The efficacy of drugs has to be demonstrated following the principal approach of statistical evaluation in controlled clinical trials. This scientifically and internationally accepted numerical approach has developed over the years to its importance, in contrast to the more pharmacologically attempt to extrapolate human efficacy of drugs from data obtained in animal experiments or, to the so-called physiological medicine, which did not allow to delineate the suitability of drugs from a given collective to the individual patient. The requirements for the clinical trial are not always met, especially not with so-called surrogate markers. In addition, concerns exist now as ever that the numerically based approach leads to average drugs and information for the "responsible adult" only, to the debit of the individual patient. The concern does not mind the clinical trial as such, which principally can be tailored to the individual as applied with pharmacogenetics. On the other hand, an unbearable situation of increased efforts towards individualization, drug tailoring, and neglect of treatment for patients with neglected diseases, respectively, is immense. The contribution of the pharmacologists is, to present those detailed information which allow proper judgement for the clinical application of drugs for all patients. Publication Types: Review

Drug Metab Rev. 2005;37(2):327-78. Related Articles, Links An interethnic comparison of polymorphisms of the genes encoding drug-metabolizing enzymes and drug transporters: experience in Singapore. Chowbay B, Zhou S, Lee EJ. Laboratory of Clinical Pharmacology, Division of Clinical Trials and Epidemiological Sciences, National Cancer Centre, Singapore. Much of the interindividual variability in drug response is attributable to the presence of single nucleotide polymorphisms (SNPs) in genes encoding drug-metabolizing enzymes and drug transporters. In recent years, we have investigated the polymorphisms in a number of genes encoding phase I and II drug-metabolizing enzymes including CYPIA1, CYP3A4, CYP3A5, GSTM1, NAT2, UGT1A1, and TPMT and drug transporter (MDR1) in three distinct Asian populations in Singapore, namely the Chinese, Malays, and Indians. Significant differences in the frequencies of common alleles encoding these proteins have been observed among these three ethnic groups. For example, the frequency of the variant A2455G polymorphism of CYP1A1 was 28% in Chinese and 31% in Malays, but only 18% in Indians. CYP3A4*4 was detected in two of 110 Chinese subjects, but absent in Indians and Malays. Many Chinese and Malays (61-63%) were homozygous for the GSTM1*0 null genotype compared with 33% of Indians. The frequency of the UGTIA1*28 allele was highest in the Indian population (35%) compared to similar frequencies that were found in the Chinese (16%) and Malay (19%) populations. More importantly, our experience over the years has shown that the pharmacogenetics of these drug-metabolizing enzymes and MDR1 in the Asian populations are different from these in the Caucasian and African populations. For example, the CYP3A4*1B allele, which contains an A-290G substitution in the promoter region of CYP3A4, is absent in all three Asian populations of Singapore studied, but occurs in more than 54% of Africans and 5% of Caucasians. There were no difference in genotype and allelic variant frequencies in exon 12 of MDR1 between the Chinese, Malay, and Indian populations. When compared with other ethnic groups, the distribution of the wild-type C allele in exon 12 in the Malays (34.2%) and Indians (32.8%) was relatively high and similar to the Japanese (38.55%) and Caucasians (41%) but different from African-Americans (15%). The frequency of wild-type TT genotype in Asians (43.5% to 52.1%) and Japanese (61.5%) was much higher than those found in Caucasians (13.3%). All the proteins we studied represent the primary hepatic or extrahepatic enzymes, and their polymorphic expression may be implicated in disease risk and the disposition of drugs or endogenous substances. As such, dose requirements of certain drugs may not be optimal for Asian populations, and a second look at the factors responsible for this difference is necessary. Publication Types: Review

Drug Metab Rev. 2005;37(3):565-74. Related Articles, Links Clinical pharmacogenetics of irinotecan (CPT-11). Ando Y, Hasegawa Y. Department of Clinical Oncology, Saitama Medical School, Saitama, Japan. yando@saitama-med.ac.jp Irinotecan (CPT-11) is now widely used, especially for colorectal and lung cancers, whereas the drug causes severe adverse drug reactions (ADR), such as leukopenia/neutropenia or diarrhea. Irinotecan undergoes drug metabolism to form an active SN-38, which is further converted to its beta-glucuronide by UDP-glucuronosyltransferase (UGT) 1A1. A variant in the promoter of UGT1A1 gene, UGT1A1*28 allele, has been extensively studied, and pharmacogenetic relationships between the variant and ADR to irinotecan have been reported. A case-control study of Japanese cancer patients demonstrated that the patients having UGT1A1*28 were at significantly increased risk of severe ADR to irinotecan. To date, genetic variations of the UGT1A1 gene is the most important hereditary factor to predict severe ADR to irinotecan. The UGT1A1*28 is the only one variant that has multiple lines of clinical evidence in multiple races, whereas genetic variations of other UGT isoforms, drug-metabolizing enzymes and drug transporters need more confirmations of its clinical significance in multiple patient groups. At present, irinotecan chemotherapy based on a patient's UGT1A1 genetic status is scientifically reasonable. Publication Types: Review

Drug News Perspect. 2004 Mar;17(2):143-8. Related Articles, Links Trends in early drug safety. Armer RE, Morris ID. Oxagen Ltd, Oxon, UK. Successful introduction of a new drug to the market is not only an extremely costly and complicated process, but also fraught with a substantial risk of failure. The number of new drugs launched each year from 1990 to 2000 has stayed relatively constant, while the cost of pharmaceutical research and development has risen by almost 2.5-fold over the same period. What is not revealed by these figures is that the chance of success for a drug candidate passing through the various hurdles in pharmaceutical development is at best 1 in 10 and has barely changed despite advancing technology in other areas of research and development. While we expect high failure rates in drug discovery, it is of substantial concern that most candidates in development on which large investments have already been made are probably not going to make any return. A major stumbling block is the absorption, distribution, metabolism, excretion and toxicology profile of drug candidates. These issues were discussed at the Society for Medicines Research symposium held September 18, 2003, in London, United Kingdom. Recent SMR symposia have focused on the ADME and pharmacokinetic aspects of drug discovery and development. Indeed, it is now uncommon for drug discovery projects not to address these issues early in their lifetimes. Although it is less common to address drug safety early in a project, it is being utilized more frequently to help select the best clinical candidates for further development. This meeting report summarizes some of the key aspects of early drug safety issues facing the drug discoverer today. Classical approaches to toxicology, p450-mediated safety, cardiovascular safety, "omics" approaches and their impact upon clinical safety will be discussed. Publication Types: Congresses

Drug News Perspect. 2004 Nov;17(9):594-605. Related Articles, Links New approaches and applications in chemical biology. Gomez A, Ingelman-Sundberg M, Johansson I, Karlgren M, Rodriguez-Antona C, Sim SC. Division of Molecular Toxicology, IMM, Karolinska Institutet, SE-171 77 Stockholm, Sweden. The 15th International Symposium on Microsomes and Drug Oxidations: Chemical Biology in the Postgenomic Era--New Approaches and Applications in Mainz, Germany, July 4-9, 2004, had 570 attendees and was nicely organized by Franz and Barbara Oesch and colleagues. At the meeting, 73 different lectures were presented and about 240 posters were shown. This review discusses most of the lectures presented at the Symposium. Copyright 2004 Prous Science. All rights reserved. Publication Types: Congresses

Drug News Perspect. 2004 Nov;17(9):615-32. Related Articles, Links New drugs and new targets. Doggrell SA. University of Queensland, School of Biomedical Sciences, QLD 4072, Australia. s_doggrell@yahoo.com At the 8th World Congress on Clinical Pharmacology and Therapeutics, held August 1-6, 2004, in Queensland, Australia, there were late-breaking news symposia on presynaptic receptors as targets in the treatment of schizophrenia; cyclooxygenase inhibition, present and future; adiposity, drug treatment and causes; G-protein-coupled receptors, important new targets; osteoporosis, causes, prevention and cures; ischemic stroke; drugs and arrhythmias, causes and cures; and the pharmacology of cardiac protection. One of the plenary lectures was of targeted cancer therapies. The new drugs and new targets for therapeutic intervention from these presentations are discussed in this report. Copyright 2004 Prous Science. All rights reserved. Publication Types: Congresses

Drug Resist Updat. 2004 Dec;7(6):325-31. Epub 2004 Dec 21. Related Articles, Links Individualized chemotherapy treatment for breast cancer: is it necessary? Is it feasible? Pusztai L, Rouzier R, Wagner P, Symmans WF. Department of Breast Medical Oncology, The University of Texas M.D. Anderson Cancer Center, Unit 424, 1515 Holcombe Boulevard, Houston, TX 77030-4009, USA. lpusztai@mdanderson.org Individualized selection of chemotherapy regimens based on the molecular characteristics of the cancer would be desirable. However, it is not currently feasible. The development of clinically useful predictors of response to chemotherapy has proven to be difficult. Recently, novel analytical tools particularly transcriptional profiling, have shown promise as potential predictive tests in several small exploratory studies. However, many of the practical challenges of clinical pharmacogenomics are the same that have plagued prognostic and predictive marker research for decades. Perhaps, the most important challenge is to prospectively design and conduct validation trials that demonstrate clinical utility by showing improved patient outcomes with the use of a proposed new test. Publication Types: Review

Drug Resist Updat. 2005 Feb-Apr;8(1-2):85-97. Related Articles, Links Mechanistic perspectives for 1,2,4-trioxanes in anti-cancer therapy. Efferth T. German Cancer Research Center, M070, Im Neuenheimer Feld 280, 69120 Heidelberg, Germany. thomas.efferth@web.de In addition to their well-known anti-malarial activity, artemisinin and its derivatives (1,2,4-trioxanes) possess potent activity against tumor cells in the nano- to micromolar range. Candidate genes that may contribute to the sensitivity and resistance of tumor cells to artemisinins were identified by pharmacogenomic and molecular pharmacological approaches. Target validation was performed using cell lines transfected with candidate genes or corresponding knockout cells. These genes are from classes with different biological function; for example, regulation of proliferation (BUB3, cyclins, CDC25A), angiogenesis (vascular endothelial growth factor and its receptor, matrix metalloproteinase-9, angiostatin, thrombospondin-1) or apoptosis (BCL-2, BAX). Artesunate triggers apoptosis both by p53-dependent and -independent pathways. Anti-oxidant stress genes (thioredoxin, catalase, gamma-glutamyl-cysteine synthetase, glutathione S-transferases) as well as the epidermal growth factor receptor confer resistance to artesunate. Cell lines over-expressing genes that confer resistance to established anti-tumor drugs (MDR1, MRP1, BCRP, dihydrofolate reductase, ribonucleotide reductase) were not cross-resistant to artesunate, indicating that this drug has a different target and is not subject to multidrug resistance. The Plasmodium translationally controlled tumor protein (TCTP) represents a known target protein of artemisinin and its derivatives in the malaria parasite. The microarray-based mRNA expression of human TCTP correlated with sensitivity to artesunate in tumor cells, suggesting that human TCTP contributes to response of tumor cells to the drug. The multi-factorial nature of cellular response to artemisinin and its derivatives may be beneficial to treat otherwise drug-resistant tumors and may explain why resistance development has not been observed in either cancer or malaria. Publication Types: Review

Drug Saf. 2004;27(15):1171-84. Related Articles, Links Linking pharmacovigilance with pharmacogenetics. Clark DW, Donnelly E, Coulter DM, Roberts RL, Kennedy MA. The New Zealand Intensive Medicines Monitoring Programme (IMMP), New Zealand Pharmacovigilance Centre, Department of Preventive and Social Medicine, Dunedin School of Medicine, Dunedin, New Zealand. david.clark@stonebow.otago.ac.nz The ability to identify individuals who are susceptible to adverse drug reactions (ADRs) has the potential to reduce the personal and population costs of drug-related morbidity. Some individuals may show an increased susceptibility to certain ADRs through genetic polymorphisms that alter their responses to various drugs. We wished to establish a methodology that would be acceptable to members of the general population and that would enable estimation of the risks that specific genetic factors confer on susceptibility to specific ADRs. Buccal swabs were selected as a minimally invasive method to obtain cells for DNA extraction. We wished to determine whether DNA of sufficient quantity and quality could be obtained to enable genotyping for two different polymorphic genes that code for enzymes that are widely involved in drug disposition. This article describes a small pilot study of methodology developed in the New Zealand Intensive Medicines Monitoring Programme (IMMP) to link prescription event monitoring (PEM) studies with pharmacogenetics. The methodology involves a nested case-control study design to investigate whether patients with genetic variants in P-glycoprotein (P-gp) and cytochrome P450 (CYP) 2C9 are more susceptible to psychiatric or visual disturbances following cyclo- oxygenase-2 inhibitor use (ADR signals identified in the IMMP database) than matched control patients taking the medication without experiencing any ADRs. It was concluded that the use of buccal swabs is acceptable to patients and provides DNA of sufficient quantity and quality for genotyping. Although no differences in the distribution of genotypes in the case and control populations were found in this small study, case-control studies investigating genetic risks for ADRs using drug cohorts from PEM studies are possible, and there are several areas where population-based studies of genetic risk factors for ADRs are needed. Examples are discussed where research in large populations is required urgently. These are: (i) genetic variations affecting P-gp function; (ii) variations affecting drugs metabolised by CYP2C9 and other polymorphic CYP enzymes; (iii) genetic variation in beta-adrenergic receptors and adverse outcomes from beta-adrenoceptor agonist therapy; and (iv) genetic variation in cardiac cell membrane potassium channels and their association with long QT syndromes and serious cardiac dysrhythmias. Such studies will help to identify factors that increase the risk of unwanted outcomes from drug therapy. They will also help to establish in what circumstances genotyping should be performed prior to commencing drug treatment and in tailoring drug treatment for individual patients.

Drug Saf. 2004;27(8):535-54. Related Articles, Links Clinical pharmacology: special safety considerations in drug development and pharmacovigilance. Atuah KN, Hughes D, Pirmohamed M. Department of Pharmacology and Therapeutics, The University of Liverpool, Liverpool, United Kingdom. The dose of a drug is a major determinant of its safety, and establishing a safe dose of a novel drug is a prime objective during clinical development. The design of pre-marketing clinical trials precludes the representation of important subpopulations such as children, the elderly and people with co-morbidities. Therefore, postmarketing surveillance (PMS) activities are required to monitor the safety profile of drugs in real clinical practice. Furthermore, individual variations in pharmacogenetic profiles, the immune system, drug metabolic pathways and drug-drug interactions are also important factors in the occurrence of adverse drug reactions. Thus, the safety of a drug is a major clinical consideration before and after it is marketed. A multidisciplinary approach is required to enhance the safety profile of drugs at all stages of development, including PMS activities. Clinical pharmacology encompasses a range of disciplines and forms the backbone of drug safety consideration during clinical drug development. In this review we give an overview of the clinical drug development process and consider its limitations. We present a discussion of several aspects of clinical pharmacology and their application to enhancing drug safety. Pharmacokinetic-pharmacodynamic modelling provides a method of predicting a clinically safe dose; consideration of drug pharmacokinetics in special populations may enhance safe therapeutics in a wider spectrum of patients, while pharmacogenetics provides the possibility of genotype-specific therapeutics. Pharmacovigilance activities are also discussed. Given the complex nature and unpredictability of type B reactions, PMS activities are crucial in managing the risks drugs pose to the general population. The various aspects of clinical pharmacology discussed make a strong case for this field as the backbone of optimising and promoting safe development and use of drugs. Publication Types: Review

Drug Ther Bull. 2004 Aug;42(8):63-4. Related Articles, Links Deciding the dose to prescribe. [No authors listed] The dose of a medicine prescribed is so much a part of everyday practice and prescribing guidance that it might appear a surprising subject for a symposium. In reality, however, many questions about choosing doses are unresolved. Here we summarise the talks given at our March 2004 symposium--Deciding the dose to prescribe--incorporating views raised in discussion.

Drugs Today (Barc). 2004 Mar;40(3):247-57. Related Articles, Links Use of pharmacogenctics to guide warfarin therapy. Voora D, McLeod HL, Eby C, Gage BF. Departments of Medicine and Pathology, Washington University School of Medicine, St Louis, Missouri 63110, USA. The Human Genome Project heralds new opportunities for pharmacogenetics, the use of genetics to individualize the application of pharmaceuticals in the practice of medicine (1-3). Single nucleotide polymorphisms (SNPs) and other genetic variants in genes responsible for absorption, metabolism and excretion have been associated with alterations in drug disposition or effect. Warfarin is a potential target for pharmacogenetics-based dosing because of its wide use, variability in individual response, high prevalence of genetic variants and severity of adverse drug reactions (4). The genotype assays for genetic variants relevant to warfarin are widely used and are being developed for commercial use (5), making the promise of a pharmacogenetics-based approach a near reality. c) 2004 Prous Science. All rights reserved

Drugs Today (Barc). 2005 Dec;41(12):799-814. Related Articles, Links Pharmacogenetics of therapies in rheumatoid arthritis. Ranganathan P. Department of Medicine, Division of Rheumatology, Washington University School of Medicine, St. Louis, Missouri 63110, USA. prangana@im.wustl.edu Rheumatoid arthritis (RA) is an inflammatory, aggressive arthritis causing irreversible joint destruction and damage when left untreated. Disease-modifying antirheumatic drugs (DMARDs) are the mainstay of treatment for RA and ameliorate not only the clinical signs and symptoms but also joint damage associated with the disease. In recent years, biological therapies have been introduced for the treatment of RA, and the effectiveness of these agents in slowing the clinical and radiographic progression in RA has been established beyond question. However, there is significant variability in the response of patients with RA to these therapies. Moreover, the biological therapies are expensive, totaling several thousand dollars in yearly patient costs. Pharmacogenomics, the study of genetic variations in drug-metabolizing enzymes and their translation to differential responses to drugs, is a nascent but rapidly evolving field. The application of pharmacogenomics to therapies used in RA, particularly the new expensive biological agents, holds great promise for tailoring therapy with these agents based on a patient's genetics. Published literature on the pharmacogenetics of commonly used DMARDs and the emerging body of literature on the pharmacogenetics of the new biological therapies in RA are the focus of this review. As evident from the contents of this review, pharmacogenomics is an exciting field which is progressing productively and rapidly. Pharmacogenomic approaches offer powerful tools to optimize drug therapy in individual patients. Copyright 2005 Prous Science

Drugs. 2004;64(16):1801-16. Related Articles, Links Drug-gene interactions between genetic polymorphisms and antihypertensive therapy. Schelleman H, Stricker BH, De Boer A, Kroon AA, Verschuren MW, Van Duijn CM, Psaty BM, Klungel OH. Department of Epidemiology and Biostatistics, Erasmus MC, Rotterdam, The Netherlands. Genetic factors may influence the response to antihypertensive medication. A number of studies have investigated genetic polymorphisms as determinants of cardiovascular response to antihypertensive drug therapy. In most candidate gene studies, no such drug-gene interactions were found. However, there is observational evidence that hypertensive patients with the 460 W allele of the alpha-adducin gene have a lower risk of myocardial infarction and stroke when treated with diuretics compared with other antihypertensive therapies. With regard to blood pressure response, interactions were found between genetic polymorphisms for endothelial nitric oxide synthase and diuretics, the alpha-adducin gene and diuretics, the alpha-subunit of G protein and beta-adrenoceptor antagonists, and the ACE gene and angiotensin II type 1 (AT(1)) receptor antagonists. Other studies found an interaction between ACE inhibitors and the ACE insertion/deletion (I/D) polymorphism, which resulted in differences in AT(1) receptor mRNA expression, left ventricular hypertrophy and arterial stiffness between different genetic variants. Also, drug-gene interactions between calcium channel antagonists and ACE I/D polymorphism regarding arterial stiffness have been reported. Unfortunately, the quality of these studies is quite variable. Given the methodological problems, the results from the candidate gene studies are still inconclusive and further research is necessary. Publication Types: Review

Dtsch Med Wochenschr. 2004 Apr 8;129(15):799. Related Articles, Links [Cardiovascular pharmacology] [Article in German] Ravens U, Erdmann E. Publication Types: Editorial

Dtsch Med Wochenschr. 2004 Apr 8;129(15):831-5. Related Articles, Links [Genetic polymorphisms in drug metabolizing enzymes--impact on treatment with beta-blockers] [Article in German] Wuttke H, Rau T, Eschenhagen T. Institut fur Experimentelle und Klinische Pharmakologie, Universitatsklinikum Hamburg-Eppendorf, Hamburg. t.eschenhagen@uke.uni-hamburg.de Publication Types: Review

Dtsch Med Wochenschr. 2004 Dec 3;129(49):2672-5. Related Articles, Links [Individualization of diagnosis and therapy] [Article in German] Ach JS, Bayertz K, Wiesing U. Forschungsstelle Bioethik, Munster. Publication Types: Review

Dtsch Med Wochenschr. 2004 Oct 29;129(44):2366-71. Related Articles, Links [Adjuvant therapy for colon cancer] [Article in German] Lordick F, Rosenberg R, Stein HJ, Peschel C, Siewert JR. III. Medizinische Klinik und Poliklinik, Technische Universitat Munchen, Munchen. f.lordick@lrz.tum.de Publication Types: Review

Dtsch Med Wochenschr. 2005 Jun 24;130(25-26):1568-72. Related Articles, Links Comment in: Dtsch Med Wochenschr. 2005 Jun 24;130(25-26):1535. [Molecular medicine--personalized medicine. Principles and state-of-the-art] [Article in German] Blum HE. Medizinische Universitatsklinik Freiburg. hubert.blum@uniklinik-freiburg.de Publication Types: Review

Dtsch Med Wochenschr. 2006 Feb 17;131(7):307-8. Related Articles, Links [Principles and perspectives -- advances and future of medicine] [Article in German] Blum HE. Publication Types: Editorial

Dtsch Med Wochenschr. 2006 Feb 17;131(7):310-3. Related Articles, Links [Pharmacogenomics: principles and perspectives] [Article in German] Mahlknecht U. Universitatsklinikum Heidelberg, Medizinische Klinik V, Abteilung fur Hamatologie/Onkologie. Ulrich.Mahlknecht@med.uni-heidelberg.de Publication Types: Review

Duodecim. 2004;120(18):2230-1. Related Articles, Links [What does the genome sequence of tuberculosis bacteria reveal to us?] [Article in Finnish] Viljanen MK.

Turun yliopisto, laaketieteellinen mikrobiologia, Turku. matti.viljanen@utu.fi Publication Types: Review

Duodecim. 2004;120(20):2399-404. Related Articles, Links [Preparing for genomic medicine] [Article in Finnish] Makela T. Helsingin biolaaketieteellinen tutkijakoulu, molekyyli- ja syopabiologian tutkimusohjelma, Biomedicum Helsinki, Helsingin yliopisto. tomi.makela@helsinki.fi Publication Types: Lectures

Duodecim. 2005;121(2):177-80. Related Articles, Links [Genetic mutation as a risk factor for a patient treated with warfarin] [Article in Finnish] Laine K, Lundgren S, Ketonen M. Turun yliopiisto ja TYKS, kliininen farmakologia, Pharmacity, Turku. karlai@utu.fi Publication Types: Case Reports

Eksp Klin Farmakol. 2005 Sep-Oct;68(5):59-67. Related Articles, Links [Pharmacogenomics: way to individual therapy] [Article in Russian] Piruzian AL. Problems pertaining to the development of individual therapy based on the achievements of modern pharmacogenetics and pharmacogenomics, as well as the safety of using drugs from various pharmacological groups in patients belonging to different ethnical groups (with the corresponding features of metabolism) are considered. The terms "pharmacogenetics" and "pharmacogenomics" are discussed in connection to the significance of genetic polymorphism (or single nucleotide polymorphism) in determining of the individual sensitivity with respect to certain drugs. Publication Types: Review

Encephale. 2005 Jul-Aug;31(4 Pt 1):437-47. Related Articles, Links [Meta-analysis of candidate genes in attention-deficit hyperactivity disorder] [Article in French] Wohl M, Purper-Ouakil D, Mouren MC, Ades J, Gorwood P. CHU Robert-Debre (AP-HP, Paris VII), 75019 Paris. Attention-deficit hyperactivity disorder (ADHD) is a common behavioral disorder observed during childhood, detected in 3% to 5% of school-age children. The disorder is characterised by marked inattention, hyperactivity, and impulsiveness. In most cases, symptoms can be treated by catecholamine-releasing drugs, such as methylphenidate. Children with ADHD are at higher risk for substance abuse and oppositional, conduct and mood disorders. Familial and adoption studies shed light on the genetic vulnerability of ADHD. Twin studies estimated the broad heritability to range between 40% and 90%. The mode of transmission is yet unknown, but is likely polygenic. Molecular genetic studies in ADHD should contribute to a greater understanding of the pathophysiology of the disorder (genetics of the vulnerability), and could help to select a more rational type of treatment (pharmacogenetic). Family-based association studies already performed are reviewed in this manuscript. Association studies, using haplotype relative risk (HRR) or transmission disequilibrium test (TDT) have focused on candidate genes which code for proteins potentially involved in the etiopathogenesis of the disorder. Genes involved in dopamine, serotonin, and noradrenalin systems have thus been assessed for their role in core features of ADHD, such as motor overactivity, inattention, and impulsiveness. According to a meta-analysis, the DAT1 gene, an obvious candidate gene in ADHD vulnerability, does not appear to be involved (OR = 1.13, p = 0.21). On the other hand, DRD4 (OR = 1.26, p = 0.01) and DRD5 (OR = 1.4, p = 0.01) are significantly associated to ADHD according to the present meta-analysis, confirming previous ones. Recent studies showed a trend for an association between one allele of the 5-HTT (considering case-control studies) and DBH (OR = 1.27, p = 0.06) genes and ADHD, but these positive findings have to be replicated. ADHD is a complex disorder with potentially many different risk factors. Genetic and phenotypic heterogeneity could explain why some association studies are positive, whereas others are negative. For instance, different developmental pathways are likely to lead to similar clinical outcomes. More clear-cut phenotypes, such as ADHD with conduct disorder, or ADHD with bipolar disorder, could be more homogenous, the genes involved being therefore more easy to detect. These phenotypes are beginning to be specifically studied in molecular genetics. In addition, the development of pharmacogenetics could help to identify predictors of clinical response for a specific type of treatment, which would be clearly helpful in clinical practice. Publication Types: Meta-Analysis

Endocrinology. 2006 Mar 23; [Epub ahead of print] Links Mini Review: Pharmacogenetics and beyond: the interaction of therapeutic response, beta-cell physiology and genetics in diabetes. Hattersley AT, Pearson ER. Peninsula Medical School, Exeter, England; Ninewells Hospital and Medical School, Dundee, Scotland. Defining the molecular genetics of diabetes gives new insights into the underlying etiology and so should help improve treatment. The genetic etiology is now known for most patients with beta-cell monogenic diabetes allowing genetic classification. We review how this genetic knowledge alters treatment. Patients with a glucose sensing beta-cell defect due to glucokinase mutations have regulated, mild fasting hyperglycaemia. Oral hypoglycaemic agents or low dose insulin rarely improve glycaemic control. Patients with HNF1alpha mutations have progressive beta-cell deterioration and need treatment. HNF1alpha patients are four times more sensitive to sulfonylureas than matched Type 2 diabetic patients. This is partly due to greater insulin secretion, reflecting that the defect in HNF1alpha deficiency precedes the KATP channel where sulfonylureas act. HNF1beta is expressed in pancreatic stem cells before differentiation into endocrine or exocrine cells so patients with HNF1beta mutations have reduced pancreatic development resulting in early-onset diabetes and exocrine dysfunction. These patients usually rapidly require insulin and are not sensitive to sulfonylureas. 35-50% of patients diagnosed with diabetes before 6 months have a mutation in Kir6.2. The mutated KATP channel in these patients does not close in response to increased ATP concentrations but can be closed when sulfonylureas bind to the SUR1 subunit of the channel by an ATP independent route. These patients are usually insulin dependent but have excellent glycaemic control on high dose sulfonylureas tablets. In conclusion the defining of molecular genetic etiology in monogenic diabetes has defined several specific beta cell defects and these are critical in determining the response to treatment.

Enferm Infecc Microbiol Clin. 2004 Jun-Jul;22(6):337-41. Related Articles, Links The genetic cohorts: facing the new challenges in infectious diseases. The HIV model. Telenti A. Institute of Microbiology, University Hospital, Lausanne, Switzerland. amalio.telenti@hospvd.ch All physicians are confronted with the diversity of susceptibility to infectious diseases or response to medication among patients. Much work has been done to characterize the virulence factors of pathogens, while less is known about the host (human) factor. Two unrelated people share about 99.9% of their DNA sequences, while the remaining 0.1% contains the genetic variants that influence how they differ in their risk of disease or response to drugs. The completion of the Human Genome Project gives a new start to developing the field of host genetic susceptibility. This review highlights ethical and practical issues on developing genetic cohorts by using the model of the Swiss HIV Cohort Study. Publication Types: Review

Environ Health Perspect. 2004 Aug;112(12):1217-24. Related Articles, Links Gene interaction network suggests dioxin induces a significant linkage between aryl hydrocarbon receptor and retinoic acid receptor beta. Toyoshiba H, Yamanaka T, Sone H, Parham FM, Walker NJ, Martinez J, Portier CJ. Laboratory of Computational Biology and Risk Analysis, National Institute of Environmental Health Sciences, Research Triangle Park, North Carolina 27709, USA. Gene expression arrays (gene chips) have enabled researchers to roughly quantify the level of mRNA expression for a large number of genes in a single sample. Several methods have been developed for the analysis of gene array data including clustering, outlier detection, and correlation studies. Most of these analyses are aimed at a qualitative identification of what is different between two samples and/or the relationship between two genes. We propose a quantitative, statistically sound methodology for the analysis of gene regulatory networks using gene expression data sets. The method is based on Bayesian networks for direct quantification of gene expression networks. Using the gene expression changes in HPL1A lung airway epithelial cells after exposure to 2,3,7,8-tetrachlorodibenzo-(Italic)p(/Italic)-dioxin at levels of 0.1, 1.0, and 10.0 nM for 24 hr, a gene expression network was hypothesized and analyzed. The method clearly demonstrates support for the assumed network and the hypothesis linking the usual dioxin expression changes to the retinoic acid receptor system. Simulation studies demonstrated the method works well, even for small samples.

Environ Health Perspect. 2004 Aug;112(12):1225-35. Related Articles, Links Valproic acid teratogenicity: a toxicogenomics approach. Kultima K, Nystrom AM, Scholz B, Gustafson AL, Dencker L, Stigson M. Department of Pharmaceutical Biosciences, Division of Toxicology, The Biomedical Center, Uppsala University, Uppsala, Sweden. Embryonic development is a highly coordinated set of processes that depend on hierarchies of signaling and gene regulatory networks, and the disruption of such networks may underlie many cases of chemically induced birth defects. The antiepileptic drug valproic acid (VPA) is a potent inducer of neural tube defects (NTDs) in human and mouse embryos. As with many other developmental toxicants however, the mechanism of VPA teratogenicity is unknown. Using microarray analysis, we compared the global gene expression responses to VPA in mouse embryos during the critical stages of teratogen action in vivo with those in cultured P19 embryocarcinoma cells in vitro. Among the identified VPA-responsive genes, some have been associated previously with NTDs or VPA effects [vinculin, metallothioneins 1 and 2 (Mt1, Mt2), keratin 1-18 (Krt1-18)], whereas others provide novel putative VPA targets, some of which are associated with processes relevant to neural tube formation and closure [transgelin 2 (Tagln2), thyroid hormone receptor interacting protein 6, galectin-1 (Lgals1), inhibitor of DNA binding 1 (Idb1), fatty acid synthase (Fasn), annexins A5 and A11 (Anxa5, Anxa11)], or with VPA effects or known molecular actions of VPA (Lgals1, Mt1, Mt2, Id1, Fasn, Anxa5, Anxa11, Krt1-18). A subset of genes with a transcriptional response to VPA that is similar in embryos and the cell model can be evaluated as potential biomarkers for VPA-induced teratogenicity that could be exploited directly in P19 cell-based in vitro assays. As several of the identified genes may be activated or repressed through a pathway of histone deacetylase (HDAC) inhibition and specificity protein 1 activation, our data support a role of HDAC as an important molecular target of VPA action in vivo.

Environ Health Perspect. 2004 Aug;112(12):1236-48. Related Articles, Links Discriminating different classes of toxicants by transcript profiling. Steiner G, Suter L, Boess F, Gasser R, de Vera MC, Albertini S, Ruepp S. Non-Clinical Drug Safety, F. Hoffmann-La Roche Ltd., Basel, Switzerland. Male rats were treated with various model compounds or the appropriate vehicle controls. Most substances were either well-known hepatotoxicants or showed hepatotoxicity during preclinical testing. The aim of the present study was to determine if biological samples from rats treated with various compounds can be classified based on gene expression profiles. In addition to gene expression analysis using microarrays, a complete serum chemistry profile and liver and kidney histopathology were performed. We analyzed hepatic gene expression profiles using a supervised learning method (support vector machines; SVMs) to generate classification rules and combined this with recursive feature elimination to improve classification performance and to identify a compact subset of probe sets with potential use as biomarkers. Two different SVM algorithms were tested, and the models obtained were validated with a compound-based external cross-validation approach. Our predictive models were able to discriminate between hepatotoxic and nonhepatotoxic compounds. Furthermore, they predicted the correct class of hepatotoxicant in most cases. We provide an example showing that a predictive model built on transcript profiles from one rat strain can successfully classify profiles from another rat strain. In addition, we demonstrate that the predictive models identify nonresponders and are able to discriminate between gene changes related to pharmacology and toxicity. This work confirms the hypothesis that compound classification based on gene expression data is feasible.

Environ Health Perspect. 2004 Aug;112(12):1249-54. Related Articles, Links Assessment of prediction confidence and domain extrapolation of two structure-activity relationship models for predicting estrogen receptor binding activity. Tong W, Xie Q, Hong H, Shi L, Fang H, Perkins R. Center for Toxicoinformatics, National Center for Toxicological Research, Food and Drug Administration, Jefferson, Arkansas 72079, USA. wtong@nctr.fda.gov Quantitative structure-activity relationship (QSAR) methods have been widely applied in drug discovery, lead optimization, toxicity prediction, and regulatory decisions. Despite major advances in algorithms and software, QSAR models have inherent limitations associated with a size and chemical-structure diversity of the training set, experimental error, and many characteristics of structure representation and correlation algorithms. Whereas excellent fit to the training data may be readily attainable, often models fail to predict accurately chemicals that are outside their domain of applicability. A QSAR's utility and, in the case of regulatory decisions, justification for usage increasingly depend on the ability to quantify a model's potential for predicting unknown chemicals with some known degree of certainty. It is never possible to predict an unknown chemical with absolute certainty. Here we report on two QSAR models based on different data sets for classification of chemicals according to their ability to bind to the estrogen receptor. The models were developed by using a novel QSAR method, Decision Forest, which combines the results of multiple heterogeneous but comparable Decision Tree models to produce a consensus prediction. We used an extensive cross-validation process to define an applicability domain for model predictions based on two quantitative measures: prediction confidence and domain extrapolation. Together, these measures quantify the accuracy of each prediction within and outside of the training domain. Despite being based on large and diverse training sets, both QSAR models had poor accuracy for chemicals within the domain of low confidence, whereas good accuracy was obtained for those within the domain of high confidence. For prediction in the high confidence domain, accuracy was inversely proportional to the degree of domain extrapolation. The model with a larger training set of 1,092, compared with 232 for the other, was more accurate in predicting chemicals at larger domain extrapolation, and could be particularly useful for rapidly prioritizing potential endocrine disruptors from large chemical universe.

Environ Health Perspect. 2004 Aug;112(12):1255-63. Related Articles, Links Biokinetics and subchronic toxic effects of oral arsenite, arsenate, monomethylarsonic acid, and dimethylarsinic acid in v-Ha-ras transgenic (Tg.AC) mice. Xie Y, Trouba KJ, Liu J, Waalkes MP, Germolec DR. Inorganic Carcinogenesis Section, Laboratory of Comparative Carcinogenesis, National Cancer Institute at the National Institute of Environmental Health Sciences Research Triangle Park, North Carolina 27709, USA. Previous research demonstrated that 12-O-tetradecanoylphorbol-13-acetate (TPA) treatment increased the number of skin papillomas in v-Ha-ras transgenic (Tg.AC) mice that had received sodium arsenite [(As(III)] in drinking water, indicating that this model is useful for studying the toxic effects of arsenic in vivo. Because the liver is a known target of arsenic, we examined the pathophysiologic and molecular effects of inorganic and organic arsenical exposure on Tg.AC mouse liver in this study. Tg.AC mice were provided drinking water containing As(III), sodium arsenate [As(V)], monomethylarsonic acid [(MMA(V)], and 1,000 ppm dimethylarsinic acid [DMA(V)] at dosages of 150, 200, 1,500, or 1,000 ppm as arsenic, respectively, for 17 weeks. Control mice received unaltered water. Four weeks after initiation of arsenic treatment, TPA at a dose of 1.25 microg/200 microL acetone was applied twice a week for 2 weeks to the shaved dorsal skin of all mice, including the controls not receiving arsenic. In some cases arsenic exposure reduced body weight gain and caused mortality (including moribundity). Arsenical exposure resulted in a dose-dependent accumulation of arsenic in the liver that was unexpectedly independent of chemical species and produced hepatic global DNA hypomethylation. cDNA microarray and reverse transcriptase-polymerase chain reaction analysis revealed that all arsenicals altered the expression of numerous genes associated with toxicity and cancer. However, organic arsenicals [MMA(V) and DMA(V)] induced a pattern of gene expression dissimilar to that of inorganic arsenicals. In summary, subchronic exposure of Tg.AC mice to inorganic or organic arsenicals resulted in toxic manifestations, hepatic arsenic accumulation, global DNA hypomethylation, and numerous gene expression changes. These effects may play a role in arsenic-induced hepatotoxicity and carcinogenesis and may be of particular toxicologic relevance.

Environ Health Perspect. 2004 Aug;112(12):A662. Related Articles, Links Toxicogenomics in risk assessment: communicating the challenges. Pettit SD. Publication Types: Editorial

Environ Health Perspect. 2004 Aug;112(12):A663-4. Related Articles, Links Regulatory acceptance of toxicogenomics data. Frueh FW, Huang SM, Lesko LJ. Publication Types: Editorial

Environ Health Perspect. 2004 Aug;112(12):A666-7. Related Articles, Links Standards for microarray data: an open letter. Ball C, Brazma A, Causton H, Chervitz S, Edgar R, Hingamp P, Matese JC, Parkinson H, Quackenbush J, Ringwald M, Sansone SA, Sherlock G, Spellman P, Stoeckert C, Tateno Y, Taylor R, White J, Winegarden N; MGED Society. Publication Types: Letter

Environ Health Perspect. 2004 Aug;112(12):A670. Related Articles, Links Encyclopedia of DNA. Dahl R. Publication Types: News

Environ Health Perspect. 2004 Aug;112(12):A671. Related Articles, Links BAC to the future. Potera C. Publication Types: News

Environ Health Perspect. 2004 Aug;112(12):A676-7. Related Articles, Links Cooperation achieves results at UNC-CH. Eubanks M. Publication Types: News

Environ Health Perspect. 2004 Aug;112(12):A678-85. Related Articles, Links Toxicogenomics data: the road to acceptance. Freeman K. Regulatory agencies believe microarray data could be extremely useful in testing prospective chemical products and investigating safety problems after chemicals have been marketed. However, it has not yet been clearly established how this information will be used by agencies in the approval of pharmaceuticals and other chemicals--or even whether companies will be required to submit microarray data. Although some private companies are already voluntarily submitting microarray data along with their drug and pesticide applications, others are hesitant to do so. Most of the stakeholders involved agree that standardization of microarray experiment procedures and of genomic signatures are key to the broad acceptance and use of these data.

Environ Health Perspect. 2004 Mar;112(4):A217. Related Articles, Links FDA eyes pharmacogenomics data. Wakefield J. Publication Types: News

Environ Health Perspect. 2004 Mar;112(4):A231. Related Articles, Links Comment on: Environ Health Perspect.

2004 Mar;112(4):417-9. Taking stock of toxicogenomics: mini-monograph offers overview. Hood E. Publication Types: Comment

Environ Health Perspect. 2004 May;112(6):740-5. Related Articles, Links Human genetics, environment, and communities of color: ethical and social implications. Sze J, Prakash S. Office of the President, University of California at San Diego, La Jolla, California, USA. A conference titled "Human Genetics, Environment, and Communities of Color: Ethical and Social Implications" and a workshop symposium titled "Human Genetics and Environmental Justice" were held by West Harlem Environmental Action, Inc., with cosponsorship by the National Institute of Environmental Health Sciences (NIEHS), the Community Outreach and Education Program of the NIEHS P30 Center for Environmental Health at the Mailman School of Public Health at Columbia University, New York, and the U.S. Environmental Protection Agency. The conference and symposium took place at Columbia University in New York City on 4-5 February 2002. Expert panels composed of public health practitioners, genetic researchers, ethicists, lawyers, social scientists, and community organizations were assembled to explore how genetic research will affect communities of color, specifically in environmental health research. The goal of the conference was to educate participants on the science and ethics of genetic research and to explore the potential benefits and pitfalls of genetic research vis-a-vis new trends in environmental health research, specifically with reference to communities of color. The goal of the symposium was to discuss the major perceptions and concerns for community-based environmental justice advocates and other communities of color regarding environmental health genetic research. The conference and symposium drew more than 300 participants and articulated important perspectives on the opportunities and challenges for environmental justice advocates and other communities of color posed by rapid advances in environmental health genetic research and toxicogenomics. Publication Types: Congresses

Environ Health Perspect. 2004 May;112(7):805-7. Related Articles, Links Toxicogenomics through the eyes of informatics: conference overview and recommendations. Olden K, Call N, Sobral B, Oakes R. National Institute of Environmental Health Sciences, National Institutes of Health, Department of Health and Human Services, Research Triangle Park, North Carolina, USA. Virginia Bioinformatics Institute, in conjunction with National Institutes of Environmental Health Sciences, hosted a conference, "Toxicogenomics through the Eyes of Informatics," in Bethesda, Maryland, USA, on 12-13 May 2003. Researchers around the world met to discuss how the application of bioinformatics tools, methodologies, and technologies will enhance our understanding of how cells and organisms respond to toxins. Conference topics included statistical methods, quantitative molecular data sets, computational algorithms for data analysis, computational modeling and simulation, challenges and opportunities in computational biology, and information technology infrastructure for data and tool management. This meeting report is a summary of conference presentations, survey results, current toxicogenomics concerns, and future directions of the toxicogenomics community. In conclusion this report discusses toxicogenomics as related to environmental agents, cell-chemical reactions, and gene-environment interactions. Publication Types: Congresses

Environ Health Perspect. 2004 May;112(7):A402. Related Articles, Links Harnessing the HGP of public health. Freeman K. Publication Types: News

Environ Health Perspect. 2004 May;112(7):A408-9. Related Articles, Links Drawing comparisons at Duke. Hood E.

Environ Health Perspect. 2004 May;112(7):A416. Related Articles, Links Hexachlorobenzene exposure: widespread toxicant produces pervasive effects. McGovern V. Publication Types: News

Environ Health Perspect. 2005 Apr;113(4):A234-5. Related Articles, Links MIT toxicogenomics research program. Eubanks M. Publication Types: News

Environ Health Perspect. 2005 Jul;113(7):818-22. Related Articles, Links Ushering in the new toxicology: toxicogenomics and the public interest. Balbus JM. Environmental Defense, Washington, DC 20009, USA. jbalbus@environmentaldefense.org New scientific tools spawned by the genomics revolution promise to improve our ability to identify causative factors in human diseases. But as these new tools elucidate the complex interactions between chemical toxins and biologic systems, the strain on traditional ways of understanding toxic effects grows. Despite major advances in the science and technology of these new toxicogenomics tools, scientific and political complexities threaten to delay the use of toxicogenomics to further the public interest or--worse--to advance its use initially to weaken the regulation and safety of widely used chemicals. To gain further insight into the scientific and political landscape of the new toxicology, we interviewed 27 experts from a variety of disciplines and sectors. Interviewees expressed widespread agreement that the new toxicology promises a significant increase in the amount of information available on toxic effects of chemicals. But the interviews show that the promise of the new toxicology will be realized only if technical and political obstacles can be overcome. Although scientific rigor is necessary for the new toxicology to move forward, the scientific and public-interest communities must ensure that inappropriate definitions of rigor, as well as proprietary interests, do not create unnecessary barriers to more effective public health protection. Publication Types: Interview

Environ Health Perspect. 2005 Jul;113(7):840-8. Related Articles, Links Personalized exposure assessment: promising approaches for human environmental health research. Weis BK, Balshaw D, Barr JR, Brown D, Ellisman M, Lioy P, Omenn G, Potter JD, Smith MT, Sohn L, Suk WA, Sumner S, Swenberg J, Walt DR, Watkins S, Thompson C, Wilson SH. Division of Extramural Research and Training, National Institute of Environmental Health Sciences, National Institutes of Health, Department of Health and Human Services, Research Triangle Park, North Carolina 27709, USA. weis@niehs.nih.gov New technologies and methods for assessing human exposure to chemicals, dietary and lifestyle factors, infectious agents, and other stressors provide an opportunity to extend the range of human health investigations and advance our understanding of the relationship between environmental exposure and disease. An ad hoc

Committee on Environmental Exposure Technology Development was convened to identify new technologies and methods for deriving personalized exposure measurements for application to environmental health studies. The committee identified a "toolbox" of methods for measuring external (environmental) and internal (biologic) exposure and assessing human behaviors that influence the likelihood of exposure to environmental agents. The methods use environmental sensors, geographic information systems, biologic sensors, toxicogenomics, and body burden (biologic) measurements. We discuss each of the methods in relation to current use in human health research; specific gaps in the development, validation, and application of the methods are highlighted. We also present a conceptual framework for moving these technologies into use and acceptance by the scientific community. The framework focuses on understanding complex human diseases using an integrated approach to exposure assessment to define particular exposure-disease relationships and the interaction of genetic and environmental factors in disease occurrence. Improved methods for exposure assessment will result in better means of monitoring and targeting intervention and prevention programs. Publication Types: Review

Environ Health Perspect. 2005 Jul;113(7):A440. Related Articles, Links The NIEHS and the National Toxicology Program: an integrated scientific vision. Portier CJ, Schwartz DA. portier@niehs.nih.gov

Environ Health Perspect. 2005 Jun;113(6):775-81. Related Articles, Links Developmentally restricted genetic determinants of human arsenic metabolism: association between urinary methylated arsenic and CYT19 polymorphisms in children. Meza MM, Yu L, Rodriguez YY, Guild M, Thompson D, Gandolfi AJ, Klimecki WT. Department of Natural Resources, Sonora Institute of Technology (ITSON), Ciudad Obregon, Sonora, Mexico. We report the results of a screen for genetic association with urinary arsenic metabolite levels in three arsenic metabolism candidate genes, PNP, GSTO, and CYT19, in 135 arsenic-exposed subjects from the Yaqui Valley in Sonora, Mexico, who were exposed to drinking water concentrations ranging from 5.5 to 43.3 ppb. We chose 23 polymorphic sites to test in the arsenic-exposed population. Initial phenotypes evaluated included the ratio of urinary inorganic arsenic(III) to inorganic arsenic(V) and the ratio of urinary dimethylarsenic(V) to monomethylarsenic(V) (D:M). In the initial association screening, three polymorphic sites in the CYT19 gene were significantly associated with D:M ratios in the total population. Subsequent analysis of this association revealed that the association signal for the entire population was actually caused by an extremely strong association in only the children (7-11 years of age) between CYT19 genotype and D:M levels. With children removed from the analysis, no significant genetic association was observed in adults (18-79 years). The existence of a strong, developmentally regulated genetic association between CYT19 and arsenic metabolism carries import for both arsenic pharmacogenetics and arsenic toxicology, as well as for public health and governmental regulatory officials.

Environ Health Perspect. 2005 Jun;113(6):A388-93. Related Articles, Links From point B to point A: applying toxicogenomics to biological inference. Freeman K.

Environ Health Perspect. 2005 Nov;113(11):1622-6. Related Articles, Links Meeting report: Structural determination of environmentally responsive proteins. Reinlib L. Division of Extramural Research and Training, National Institute of Environmental Health Sciences, National Institutes of Health, U.S. Department of Health and Human Services, Research Triangle Park, North Carolina 27709-2233, USA. reinlib@niehs.nih.gov The three-dimensional structure of gene products continues to be a missing lynchpin between linear genome sequences and our understanding of the normal and abnormal function of proteins and pathways. Enhanced activity in this area is likely to lead to better understanding of how discrete changes in molecular patterns and conformation underlie functional changes in protein complexes and, with it, sensitivity of an individual to an exposure. The National Institute of Environmental Health Sciences convened a workshop of experts in structural determination and environmental health to solicit advice for future research in structural resolution relative to environmentally responsive proteins and pathways. The highest priorities recommended by the workshop were to support studies of structure, analysis, control, and design of conformational and functional states at molecular resolution for environmentally responsive molecules and complexes; promote understanding of dynamics, kinetics, and ligand responses; investigate the mechanisms and steps in posttranslational modifications, protein partnering, impact of genetic polymorphisms on structure/function, and ligand interactions; and encourage integrated experimental and computational approaches. The workshop participants also saw value in improving the throughput and purity of protein samples and macromolecular assemblies; developing optimal processes for design, production, and assembly of macromolecular complexes; encouraging studies on protein-protein and macromolecular interactions; and examining assemblies of individual proteins and their functions in pathways of interest for environmental health.

Environ Health Perspect. 2006 Jan;114(1):4-9. Related Articles, Links Recent applications of DNA microarray technology to toxicology and ecotoxicology. Lettieri T. Laboratory of Molecular Ecotoxicology, Inland and Marine Water Unit, Institute for Environment and Sustainability, Joint Research Centre of the European Commission, Ispra, Italy. teresa.lettieri@jrc.it Gene expression is a unique way of characterizing how cells and organisms adapt to changes in the external environment. The measurements of gene expression levels upon exposure to a chemical can be used both to provide information about the mechanism of action of the toxicant and to form a sort of "genetic signature" for the identification of toxic products. The development of high-quality, commercially available gene arrays has allowed this technology to become a standard tool in molecular toxicology. Several national and international initiatives have provided the proof-of-principle tests for the application of gene expression for the study of the toxicity of new and existing chemical compounds. In the last few years the field has progressed from evaluating the potential of the technology to illustrating the practical use of gene expression profiling in toxicology. The application of gene expression profiling to ecotoxicology is at an earlier stage, mainly because of the the many variables involved in analyzing the status of natural populations. Nevertheless, significant studies have been carried out on the response to environmental stressors both in model and in nonmodel organisms. It can be easily predicted that the development of stressor-specific signatures in gene expression profiling in ecotoxicology will have a major impact on the ecotoxicology field in the near future. International collaborations could play an important role in accelerating the application of genomic approaches in ecotoxicology. Publication Types: Review

Environ Health Perspect. 2006 Jan;114(1):92-9. Related Articles, Links Gene expression analysis of the hepatotoxicant methapyrilene in primary rat hepatocytes: an interlaboratory study. Beekman JM, Boess F, Hildebrand H, Kalkuhl A, Suter L. Schering AG, Berlin, Germany. johanna.beekman@schering.de Genomics technologies are used in several disciplines, including toxicology. However, these technologies are relatively new, and their applications require further investigations. When investigators apply these technologies to in vitro experiments, two major issues need to be clarified: a) can in vitro toxicity studies, in combination with genomics analyses, be used to predict the toxicity of a compound; and b) are the generated toxicogenomics data reproducible between laboratories? These questions were addressed by an interlaboratory study with laboratories of four pharmaceutical companies. We evaluated gene expression patterns from cultured rat primary hepatocytes after a 24-hr incubation with methapyrilene (MP). Extensive data analysis showed that comparison of genomics data from different sources is complex because both experimental and statistical variability are important confounding factors. However, appropriate statistical tools allowed us to use gene expression profiles to distinguish high-dose-treated cells from vehicle-treated cells. Moreover, we correctly identified MP in an independently generated in vitro database, underlining that in vitro toxicogenomics could be a predictive tool for toxicity. From a mechanistic point of view, despite the observed site-to-site variability, there was good concordance regarding the affected biologic processes. Several subsets of regulated genes were obtained by analyzing the data sets with one method or using different statistical analysis methods. The identified genes are involved in cellular processes that are associated to the exposure of primary hepatocytes to MP. Whether they are specific for MP and are cause or consequence of the toxicity requires further investigations.

Environ Health Perspect. 2006 Jan;114(1):A14. Related Articles, Links Environmental genomics: an opportunity for the NIEHS. Schwartz DA. NIEHS and NTP, Durham, NC, USA. david.schwartz@niehs.nih.gov

Environ Pollut. 2004 Sep;131(1):137-45. Related Articles, Links A method for diagnosis of plant environmental stresses by gene expression profiling using a cDNA macroarray. Tamaoki M, Matsuyama T, Nakajima N, Aono M, Kubo A, Saji H. Biodiversity Conservation Research Project, National Institute for Environmental Studies, 16-2 Onogawa, Tsukuba, Ibaraki 305-8506, Japan. mtamaoki@nies.go.jp Plants in the field are subjected to numerous environmental stresses. Lengthy continuation of such environmental stresses or a rapid increase in their intensity is harmful to vegetation.

Assessments of the phytotoxicity of various stresses have been performed in many countries, although they have largely been based on estimates of leaf injury. We developed a novel method of detecting plant stresses that is more sensitive and specific than those previously available. This method is based on the detection of mRNA expression changes in 205 ozone-responsive Arabidopsis expressed sequence tags (ESTs) by cDNA macroarray analysis. By using this method, we illustrated shifts in gene expression in response to stressors such as drought, salinity, UV-B, low temperature, high temperature, and acid rain, as distinct from those in response to ozone. We also made a mini-scale macroarray with 12 ESTs for diagnosis of the above environmental stresses in plants. These results illustrate the potential of our cDNA macroarray for diagnosis of various stresses in plants.

Environ Pollut. 2005 Nov;138(2):307-15. Related Articles, Links A biomarker model of sublethal genotoxicity (DNA single-strand breaks and adducts) using the sentinel organism Aporrectodea longa in spiked soil. Martin FL, Piearce TG, Hewer A, Phillips DH, Semple KT. Department of Biological Sciences, Institute of Environmental and Natural Sciences, Lancaster University, Lancaster LA1 4YQ, UK. f.martin@lancaster.ac.uk There is a need to develop risk biomarkers during the remediation of contaminated land. We employed the earthworm, Aporrectodea longa (Ude), to determine whether genotoxicity measures could be applied to this organism's intestinal tissues. Earthworms were added, for 24h or 7 days, to soil samples spiked with benzo[a]pyrene (B[a]P) and/or lindane. After exposure, intestinal tissues (crop/gizzard or intestine) were removed prior to the measurement in disaggregated cells of DNA single-strand breaks (SSBs) by the alkaline comet assay. Damage was quantified by comet tail length (CTL, microm). B[a]P 24-h exposure induced dose-related increases ($P<0.0001$) in SSBs. Earthworm intestine was significantly ($P<0.0001$) more susceptible than crop/gizzard to B[a]P and/or lindane. However, both tissues appeared to acquire resistance following 7-day exposure. B[a]P-DNA adducts, measured by (32)P-postlabelling, showed a two-adduct-spot pattern. This preliminary investigation suggests that earthworm tissues may be incorporated into genotoxicity assays to facilitate hazard identification within terrestrial ecosystems.

Environ Sci Technol. 2005 Aug 1;39(15):5893-9. Related Articles, Links Microarray analysis of toxicogenomic effects of peracetic acid on Pseudomonas aeruginosa. Chang W, Small DA, Toghrol F, Bentley WE. Center for Biosystems Research, University of Maryland Biotechnology Institute, College Park, Maryland 20742, USA. Hospital-acquired (nosocomial) infection (HAI) represents a serious threat to public health, both in terms of human casualty and in terms of economic impact. On an annual basis, 2 million individuals require prolonged hospitalization, and an estimated 90 000 patients die due to HAI. Economic damages are reported to exceed $4.5 billion, annually. While many disinfectants, including peracetic acid, have been employed to eradicate infectious bacteria, a lack of understanding their mode of action and the corresponding defense mechanisms hinders successful antimicrobial application. We report here the first transcriptome analysis of the response of Pseudomonas aeruginosa, a pathogen infecting those with cystic fibrosis, upon 20 min exposure to a sublethal concentration (1 mM) of peracetic acid. As a result, we identified that 570 out of a total of 5570 P. aeruginosa genes showed statistically significant transcript level changes. Our findings indicate that (i) many genes associated with cellular protective processes were induced, (ii) the transcription of genes involved in primary metabolic pathways was repressed, and (iii) the transcription of genes encoding membrane proteins and small molecule transporters was altered. We also observed that genes within operons were highly cotranscribed in this study. Finally, this global transcriptional profile can help identify signature genes that are also activated with other oxidative disinfectants, which may be used to design new more effective treatments or more efficaciously apply existing compounds.

Environ Sci. 2004;11(6):325-35. Related Articles, Links Construction of a data dependent analysis (DDA) yeast cDNA microarray experiment for use in toxicogenomics. Mizukami S, Suzuki Y, Kitagawa E, Momose Y, Kim HJ, Iwahashi H. National Institute of Advanced Industrial Science and Technology (AIST), Central 6, 1-1-1, Higashi, Tsukuba, Ibaraki 305-8566, Japan. DNA microarrays are becoming increasingly popular in toxicogenomic studies. It is common knowledge that multiple repeats of microarray experiments have to be performed with multiple samples to get reliable data, due to experimental variations (both technical and biological) contained in microarray experiments. However, the use of multiple samples and replicate experiments is not practical in the field of environmental toxicology, since environmental samples are limited and microarray experiments are expensive. Thus it is desirable to obtain reliable data from a minimum number of repeats of microarray experiments. To further establish and extend gene expression profiling for toxicogenomics using microarrays, it is necessary to establish an analytical method of microarrays for toxicogenomics. In this study, we attempted to construct a "Data Dependent Analysis (DDA)" yeast cDNA microarray experiment from 100 microarray datasets in order to get reliable data from one microarray experiment.

Epilepsia. 2004 Nov;45(11):1429-42. Related Articles, Links Genetic association studies in epilepsy: "the truth is out there". Tan NC, Mulley JC, Berkovic SF. Epilepsy Research Centre and Department of Medicine (Neurology), University of Melbourne, Australia. Success has been achieved in identifying many mutations in rare monogenic epilepsy syndromes by using linkage analysis, but dissecting the genetic basis of common epilepsy syndromes has proven more difficult. Common epilepsies are genetically complex disorders believed to be influenced by variation in several susceptibility genes. Association studies can theoretically identify these genes, but despite more than 50 association studies in epilepsy, no consistent or convincing susceptibility genes have emerged, leading to scepticism about the association-study approach. We review the results of existing association studies in focal epilepsies, generalized epilepsies, febrile seizures, and epilepsy pharmacogenetics. By using an illustrative example, we discuss how methodologic issues of sample size, selection of appropriate controls, population stratification, and significance thresholds can lead to bias and false-positive associations; the importance of biologic plausibility also is emphasized. Newer methodologic refinements for association studies, such as use of two control groups, genomic control, haplotyping, and use of two independent datasets, are discussed. A summary of existing guidelines and a checklist for planning and appraising such association studies in epilepsy is presented. We remain cautiously optimistic that with methodologic refinements and multicenter collaborations with large sample sizes, association studies will ultimately be useful in dissecting the genetic basis of common epilepsy syndromes. Publication Types: Multicenter Study Review

Epilepsia. 2005 Feb;46(2):224-35. Related Articles, Links Potential role of drug transporters in the pathogenesis of medically intractable epilepsy. Kwan P, Brodie MJ. Division of Neurology, Department of Medicine and Therapeutics, The Chinese University of Hong Kong, Prince of Wales Hospital, Shatin, Hong Kong. patrickkwan@cuhk.edu.hk The pathogenesis underlying pharmacoresistance in epilepsy is unclear. One of the candidate mechanisms that has attracted growing interest is the limitation of antiepileptic drug (AED) access to the seizure focus by a range of efflux transporters, the prototype of which is P-glycoprotein (P-gp). P-gp is encoded by the multidrug resistance (MDR1 or ABCB1) gene. Predominantly expressed in organs with excretory functions and at blood-tissue barriers, P-gp is thought to act as a physiologic defense by extruding xenobiotics from mammalian cells and affording protection of sensitive organs. The high level of P-gp in the cerebrovascular endothelium is believed to contribute to the functionality of the blood-brain barrier. Overexpression of P-gp causes multidrug resistance in certain cancers. It has been hypothesized that overexpression of P-gp and other efflux transporters in the cerebrovascular endothelium, in the region of the epileptic focus, also may lead to drug resistance in epilepsy. This hypothesis is supported by the findings of elevated expression of efflux transporters in epileptic foci in patients with drug-resistant epilepsy, induction of expression by seizures in animal models, and experimental evidence that some commonly used AEDs are substrates. Conflicting reports suggest a possible association between variants of the MDR1 gene and medical intractability in epilepsy. Further studies to delineate the exact role, if any, of P-gp and other efflux transporters in drug-resistant epilepsy are warranted. Publication Types: Review

Epilepsia. 2005 Jun;46(6):858-77. Related Articles, Links Drug resistance in epilepsy: putative neurobiologic and clinical mechanisms. Schmidt D, Loscher W. Epilepsy Research Group, Berlin, Germany. dbschmidt@t-online.de Drug-resistant epilepsy with uncontrolled severe seizures despite state-of-the-art medical treatment continues to be a major clinical problem for up to one in three patients with epilepsy. Although drug resistance may emerge or remit in the course of epilepsy or its treatment, in most patients, drug resistance seems to be continuous and to occur de novo. Unfortunately, current antiepileptic drugs (AEDs) do not seem to prevent or to reverse drug resistance in most patients, but add-on therapy with novel AEDs is able to exert a modest seizure reduction in as many as 50% of patients in short-term clinical trials, and a few become seizure free during the trial. It is not known why and how epilepsy becomes drug resistant, while other patients with seemingly identical seizure types can achieve seizure control with medication. Several putative mechanisms underlying drug resistance in epilepsy have been identified in recent years. Based on experimental and clinical studies, two major neurobiologic theories have been put forward: (a) removal of AEDs from the epileptogenic tissue through excessive expression of multidrug transporters, and (b) reduced drug-target sensitivity in epileptogenic brain tissue. On the clinical side, genetic and clinical features and structural brain lesions have been associated with drug resistance in epilepsy. In this article, we review the laboratory and clinical evidence to date supporting the drug-transport and the drug-target hypotheses and provide directions for future research, to define more clearly the role of these hypotheses in the clinical spectrum of drug-resistant epilepsy. Publication Types: Review

Epilepsia. 2005 May;46(5):643-7. Related Articles, Links Lack of association between the C3435T polymorphism in the human multidrug resistance (MDR1) gene and response to antiepileptic drug treatment. Sills GJ, Mohanraj R, Butler E, McCrindle S, Collier L, Wilson EA, Brodie MJ. Epilepsy Unit, Section of Clinical Pharmacology and Stroke Medicine, University Division of Cardiovascular and Medical Sciences, Western Infirmary, Glasgow, Scotland. g.j.sills@clinmed.gla.ac.uk PURPOSE: P-glycoprotein (P-gp) has been implicated in the causation of refractory epilepsy. The expression and efflux efficiency of P-gp is influenced by a polymorphism (C3435T) in the encoding gene (MDR1). Recent evidence suggests that the homozygous C-variant, which is associated with higher expression and increased activity of P-gp, is more common in patients with pharmacoresistant epilepsy. We have investigated the prevalence of this polymorphism in a series of patients attending a specialist epilepsy clinic. METHODS: DNA samples were obtained from 400 patients, irrespective of seizure type or drug treatment. Genotype of the C3435T polymorphism was determined by traditional polymerase chain reaction (PCR) followed by restriction digest. Classification of response to treatment was determined in a blinded fashion by an independent physician. Results were expressed as genotype and allele frequencies per response group and compared by logistic regression analysis. RESULTS: In total, 170 patients were classified as responders, with > or =12 months seizure freedom on current treatment. The remaining 230 patients were classified as nonresponders. Comparison of responders and nonresponders revealed no significant difference in allele frequency (C vs. T; odds ratio, 1.03; 95% CI, 0.78-1.37; p = 0.83) or genotype frequency (CC vs TT; odds ratio, 1.07; 95% CI, 0.60-1.91; p = 0.81). Subanalyses of individual seizure types were similarly unremarkable. CONCLUSIONS: This study failed to corroborate a previously reported association between the C3435T polymorphism in the human MDR1 gene and pharmacoresistant epilepsy. Whether the C3435T polymorphism can act as a marker for the natural history of treated epilepsy remains to be determined.

Epilepsia. 2005;46 Suppl 10:31-2. Related Articles, Links Response to antiepileptic drug therapy: winners and losers. Brodie MJ. Epilepsy Unit, Division of Cardiovascular and Medical Sciences, Western Infirmary, Glasgow, Scotland, U.K. Martin.J.Brodie@clinmed.gla.ac.uk Recent evidence suggests that the vast majority of people with epilepsy will respond to their first or second treatment regimen or will be refractory de novo. Two patients with symptomatic epilepsy secondary to underlying cortical dysplasias are presented to illustrate these different scenarios. Clinical observations can provide insights to the processes underlying pharmacoresistance. Publication Types: Case Reports

Epilepsia. 2005;46 Suppl 10:33-8. Related Articles, Links Genetics of drug resistance. Sisodiya SM. Department of Clinical and Experimental Epilepsy, Institute of Neurology, UCL, Queen Square, London, United Kingdom. sisodiya@ion.ucl.ac.uk Drug resistance in epilepsy affects about a third of patients and is an important clinical problem, associated with increased morbidity and mortality. It is important to consider carefully the definition of drug resistance. Recent interest in the field has focused on the potential molecular mechanisms underlying drug resistance. Environmental and seizure-related acquired causes are likely to contribute to the multifaceted basis of resistance in most cases. Genetic causes have attracted particular attention, partly because they may allow prediction of drug resistance and, potentially, rational treatment strategies. Gene mutations, however, are unlikely to cause many cases of drug resistance. However, common variation in genes probably will turn out to generate an important contribution to drug resistance phenomena. Associations between common variations in a number of genes and clinical drug resistance have now been published. However, to date, none of these associations has been unequivocally replicated by others to the extent that the original association has been accepted. Some of these associations are considered. Despite this apparently uninspiring record, the genetics of drug resistance are likely to prove productive in the near future, but their pursuit will require painstaking studies and multicenter collaboration. Publication Types: Review

Epilepsy Behav. 2004 Oct;5(5):621-6. Related Articles, Links Ethical implications in genetic counseling and family studies of the epilepsies. Godard B, Cardinal G. Faculty of Medicine and Research Centre for Public Law, Universite de Montreal, Montreal, Canada H3C 3J7. beatrice.godard@umontreal.ca <beatrice.godard@umontreal.ca> Most of the inherited epilepsies do not follow a Mendelian inheritance pattern but rather are complex disorders. This leads us to reconsider the traditional ethical framework applying to genetics, which is still based largely on the understanding of Mendelian inheritance, to ethically use the genetic tests likely to be forthcoming for the prevention and surveillance of epilepsies. This article is a review of the ethical issues raised by family studies of the epilepsies, in both a clinical and a research context. These issues include the use of genetic tests, the scope of genetic counseling, the upholding of the risk-benefit ratio in pharmacogenetics, as well as those related to the availability of treatments, health professionals' changing responsibilities, and the communication within families. A reasonable approach calls for a case-by-case determination of whether the benefit and harm of genetic testing outweigh benefit and harm of protecting autonomy and nonmaleficence. Publication Types: Review

Epilepsy Behav. 2005 Aug;7(1):18-36. Related Articles, Links The relationship between the pharmacology of antiepileptic drugs and human gene variation: an overview. Ferraro TN, Buono RJ. Departments of Psychiatry and Pharmacology, University of Pennsylvania, Philadelphia, PA 19104, USA. tnf@mail.med.upenn.edu Individual differences in clinical responsiveness to antiepileptic drugs are due to a complex interaction between environmental factors and genetic variation. Considerable interest has arisen in exploiting advances in molecular genetics to improve drug therapy for epilepsy and many other diseases; however, practical application of pharmacogenetics has been difficult to realize. Attempts to define gene variants that are associated with therapeutic (or adverse) effects of antiepileptic drugs rely currently on the prior identification of candidate genes and the subsequent evaluation of the distribution of allelic variants between individuals who have a "good" versus a "poor" clinical response. Many factors can adversely affect interpretation of such data, and careful consideration must be given to the design of genetic association studies involving candidate genes. Candidate genes may be identified in a number of ways; however, for studies of drugs, application of knowledge derived from basic pharmacology can suggest focused and testable hypotheses that are based on the fundamental principles of drug action. Thus, studies of genetic variation as they relate to proteins involved in antiepileptic drug kinetics and dynamics will identify key polymorphisms in endogenous molecules that determine degrees of drug efficacy and toxicity. Delineation of these effects in the coming years will promote enhanced success in the treatment of epilepsy. Publication Types: Review

Epilepsy Curr. 2005 Nov-Dec;5(6):236-8. Links Pharmacogenetics of epilepsy: one step forward? Sills GJ.

Essent Psychopharmacol. 2005;6(4):193-208. Related Articles, Links Genetics and psychopharmacology: prospects for individualized treatment. Nnadi CU, Goldberg JF, Malhotra AK. Department of Psychiatry Research, Zucker Hillside Hospital, Glen Oaks, New York, USA. This article provides a clear and succinct description of the components of inheritance, such as trait transmission, genetic variability, and gene interaction. Genetic sequences constitute the prime focus of pharmacogenetic studies. Variations in drug-metabolizing enzyme systems tend to be monogenic, whereas the pharmacologic effects of medications appear to be polygenic, i.e., complex phenotypes shaped by the interaction of genes and environment. Translated into clinical terms, a history of a good response to a drug in a close relative of a patient is presumed to predict a good response to the same medication by the patient. This seems to hold for antidepressants, antipsychotics, and lithium, but the evidential studies generally have meaningful limitations. Bit by bit, information about the relationship between particular genetic formations and the effectiveness of these medications as well as their side effects, is appearing. The authors cite a number of examples, one such being an association between impaired antidepressant activity and the short allele of SLC6A4. This research promises to strengthen the accuracy, effectiveness, safety, and cost of our psychopharmacological practices. Publication Types: Review

Eur J Anaesthesiol. 2004 Jul;21(7):505-8. Related Articles, Links Microarrays: new pharmacogenomic tools for the twenty-first century. Sweeney BP. Publication Types: Editorial

Eur J Cancer. 2004 Nov;40(17):2560-91. Related Articles, Links Gene expression microarray technologies in the development of new therapeutic agents. Clarke PA, te Poele R, Workman P. Cancer Research UK Centre for Cancer Therapeutics, The Institute of Cancer Research, Haddow Laboratories, Sutton,

Surrey SM2 5NG, UK. We review in detail how gene expression microarray technology is benefiting all phases of the discovery, development and subsequent use of new cancer therapeutics. Global gene expression profiling is valuable in cancer classification, elucidation of biochemical pathways and the identification of potential targets for novel molecular therapeutics. We exemplify the value in tissue culture and animal models of cancer, as well as in clinical studies. The power of expression profiling alongside gene knockout or knockdown methods such as RNA interference is illustrated. The use of basal or constitutive gene expression profiling to understand and predict drug sensitivity or resistance is described. The ability of expression profiling to define detailed molecular signatures of drug action is emphasised. The approach can identify on-target and off-target effects. It can be used to identify molecular biomarkers for proof of concept studies, pharmacodynamic endpoints and prognostic markers for predicting outcome and patient selection. Publication Types: Review

Eur J Clin Pharmacol. 2004 Jul;60(5):329-36. Epub 2004 May 28. Related Articles, Links Impact of polymorphisms of cytochrome-P450 isoenzymes 2C9, 2C19 and 2D6 on plasma concentrations and clinical effects of antidepressants in a naturalistic clinical setting. Grasmader K, Verwohlt PL, Rietschel M, Dragicevic A, Muller M, Hiemke C, Freymann N, Zobel A, Maier W, Rao ML. Department of Psychiatry, University of Bonn, Sigmund-Freud-Strasse 25, 53105 Bonn, Germany. OBJECTIVE: This evaluation focuses on polymorphisms of the cytochrome-P450 (CYP) isoenzymes 2C9, 2C19 and 2D6 and their association with plasma concentrations within a typical clinical setting. Side effects and treatment response were analysed in an exploratory approach in poor and ultra-rapid metabolisers. PATIENTS AND METHODS: We analysed 136 Caucasian depressed inpatients treated with amitriptyline, citalopram, clomipramine, doxepin, fluvoxamine, mirtazapine, paroxetine, sertraline and venlafaxine, who underwent weekly plasma concentration measurements, assessment of the severity of illness and side effects during their stay in the hospital. Patients were genotyped with respect to CYP2C9 alleles *1 and *2, the CYP2C19 alleles *1, *2 and *3 and the CYP2D6 alleles *1 to *9 and CYP2D6 gene duplication. RESULTS: CYP2D6 poor metaboliser genotype and co-medication with inhibitors of CYP2D6 were associated with higher plasma concentrations than the drug-specific median plasma concentration when normalised to dose; plasma concentrations of CYP2C19 extensive metabolisers and smokers were significantly lower than the drug-specific median. Five of the six CYP2D6 poor metabolisers experienced side effects. Response was not associated with plasma concentrations above or below the lower limit of a presumed therapeutic range. CONCLUSION: These data indicate a significant influence of the CYP2D6 genotype, minor influence of the CYP2C19 genotype and no influence of the CYP2C9 genotype on plasma concentrations of patients taking mainly second-generation antidepressants. Because of the good tolerability of the latter and the flat dose-response relationship, genotyping should only be considered in cases of suspected side effects. Publication Types: Clinical Trial

Eur J Clin Pharmacol. 2004 May;60(3):165-71. Epub 2004 Mar 25. Related Articles, Links Cytochrome P450 2C9 phenotyping using low-dose tolbutamide. Jetter A, Kinzig-Schippers M, Skott A, Lazar A, Tomalik-Scharte D, Kirchheiner J, Walchner-Bonjean M, Hering U, Jakob V, Rodamer M, Jabrane W, Kasel D, Brockmoller J, Fuhr U, Sorgel F. Department of Pharmacology, Clinical Pharmacology, University of Cologne, Gleueler Strasse 24, 50931 Cologne, Germany. alexander.jetter@medizin.uni-koeln.de OBJECTIVES: The hypoglycaemic drug tolbutamide is used for assessment of CYP2C9 activity in vivo. However, therapeutically active doses of 500 mg bear the risk of hypoglycaemia, and a tolbutamide-derived parameter based on a single plasma or urine concentration reflecting CYP2C9 activity accurately is lacking. METHODS: We examined tolbutamide and its metabolites 4'-hydroxy-tolbutamide and carboxytolbutamide in plasma and urine of 26 healthy, male volunteers up to 24 h after intake of 125 mg tolbutamide using liquid chromatography-tandem mass spectrometry. CYP2C9 genotypes were determined by sequencing of exons 3 and 7. Raw plasma and urine data were compared with pharmacokinetic parameters, CYP2C9 genotypes, and data from a study in 23 volunteers with all six CYP2C9*1-*3 combinations who received 500 mg tolbutamide. RESULTS: Plasma clearance and tolbutamide plasma concentrations 24 h after drug intake reflected the genotypes: 0.85 l/h and 1.70 microg/ml (95% confidence interval, CI, 0.80-0.89 l/h and 1.50-1.90 microg/ml) for CYP2C9*1 homozygotes (n=15), 0.77 l/h and 2.14 microg/ml (95%CI, 0.67-0.88 l/h and 1.64-2.63 microg/ml) for *1/*2 genotypes (n=7), 0.60 l/h and 3.13 microg/ml (95%CI, 0.58-0.62 l/h and 2.68-3.58 microg/ml) for *1/*3 genotypes (n=3), and 0.57 l/h and 3.27 microg/ml in the single *2/*2 carrier. Natural logarithms of tolbutamide plasma concentrations 24 h after intake correlated to plasma clearance (r(2)=0.84, P<0.0000001). This correlation was confirmed in the comparison data set (r(2)=0.97, P<0.0000001). CONCLUSIONS: A low dose of 125 mg tolbutamide can safely and accurately be used for CYP2C9 phenotyping. As a simple metric for CYP2C9 activity, we propose to determine tolbutamide in plasma 24 h after drug intake.

Eur J Clin Pharmacol. 2005 Aug;61(7):491-7. Epub 2005 Jul 16. Related Articles, Links Polymorphism of CYP2D6, CYP2C19, CYP2C9 and CYP2C8 in the Faroese population. Halling J, Petersen MS, Damkier P, Nielsen F, Grandjean P, Weihe P, Lundgren S, Lundblad MS, Brosen K. Clinical Pharmacology, Faculty of Health Sciences, Institute of Public Health, University of Southern Denmark, Winslovparken 19, 5000 Odense C, Denmark. jhalling@health.sdu.dk OBJECTIVE: The purpose of the study was to study the distribution of poor and extensive metabolizers of CYP2C19 and CYP2D6 and to genotype for CYP2C8 and CYP2C9 among 312 randomly selected Faroese.METHODS AND RESULTS: The participants were phenotyped for CYP2D6 with the use of sparteine. The distribution of the sparteine metabolic ratio (sparteine/didehydrosparteines) was bimodal, and 14.5% (n=44; 95% CI: 10.7--18.9%) of the subjects were phenotyped as poor metabolizers. The frequency of poor metabolizers was higher (P=0.0002; chi(2) test) among the Faroese than in other European populations (7.4%). Genotype analyses for the CYP2D6*3, *4, *6 and *9 alleles were performed using real-time polymerase chain reaction (PCR) (TaqMan, Foster City, CA, USA), and we found 14.6% (n=45) (95% CI: 10.8--19.0%) with deficient CYP2D6 genes

(*3/*4, *4/*4, *4/*6, *6/*6) in the Faroese population. The subjects were phenotyped for CYP2C19 with the use of mephenytoin and 10 subjects, i.e., 3.2% (95% CI: 1.6--5.9%) were phenotyped as poor metabolizers. Genotype analysis for the CYP2C19*2 and *3 alleles was performed by means of PCR analysis, and 2.9% (n=9) (95% CI: 1.3-5.4%) of the Faroese were found to have a deficient CYP2C19 gene all explained by the CYP2C19*2/*2 genotype. The allele frequencies of the CYP2C9*2 and CYP2C9*3 alleles were 8.8% (95% CI: 6.7--11.4%) and 5.3% (95% CI: 3.7--7.4%), respectively, while the CYP2C8*3 allele frequency was 6.9% (95% CI: 5.0--9.2%). Real-time PCR (TaqMan) was used for both CYP2C9 and CYP2C8 genotype analyses.CONCLUSION: The frequency of CYP2D6 poor metabolizers is twofold higher among the Faroese population than other Caucasians, while the frequencies of Faroese subjects with decreased CYP2C19, CYP2C8 and CYP2C9 enzyme activity are the same as seen in other Caucasian populations. A possible consequence might be a higher incidence of side effects among Faroese patients taking pharmaceuticals that are CYP2D6 substrates.

Eur J Clin Pharmacol. 2005 Mar;61(1):15-8. Epub 2005 Jan 27. Related Articles, Links CYP2C8 polymorphism frequencies among malaria patients in Zanzibar. Cavaco I, Stromberg-Norklit J, Kaneko A, Msellem MI, Dahoma M, Ribeiro VL, Bjorkman A, Gil JP. Centre for Molecular and Structural Biomedicine, Universidade do Algarve, Campus de Gambelas, Faro, 8000-117, Portugal. OBJECTIVE: The determination of the prevalence of the CYP2C8 main alleles in a typical set of malaria patients in Zanzibar, as these patients represent a typical population exposed to amodiaquine, an antimalarial mainly metabolized by CYP2C8. Also, to determine for the first time the frequencies of CYP2C8 alleles in native African populations. METHODS: Polymerase chain reaction-restriction fragment polymorphism for the identification of CYP2C8*1, CYP2C8*2, CYP2C8*3 and CYP2C8*4 on a random population of 165 unrelated malaria patients. RESULTS: The allele frequencies found were: CYP2C8*1 (wild type, 83.4%), CYP2C8*2 (13.9%), CYP2C8*3 (2.1%) and CYP2C8*4 (0.6%). In terms of genotypes, 70.4% of the patients showed the CYP2C8*1/ CYP2C8*1 genotypes, while heterozygous between the wild type and other minor alleles were seen in 26.0%. Finally, 3.6% of the patients were homozygous for slow metabolizer alleles. The frequencies observed are equivalent to those documented for African-Americans. CONCLUSIONS: CYP2C8 non-wild type alleles have a significant prevalence in the East African population studied. The consequent frequency of 3.6% of patients homozygous for slow metabolizer alleles represent a significant fraction of the population potentially in higher risk of adverse effects due to a less efficient metabolism of amodiaquine. As approximately 10(6) first-line treatments are currently performed in Zanzibar per year, this represents a non-negligible absolute number of amodiaquine exposures. This information constitutes a background for the pharmacovigilance programs presently being employed in Zanzibar. Publication Types: Clinical Trial

Eur J Clin Pharmacol. 2005 Mar;61(1):19-23. Epub 2005 Jan 21. Related Articles, Links The effect of the CYP2C19 genotype on the hydroxylation index of omeprazole in South Indians. Rosemary J, Adithan C, Padmaja N, Shashindran CH, Gerard N,

Krishnamoorthy R. Department of Pharmacology, Pharmacogenomics Laboratory, Jawaharlal Institute of Postgraduate Medical Education and Research (JIPMER), Pondicherry, 605 006, India. To investigate the relationship between CYP2C19 genotypes and the hydroxylation index (HI) of omeprazole in the South Indian population. Healthy unrelated South Indian subjects (n=300) were separated into three groups based on their CYP2C19 genotypes. They were administered a single oral dose of 20 mg omeprazole, and venous blood was collected 3 h later. Plasma was assayed using reversed-phase high-performance liquid chromatography, and the omeprazole HI was calculated. The means of HIs in individuals with CYP2C19*1/*1 (n=124), *1/*2 (n=129) and *2/*2,*2/*3 (n=47) were 2.4, 5.3 and 22.5, respectively, and were found to be significantly different between any two groups (P<0.0001). A good correlation was established between CYP2C19 genotype and omeprazole HI (r=0.54, 95% CI 0.45-0.62; P<0.0001). Of the 300 subjects, 42 (14.0%; 95% CI 10.1-17.9) were phenotypic poor metabolizers (PMs), but only 33 of them had two mutant alleles and the remaining 9 PMs had at least one wild-type allele. Among the 258 extensive metabolizers, 14 had two mutant alleles. The prevalence of PMs in the South Indian population was 14.0%, which is similar to that in North Indians and Orientals but significantly higher than in Caucasians and Africans. A genotype-phenotype relationship was established between the CYP2C19 genotype and HI of omeprazole, but 7.7% of subjects deviated from expected genotype-phenotype associations. This could be due to an additional mutation, either in the exons/introns or in the 5'-regulatory region of the CYP2C19 gene. Publication Types: Clinical Trial

Eur J Clin Pharmacol. 2005 Mar;61(1):25-34. Epub 2005 Feb 4. Related Articles, Links Haplotype structures of EPHX1 and their effects on the metabolism of carbamazepine-10,11-epoxide in Japanese epileptic patients. Nakajima Y, Saito Y, Shiseki K, Fukushima-Uesaka H, Hasegawa R, Ozawa S, Sugai K, Katoh M, Saitoh O, Ohnuma T, Kawai M, Ohtsuki T, Suzuki C, Minami N, Kimura H, Goto Y, Kamatani N, Kaniwa N, Sawada J. Project team for Pharmacogenetics, National Institute of Health Sciences, 1-18-1 Kamiyoga, Setagaya-ku, Tokyo, 158-8501, Japan. OBJECTIVE: Microsomal epoxide hydrolase (mEH) is an enzyme that detoxifies reactive epoxides and catalyzes the biotransformation of carbamazepine-10,11-epoxide (CBZ-epoxide) to carbamazepine-10,11-diol (CBZ-diol). Utilizing single nucleotide polymorphisms (SNPs) of the EPHX1 gene encoding mEH, we identified the haplotypes of EPHX1 blocks and investigated the association between the block haplotypes and CBZ-epoxide metabolism. METHODS: SNPs of EPHX1 were analyzed by means of polymerase chain reaction amplification and DNA sequencing using DNA extracted from the blood leukocytes of 96 Japanese epileptic patients, including 58 carbamazepine-administered patients. The plasma concentrations of CBZ and its four metabolites were determined using high-performance liquid chromatography. RESULTS: From sequencing all 9 exons and their surrounding introns, 29 SNPs were found in EPHX1. The SNPs were separated into three blocks on the basis of linkage disequilibrium, and the block haplotype combinations (diplotypes) were assigned. Using plasma CBZ-diol/CBZ-epoxide ratios (diol/epoxide ratios) indicative of the mEH activity, the effects of the diplotypes in each EPHX1 block were analyzed on CBZ-epoxide metabolism. In block 2, the diol/epoxide ratios increased significantly depending on the number of haplotype *2 bearing Y113H (P=0.0241). In block 3, the ratios decreased depending on the number of haplotype *2 bearing H139R (P=0.0351). Also, an increasing effect of a *1 subtype, *1c, was observed on the ratio. CONCLUSION: These results show that some EPHX1 haplotypes are associated with altered CBZ-epoxide metabolism. This is the first report on the haplotype structures of EPHX1 and their potential in vivo effects. Publication Types: Clinical Trial

Eur J Clin Pharmacol. 2006 Jan 12;:1-5 [Epub ahead of print] Related Articles, Links Lack of effect of growth hormone replacement therapy on CYP1A2 and xanthine oxidase activities in growth hormone-deficient children. Mayayo-Sinues E, Fanlo A, Sinues B, Mayayo E, Labarta JI, Garcia de Jalon A, Ferrandez-Longas A. Department of Pharmacology, Medicine School, University of Zaragoza, Domingo Miral s/n, 50009, Zaragoza, Spain, bsinues@unizar.es. BACKGROUND AND OBJECTIVES: The recombinant human growth hormone (rhGH) is being increasingly used for a number of metabolic alterations. GH is the main regulator of several hepatic drug metabolizing enzymes in rodents. In addition, GH could play a major role in defining the interface between pharmacogenetics and development. However, little is known about the effect of GH on the activity of hepatic enzymes in children. The aim of this study was to determine the effect of rhGH replacement therapy for 4 weeks on CYP1A2 and xanthine oxidase (XO) activities in children. METHODS: We used caffeine as a probe drug to assess the enzyme activities at two points in time: before starting GH treatment (day 0) and after 4 weeks on rhGH therapy (day A). A total of 31 GH-deficient children (age range: 4.1-13.1 years, mean age: 9.88+/-2.89 years) participated. Urinary concentrations of caffeine and metabolites were determined by high-performance liquid chromatography (HPLC) to calculate the metabolite ratios: (AFMU+1X+1U)/17U for CYP1A2 and 1U/(1X+1U) for XO. RESULTS: Four weeks of GH substitution did not importantly alter the markers of the enzyme activities measured in this study. Median values and 95% confidence intervals (CI) at baseline were 5.17 (3.87-5.59) for the CYP1A2 ratio and 0.62 (0.56-0.65) for the XO ratio. These values, after treatment, were 4.57 (3.90-5.97) for the CYP1A2 marker and 0.62 (0.59-0.67) for the XO ratio. Data comparison between periods showed lack of statistically significant differences (P>0.05). The relative changes measured by the ratios of medians and 90% CI were 1.14 (0.90-1.31) and 0.99 (0.94-1.06) for CYP1A2 and XO, respectively. CONCLUSIONS: The absence of significant changes in the markers of enzyme activities CYP1A2 and XO suggests that rhGH replacement therapy of GH-deficient children for 4 weeks could not noticeably modify the efficacy or toxicity of substrates of these metabolic enzymes. y publisher]

Eur J Hum Genet. 2005 Sep;13(9):1055-62. Related Articles, Links Communication of pharmacogenetic research results to HIV-infected treated patients: standpoints of professionals and patients. Moutel G, Duchange N, Raffi F, Sharara LI, Theodorou I, Noel V, de Montgolfier S, Callies I, Bricaire F, Herve C, Leport C; APROCO-COPILOTE Study Group. Laboratoire d'Ethique Medicale et Medecine Legale and Institut International de Recherche en Ethique Biomedicale, Faculte de Medecine Paris 5. 45 rue des Saints-Peres, Paris 75006, France. moutel@necker.fr The aim of pharmacogenetic studies is to adapt therapeutic strategies to individual genetic profiles, thus maximising their efficacy and minimising the likelihood of adverse side effects. Since the advent of personalised medicine, the issue of communicating research results to participants has become increasingly important. We addressed this question in the context of HIV infection, as patients and associations are particularly concerned by research and therapeutic advances. We explored the standpoints of both research professionals and participants involved in a pharmacogenetic study conducted in a cohort of HIV-infected patients. The setting of the research protocol was followed over a 2-year period. Participants' standpoints were collected through a questionnaire and interviews were conducted with research professionals. Of 125 participants, 76% wished to receive individual results and 71% wished to receive collective results; 39% did not know when results might be expected. Communication of global research results is a principle that is generally accepted by professionals. Concerning individual feedback, the professionals felt that it was necessary if it could be of direct benefit to the participant, but they expressed doubts for situations with no recognised benefit. Our results highlight the necessity to consider this issue in greater detail. We suggest the need to anticipate the debates concerning individual feedback, to differentiate between situations and the importance of further investigations on the opportunities and modalities of communication. Finally, our work emphasised the opposite pressures between the pursuit of scientific knowledge and the therapeutic orientation of clinical trials.

Eur J Intern Med. 2005 Nov;16(7):492-5. Related Articles, Links Pseudocholinesterase polymorphism in an Irish population. Adebayo GI, Williams J, Healy S. Department of Medicine, Garavogue Centre, Level 3, Sligo General Hospital, The Mall, Sligo, Ireland. BACKGROUND: Pseudocholinesterase polymorphism, as an example of pharmacogenetics with important clinical implications, has been widely studied and documented. However, data on a sample Irish population is lacking. We sought to provide this. METHOD: In an assay involving Ellman's reaction, pseudocholinesterase activity, alone and with dibucaine or fluoride as an inhibitor, was quantified using propionylthiocholine iodide as substrate. RESULTS: Pseudocholinesterase activities of 1.13-12.71 U/ml (mean +/- SD 6.74 +/- 2.04 U/ml) showed a normal distribution among our 116 healthy, non-medicated volunteers, aged 11-80 years (30.7 +/- 10.5 years) and weighing 46-114.6 kg (66.8 +/- 11.4 kg). However, dibucaine numbers from an inhibition study yielded a trimodal pattern consistent with the hypothesis of two allelic genes. Using an established nomenclature, 92 (79.3%) of our volunteers were homozygous for the usual form of the enzyme (E1uE1u). Of the 13 genotyped as E1uE1a, it is possible that 3 were misclassified and are probably E1kE1a. Only one volunteer was homozygous for the atypical form of the enzyme, with activity of 1.13 U/ml and dibucaine and fluoride number of 18.2 and 82.8, respectively. CONCLUSION: The continuous variation in pseudocholinesterase activity and the trimodal pattern of dibucaine numbers are both in accord with observations in other population groups. Although dibucaine number yields a trimodal pattern, its use could lead to misclassification of some E1kE1a as E1uE1a. ature. 2006 Jan 19;439(7074):353-7. Epub 2005 Nov 6. Related Articles, Links Comment in: Nature. 2006 Jan 19;439(7074):274-5. Oncogenic pathway signatures in human cancers as a guide to targeted therapies. Bild AH, Yao G, Chang JT, Wang Q, Potti A, Chasse D, Joshi MB, Harpole D, Lancaster JM, Berchuck A, Olson JA Jr, Marks JR, Dressman HK, West M, Nevins JR. Institute for Genome Sciences and Policy, Duke University, Durham, North Carolina 27708, USA. The development of an oncogenic state is a complex process involving the accumulation of multiple independent mutations that lead to deregulation of cell signalling pathways central to the control of cell growth and cell fate. The ability to define cancer subtypes, recurrence of disease and response to specific therapies using DNA microarray-based gene expression signatures has been demonstrated in multiple studies. Various studies have also demonstrated the potential for using gene expression profiles for the analysis of oncogenic pathways. Here we show that gene expression signatures can be identified that reflect the activation status of several oncogenic pathways. When evaluated in several large collections of human cancers, these gene expression signatures identify patterns of pathway deregulation in tumours and clinically relevant associations with disease outcomes. Combining signature-based predictions across several pathways identifies coordinated patterns of pathway deregulation that distinguish between specific cancers and tumour subtypes. Clustering tumours based on pathway signatures further defines prognosis in respective patient subsets, demonstrating that patterns of oncogenic pathway deregulation underlie the development of the oncogenic phenotype and reflect the biology and outcome of specific cancers. Predictions of pathway deregulation in cancer cell lines are also shown to predict the sensitivity to therapeutic agents that target components of the pathway. Linking pathway deregulation with sensitivity to therapeutics that target components of the pathway provides an opportunity to make use of these oncogenic pathway signatures to guide the use of targeted therapeutics.

Eur J Paediatr Neurol. 2006 Mar 9; [Epub ahead of print] Related Articles, Links The potential of pharmacogenetics in the treatment of epilepsy. Depondt C. Service de Neurologie, Hopital Erasme, Universite Libre de Bruxelles, Route de Lennik 808, 1070 Anderlecht, Belgium. Pharmacogenetics studies how genetic variants influence individual drug responses. Although pharmacogenetics is currently the subject of intensive research in several disease domains, it remains relatively unexplored in the field of epilepsy. Drug treatment of epilepsy is characterized by unpredictability of efficacy, adverse drug reactions and optimal doses in individual patients. Moreover, a substantial fraction of patients develop drug refractory epilepsy despite optimal treatment. Insights in the pathogenesis of epilepsy and the mechanisms of action of antiepileptic drugs (AEDs) have improved our understanding of the genetic determinants of AED response. The first reports in epilepsy pharmacogenetics are becoming available, and large-scale pharmacogenetic studies are now possible thanks to recent advances in genetics and decreasing genotyping costs. It is hoped that ultimately, findings in epilepsy pharmacogenetics will lead to a more efficacious and less harmful treatment of epilepsy, development of more effective AEDs and facilitation of clinical trials of new AEDs. However, although pharmacogenetics will undoubtedly improve our insight into the mechanisms underlying response to AEDs and perhaps into the pathogenesis of drug refractory epilepsy, clinical application of any findings is expected to be a long process, and considerable practical and theoretical hurdles need to be overcome before pharmacogenetic information will prove of any major utility in the clinical setting. This review addresses current knowledge on genetic factors contributing to AED response and discusses the potential of epilepsy pharmacogenetics in the clinical treatment of epilepsy and new AED development. y publisher]

Eur J Pain. 2005 Apr;9(2):101-4. Related Articles, Links Genetics and variability in opioid response. Stamer UM, Bayerer B, Stuber F. Department of Anaesthesiology and Intensive Care Medicine, Rheinische Friedrich-Wilhelms-Universitat Bonn, Sigmund-Freud-Str. 25, 53105 Bonn, Germany. ulrike.stamer@ukb.uni-bonn.de The human genome project has revealed data on genomic variation which may influence the pharmacological responses. In pain therapy, the genetic background influencing the efficacy of opioid therapy is of special interest. Screening for variations in expression of drug metabolizing enzymes has been suggested as a potential tool for improving patient therapy. CYP2D6 genetic variability is supposed to be a major factor of adverse drug reaction, possibly influencing hospital stay and total costs. Further candidate genes involved in pain perception, pain processing and pain management like opioid receptors, transporters and other targets of pharmacotherapy are under investigation. Aspects of genetic differences influencing efficacy, side effects and adverse outcome of pharmacotherapy will be of importance for future pain management. Publication Types: Review

Eur J Pharm Sci. 2006 Jan;27(1):54-61. Epub 2005 Sep 23. Related Articles, Links Pharmacogenetics of cyclophosphamide in patients with hematological malignancies. Xie H, Griskevicius L, Stahle L, Hassan Z, Yasar U, Rane A, Broberg U, Kimby E, Hassan M. Department of Laboratory Medicine, Division of Clinical Pharmacology, Karolinska Institutet, SE 141-86 Stockholm, Sweden. PURPOSE: A high degree of interindividual variation in cyclophosphamide (CPA) pharmacokinetics was reported in certain cancer patient groups. To better understand the mechanisms underlying the variation in CPA metabolism, we have investigated the pharmacokinetics of CPA and its active metabolite 4-hydroxycyclophosphamide (4-OH-CPA) in patients with hematological tumors. The pharmacokinetics of CPA and its active metabolite were related to the genotype of CYP2B6, CYP2C9 and CYP2C19. The influence of liver function on CPA metabolism was also evaluated. METHODS: Twenty-nine patients with hematological malignancies (MM, ALL or NHL) treated with a conventional CPA dose (1g/m(2)) were recruited to this study. Blood samples were collected before, during and after CPA treatment. HPLC was used to measure plasma concentrations of CPA and 4-OH-CPA. Patients were genotyped for the CYP2B6 G516T, CYP2C9*2, CYP2C9*3, CYP2C19*2 and CYP2C19*3 alleles. Serum bilirubin levels were measured before the treatment. Data was analyzed individually and by population pharmacokinetic methods, using non-linear mixed effect modeling. RESULTS: The interindividual variability in exposure to CPA, 4-OHCPA and 4-OH-CPA/CPA was 5.8-, 3.3- and 10.3-fold, respectively. A positive correlation between half-lives of CPA and 4-OH-CPA was found while a significant negative correlation between AUCs of CPA and 4-OH-CPA was detected. In the population analysis, the CYP2B6 G516T variant allele contribution to CPA clearance was about twice as the contribution from the wild type gene while the genotype of CYP2C9 and CYP2C19 did not influence clearance. A negative correlation was observed between bilirubin level and CPA bioactivation. CONCLUSION: This study demonstrates for the first time that the presence of the CYP2B6 G516T mutation increases the rate of 4-OH-CPA formation in patients with hematological malignancies. The liver function prior therapy as assessed by s-bilirubin influences CPA metabolism. Publication Types: Clinical Trial

Eur J Pharmacol. 2004 Oct 1;500(1-3):267-80. Related Articles, Links Erratum in: Eur J Pharmacol. 2005 Jan 4;506(3):297. Advances in pharmacogenomics and individualized drug therapy: exciting challenges that lie ahead. Nebert DW, Vesell ES. Division of Human Genetics, Department of Pediatrics and Molecular Developmental Biology, University of Cincinnati Medical Center, P.O. Box 670056, Cincinnati OH 45267-0056, USA. dan.nebert@uc.edu Between the 1930s and 1990s, several dozen predominantly monogenic, high-penetrance disorders involving pharmacogenetics were described, fueling the crusade that gene-drug interactions are quite simple. Then, in 1990, the Human Genome Project was established; in 1995, the term pharmacogenomics was introduced; finally, the complexities of determining an unequivocal phenotype, as well as an unequivocal genotype, have recently become apparent. Since 1965, more than 1000 reviews on this topic have painted an overly optimistic picture-suggesting that the advent of individualized drug therapy used by the practicing physician is fast approaching. For many reasons listed here, however, we emphasize that these high expectations must be tempered. We now realize that the nucleotide sequence of the genome represents only a starting point from which we must proceed to a more difficult stage: knowledge of the function encoded and how this affects the phenotype. To achieve individualized drug therapy, a high level of accuracy and precision is required of any clinical test proposed in human patients. Finally, we suggest that metabonomics, perhaps in combination with proteomics, might complement genomics in eventually helping us to achieve individualized drug therapy. Publication Types: Review

Eur J Pharmacol. 2005 Dec 19;527(1-3):1-22. Epub 2005 Nov 28. Related Articles, Links Pharmacogenomics and cardiovascular drugs: need for integrated biological system with phenotypes and proteomic markers. Siest G, Marteau JB, Maumus S, Berrahmoune H, Jeannesson E, Samara A, Batt AM, Visvikis-Siest S. Inserm U525 Equipe 4, Universite Henri Poincare Nancy I, 30 rue Lionnois Faculte de Pharmacie, 54000 Nancy, France. gerard.siest@pharma.uhp-nancy.fr Personalized medicine is based on a better knowledge of biological variability, considering the important part due to genetics. When trying to identify involved genes and their products in differential cardiovascular drug responses, a five-step strategy is to be followed: 1) Pharmacokinetic-related genes and phenotypes (2) Pharmacodynamic targets, genes and products (3) Cardiovascular diseases and risks depending on specific or large metabolic cycles (4) Physiological variations of previously identified genes and proteins (5) Environment influences on them. After summarizing the most well-known genes involved in drug metabolism, we will take as example of drugs, the statins, considered as very important drugs from a Public-Health standpoint, but also for economical reasons. These drugs respond differently in human depending on multiple polymorphisms. We will give examples with common ApoE polymorphisms influencing the hypolipemic effects of statins. These drugs also have pleiotropic effects and decrease inflammatory markers. This illustrates the need to separate clinical diseases phenotypes in specific metabolic pathways, which could propose other classifications, of diseases and related genes. Hypertension is also a good example of clinical phenotype which should be followed after various therapeutic approaches by genes polymorphisms and proteins markers. Gene products are under clear environmental expression variations such as age, body mass index and obesity, alcohol, tobacco and dietary interventions which are the first therapeutical actions taken in cardiovascular diseases. But at each of the five steps, within a pharmacoproteomic strategy, we also need to use available information from peptides, proteins and metabolites, which usually are the gene products. A profiling approach, i.e., dealing with genomics, but now also with proteomics, is to be used. In conclusion, the profiling, as well as the large amount of data, will more than before render necessary an organized interpretation of DNA, RNA as well as proteins variations, both at individual and population level. Publication Types: Review

Eur J Surg Suppl. 2002;(587):70-6. Related Articles, Links Pharmacogenomics in gastrointestinal disorders. Schreiber S, Costello CM. From the 1st Department of Medicine, Christian-Albrechts-University, Kiel, Germany. s.schreiber@mucosa.de Genomic techniques offer new approaches to the investigation of the aetiology and pathophysiology of intestinal disorders. An important field that is relevant to treatment is the pharmacogenetic investigation of gene variations that may predict response to certain drugs in order to target these drugs more precisely. For the surgeon the perioperative situation will be here of great interest. To date only about 8000 of the estimated 30,000-50,000 human genes have been characterised, so the use of techniques for global analysis of gene expression may allow the identification of new pathways or molecules. In can be anticipated that genomic methods will profoundly influence the treatment of gastrointestinal disorders and will lead to new insights into both aetiology and pathophysiology of chronic intestinal inflammation. Publication Types: Review

Eur Neuropsychopharmacol. 2005 Mar;15(2):143-51. Related Articles, Links Pharmacogenetics of treatment in first-episode schizophrenia: D3 and 5-HT2C receptor polymorphisms separately associate with positive and negative symptom response. Reynolds GP, Yao Z, Zhang X, Sun J, Zhang Z. Department of Mental Health, Queen's University Belfast, Whitla Medical Building, 97 Lisburn Road, Belfast BT9 7BL, UK. g.reynolds@qub.ac.uk We have been studying the pharmacogenetic correlates of side effects and early response to antipsychotic treatment in a series of

Chinese Han first-episode drug-naive patients with schizophrenia. Here, we report the association of three functional polymorphisms of receptor genes on initial symptom severity and outcome in these patients. We studied the dopamine D3 receptor ser9gly, the dopamine D2 receptor Taq IA and the 5-HT2C receptor promoter -759C/T polymorphisms in 117 patients who had symptoms assessed by Positive and Negative Syndrome Scale (PANSS) on admission and following 10-week antipsychotic treatment, primarily with risperidone or chlorpromazine. The D2 polymorphism was found not to be significantly associated with baseline levels or changes in total PANSS in these patients. The D3 genotype is associated with the change in total PANSS ($p<0.01$), an effect reflecting positive and general (each $p<0.01$) but not negative symptom improvement. However, symptom improvement at 10 weeks strongly correlates with total PANSS score on admission, in which the greater improvement is seen with the more severe initial symptom score. The D3 genotype is also related to severity on admission, i.e. to total baseline PANSS ($p<0.05$), including baseline PANSS score as a covariate, the association of the genotype to change over 10 weeks remains significant for total PANSS ($p<0.05$) and for positive and general, but not negative, symptom scores. The 5-HT2C promoter polymorphism was also associated with improvement in PANSS ($p<0.05$), but reflecting effects on negative and general, but not positive, symptom scores. This polymorphism was not associated with PANSS score on admission, although after controlling for the effect of this parameter on 10-week outcome, a stronger association with change in total PANSS ($p<0.01$) was apparent, again reflecting improvements in negative and general symptoms but not changes in positive symptoms.

Eur Neuropsychopharmacol. 2006 Feb 1; [Epub ahead of print] Related Articles, Links Association study of two serotonin 1A receptor gene polymorphisms and fluoxetine treatment response in Chinese major depressive disorders. Yu YW, Tsai SJ, Liou YJ, Hong CJ, Chen TJ. Yu's Psychiatric Clinic, Kaohsiung, Taiwan. The firing rate of dorsal raphe serotonergic neurons is modulated by somatodendritic 5-hydroxytryptamine 1A (HTR1A) autoreceptors. Evidence from animal and clinical studies has suggested that desensitization of HTR1A is implicated in the antidepressant therapeutic mechanism of selective serotonin reuptake inhibitors (SSRIs). Recent studies, including our recent findings, have reported that a functional HTR1A C-1019G polymorphism in the promoter region, as well as a nonsynonymous polymorphism, Gly272Asp, may be associated with SSRI pharmacogenetics. In this study, we tested whether Gly272Asp genetic variants are related to a 4-week fluoxetine antidepressant effect in 222 Chinese major depressive patients. We also tested the linkage disequilibrium (LD) measurement between HTR1A Gly272Asp and C-1019G polymorphisms, and haplotype analysis was conducted to assess the association between the two markers within the HTR1A gene and fluoxetine antidepressant response. The results show that the HTR1A Gly272Asp polymorphism was not associated with fluoxetine therapeutic response. The two markers are in strong LD and the HTR1A haplotype of the two polymorphisms is associated with fluoxetine therapeutic response. This association is gender-specific and mostly arises from the effect of HTR1A C-1019G polymorphism: female patients with -

1019C/C genotype showed a better response than -1019G carriers. These findings need to be confirmed in other ethnic populations. y publisher]

Evid Based Cardiovasc Med. 2001 Dec;5(4):109-10. Related Articles, Links Pharmacogenetics in Evidence-based practice--what to watch for. Kilborn M. Publication Types: Editorial rug Metab. 2005 Dec;6(6):553-68. Related Articles, Links Improving cancer therapeutics by molecular profiling. Corchero J, Fernandez-Salguero PM. Departamento de Bioquimica y Biologia Molecular, Facultad de Ciencias, Universidad de Extremadura, Avenida de Elvas s/n 06071 Badajoz, Spain. The individualized medicine aims to identify the molecular basis of the individual's response to different therapeutic treatments. Individualized medicine is very relevant for human diseases such as cancer and it has become a major task to accomplish more efficient and specific therapeutics. An individualized response to treatment could underline therapeutic success or failure and, even more, could support the rationale for good or bad prognosis. The use of up to date genomic approaches is changing the way we understand modern medicine in terms of drug efficacy, toxicity and diagnosis. Results from genetic polymorphism studies, gene expression profiling and epigenetics illustrate how pharmacogenomic testing will contribute to the goal of individualized medicine. Antineoplastic drugs are designed to block the anomalous activity of specific molecules (therapeutic targets) that regulate cellular processes such as cell cycle. Understanding the relationship between molecular changes in therapeutic targets and enhanced antitumoral response or chemotherapeutic resistance is crucial to establish the clinical relevance of genomic approaches. The goal of this review is to discuss the basic and the clinical significance of genomic research on drug targets and its impact on the early diagnosis and treatment of cancer. We will also assess how these methodologies could contribute to individualized medicine in oncology. A special focus will be put on oncogenes and tumor suppressor genes. Aspects such as drug efficacy, side effects and the diagnostic value of antineoplastic pharmacogenomic research will be also considered. Publication Types: Review

Exp Physiol. 2005 May;90(3):283-9. Epub 2005 Mar 18. Related Articles, Links Cardiovascular pharmacogenomics. Johnson JA, Cavallari LH. UF Center for Pharmacogenomics, University of Florida, Gainesville, FL, USA. johnson@cop.ufl.edu There is large interpatient variability in the response to drugs, including cardiovascular drugs. Thus, while some patients achieve the desired therapeutic response from their drug therapy, others do not. There is also a subset of patients who will experience adverse effects, which can range from bothersome to life threatening. Research in recent years has provided compelling evidence that in many cases, genetics contributes importantly to this variable drug response. Thus, pharmacogenomics is a field focused on unravelling the genetic determinants of variable drug response. Examples from the literature of genetic associations with drug efficacy and toxicity are described to provide insight into the field, including the roles of genetic variability in drug-metabolizing enzymes and drug targets. There is also a detailed discussion of the experimental approaches used in cardiovascular pharmacogenomics. Current research is largely focused on a limited candidate gene approach, which allows for description of significant genetic associations with variable response, but often does not explain the genetic basis of variable drug response enough to be useful clinically. As such, there is a move towards genome-wide approaches, and the various technologies available to obtain genomic data are discussed. Cardiovascular pharmacogenomics has the potential for leading to improvements in the use of cardiovascular drug therapy, through selection of the most appropriate drug therapy in an individual based on their genetic information. It will probably be a decade or more before genetic information is widely used in drug therapy decisions, but it seems clear that important findings in the area will continue to expand and the experimental approaches will continue to evolve. Publication Types: Review

Expert Opin Drug Deliv. 2005 Jul;2(4):683-705. Related Articles, Links Role of efflux pumps and metabolising enzymes in drug delivery. Katragadda S, Budda B, Anand BS, Mitra AK. University of Missouri-Kansas City, Division of Pharmaceutical Sciences, School of Pharmacy, 64110-2499, USA. The impact of efflux pumps and metabolic enzymes on the therapeutic activity of various drugs has been well established. The presence of efflux pumps on various tissues and tumours has been shown to regulate the intracellular concentration needed to achieve therapeutic activity. The notable members of efflux proteins include P-glycoprotein, multi-drug resistance protein and breast cancer resistance protein. These efflux pumps play a pivotal role not only in extruding xenobiotics but also in maintaining the body's homeostasis by their ubiquitous presence and ability to coordinate among themselves. In this review, the role of efflux pumps in drug delivery and the importance of their tissue distribution is discussed in detail. To improve pharmacokinetic parameters of substrates, various strategies that modulate the activity of efflux proteins are also described. Drug metabolising enzymes mainly include the cytochrome P450 family of enzymes. Extensive drug metabolism due to the this family of enzymes is the leading cause of therapeutic inactivity. Therefore, the role of metabolising enzymes in drug delivery and disposition is extensively discussed in this review. The synergistic relationship between metabolising enzymes and efflux proteins is also described in detail. In summary, this review emphasises the urgent need to make changes in drug discovery and drug delivery as efflux pumps and metabolising enzymes play an important role in drug delivery and disposition. Publication Types: Review

Expert Opin Drug Saf. 2004 May;3(3):231-48. Related Articles, Links Risk-benefit of antiemetics in prevention and treatment of chemotherapy-induced nausea and vomiting. Herrstedt J. Department of Oncology, Copenhagen University Hospital, Herlev, Denmark. jrhe@herlevhosp.kbhamt.dk The development of effective antiemetic prophylaxis is one of the most significant steps forward in the area of supportive care. Fifteen years ago, patients receiving chemotherapy had to face the fact that nausea and vomiting were inevitable adverse effects, which could only be partially prevented by treatment with antiemetics such as dopamine (DA) D2 receptor antagonists and corticosteroids. The first group of drugs specifically developed as antiemetics was the serotonin (5-hydroxytryptamine [5-HT](3)) receptor antagonists. These drugs have dramatically improved prophylaxis of chemotherapy-induced emesis, particularly when used in combination with a corticosteroid. This combination has resulted in a significant decrease in the number of patients vomiting, whereas the improvement in the prophylaxis of nausea has been less successful. Another group of antiemetics, the neurokinin (NK) 1 receptor antagonists, has recently been developed, and the first drug in this class, aprepitant, has been approved by the FDA and the EU authorities. Studies have showed that patients benefit from the use of this drug in combination with standard antiemetic therapy (5-HT 3 receptor antagonist plus a corticosteroid), both in the acute and delayed phase of nausea and vomiting induced by cisplatin-based chemotherapy. This development has not only led to improved efficacy but also to a decreased risk associated with the use of antiemetics. One of the problems with traditional antiemetics, for example, the DA D2 receptor antagonists, is the risk of unpleasant adverse effects including restlessness and dystonic reactions. To avoid these adverse effects, combination with benzodiazepines or antihistamines was necessary, often resulting in sedation. Modern research also includes pharmacogenomic investigations. This has led to speculation about the importance of drug-drug interactions involving antiemetics through competition for metabolism by the cytochrome P450 isoenzymes. The worst possible interaction would be a decrease in the effect of different cytotoxins but there is no evidence that such interactions are of importance in daily clinical practice. Guidelines are useful tools in the optimisation of antiemetic prophylaxis but, unfortunately, implementation of the evidence-based recommendations is far from successful. A prerequisite for further optimisation of antiemetic prophylaxis is updating of the guidelines, including recommendations for the use of NK 1 receptor antagonists (aprepitant), followed by implementation of these recommendations in the clinic. Future research must include 'the difficult trials' focusing on the remaining groups of patients with severe chemotherapy-induced nausea and vomiting, including patients with refractory and breakthrough emesis. Publication Types: Review

Expert Opin Pharmacother. 2005 Aug;6(9):1463-76. Related Articles, Links Personalised medicine for cancer: from drug development into clinical practice. Jain KK. Jain PharmaBiotech, Blaesiring 74057 Basel, Switzerland. jain@pharmabiotech.ch Personalised management of cancer means the prescription of specific therapeutics that are best suited for an individual patient and the type of tumour. Molecular diagnostics influences cancer management in several ways that aid personalisation. These technologies are enabling the classification of cancer, using molecular profiles, as a basis for more effective personalised therapies. Using microarrays, classification of a cancer based on the gene expression profile is important for personalising cancer therapy. Molecular imaging, such as by positron emission tomography, enables determination of tumour response to drug action at the molecular level. The combination of diagnostics with therapeutics--an important feature of personalised cancer therapy--is facilitated by the use of monoclonal antibodies and nanobiotechnology. Development of drug resistance--an important problem in cancer management--varies according to the anticancer agent, type of tumour and individual patient. There are no universal strategies to overcome drug resistance in cancer. Various efforts to deal with this problem should be tailored to each patient, and examples are given in this review. A better understanding of cancer biology will facilitate rational drug discovery for cancer, by linking the various pathways involved to targeted therapies. Oncoproteomics will play an important role in the development of personalised cancer therapy. Use of pharmacogenomic technologies in early clinical trials is enabling rapid assessment of the efficacy of anticancer agents, and reducing the time of drug development. Application of pharmacogenetics will reduce the adverse effect of anticancer drugs. Cell/gene therapies, cancer vaccines and RNA interference will facilitate the development of personalised cancer therapy.

Expert Opin Pharmacother. 2005 Dec;6(15):2577-91. Related Articles, Links The PPAR genes, cardiovascular disease and the emergence of PPAR pharmacogenetics. Cresci S. Department of Medicine, Washington University School of Medicine, 660 South Euclid Avenue, Campus Box 8086, Saint Louis, MO 63110-1093, USA. scresci@im.wustl.edu The peroxisome proliferator-activated receptors (PPARs) comprise a group of related transcription factors that serve to regulate a number of cellular processes that are central to cardiovascular health and disease. Two large bodies of work strongly implicate the PPARs as key factors in normal cardiovascular physiology and in cardiovascular pathophysiology: i) studies demonstrating associations between PPAR and abnormal cardiovascular phenotypes; and ii) pharmacological studies assessing the effects of specific PPAR agonists in clinical trials. With the abundance of data available from these studies as a background, PPAR pharmacogenetics has become a promising and rapidly-advancing field. This review summarises the current state of understanding of PPAR pharmacogenetics and its profound implications for the individualisation of therapy for patients with a diverse group of cardiovascular diseases.

Expert Opin Pharmacother. 2005 Dec;6(15):2593-605. Related Articles, Links Does pharmacogenetics have the potential to allow the individualisation of immunosuppressive drug dosing in organ transplantation? MacPhee IA, Fredericks S, Holt DW. Cellular and Molecular Medicine, Renal Medicine, St. George's Hospital, University of London, Cranmer Terrace, London, SW17 0RE, UK. imacphee@sgul.ac.uk The immunosuppressive drugs used in organ transplantation have a narrow therapeutic index, with rejection occurring as a consequence of underdosing and infection, malignancy and a number of drug-specific side effects with excessive dosing. Significant heterogeneity in the dose of drug required to achieve therapeutic blood concentrations adds to the complexity of the problem, which has been partly resolved by therapeutic drug monitoring. Single nucleotide polymorphisms have been identified in genes encoding metabolic enzymes, drug efflux pumps and drug targets for most of the drugs in widespread use. A pharmacogenetic approach to immunosuppressive drug prescribing remains to be tested. Based on current evidence, the most promising strategy would be use of the cytochrome P450 3A5 expresser genotype to guide initial dosing with tacrolimus.

Expert Opin Pharmacother. 2005 Dec;6(15):2607-16. Related Articles, Links Pharmacogenetics of colorectal cancer. Marsh S. Division of Oncology, Washington University School of Medicine, 660 South Euclid Ave, Campus Box 8069, St Louis, MO 63110, USA.

smarsh@im.wustl.edu Colorectal cancer is one of the most common types of cancer in both men and women. Multiple chemotherapy combinations exist; however, there is currently no strategy for individualised therapy selection prior to treatment. Genetic polymorphisms in genes involved in the metabolism, transport or targets for the commonly used chemotherapy drugs (5-fluorouracil, irinotecan and oxaliplatin) have been described. Many require validation in large prospective trials before they can be used as markers for outcome and/or toxicity. This review describes the data available on polymorphisms in key genes that are associated with chemotherapy toxicity and response in colorectal cancer.

Expert Opin Pharmacother. 2005 Jul;6(8):1305-12. Related Articles, Links The role of common variation in drug transporter genes in refractory epilepsy. Soranzo N, Goldstein DB, Sisodiya SM. Department of Biology, University College London, Queen Square, London, UK. Resistance to antiepileptic drugs (AEDs) is one of the most serious clinical problems in epilepsy, and along with AED teratogenicity, perhaps the major concern of epilepsy pharmacogenetics. Studying the genetics of drug resistance in epilepsy is important, as it may identify or confirm key mechanisms underlying this phenomenon that have real clinical importance; it might also offer insights into its prediction and management. Drug resistance in epilepsy is likely to be multifactorial: overactivity of multi-drug transporters provides one likely underlying mechanism through lowering of AED concentration in the epileptogenic focus. Genetic association studies may provide a tool to assess this 'transporter' hypothesis by determining whether differences between individuals contribute to resistance phenotypes. Most of these studies have investigated one variant in the ABCB1 gene, and have provided, thus far, inconclusive evidence. This review also considers current knowledge of the role of genetic polymorphisms in multi-drug transporters in pharmacoresistant epilepsy, to highlight possible confounding factors affecting the implementation and interpretation of association studies in this field.

Expert Opin Pharmacother. 2006 Feb;7(2):119-33. Related Articles, Links Pharmacogenetics for off-patent antipsychotics: reframing the risk for tardive dyskinesia and access to essential medicines. Ozdemir V, Aklillu E, Mee S, Bertilsson L, Albers LJ, Graham JE, Caligiuri M, Lohr JB, Reist C. VA Long Beach Healthcare System, Southern California Institute for Research and Education, Department of Psychiatry and Human Behavior, College of Medicine, University of California, Irvine, Long Beach, CA 90822, USA. pgxethics@hotmail.com First-generation antipsychotics (FGAs) induce tardive dyskinesia, a debilitating involuntary hyperkinetic movement disorder, in 20-50% of individuals with a psychotic illness during chronic treatment. There is presently no curative treatment or definitive predictive test for tardive dyskinesia. The authors note that the three antipsychotic drugs enlisted in the most recent (14th) World Health Organization Model List of Essential Medicines--chlorpromazine, fluphenazine and haloperidol--belong to the FGA therapeutic class. In this regard, the need to choose between the competing objectives of ensuring global access to affordable and efficacious medicines, such as FGAs, and the formidable long-term risk for tardive dyskinesia, may create an ethical conundrum. Pharmacogenetics has thus far been conceptually framed as a tool to individualize therapy with new drugs under patent protection. However, the authors suggest that pharmacogenetics may also improve access to pharmacotherapy through the reintroduction of affordable second-line generic drugs or FGAs with suboptimal safety, as first-line therapy, in targeted subpopulations in whom they present a lower risk for tardive dyskinesia. To impact positively on global public health and distributive justice, a directory complementary to the essential medicines library--one that enlists the 'essential biomarkers' required for optimal pharmacotherapy--may benefit patients who do not have adequate access to new antipsychotic medications. This review discusses pharmacogenetic associations of tardive dyskinesia that are in part supported by meta-analyses and the oxidative stress-neuronal degeneration hypothesis.

Expert Rev Anti Infect Ther. 2003 Jun;1(1):75-81. Related Articles, Links Optimized antiretroviral therapy: the role of therapeutic drug monitoring and pharmacogenomics. van Heeswijk RP. Clinical Investigation Unit, Division of Infectious Diseases, The Ottawa Hospital, 501 Smyth Road, Ottawa, ON, K1H 8L6, Canada. rvanheeswijk@ottawahospital.on.ca. The identification of relationships between plasma concentrations of protease inhibitors and later, the non-nucleoside reverse transcriptase inhibitors and their efficacy and toxicity has caused a growing interest in the concept of therapeutic drug monitoring in the treatment of HIV infection. Some evidence suggests a beneficial effect of therapeutic drug monitoring of protease inhibitors. More recently, plasma protease inhibitor concentrations have been combined with viral susceptibility into one parameter, the inhibitory quotient, which may be a better predictor of the response to therapy, especially in pretreated patients. This paper reviews the current literature on therapeutic drug monitoring and the inhibitory quotient in the management of HIV infection and speculates on the future role of pharmacogenomics in this therapeutic area. Publication Types: Review

Expert Rev Anticancer Ther. 2005 Jun;5(3):415-7. Related Articles, Links 6th International Symposium and expert workshops on Leukemia and Lymphoma. 17-19 March, 2005, Amsterdam, The Netherlands. Kaspers GJ. Division of Oncology-Hematology, Department of Pediatrics, VU University Medical Center, De Boelelaan 1117, NL-1081 HV Amsterdam, The Netherlands. gjl.kaspers@vumc.nl Publication Types: Congresses

Expert Rev Mol Diagn. 2004 Nov;4(6):761-77. Related Articles, Links QA/QC: challenges and pitfalls facing the microarray community and regulatory agencies. Shi L, Tong W, Goodsaid F, Frueh FW, Fang H, Han T, Fuscoe JC, Casciano DA. US Food and Drug Administration, Center for Toxicoinformatics, Division of Systems Toxicology, National Center for Toxicological Research, HFT-020, 3900 NCTR Road, Jefferson, AR 72079, USA. Leming.Shi@fda.hhs.gov The scientific community has been enthusiastic about DNA microarray technology for pharmacogenomic and toxicogenomic studies in the hope of advancing personalized medicine and drug development. The US Food and Drug Administration has been proactive in promoting the use of pharmacogenomic data in drug development and has issued a draft guidance for the pharmaceutical industry on data submissions. However, many challenges and pitfalls are facing the microarray community and regulatory agencies before microarray data can be reliably applied to support regulatory decision making. Four types of factors (i.e., technical, instrumental, computational and interpretative) affect the outcome of a microarray study, and a major concern about microarray studies has been the lack of reproducibility and accuracy. Intralaboratory data consistency is the foundation of reliable knowledge extraction and meaningful crosslaboratory or crossplatform comparisons; unfortunately, it has not been seriously evaluated and demonstrated in every study. Profound problems in data quality have been observed from analyzing published data sets, and many laboratories have been struggling with technical troubleshooting rather than generating reliable data of scientific significance. The microarray community and regulatory agencies must work together to establish a set of consensus quality assurance and quality control criteria for assessing and ensuring data quality, to identify critical factors affecting data quality, and to optimize and standardize microarray procedures so that biologic interpretation and decision-making are not based on unreliable data. These fundamental issues must be adequately addressed before microarray technology can be transformed from a research tool to clinical practices. Publication Types: Review

Expert Rev Mol Diagn. 2005 Nov;5(6):947-53. Related Articles, Links Pyrosequencing: nucleotide sequencing technology with bacterial genotyping applications. Clarke SC. Portsmouth City Primary Care Trust, Finchdean House, Portsmouth, PO3 6DP, UK. stuartcclarke@hotmail.com Pyrosequencing is a relatively new method for real-time nucleotide sequencing. It has rapidly found applications in DNA sequencing, genotyping, single nucleotide polymorphism analysis, allele quantification and whole-genome sequencing within the areas of microbiology, clinical genetics and pharmacogenetics. It is fast becoming a real alternative to the traditional Sanger sequencing method although, at present, read lengths are normally limited to approximately 70 nucleotides. The pyrosequencing method involves four main stages: first, target DNA is amplified using PCR; second, double-stranded DNA is converted to single-stranded DNA templates; third, oligonucleotide primers are hybridized to a complementary sequence of interest; and, finally, the pyrosequencing reaction itself, in which a reaction mixture of enzymes and substrates catalyses the synthesis of complementary nucleotides. Data are shown as a collection of signal peaks in a pyrogram. Pyrosequencing is increasingly used for bacterial detection, identification and typing, and, recently, a commercial system became available for the identification of bacterial isolates. Pyrosequencing can also be partially or fully automated, thus enabling the high-throughput analysis of samples. Wider use of pyrosequencing may occur in the future if longer nucleotide reads are made possible, which will enable its expansion into larger nucleotide sequencing such as multilocus sequence typing and whole-genome sequencing.

Expert Rev Mol Diagn. 2005 Sep;5(5):643-8. Related Articles, Links FDA perspectives on pharmacogenetic testing. Harper CC, Philip R, Robinowitz M, Gutman SI. Center for Devices and Radiological

Health, Office of In Vitro Diagnostic Device Evaluation and Safety, US Food and Drug Administration, HFZ-440, 2098 Gaither Rd, Rockville, MD 20850, USA. courtney.harper@fda.hhs.gov The field of pharmacogenetic testing is emerging as a topic of interest for many, due to its potential to improve patient care and optimize therapeutic development. The US Food and Drug Administration is interested in incorporating pharmacogenetics into development activities whenever appropriate to protect and promote public health. This article is intended to reflect the opinions of the Office of In vitro Diagnostic Device Evaluation and Safety in the Center for Devices and Radiological Health on some issues associated with developing in vitro diagnostic devices for use in pharmacogenetics. General points and potential issues related to the analytical and clinical validation of these types of devices will be discussed.

Expert Rev Mol Diagn. 2005 Sep;5(5):755-67. Related Articles, Links Molecular diagnosis of ATP-binding cassette transporter-related diseases. Schuierer MM, Langmann T. University of Regensburg, Institute of Pathology, Franz-Josef-Strauss Allee 11, D-93053, Germany. marion.schuierer@klinik.uni-regensburg.de ATP-binding cassette (ABC) transporters are involved in a variety of physiologic processes such as xenobiotic defense, lipid metabolism, ion homeostasis and immune functions. A large number of ABC proteins have been causatively linked to rare and common human genetic diseases including familial high-density lipoprotein deficiency, retinopathies, cystic fibrosis, diabetes and cardiomyopathies. Furthermore, genetic variations in ABC transporter genes and dysregulated expression patterns of these molecules significantly contribute to drug resistance in human cancer cells and alter the pharmacokinetic properties of a variety of drugs. In order to analyze DNA sequence alterations or define disease-associated mRNA expression patterns of the complete ABC transporter superfamily, novel high-throughput molecular methods such as quantitative real-time PCR and DNA microarray analysis are emerging. The aim of this review is to provide an overview and to present some examples of human ABC transporters involved in monogenic diseases, cancer and pharmacogenetics. Methodologic aspects of molecular diagnostics applied to analyze genetic variations, mRNA and protein expression levels and functional characteristics of ABC transporters are discussed.

Expert Rev Mol Diagn. 2006 Mar;6(2):145-52. Related Articles, Links Affymetrix GeneChip system: moving from research to the clinic. Ragoussis J, Elvidge G. Genomics Laboratory, Wellcome Trust Centre for Human Genetics, Oxford University, Oxford, OX3 7BN, UK. ioannis.ragoussis@well.ox.ac.uk Affymetrix Inc.'s GeneChip technology has become the industry standard in microarray-based research. Due to the high density of content per array that can be achieved today (an industry leading 6.5 million features) the GeneChips can be used for high-throughput mutation detection, single nucleotide polymorphism genotyping, expression profiling and detection of chromosomal aberrations. This in turn opens the way for clinical applications in genetics, cytogenetics, pharmacogenetics, oncology and pathogen recognition. Establishing standards is a central issue in improving data quality and, in combination with automatic, easy-to-interpret reports, will form the basis of the clinical applicability. Future pricing policies and the resolving of ethical considerations will also dictate the technology's full translation from research into clinical laboratories.

Expert Rev Mol Diagn. 2006 Mar;6(2):193-205. Related Articles, Links Pharmacogenetics in clinical practice: considerations for testing. Constable S, Johnson MR, Pirmohamed M. Department of Pharmacology and Therapeutics, Ashton Street Medical School, University of Liverpool, Ashton Street, Liverpool, L69 3GE, UK. s.constable@liverpool.ac.uk Pharmacogenetics is a rapidly evolving field that will undoubtedly lead to the development of pharmacogenetic tests. Such tests will need to be assimilated into healthcare systems, but represent a further call on scarce healthcare resources. Therefore, in order for a pharmacogenetic test to fulfill its potential beyond the laboratory and into the clinical environment, it must prove itself on a wide range of multifaceted criteria. The test must have proven and reproducible analytical and clinical validity, and stand up to critical appraisal of clinical utility and cost-effectiveness. Pharmacogenetic testing can be considered to be a form of screening, and the experience that has been gained to date in evaluating other forms of screening tests may prove beneficial in evaluating pharmacogenetic technology. It is essential that the goals of pharmacogenetic testing are defined as early as possible to ensure that appropriate studies can be designed to provide the evidence base, and thereby enable appropriate evaluation of the technology by clinicians and healthcare administrators for incorporation into clinical practice. This review focuses on issues that will need to be considered in the scientific assessment of pharmacogenetic testing.

FDA Consum. 2005 Jan-Feb;39(1):36-7. Related Articles, Links Genetics play role in response to asthma drugs. [No authors listed]

FDA Consum. 2005 Jul-Aug;39(4):10-5. Related Articles, Links Does sex make a difference? Bren L.

FDA Consum. 2005 Jul-Aug;39(4):4. Related Articles, Links Personalized medicine. [No authors listed] Publication Types: News

FDA Consum. 2005 Mar-Apr;39(2):2. Related Articles, Links First-of-a-kind genetic lab test. [No authors listed] Publication Types: News

Fertil Steril. 2004 Mar;81 Suppl 2:4-8. Related Articles, Links Mining the human genome for new health therapies. Zilberstein M. USA. The completion of the Human Genome Project heralds advances in determining the foundations of disease and in developing new therapeutic treatments. Tests already exist for the detection of some genetic abnormalities that can cause disease, and more are being developed. In the future, pharmacogenetics will be used to tailor treatment to specific patients.

Fertil Steril. 2004 May;81(5):1187-93. Related Articles, Links Monitoring plasma concentrations to individualize treatment with clomiphene citrate. Rostami-Hodjegan A, Lennard MS, Tucker GT, Ledger WL. Department of Molecular Pharmacology and Pharmacogenetics, University of Sheffield, Sheffield, United Kingdom. a.rostami@sheffield.ac.uk OBJECTIVE: Recent reports have indicated that a number of individual patient characteristics are responsible for the success or failure of clomiphene citrate treatment. However, a priori individualization of doses in different patients has not been investigated. We examined the thesis that wide variability in the metabolism of the active component (zuclomiphene) contributes to variability in response. METHODS: The dose-response relationship of clomiphene was established from a meta-analysis of data from 13 published reports. Limited data relating plasma drug concentrations to treatment outcome were examined to determine whether insufficient systemic exposure at a fixed dosage might contribute to therapeutic failure. RESULTS: A fixed-dosage regimen of 50 mg clomiphene per day is likely to cause ovulation in only 46% of patients; subsequent increment in dosage increases the number of responders but at the expense of considerable delay in individualization of treatment. Case reports indicated that dosage based on plasma drug concentration monitoring could improve patient management, and an algorithm is proposed to facilitate treatment. CONCLUSIONS: Prospective studies of clomiphene citrate should be performed to confirm the hypothesis that the monitoring of plasma zuclomiphene concentrations can significantly accelerate dose individualization and improve the therapeutic outcome with this "orphan" drug.

Fetal Pediatr Pathol. 2004 Jul-Aug;23(4):211-29. Related Articles, Links Developmental renal pathology: its past, present, and future. Rodriguez MM. University of Miami, School of Medicine, Jackson Children's Hospital, Department of Pathology, 1611 NW 12 Avenue, Miami, FL 33184, USA. mrodrig2@med.miami.edu Congenital anomalies of the kidney and urinary tract are responsible for approximately 40% of cases of childhood end-stage renal failure in the United States. This article describes the spectrum of developmental renal lesions in children (including renal agenesis, dysplasias, hereditary hydronephrosis, autosomal recessive and dominant polycystic kidneys, vesicoureteral reflux, diabetic embryopathy, some teratogenic drugs affecting renal development, and syndromes associated with renal dysplasias). The article quotes some historic references that established the foundation for further studies; reviews the embryology, pathology, postnatal renal development, and its possible consequences of renal function; as well as recent advances in fetal ultrasonography and molecular biology with some novel treatment and diagnostic modalities. Finally, an attempt is made to predict several future avenues in pharmacogenetics that are being built currently and that will allow a better prognosis for many children with congenital renal conditions. Publication Types: Review

Fiziol Cheloveka. 2004 Mar-Apr;30(2):76-85. Related Articles, Links [Pharmacological ethnic metabolic safety. Communication II] [Article in Russian] Piruzian LA, Mikhailovskii EM.

Food Drug Law J. 2004;59(4):519-35. Related Articles, Links Legal implications of pharmacogenomics regarding drug trials, drug labeling, and genetic testing for drug prescription: an international approach. Mandry T. Pharmacogenomics applies genomic technology to discover and develop drugs as well as to treat patients more effectively. This article addresses legal questions raised by pharmacogenomics, from drug development to drug use. Part II defines pharmacogenomics in further detail and explains the use of pharmacogenomics in drug development. Part III identifies potential legal questions raised by this approach to drug development and delivery. Parts IV to VIII offer possible solutions to these potential problems, analyzing the law in both the United States and the European Union (EU).

Fortune. 2005 Mar 7;151(5):60. Related Articles, Links The pharma of tomorrow. Haseltine W. Publication Types: News

Free Radic Biol Med. 2005 Jul 15;39(2):152-63. Epub 2005 Mar 30. Related Articles, Links Pharmacogenomic profiling of an oxidative stress-mediated spongiform encephalopathy. Golden TR, Hubbard A, Morten KJ, Hinerfeld D, Melov S. Buck Institute for Age Research, 8001 Redwood Boulevard, Novato, CA 94945, USA. The majority of cellular superoxide is generated in the mitochondria as a by-product of normal oxidative metabolism. In the mitochondria, superoxide is detoxified by manganese superoxide dismutase (SOD2). Mice lacking SOD2 demonstrate a multifaceted neonatal lethal phenotype, including a spongiform encephalopathy that is preventable through antioxidant treatment. The molecular events behind the observed pathology in the cortex of these mice are unknown. We hypothesized that the lack of SOD2 would result in significant changes in cortical gene expression and that therapeutically beneficial antioxidant treatment would normalize the expression of some genes, providing insight into the mechanism by which mitochondrial oxidative stress results in neurodegeneration. We report the identification of gene expression profiles associated with this paradigm, which characterize the degree of response to the pharmacologic intervention. We have identified specific pathways targeted by endogenous oxidative stress, including glutathione metabolism, iron metabolism, and cell-survival pathways centering on the kinase AKT. The normalization of expression of some of these pathways by antioxidant treatment suggests approaches to treating disease in which endogenous oxidative stress plays a role.

Front Biosci. 2005 Sep 1;10:2892-903. Related Articles, Links Androgen metabolic genes in prostate cancer predisposition and progression. Makridakis NM, Buchanan G, Tilley W, Reichardt JK. Department of Biochemistry and Molecular Biology, Institute for Genetic Medicine, USC Keck School of Medicine, 2250 Alcazar Street, Los Angeles, CA 90089-9075, USA. Significant evidence implicates androgens in prostate cancer etiology. We review recent data with regard to the association between several allelic variants of specific androgen-metabolic genes and the predisposition to prostate cancer. We also review the emerging evidence regarding the role of genetic variants of these genes as well as the androgen receptor in prostate cancer progression. Based on the prostate cancer paradigm, we propose that a multidisciplinary attack on the problem--involving biochemistry, genetics, pharmacogenetics, endocrinology and molecular epidemiology--may be important for the understanding and successful treatment of complex (in terms of etiology) human diseases.

Fukuoka Igaku Zasshi. 2004 Oct;95(10):253. Related Articles, Links [Correlation between 21st century COE of Center for Frontier Research Education on Lifestyle-Related Disease based on the large-scale cohort study and Kyushu University Hospital] [Article in Japanese] Nawata H. Department of Medicine and Bioregulatory Science, Graduate School of Medical Sciences, Kyushu University.

Fundam Clin Pharmacol. 2004 Dec;18(6):705-8. Related Articles, Links

Pharmacogenomics in cardiovascular clinical trials. Shah R, Darne B, Atar D, Abadie E, Adams KF, Zannad F; 5th Cardiovascular Clinical Trialists Workshop. CIC INSERM-CHU, Hopital Jeanne d'Arc, 54200 Dommartin Les Toul, France. Genomics - having quickly emerged as the central discipline in basic science and biomedical research - is poised to take the center stage in clinical medicine as well over the next few decades. Although there is no specific regulatory guideline on the application of pharmacogenetics to drug development, some recommendations are already included in several published guidelines on drug development. The patients more likely to provide the most valuable information on the specific contribution of a given gene or its variant are those who fail to respond to a drug ('therapeutic failures') and those who develop toxicity to the drug. However, before drawing definite conclusions on subgroups following pharmacogenomic analyses, one must be aware of disease classification, data collection, and how much is known about the disease process. It seems reasonable to collect genomic DNA from all patients enrolled in clinical drug trials (along with appropriate consent to permit pharmacogenetic studies) for the purpose of post hoc analyses. One exception to post hoc genomic analysis is when patients with a specific genotype are excluded from randomization into a clinical trial. Physicians will need to understand the concept of genetic variability, its interactions with the environment (e.g. drug-drug or drug-disease interactions), and its implication for patient care.

G Ital Med Lav Ergon. 2004 Oct-Dec;26(4):302-10. Related Articles, Links [New effect biomarkers] [Article in Italian] De Palma G, Corradi M, Mutti A, Baccarelli A, Pesatori A, Bertazzi PA. Dipartimento di Clinica Medica, Nefrologia e Scienze della Prevenzione, Universita degli Studi di Parma. The major research goals for researchers developing biomarkers of effect are the development and validation of biomarkers that permit the prediction of the risk of disease in individuals and groups. One important objective is to prevent human cancer. This article reviews the most recent analytical methodologies, validation studies and field trials together with auditing and quality assessment of the necessary data based on scientific grounds. Consideration is given to new developments in the relatively young field of toxicogenomics, possibly leading to the identification of early changes that may lead to both cancer and non-cancer end points. Although the creation and development of reliable databases integrating information from genomic and proteomic research programmes should offer a contribution to the prediction of risks and prevention of diseases related to chemical exposure, the most promising future application of these technologies lies in the molecular diagnosis of diseases whose nosography will probably be redefined. Publication Types: Review

Gan To Kagaku Ryoho. 2005 Nov;32(12):1886-90. Related Articles, Links [Pharmacogenomic data for personalized medicines] [Article in Japanese] Yamazaki H. Laboratory of Drug Metabolism and Pharmacokinetics, Showa Pharmaceutical University. FDA issued guidance for industry regarding pharmarcogenomic data submission this year. Polymorphic cytochrome P450 2D6 and thiopurine S-methyltransferase in patients are now considered biomarkers for drugs which are predominantly metabolized by these enzymes. This article reviews current efforts to treat pharmacogenomic data for new drug development and personalized medicines. Publication Types: Review

Gan To Kagaku Ryoho. 2005 Nov;32(12):1895-901. Related Articles, Links [Genetic alterations and chemoresistance] [Article in Japanese] Akiyama S. Dept. of Molecular Oncology, Field of Oncology, Course of Advanced Therapeutics, Graduate School of Medical and Dental Sciences, Kagoshima University. Molecular targeting agents will likely play an increasing role in the management of cancer.However, resistance to anti-neoplastic drugs remains a serious obstacle to successful cancer treatment. Analysis of SNPs and microarray technologies should enable us to predict toxic responses and sensitivities to anticancer agents of each patient, and the prediction may permit patient-specific anticancer agents and dosages that reduce the risk of acute toxicity and emergence of drug-resistant tumors. The relationships are reviewed between the chemoresistance(chemosensitivity) and polymorphisms, tumor gene expression profiles or mutations of targeted molecules that confer resistance to molecular target therapy. Publication Types: Review

Gan To Kagaku Ryoho. 2005 Nov;32(12):1902-7. Related Articles, Links [Polygenetic pharmacogenomic strategies to identify drug sensitivity biomarkers] [Article in Japanese] Nishiyama M. Dept. of Translational Cancer Research, Research Institute for Radiation Biology and Medicine, Hiroshima University. Pharmacogenomics is a large-scale systematic approach using a variety of genomic technologies to discover drug response determinants and promote a better understanding of the genetic and molecular basis underlying variable drug response among patients. However, few critical prediction markers of drug response have been validated to date. Drug sensitivity is determined by multiple genes:drugs are often involved in complex metabolic pathways before they produce anti-cancer activity, and the related genes do not act in isolation. Although the worldwide research on the human genome exerts a major impact on medical science and advanced medicine, the detailed function and interaction of most genes remain unclear. There is clear evidence that a variety of genes are closely associated with cellular drug sensitivity, but most of the regulatory mechanisms of their expressions are poorly understood. To understand the drug sensitivity mechanism and identify the key biomarkers, recent attention has focused on the transcriptional mechanisms of drug sensitivity genes and their network. These approaches in genome research and the functional analysis may revolutionize the anticancer chemotherapy world. The possible contribution of new challenges and problems of the day were reviewed while showing recent findings on the analyses of 5-FU metabolic pathway and the key gene DPYD as an example. Publication Types: Review

Gan To Kagaku Ryoho. 2005 Nov;32(12):1908-13. Related Articles, Links [SNPs associated with adverse effects] [Article in Japanese] Isomura M, Miki Y. Genome Center of the Japanese Foundation for Cancer Research. In recent years, pharmacogenomics have received much attention from the increased expectations for so-called order-made medicine. It is experientially clear that inter-individual differences exist in the degree of efficacy and occurrence of adverse effects. These inter-individual differences are observed not only among anticancer chemotherapeutics but in almost all drugs. Several studies have revealed that genetic factors are involved in these inter-individual differences. To date, the relationships have been revealed between adverse effects of some anticancer drugs and polymorphisms of drug metabolizing genes. Such relationships include 5-FU and DPYD gene, methotorexate and MTHFR gene, irinotecan and UGT 1A1 gene and 6-MP and TPMT gene. By using information on these polymorphisms, it will be possible to predict the occurrence of adverse effects before using anticancer drugs. In particular, information on polymorphisms related to the possibly adverse effects of irinotecan is now given in its package leaflet. This means that order-made medicine is a step closer. In this review, we discuss the relationships between polymorphisms of genes and the adverse effects of anticancer drugs. Furthermore, we want to suggest the direction of further pharmacogenomic studies with an eye to the realization of order-made medicine. Publication Types: Review

Gastroenterology. 2004 May;126(6):1533-49. Related Articles, Links Clinical relevance of advances in genetics and pharmacogenetics of IBD. Ahmad T, Tamboli CP, Jewell D, Colombel JF. Gastroenterology Unit, University of Oxford, Gibson Laboratories, Radcliffe Infirmary, Oxford, United Kingdom UK. Crohn's disease and ulcerative colitis result from an inappropriate response of the mucosal immune system to the normal enteric flora in a genetically susceptible individual. During the past decade, exciting progress has been made in our understanding of the contribution of genetics to inflammatory bowel disease susceptibility and phenotype. This article reviews recent advances in the genetics of inflammatory bowel disease and explores how they might impact on clinical practice. Current knowledge of the genetic basis for disease susceptibility, phenotype, and response to therapy is explored and the factors currently limiting the translation of this knowledge to clinical practice is discussed. Publication Types: Review

Genet Med. 2004 Jul-Aug;6(4):165-72. Related Articles, Links Genetic testing: hope or hype? Epstein CJ. Department of Pediatrics, University of California-San Francisco, 533 Parnassus, San Francisco, CA 94143-0748, USA. Publication Types: Addresses

Genet Med. 2005 Feb;7(2):97-104. Related Articles, Links CYP2C9 gene variants, drug dose, and bleeding risk in warfarin-treated patients: a HuGEnet systematic review and meta-analysis. Sanderson S, Emery J, Higgins J. Department of Public Health and Primary Care, University of Cambridge and Cambridge Genetics Knowledge Park, Cambridge, UK. PURPOSE: Two common variant alleles of the cytochrome CYP2C9 (CYP2C9*2 and CYP2C9*3) lead to reduced warfarin metabolism in vitro and in vivo. The study objective was to examine the strength and quality of existing evidence about CYP2C9 gene variants and clinical outcomes in warfarin-treated patients. METHODS: The study was a systematic review and meta-analysis. Multiple electronic databases were searched, references identified from bibliographies were sought, and experts and authors of primary studies were also contacted. Strict review inclusion criteria were determined. Three reviewers independently extracted data using prepiloted proformas. RESULTS: In all, 11 studies meeting review inclusion criteria were identified (3029 patients). Nine were included in the meta-analyses (2775 patients). Random effects meta-analyses were performed; statistical heterogeneity and inconsistency was assessed. Twenty percent of patients studied carry a variant allele: CYP2C9*2 12.2% (9.7%-15.0%) and CYP2C9*3, 7.9% (6.5%-9.7%). Mean difference in daily warfarin dose: for CYP2C9*2, the reduction was 0.85 mg (0.60-1.11 mg), a 17% reduction. For CYP2C9*3, the reduction was 1.92 mg (1.37-2.47 mg), a 37% reduction. For CYP2C9*2 or *3, the reduction was 1.47 mg (1.24-1.71 mg), a 27% reduction. The relative bleeding risk for CYP2C9*2 was 1.91 (1.16-3.17) and for CYP2C9*3 1.77 (1.07-2.91). For either variant, the relative risk was 2.26 (1.36-3.75). CONCLUSIONS: Patients with CYP2C9*2 and CYP2C9*3 alleles have lower mean daily warfarin doses and a greater risk of bleeding. Testing for gene variants could potentially alter clinical management in patients commencing warfarin. Evidence for the clinical utility and cost-effectiveness of genotyping is needed before routine testing can be recommended. Publication Types: Meta-Analysis Review

Genetics. 2005 Jun;170(2):919-28. Epub 2005 Mar 31. Related Articles, Links Theoretical basis for the identification of allelic variants that encode drug efficacy and toxicity. Lin M, Wu R. Department of Statistics, University of Florida, Gainesville, 32611, USA. Almost all drugs that produce a favorable response (efficacy) may also produce adverse effects (toxicity). The relative strengths of drug efficacy and toxicity that vary in human populations are controlled by the combined influences of multiple genes and environmental influences. Genetic mapping has proven to be a powerful tool for detecting and identifying specific DNA sequence variants on the basis of the haplotype map (HapMap) constructed from single-nucleotide polymorphisms (SNPs). In this article, we present a novel statistical model for sequence mapping of two different but related drug responses. This model is incorporated by mathematical functions of drug response to varying doses or concentrations and the statistical device used to model the correlated structure of the residual (co)variance matrix. We implement a closed-form solution for the EM algorithm to estimate the population genetic parameters of SNPs and the simplex algorithm to estimate the curve parameters describing the pharmacodynamic changes of different genetic variants and matrix-structuring parameters. Extensive simulations are performed to investigate the statistical properties of our model. The implications of our model in pharmacogenetic and pharmacogenomic research are discussed.

Genewatch. 2004 Jul-Aug;17(4):6-10. Related Articles, Links The wild genetic goose chase: Neil Holtzman talks about genetics and medicine [interview by Brandon Keim]. Holtzman N. Council for Responsible Genetics, USA.

Genewatch. 2005 Jul-Aug;18(4):8-10. Related Articles, Links The new racial economy: making a silk purse out of the sow's ear of racial distinctions. Balaban E. McGill University, Canada.

Genewatch. 2005 Nov-Dec;18(6):6-9, 18. Related Articles, Links BiDil: false promises: faulty statistics and reasoning have lead to the first "racial medicine". Kahn J. Hamline University School of Law, USA.

Genome Biol. 2004;5(6):108. Epub 2004 May 28. Related Articles, Links Pharmacogenomics arrives. Petsko GA. Rosenstiel Basic Medical Sciences

Research Center, Brandeis University, Waltham, MA 02454-9110, USA. petsko@brandeis.edu Publication Types: Review

Genome Res. 2005 Jan;15(1):67-77. Related Articles, Links Identification of polymorphic motifs using probabilistic search algorithms. Basu A, Chaudhuri P, Majumder PP. Human Genetics Unit, Indian Statistical Institute, Kolkata, 700108 India. The problem of identifying motifs comprising nucleotides at a set of polymorphic DNA sites, not necessarily contiguous, arises in many human genetic problems. However, when the sites are not contiguous, no efficient algorithm exists for polymorphic motif identification. A search based on complete enumeration is computationally inefficient. We have developed probabilistic search algorithms to discover motifs of known or unknown lengths. We have developed statistical tests of significance for assessing a motif discovery, and a statistical criterion for simultaneously estimating motif length and discovering it. We have tested these algorithms on various synthetic data sets and have shown that they are very efficient, in the sense that the "true" motifs can be detected in the vast majority of replications and in a small number of iterations. Additionally, we have applied them to some real data sets and have shown that they are able to identify known motifs. In certain applications, it is pertinent to find motifs that contain contrasting nucleotides at the sites included in the motif (e.g., motifs identified in case-control association studies). For this, we have suggested appropriate modifications. Using simulations, we have discovered that the success rate of identification of the correct motif is high in case-control studies except when relative risks are small. Our analyses of evolutionary data sets resulted in the identification of some motifs that appear to have important implications on human evolutionary inference. These algorithms can easily be implemented to discover motifs from multilocus genotype data by simple numerical recoding of genotypes.

Gesundheitswesen. 2005 Apr;67(4):257-63. Related Articles, Links [Pharmacogenetics in future medical care -- implications for patients and physicians] [Article in German] Rogausch A, Brockmoller J, Himmel W. Bereich Humanmedizin, Abteilung Allgemeinmedizin, Georg-August-Universitat Gottingen. arogaus@gwdg.de PURPOSE: Since public acceptance of pharmacogenetic testing will largely influence their implementation in routine medical care, common implications of pharmacogenetic testing from patients', physicians' and scientists' perspective are reviewed. METHODS: Broad literature review (MEDLINE; MeSH terms: Pharmacogenetics, Delivery of Health Care, Ethics, Attitude, Patient Acceptance of Health Care) of empirical and theoretical studies describing psychological, family-related, social, and ethical consequences of pharmacogenetic testing to describe relevant aspects for further empirical studies. RESULTS: Apart from anticipated benefit, acceptance of pharmacogenetic testing might be influenced by the following: Expectation of negative psychosocial consequences, fear of discrimination or violation of privacy. Due to its great complexity, understanding of test results and explanation of their impact pose new challenges for physician-patient relations. Since most studies are conceptual, empirical studies exploring attitudes of patients/physicians and determining medical as well as economic value of pharmacogenetic testing are imperative. Publication Types: Review

GMHC Treat Issues. 2004 Jan-Feb;18(1-2):1-5. Related Articles, Links HIV and host genetics. Complexity and contradiction. Huff B. Publication Types: Newspaper Article

Gut. 2006 Mar 16; [Epub ahead of print] Related Articles, Links Pharmacogenetics during standardised initiation of thiopurine therapy in inflammatory bowel disease. Hindorf U, Lindqvist M, Peterson C, Soderkvist P, Strom M, Hjortswang H, Pousette A, Almer S. Division of Gastroenterology, Faculty of Medicine, Lund University, Sweden. BACKGROUND: Firm recommendations regarding the way thiopurine drugs are introduced and the use of TPMT and metabolite measurements during treatment in inflammatory bowel disease (IBD) are lacking. AIM: To evaluate pharmacokinetics and tolerance after initiation of thiopurine therapy with a fixed dosing schedule in patients with IBD. PATIENTS: Sixty consecutive patients with Crohn's disease (n=33) or ulcerative colitis (n=27) were included in a 20-week open and prospective study. METHODS: Thiopurine therapy was introduced according to a predefined dose escalation schedule reaching a daily target dose at week 3 of 2.5 mg azathioprine or 1.25 mg 6-mercaptopurine per kg bodyweight. TPMT and ITPA genotypes, TPMT activity, TPMT gene expression, and thiopurine metabolites were determined. Clinical outcome and occurrence of adverse events were monitored. RESULTS: Twenty-seven patients completed the study per protocol, while 33 were withdrawn from the study [early protocol violation (n=5), TPMT deficiency (n=1), thiopurine-related adverse events (n=27)]. Sixty-seven percent of patients with adverse events tolerated long- term treatment on a lower dose (median: 1.32 mg azathioprine/ kg bodyweight). TPMT activity did not change during the 20 week course of the study but a significant decrease in TPMT gene expression was found (TPMT/huCYC ratio; p=0.02). Patients with meTIMP concentrations >11450 pmol/8x108 RBC during steady-state at week 5 had an increased risk of developing myelotoxicity (OR 45.0; p=0.015). CONCLUSION: After initiation of thiopurine therapy by a fixed dosing schedule, no general induction of TPMT enzyme activity occurred, however TPMT gene expression decreased. The developments of different types of toxicity were unpredictable, but we found that measurement of meTIMP early in the steady-state phase help to identify patients at risk of developing myelotoxicity. y publisher]

Gynecol Endocrinol. 2005 Jan;20(1):36-44. Related Articles, Links Human races and pharmacogenomics of effective bone treatments. Massart F. Pediatric Division, Department of Reproductive Medicine and Child Development, University of Pisa, Italy. Osteoporosis and its complications represent one of the most important causes of morbidity and mortality around the world. Moreover, its management presents an important economic problem. Although osteoporosis is a worldwide health problem, there are many differences in ethnic groups regarding disease morbidity and drug treatment efficacy. This review analyzed clinical response data of two major osteoporotic treatments (vitamin D and estrogens) regarding four major human races (Asian, Caucasian, Hispanic and Negroid). From clinical studies, Asians seem to be more vitamin-D-sensitive while Caucasians appear more estrogen-sensitive than other human races. Different drug responses may be related to allelic variants in their signaling genes such as those for the vitamin D receptor (VDR) and estrogen receptor-alpha (ER alpha). Some polymorphisms of VDR and ER alpha loci appear to be genetic determinants of osteoporotic risk: ApaI-BsmI-TaqI, FokI variants and poly(A) repeats in VDR; PvuII-XbaI variants and (TA) repeats in ER alpha. Also, because of specific ethnic allele distributions, these VDR and ER alpha polymorphisms may be involved in race differences of osteoporosis treatment responses. Future studies and preventive strategies for the management of osteoporosis need to take into account these racial and genetic factors. Publication Types: Review

Harefuah. 2005 Oct;144(10):711-6, 750. Related Articles, Links [Pharmacogenetics: towards personalized medicine] [Article in Hebrew] Gurwitz D, Rehavi M. Department of Human Genetics and Molecular Medicine, Sackler Faculty of Medicine, Tel Aviv University, Tel Aviv, Israel. gurwitz@post.tau.ac.il For 50 years, pharmacogenetics has been studying the genetic basis for variability in drug response between individual patients, both with respect to drug toxicity and drug efficacy. Following the completion of The Human Genome Project about three years ago, and the development of technologies allowing rapid identification of polymorphic alleles using DNA chips, pharmacogenetics would soon allow the introduction of personalized medicine. For most medical disciplines, this would allow pharmacotherapy according to each patient's individual genetic data. This would allow a reduction in the rates of adverse drug reactions, currently responsible by American and European estimates for about 6% of new admissions to internal medicine wards, and causing more morbidity annually than road accidents or breast cancer. The purpose of this review is to delineate the principles of pharmacogenetics, focusing on the aspects closest to implementation in the clinic: the polymorphism of liver CYP450 metabolic enzymes, mostly CYP2D6 and CYP2C19. We shall also review current efforts to better understand the scope of human genome diversity, and present several examples for variability in drug efficacy and genetic polymorphism of drug target genes. Education of health professionals in pharmacogenetics as part of their pharmacology curricula, and explaining its potential to the general public, would be indispensable for the success of personalized medicine. Publication Types: Review

Harv Health Lett. 2005 Nov;31(1):4. Related Articles, Links Genetics begets genomics: tailor-made medicine. [No authors listed]

Harv Heart Lett. 2004 May;14(9):4. Related Articles, Links Is your daily aspirin falling down on the job? Not everyone gets the full effect of aspirin. A new test can show if it's working for you. [No authors listed]

Harv Heart Lett. 2005 Nov;16(3):1-2. Related Articles, Links Gray area for new heart failure drug. Although the FDA approved BiDil for blacks with heart failure, it may work in anyone. [No authors listed]

Hautarzt. 2005 Jan;56(1):44-7. Related Articles, Links [Pharmacogenetics: Important aspects for dermatology] [Article in German] Merk HF. Universitat-Hautklinik, Klinik fur Dermatologie and Allergologie der RWTH Aachen. hans.merk@post.rwth-aachen.de Pharmacogenetics, pharmacogenomics or metabonomics are terms reflecting a new trend in pharmacology taking into consideration individual factors which influence the effects of drugs. Examples in dermatology include glucose-6-phosphate dehydrogenase-polymorphism (DADPS), dihydropyrimidine dehydrogenase-deficiency (5-Fluoruracil), thiopurine-S-methyltransferase-deficiency (azathioprine), cytochrome P450 isoenzymes and transferases (drug allergy and allergic contact dermatitis), and intolerant reactions to NSAIDs. Publication Types: Review

Health Educ Behav. 2005 Oct;32(5):668-75. Related Articles, Links Contributions of public health to genetics education for health care professionals. Burke W. Department of Medical History and Ethics, University of Washington, Seattle, WA 98195-7120, USA. wburke@u.washington.edu With growing knowledge about the role of genetics in health, genetics education for health care professionals has taken on increasing importance. Many efforts are under way to develop new genetics curricula. Although such efforts are primarily the responsibility of health professional schools and professional societies, the public health system is an important stakeholder, and different sectors of public health have opportunities to enhance educational efforts. These include the development of authoritative information sources about the clinical utility of genetic susceptibility and pharmacogenetic tests, creation of networks that link professionals in underserved regions to educational materials and consultative backup, and sponsorship of forums for multidisciplinary discussion of controversial issues. Public health input can help to ensure an appropriate emphasis on health outcomes as new genomic tests and technologies come into use, thus helping to protect society from the social and medical costs of genetic tests with limited clinical value.

Health Policy. 2005 Feb;71(2):233-41. Related Articles, Links A lay prescription for tailor-made drugs--focus group reflections on pharmacogenomics. Almarsdottir AB, Bjornsdottir I, Traulsen JM. Faculty of Pharmacy, University of Iceland, Hagi, Hofsvallagata 53, IS-107 Reykjavik, Iceland. annaba@hi.is This study explores the lay view of pharmaceutical research and development--specifically pharmacogenomics. Forty-two persons participated in eight focus groups in Iceland. Participants were asked to comment on a future scenario consisting of predictions made by researchers concerning the consequences of the Human Genome Project over the next 40 years, and asked to give advice to politicians and the pharmaceutical industry. A dominating theme in the focus groups was the expectation that drugs developed based on pharmacogenomics will be more expensive than conventional mass produced drugs and concerns were voiced that this new technology would lead to inequalities locally and globally.

Health Serv Res. 2000 Dec;35(5 Pt 3):128-40. Related Articles, Links Implications of the genetics revolution for health services research: pharmacogenomics and improvements in drug therapy. Phillips KA, Veenstra DL, Sadee W. OBJECTIVE: To review the societal and economic implications of the use of genetic information to individualize drug therapies. Although studies have begun to address the ethical issues raised by the use of genetic information , few have examined the implications of pharmacogenomics f rom the perspective of health services research. PRINCIPAL FINDINGS: We propose a research agenda for health services research in three areas: (1) to evaluate the effectiveness and cost-effectiveness of pharmacogenomics; (2) to evaluate the effect of pharmacogenomics from the perspective of patients, providers, insurers, industry, and government ; and (3) to evaluate the ethical and societal implications of pharmacogenomics. Throughout the article we use the example of HIV genotyping as an illustration of how genetic technology is disseminated and used. CONCLUSION: More research is needed on the societal and economic implications of pharmacogenomics to inform the clinical and policy decisions about its use that will be increasingly urgent in the future. Publication Types: Review

Heart Rhythm. 2005 Nov;2(2 Suppl):S30-7. Related Articles, Links Drug-induced torsades de pointes: the evolving role of pharmacogenetics. Fitzgerald PT, Ackerman MJ. Department of Pediatric and Adolescent Medicine/Division of Pediatric Cardiology, Mayo Clinic College of Medicine, 200 First Street SW, Rochester, MN 55905, USA. Drug-induced torsades de pointes (TdP) is a rare, but potentially lethal, unwanted effect of drugs, including many commonly prescribed noncardiac drugs. Despite its low frequency, drug-induced TdP has generated a great deal of angst among physicians and pharmaceutical companies as well as tragedy, albeit rare, among patients. Although in retrospect many patients who died suddenly as a result of drug-induced TdP had identifiable risk factors, prediction in individual cases remains problematic. Over the past decade, tremendous progress has been made with respect to elucidating the fundamental pathogenic mechanisms that underlie drug-induced TdP. The vast majority of drugs associated with "QT liability" and the potential for drug-induced TdP, including all of the drugs removed from the market because of this side effect, are "HERG (human ether-a-go-go-related gene) blockers." These drugs inhibit the KCNH2-encoded HERG potassium channel, which is one of the critical repolarizing forces involved in the exquisite orchestration of the heart's action potential. Consequently, myocyte repolarization is potentially delayed as evidenced by prolongation of the QT interval, thus providing the substrate for drug-induced TdP. Rare mutations in KCNH2 provide the pathogenic substrate for type 2 congenital long QT syndrome (LQTS), thus placing this cardiac potassium channel squarely in the intersection between congenital LQTS (the "Rosetta stone" of the heritable channelopathies) and acquired LQTS (drug-induced TdP). In addition, common polymorphisms residing in the LQTS-causing channel genes may confer heightened arrhythmogenic susceptibility and contribute to the makings of a vulnerable host. This review focuses on the present strategy of identifying "at-risk compounds" and the potential future strategy involving pharmacogenetics to pinpoint "at-risk hosts" in an effort to curb this rare, unintended, but potentially life-threatening side effect.

Heart. 2005 May;91(5):563-4. Related Articles, Links Warfarin: a case history in pharmacogenetics. Hall AM, Wilkins MR. Both hereditary and environmental factors contribute to inter-individual variability in drug response. The considerable interest in the role of genes has to be balanced with the contribution of external influences. Warfarin provides a useful case study of the need to integrate both genetic and non-genetic information when selecting the right dose for a patient. This article discusses the latest data on genotype and warfarin sensitivity and the efforts to incorporate this information into normograms. Exploring the genetics of warfarin response will lead not only to safer prescribing but elucidate the mechanism of action of warfarin and enable the development of new anticoagulant drugs. Publication Types: Editorial

Hematology (Am Soc Hematol Educ Program). 2004;:118-45. Related Articles, Links Childhood and adolescent lymphoid and myeloid leukemia. Pui CH, Schrappe M, Ribeiro RC, Niemeyer CM. Department of Hematology-Oncology, St. Jude Children's Research Hospital, Memphis, TN 38105-2794, USA. Remarkable progress has been made in the past decade in the treatment and in the understanding of the biology of childhood lymphoid and myeloid leukemias. With contemporary improved risk assessment, chemotherapy, hematopoietic stem cell transplantation and supportive care, approximately 80% of children with newly diagnosed acute lymphoblastic leukemia and 50% of those with myeloid neoplasm can be cured to date. Current emphasis is placed not only on increased cure rate but also on improved quality of life. In Section I, Dr. Ching-Hon Pui describes certain clinical and biologic features that still have prognostic and therapeutic relevance in the context of contemporary treatment programs. He emphasizes that treatment failure in some patients is not due to intrinsic drug resistance of leukemic cells but is rather caused by suboptimal drug dosing due to host compliance, pharmacodynamics, and pharmacogenetics. Hence, measurement of minimal residual disease, which accounts for both the genetic (primary and secondary) features of leukemic lymphoblasts and pharmacogenomic variables of the host, is the most reliable prognostic indicator. Finally, he contends that with optimal risk-directed systemic and intrathecal therapy, cranial irradiation may be omitted in all patients, regardless of the presenting features. In Section II, Dr. Martin Schrappe performs detailed analyses of the prognostic impact of presenting age, leukocyte count, sex, immunophenotype, genetic abnormality, early treatment response, and in vitro drug sensitivity/resistance in childhood acute lymphoblastic leukemia, based on the large database of the Berlin-Frankfurt-Munster consortium. He also succinctly summarizes the important treatment components resulting in the improved outcome of children and young adolescents with this disease. He describes the treatment approach that led to the improved outcome of adolescent patients, a finding that may be applied to young adults in the second and third decade of life. Finally, he believes that treatment reduction under well-controlled clinical trials is feasible in a subgroup of patients with excellent early treatment response as evidenced by minimal residual disease measurement during induction and consolidation therapy. In Section III, Dr. Raul Ribeiro describes distinct morphologic and genetic subtypes of acute myeloid leukemia. The finding of essentially identical gene expression profiling by DNA microarray in certain specific genetic subtypes of childhood and adult acute myeloid leukemia suggests a shared leukemogenesis. He then describes the principles of treatment as well as the efficacy and toxicity of various forms of postremission therapy, emphasizing the need of tailoring therapy to both the disease and the age of the patient. Early results suggest that minimal residual disease measurement can also improve the risk assessment in acute myeloid leukemia, and that cranial irradiation can be omitted even in those with central-nervous-system leukemia at diagnosis. In Section IV, Dr. Charlotte Niemeyer describes a new classification of myelodysplastic and myeloproliferative diseases in childhood, which has greatly facilitated the diagnosis of myelodysplastic syndromes and juvenile myelomonocytic leukemia. The recent discovery of somatic mutations in PTPN11 has improved the understanding of the pathobiology and the diagnosis of juvenile myelomonocytic leukemia. Together with the findings of mutations in RAS and NF1 in the other patients, she suggests that pathological activation of RAS-dependent pathways plays a central role in the leukemogenesis of this disease. She then describes the various treatment approaches for both juvenile myelomonocytic leukemia and myelodysplastic syndromes in the US and Europe, emphasizing the differences between childhood and adult cases for the latter group of diseases. She also raises some controversial issues regarding treatment that will require well-controlled international clinical trials to address. Publication Types: Review

Hepatobiliary Pancreat Dis Int. 2005 Aug;4(3):332-8. Related Articles, Links Individualized immunosuppression: new strategies from pharmacokinetics, pharmacodynamics and pharmacogenomics. Chen G, Dong JH. Army Institute of Hepatobiliary Surgery, Southwest Hospital, Third Military Medical University, Chongqing 400038, China. jhdong@hbsky.org BACKGROUND: The ultimate goal of transplantation is the donor-specific immune tolerance, but at least in the first 15 to 20 years of this century, immunosuppressive agents are still the determinant of clinical outcome of transplant recipients. Individualizing patient's immunosuppression to optimize the balance between therapeutic efficacy and the occurrence of adverse events poses a great challenge to physicians. DATA SOURCES: The data in this article were taken mostly from MEDLINE (2000-2004), part of which were from the research of the authors. RESULTS: Individualized immunosuppression remains a problem because of the narrow therapeutic index and wide inter- and intra-patient variation of commonly used immunosuppressants. Recent progress in study of pharmacokinetics and pharmacodynamics improved the clinical outcome of transplant recipients. More importantly, the emergence of pharmacogenomics might provide a promising and complementary tool for traditional therapeutic drug monitoring (TDM). CONCLUSIONS: Individualizing organ recipient's immunosuppression to balance the therapeutic efficacy and the adverse events represents a great challenge to transplant clinicians. Pharmacogenomics shows great promise for an interesting and hopefully better future. Publication Types: Review

Hepatobiliary Pancreat Dis Int. 2005 May;4(2):213-9. Related Articles, Links Predictive factors for sustained response to interferon treatment in patients with chronic hepatitis C: a randomized, open, and multi-center controlled trial. Xie Y, Xu DZ, Lu ZM, Luo KX, Jia JD, Wang YM, Zhao GZ, Zhang SL, Zhang DZ. Ninth Clinical Department, Beijing Ditan Hospital, Beijing 100011, China. xieyao@public.bta.net.cn BACKGROUND: This study was undertaken to investigate the predictive factors of sustained viral response in roferon-A or pegasys treated chronic hepatitis C patients after logistic regression analysis of the factors that might be associated with the therapeutic effects of interferon (IFN). METHODS: All patients enrolled into this randomized, open and multi-center controlled trial were divided into two groups randomly and treated with pegasys and roferon-A for 24 weeks, then followed up for another 24 weeks. Before treatment, hepatitis C virus (HCV) genotype was determined, and HCV-RNA in serum was detected before and at the end of treatment and follow-up. HCV-RNA turning negative was considered the major index for evaluating the therapeutic effect. The clinical characteristics including gender, age, infection route of HCV, treatment with IFN, platelet count, AST/ALT ratio and treatment drugs were analyzed by logistic regression. RESULTS: Intention to treat (ITT) and per-protocol (PP) population groups have 208 and 197 patients respectively. In the PP group, after treatment for 24 weeks, the response rates of female patients aged less than 50 years, infected through non-transfusion, relapsed after IFN treatment, and presented with a AST/ALT ratio</=1, virus load less than 8 x 10(5) IU/ml, and non genotype 1 HCV infection, and treated finally with pegasys were higher than those of male patients, aged more than 50 years, infected by transfusion, treated firstly with IFN, presented with a AST/ALT ratio>/=1, virus load equal or more than 8 x 10(5) IU/ml, and genotype 1 infection, and treated finally with roferon-A. But, at the end of follow-up, the patients with a AST/ALT ratio>/=1 and virus load more than 8 x 10(5) IU/ml had a higher rate of sustained response than did those with a AST/ALT ratio</=1 and virus load less than 8 x 10(5) IU/ml. Logistic regression analysis and control of the promiscuous factors showed that the genotype of HCV was not related to the response rate at the end of treatment (OR 0.604, 95% CI 0.271-1.349, P=0.219), but was the independent predictive factor of virus sustained response to IFN treatment (OR 0.408, 95% CI 0.189-0.881, P=0.023). The form of IFN was significantly related to viral response at the end of treatment (OR 0.105, 95% CI 0.052-0.212, P<0.001), and pegasys were an intensely predictive factor for sustained response(OR 0.255, 95% CI 0.123-0.529, P<0.001). CONCLUSION: HCV genotype and pegasys are the predictive factors for IFN response to the IFN treatment of patients with chronic hepatitis C. Publication Types: Clinical Trial Multicenter Study Randomized Controlled Trial

Hopkins HIV Rep. 2004 May;16(3):1-7. Related Articles, Links Genes, ethnicity, and efavirenz response: clinical pharmacology update from the 11th CROI. Andrade A, Flexner C. Publication Types: Congresses Newspaper Article

Hosp Health Netw. 2005 Jun;79(6):84. Related Articles, Links Standardized microarrays could lead to medical care tailored to each person. [No authors listed] Publication Types: News

Hosp Med. 2004 Oct;65(10):594-8. Related Articles, Links Pharmacogenetics and cardiovascular disease management. Weston CF. Department of Cardiology, Singleton Hospital, Swansea. Patients differ in their response to drugs. Part of this variability may reflect genetically-determined characteristics of target genes or metabolizing enzymes. A knowledge of an individual's genetic makeup could allow drug therapy to be targeted at those most likely to benefit. Publication Types: Review

Hum Exp Toxicol. 2005 Jan;24(1):35-40. Related Articles, Links Toxicogenomics: regulatory perspective on current position.

Battershill JM. Department of Health, Skipton House, Elephant and Castle, London, UK. jon.battershill@dh.gsi.gov.uk Published studies on the utility of toxicogenomic approaches (transcriptomics, proteomics and metabonomics) in screening for toxicological mechanisms and evaluation of dose response effects have been reviewed. The information supports the use of transcriptomics to screen for specific toxicological mechanisms for which there is an a priori hypothesis, although in some areas such as mutagenicity testing, toxicogenomics appear to have limited value for identifying mutagens. Data from such screening approaches cannot be used to exclude the possibility of toxicity. Targeted transcriptomics might be valuable for screening for specific mechanisms of toxicity considered to be irrelevant for assessing risk to humans, which would help to reduce the need for detailed testing of some chemicals. An integrated approach is suggested where data from more than one toxicogenomic approach could be used as an adjunct to conventional toxicology to assess dose-response in toxicological tests. An outline preliminary proposal for use by regulators is suggested although it is noted that more data are required before this could be formally used in a decision-making process. Publication Types: Review

Hum Genomics. 2004 Aug;1(5):375-80. Related Articles, Links Human pharmacogenomics: the development of a science. Kalow W. Department of Pharmacology, University of Toronto, Toronto M5S 1A8, Canada. w.kalow@utoronto.ca Until about 50 years ago, the altering of a normal drug effect by a genetic deficiency was only rarely observed. Here, my discovery of the genetic variant of butyrylcholinesterase affecting succinylcholine action is described in some detail. Such discoveries led to the combination of the two older sciences, genetics and pharmacology, thereby forming pharmacogenetics. After the discovery of similar examples in the years that followed, pharmacogenetics expanded on the basis of two discoveries. First, the common occurrence of interethnic differences in drug response and, secondly, the fact that most pharmacological differences were multigenic. New methodologies brought a transition to pharmacogenomics; this included detection of clinically important genetic variants and has uncovered potentially new drug targets. The arrival of personalised medicine--where a patient's genes determine the choice of drug to be administered--can be hoped to gradually improve drug safety and efficacy. Efforts to reach this level of perfection are, however, dogged by uncertainties. Publication Types: Historical Article

Hum Genomics. 2004 Jan;1(2):111-25. Related Articles, Links Pharmacogenetics of lipid diseases. Ordovas JM. Nutrition and Genomics Laboratory, Jean Mayer-United States Department of Agriculture, Human Nutrition Research Center on Aging at Tufts University, Boston, MA 02111, USA. jose.ordovas@tufts.edu The genetic basis for most of the rare lipid monogenic disorders have been elucidated, but the challenge remains in determining the combination of genes that contribute to the genetic variability in lipid levels in the general population; this has been estimated to be in the range of 40-60 per cent of the total variability. Therefore, the effect of common polymorphisms on lipid phenotypes will be greatly modulated by gene-gene and gene-environment interactions. This approach can also be used to characterise the individuality of the response to lipid-lowering therapies, whether using drugs (pharmacogenetics) or dietary interventions (nutrigenetics). In this regard, multiple studies have already described significant interactions between candidate genes for lipid and drug metabolism that modulate therapeutic response-although the outcomes of these studies have been controversial and call for more rigorous experimental design and analytical approaches. Once solid evidence about the predictive value of genetic panels is obtained, risk and therapeutic algorithms can begin to be generated that should provide an accurate measure of genetic predisposition, as well as targeted behavioural modifications or drugs of choice and personalized dosages of these drugs. Publication Types: Review

Hum Genomics. 2004 Nov;1(6):444-55. Related Articles, Links Emerging strategies and applications of pharmacogenomics. Milos PM, Seymour AB. Discovery Pharmacogenomics, Pfizer Global Research and Development, Eastern Point Road, Groton, CT 06340, USA. Patrice_m_milos@groton.pfizer.com The rapid pace of genomic science advancements, including the completion of the human genome sequence, the extensive cataloguing of genetic variation and the acceleration of technologies to assess such variation, combined with clinical programmes with rich phenotypic data, serve as the foundation for the design and execution of pharmacogenomic studies which have an impact on the pharmaceutical pipeline from early discovery through to the marketplace. The authors discuss the required infrastructure to support pharmacogenomic studies and provide insight into the strategies and practical application to influence decision making in the pharmaceutical setting. Further, the influence of pharmacogenomics is currently affecting patient care in the oncology area and is highlighted as evident impact in the marketplace. Publication Types: Review

Hum Genomics. 2005;2(1):28-38. Related Articles, Links Trick or treat: The effect of placebo on the power of pharmacogenetic association studies. Singer C, Grossman I, Avidan N, Beckmann JS, Pe'er I. Department of Molecular Genetics, Weizmann Institute of Science, Rehovot, Israel. The genetic mapping of drug-response traits is often characterised by a poor signal-to-noise ratio that is placebo related and which distinguishes pharmacogenetic association studies from classical case-control studies for disease susceptibility. The goal of this study was to evaluate the statistical power of candidate gene association studies under different pharmacogenetic scenarios, with special emphasis on the placebo effect. Genotype/phenotype data were simulated, mimicking samples from clinical trials, and response to the drug was modelled as a binary trait. Association was evaluated by a logistic regression model. Statistical power was estimated as a function of the number of single nucleotide polymorphisms (SNPs) genotyped, the frequency of the placebo 'response', the genotype relative risk (GRR) of the response polymorphism, the strategy for selecting SNPs for genotyping, the number of individuals in the trial and the ratio of placebo-treated to drug-treated patients. We show that: (i) the placebo 'response' strongly affects the statistical power of association studies - even a highly penetrant drug-response allele requires at least a 500-patient trial in order to reach 80 per cent power, several-fold more than the value estimated by standard tools that are not calibrated to pharmacogenetics; (ii) the power of a pharmacogenetic association study depends primarily on the penetrance of the response genotype and, when this penetrance is fixed, power decreases for larger placebo effects; (iii) power is dramatically increased when adding markers; (iv) an optimal study design includes a similar number of placebo- and drug-treated patients; and (v) in this setting, straightforward haplotype analysis does not seem to have an advantage over single marker analysis.

Hum Mol Genet. 2004 Jul 1;13(13):1353-9. Epub 2004 May 5. Related Articles, Links Corticosteroid pharmacogenetics: association of sequence variants in CRHR1 with improved lung function in asthmatics treated with inhaled corticosteroids. Tantisira KG, Lake S, Silverman ES, Palmer LJ, Lazarus R, Silverman EK, Liggett SB, Gelfand EW, Rosenwasser LJ, Richter B, Israel E, Wechsler M, Gabriel S, Altshuler D, Lander E, Drazen J, Weiss ST. Channing Laboratory, Brigham and Women's Hospital and Harvard Medical School, Boston, MA 02115, USA. Corticosteroids mediate a variety of immunological actions and are commonly utilized in the treatment of a wide range of diseases. Unfortunately, therapy with this class of medications is associated with a large proportion of non-responders and significant side effects. Inhaled corticosteroids are the most commonly used asthma controller therapy. However, asthmatic response to corticosteroids also varies widely between individuals. We investigated the genetic contribution to the variation in response to inhaled corticosteroid therapy in asthma. The association of longitudinal change in lung function and single nucleotide polymorphisms from candidate genes crucial to the biologic actions of corticosteroids were evaluated in three independent asthmatic clinical trial populations utilizing inhaled corticosteroids as the primary therapy in at least one treatment arm. Variation in one gene, corticotropin-releasing hormone receptor 1 (CRHR1) was consistently associated with enhanced response to therapy in each of our three populations. Individuals homozygous for the variants of interest manifested a doubling to quadrupling of the lung function response to corticosteroids compared with lack of the variants (P-values ranging from 0.006 to 0.025 for our three asthmatic populations). As the primary receptor mediating the release of adrenocorticotropic hormone, which regulates endogenous cortisol levels, CRHR1 plays a pivotal, pleiotropic role in steroid biology. These data indicate that genetic variants in CRHR1 have pharmacogenetic effects influencing asthmatic response to corticosteroids, provide a rationale for predicting therapeutic response in asthma and other corticosteroid-treated diseases, and suggests this gene pathway as a potential novel therapeutic target. Copyright 2004 Oxford University Press

Hum Mol Genet. 2005 Dec 1;14(23):3595-603. Epub 2005 Oct 20. Related Articles, Links Polymorphism discovery in 51 chemotherapy pathway genes. Freimuth RR, Xiao M, Marsh S, Minton M, Addleman N, Van Booven DJ, McLeod HL, Kwok PY. Department of Medicine, Washington University School of Medicine, St. Louis, MO, USA. Candidate gene pharmacogenetic studies offer a strategy for the rapid assessment of putative predictive markers. As a first step toward studying the pharmacogenetics of cancer chemotherapy, 51 candidate genes from the pathways of antineoplastic agents were resequenced to identify common genetic polymorphisms that might alter therapeutic response or toxicity. Forty DNA samples were screened from each of three population groups: African-Americans, Asian-Americans and European-Americans. Nearly 378 kb of genomic sequence was obtained from each sample. Nine hundred and four variants were identified, including 139 coding single nucleotide polymorphisms (cSNPs). Three hundred and fifty-six (40%) polymorphisms were common to all three populations and 366 (41%) were population specific. Three hundred and forty-six (38%) variants were novel polymorphisms that were not present in the three public databases that were examined. One hundred and eleven (35%) of the 319 non-synonymous cSNPs that were identified by either resequencing or database mining were predicted by PolyPhen to be either possibly or probably damaging. For the non-synonymous cSNPs identified by resequencing, both the number of cSNPs found and the maximum estimated allele frequency decreased with increasing predicted severity. These results provide experimental validation and estimated allele frequencies for polymorphisms in three common ethnic groups and facilitate applied pharmacogenetic studies of anticancer drugs.

Hum Mol Genet. 2005 Jun 15;14(12):1671-7. Epub 2005 May 6. Related Articles, Links Molecular properties and pharmacogenetics of a polymorphism of adenylyl cyclase type 9 in asthma: interaction between beta-agonist and corticosteroid pathways. Tantisira KG, Small KM, Litonjua AA, Weiss ST, Liggett SB. Channing Laboratory, Brigham and Women's Hospital and Harvard Medical School, Boston, MA 02115, USA. In asthma, the response to beta-agonists acting at beta2-adrenergic receptors (beta2AR) displays extensive interindividual variation. One effector for airway beta2AR, adenylyl cyclase type 9 (AC9), was considered a candidate locus for predicting beta-agonist efficacy in the absence and presence of corticosteroid treatment. One non-synonymous AC9 polymorphism has been identified, which results in substitution of Met for Ile at amino acid 772. Under standard culture conditions in stably transfected cells, we found decreased catalytic activity of Met772. However, cells cultured in the presence of glucocorticoid expressing Met772 had a significantly increased albuterol-stimulated adenylyl cyclase response (approximately 80%) when compared with those expressing Ile772 (approximately 20%, P=0.02). An equivalent increase in beta2AR expression was observed in both lines due to glucocorticoid, but AC9 expression was unaffected. The hypothesis that Met772-AC9 is associated with an improved albuterol bronchodilator response in asthmatics was investigated in 436 asthmatic children who were followed for 4 years and randomized to receive placebo or the inhaled corticosteroid budesonide. Met772 carriers on budesonide showed a significant improvement in forced expiratory volume in 1 s (P=0.005). Moreover, a highly significant interaction (P=0.002) was found for budesonide treatment and the AC9 polymorphism. These in vitro and human association studies are consistent with this AC9 polymorphism altering albuterol responsiveness in the context of concomitant inhaled corticosteroid administration, which is a common asthma regimen. The Met772-AC9 polymorphism represents one of most likely several multi-gene polymorphisms along the receptor-relaxation axis, which together may provide for a composite pharmacogenetic index for asthma therapy. Publication Types: Clinical Trial Randomized Controlled Trial

Hum Mol Genet. 2005 Oct 15;14 Spec No. 2:R207-14. Related Articles, Links Pharmacogenetics/genomics and personalized medicine. Sadee W, Dai Z. Department of Pharmacology, Comprehensive Cancer Center, College of Medicine and Public Health, The Ohio State University, Columbus, OH 43210-1239, USA. sadee-1@medctr.osu.edu Despite the marked advances in drug therapy, some patients do not respond favorably or suffer severe adverse drug effects. Pharmacogenetic studies have shown that polymorphisms of drug metabolizing enzymes, transporters and receptors contribute to variable drug response. Owing to the complexity of drug actions, a broader genomics approach aims at finding new drug targets and optimizing therapy for the individual patient. However, pharmacogenomics has made only a few inroads into clinical practice to date. This review evaluates obstacles that need to be overcome. These include the complexity of mechanisms underlying drug response, given singly or in combination, uncertainty about the genetic underpinnings of complex diseases, such as cancer, diabetes, cardiovascular and mental disorders and a lack of quantitative understanding of the scope of genetic variations, even for well-studied genes. By resolving these hurdles, pharmacogenomics will yield significant, but incremental, therapeutic advances paving the way towards personalized health care. Publication Types: Evaluation Studies Review

Hum Mol Genet. 2006 Mar 1;15(5):797-805. Epub 2006 Jan 24. Related Articles, Links ABCB1/MDR1 gene determines susceptibility and phenotype in ulcerative colitis: discrimination of critical variants using a gene-wide haplotype tagging approach. Ho GT, Soranzo N, Nimmo ER, Tenesa A, Goldstein DB, Satsangi J. Molecular Medicine Unit and Gastrointestinal Unit, University of Edinburgh, Western General Hospital, Edinburgh, UK. gwotzerho@aol.com Several lines of evidence suggest a role for the multidrug resistance gene (ABCB1/MDR1) and its product, P-glycoprotein 170, in the pathogenesis of inflammatory bowel disease (IBD). In addition, P-glycoprotein activity determines bioavailability of many drugs used regularly in many medical specialties, and ABCB/MDR1 variation appears to be a critical pharmacogenetic determinant. We have utilized a gene-wide haplotype tagging approach to further define the identity of germ-line variations in the ABCB1/MDR1 gene contributing to IBD susceptibility. Six haplotype tagging single nucleotide polymorphisms (tSNPs) representing the haplotypic variations of the ABCB1/MDR1 gene were identified initially following the characterization of the haplotype structure of this gene in 24 Centre d'Etude du Polymorphisme Humain Caucasian trios. Genotyping was performed in 249 ulcerative colitis (UC) and 179 Crohn's disease (CD) patients and 260 healthy controls. Using log-likelihood analysis, we observed a highly significant association between the common haplotypes and UC (P=4.22 x 10(-7)) but not CD (P=0.22). This significant association was critically dependent on one tSNP, intronic variant rs3789243. All haplotypes with this variant retained a highly significant association (P=3.2 x 10(-7)-3.6 x 10(-12)), whereas significance was lost when rs3789243 was dropped in systematic haplotypic analysis. The effect of this tSNP was independent of C3435T

SNP, previously suggested to be the critical variant in disease susceptibility and drug transport. The association with UC was shown to be strongest with the phenotype of extensive disease (P=1.7 x 10(-7)). This 'candidate gene' approach provides compelling evidence to support the contribution of the ABCB1/MDR1 gene in determining risk to UC but not to CD and provides new insights into the localization of the critical susceptibility determinants within the gene. In addition, these findings have potentially important implications in the application of pharmacogenetics across a range of common diseases, including HIV, epilepsy and colorectal cancer.

Hum Mutat. 2004 Jun;23(6):534-9. Related Articles, Links PromoLign: a database for upstream region analysis and SNPs. Zhao T, Chang LW, McLeod HL, Stormo GD. Department of Genetics, Washington University School of Medicine, St. Louis, Missouri 63110, USA. The study of transcriptional regulation at the genomic level has been hindered by the lack of functional annotation in the putative regulatory regions. Phylogenetic footprinting, in which cross-species sequence alignment among orthologous genes is applied to locate conserved sequence blocks, is an effective strategy to attack this problem. Single nucleotide polymorphisms (SNPs) in transcription factor (TF) binding sites contribute to the heterogeneity of TF binding sites and might disrupt or enhance their regulatory activity. The correlation of SNPs with the TF sites will not only help in functional evaluation of SNPs, but will also help in the study of transcription regulation by focusing attention on specific TF sites. PromoLign (http://polly.wustl.edu/promolign/main.html) is an online database application that presents SNPs and TF binding profiles in the context of human-mouse orthologous sequence alignment with a hyperlinked graphical interface. PromoLign could be applied to a variety of SNPs and transcription related studies, including association genetics, population genetics, and pharmacogenetics. Copyright 2004 Wiley-Liss, Inc.

Hum Mutat. 2005 Feb;25(2):110-7. Related Articles, Links PolyMAPr: programs for polymorphism database mining, annotation, and functional analysis. Freimuth RR, Stormo GD, McLeod HL. Department of Medicine, Washington University School of Medicine, St. Louis, Missouri 63110, USA. Pharmacogenomic and disease-association studies rely on identifying a comprehensive set of polymorphisms within candidate genes. Public SNP databases are a rich source of polymorphism data, but mining them effectively requires overcoming at least four challenges: ensuring accurate annotations for genes and polymorphisms, eliminating both inter- and intra-database redundancy, integrating data from multiple public sources with data generated locally, and prioritizing the variants for further study. PolyMAPr (Polymorphism Mining and Annotation Programs)' was developed to overcome these challenges and to improve the efficiency of database mining and polymorphism annotation. PolyMAPr takes as input a file containing a list of genes to be processed and files containing each annotated gene sequence. Polymorphic sequences obtained from public databases (dbSNP, CGAP, and JSNP) or through local SNP discovery efforts, as well as oligonucleotide sequences (e.g., PCR primers), are mapped to the annotated gene sequences and named according to suggested nomenclature guidelines. The functional effects of nonsynonymous coding-region SNPs (cSNPs) and any variants that might alter exon splicing enhancer (ESE) sites, putative transcription factor binding sites, or intron-exon splice sites are predicted. The output files are accessible though a browser interface. In addition, the results are also provided in Extensible Markup Language (XML) format to facilitate uploading them into a local relational database. PolyMAPr increases the efficiency of mining public databases for genetic variants within candidate genes and provides a mechanism by which data from multiple sources (both public and private) can be uniformly integrated, thereby significantly reducing the effort required to obtain a comprehensive set of polymorphisms for pharmacogenomic and disease-association studies. PolyMAPr can be obtained from http://pharmacogenomics.wustl.edu. (c) 2005 Wiley-Liss, Inc.

Hum Mutat. 2005 Oct;26(4):394-5. Related Articles, Links Thromboxane synthase (TBXAS1) polymorphisms in African-American and Caucasian populations: evidence for selective pressure. Ulrich CM, Carlson CS, Sibert J, Poole EM, Yu JH, Wang LH, Sparks R, Potter JD, Bigler J. Fred Hutchinson Cancer Research Center, Cancer Prevention Program, University of Washington, Seattle, Washington 98109-1024, USA. nulrich@fhcrc.org Thromboxane synthase (TBXAS1), a cytochrome P450 enzyme, converts prostaglandin H2 into thromboxane A2, a potent vasoconstrictor and inducer of platelet aggregation. Thromboxane A2 has been implicated in modulating cell cytotoxicity and in tumor growth and metastasis. Twelve coding-region variants were identified in the human TBXAS1 gene in 48 African-American and 46 Caucasian individuals, of which eight were amino-acid substitutions. The latter were confirmed in an independent Caucasian population (n=94 unrelated individuals). We performed an evolutionary analysis of patterns of nucleotide diversity and identified patterns of amino acid replacement in human-mouse comparisons consistent with purifying selection on an inter-species time scale using the McDonald-Kreitman test. We also observed patterns of nucleotide diversity within humans consistent with purifying selection acting on existing polymorphism using Tajima's D within coding regions. These evolutionary tests suggest that some of the rare coding variations observed in the human population are deleterious. We used two sequence-homology-based software programs and molecular modeling to predict the potential impact of these polymorphisms on TBXAS1 function. The c.772C>T (p.Lys258Glu), c.1249C>G (p.Gln417Glu), and c.1348G>A (p.Glu450Lys) substitutions are predicted as most likely to alter protein function; another, c.1352C>A (p.Thr451Asn), may also affect function. Given the evolutionary evidence, these variants may be functional and therefore of relevance for disease endpoints related to inflammation and angiogenesis, as well as for the pharmacogenetics of non-steroidal anti-inflammatory drugs. (c) 2005 Wiley-Liss, Inc.

IDrugs. 2004 Dec;7(12):1090-3. Related Articles, Links Modern Drug Discovery and Development. 18-19 October 2004, San Diego, CA, USA. Xu J. BioMinerva Group, 11553 Hadar Drive, San Diego, CA 92126, USA. jxu4@san.rr.com Industrial and academic experts with diverse backgrounds attended the Modern Drug Discovery and Development conference, organized by GTCbio, a subsidiary of

Global Technology Community LLC. The conference covered a broad range of topics in drug discovery and development, including: target discovery and identification, lead discovery and identification, drug metabolism and toxicity, drug process and development, and application of genomics, proteomics, pharmacogenomics and bioinformatics in accelerating drug discovery and development. This report focuses on investigational drugs discussed at the conference. Publication Types: Congresses

IDrugs. 2004 Jul;7(7):644-7. Related Articles, Links Therapeutic insight 2004. 3-4 May 2004, Jersey City, NJ, USA. Nicoletti A. Defined Health, 55 Essex Street, Millburn NJ 07041, USA. aileennicoletti@definedhealth.com Publication Types: Congresses

IDrugs. 2004 Jun;7(6):543-7. Related Articles, Links Cambridge Healthtech Institute fourth annual conference in structure-based drug design. McInnes C. Cyclacel Ltd, Dundee Technopole, James Lindsay Place, Dundee, DD1 5JJ, Scotland, UK. cmcinnes@cyclacel.com The CHI-sponsored fourth annual meeting, held at the Sheraton hotel in Boston, USA, was attended by approximately 120 delegates, mainly from the pharmaceutical and biotechnology industries. The theme of the conference focused on new developments and validation of current techniques in structure-based drug design, as well as the successful application of these methods in drug development. Publication Types: Congresses

IDrugs. 2004 Sep;7(9):833-5. Related Articles, Links Federation of the European Pharmacological Societies-fourth annual meeting. Part II. 14-17 July 2004, Porto. Portugal. Urch C. St Mary's Hospital, Department Pharmacology, University College London, Gower Street, London, WC1E 6BT UK. c.urch@ucl.ac.uk The aims of this Federation of European Pharmacological Societies (EPHAR) meetings are to broaden the understanding of fundamental pharmacology. Rather than present clinically relevant novel therapeutics, most symposia and posters presented data exploring the role of receptors, transmitters and potential agents within a basic science framework. The opening plenary session was given by Sir James Black, and the main meeting revolved around parallel symposia and poster sessions. Most presenters gave a broad overview of the current understanding, with less emphasis on individual compounds, while others developed a theme exploring specific agonists/antagonists and experimental models. Publication Types: Congresses

IDrugs. 2005 Aug;8(8):648-50. Related Articles, Links The impact of FDA guidance on pharmacogenomic data submissions on drug development. Little S. DxS Ltd, Manchester, UK. stephen.little@dxsgenotyping.com After a long wait, the US Food and Drug Administration (FDA) finally released the much anticipated 'Guidance on Pharmacogenomic Data Submissions on Drug Development' in March 2005, but what impact will this have on the drug industry as a whole? It is becoming increasingly apparent that the field of pharmacogenomics can add value to both clinical trial design and the drug development process, but uptake by the pharmaceutical industry has so far been variable between companies. The opinion of the FDA is that the use of pharmacogenomics in drug development is a 'good thing' and one that it wishes to promote, hence, this new guidance is designed to assist drug companies to adopt pharmacogenomic technology in clinical development, and covers both targeted and exploratory aspects. While targeted pharmacogenomics must be included as part of any regulatory submission, exploratory approaches may be submitted voluntarily with assurances from the FDA that any such submissions will not be used to make regulatory decisions. With this regulatory framework now in place it is only a matter of time before it is known how the industry reacts and the impact it will have on drug development.

IDrugs. 2005 Jan;8(1):25-8. Related Articles, Links Clinical Trials in CNS--SMi Conference. Harris S. Thomson Scientific, Middlesex House, 34-42 Cleveland Street, London, W1T 4JE, UK. sarah.harris@thomson.com Publication Types: Congresses

IDrugs. 2005 Jul;8(7):555-9. Related Articles, Links European Atherosclerosis Society--75th congress. Gomaraschi M. University of Milan, Center E Grossi Paoletti, Institute of Pharmacological Sciences, Via Balzaretti 9, 20133 Milan, Italy. monica.gomaraschi@tiscali.it The 75th European Atherosclerosis Society congress, held in Prague, Czech Republic, at the end of April 2005, was a large, well-attended meeting of international scientists with specialist interest in the field of cardiovascular diseases. Few new drugs emerged at the meeting as treatment options for cardiovascular diseases, however, many interesting basic and clinical data were presented that will eventually lead to better and improved cardiovascular therapies. This report is focused on recent advances in statin therapy (the TNT study and the role of pharmacogenetics in predicting individual response to statin therapy); clinical evidence of the combination therapy of ezetimibe + simvastatin; phase III clinical data on the selective cannabinoid type I receptor blocker rimonabant (sanofi-aventis); the role of peroxisome proliferator-activated receptor a agonists in the treatment of the metabolic syndrome; and the rationale for, and the recent advances in high-density lipoprotein-targeted therapy. Publication Types: Congresses

IEEE Eng Med Biol Mag. 2005 Jul-Aug;24(4):81-7. Related Articles, Links Engineering genomics. RNA antagonists--a new class of antisense drugs. Orum H. CSO Santaris Pharma A/S,, Horsholm, Denmark. hoe@santaris.com Publication Types: Review

Immunol Allergy Clin North Am. 2005 Nov;25(4):723-42. Related Articles, Links Asthma pharmacogenomics. Hawkins GA, Weiss ST, Bleecker ER. Center for Human Genomics, Wake Forest University School of Medicine, Medical Center Boulevard, Winston-Salem, NC 27157, USA. ghawkins@wfubmc.edu It is expected that future treatments will be preceded by genetic tests to prescribe the most effect asthma medication while lowering the risk of adverse side effects. However, it will not be necessary to describe all the genetic determinants affecting drug response to apply pharmacogenomics to asthma therapy. Whether pharmacogenomics becomes common practice may not depend on the availability of tests, but on factors such as affordability, ease of application, and ease of interpreting the results.

Indian J Pediatr. 2004 Aug;71(8):721-7. Related Articles, Links Newer drugs for asthma. Singh M. Advanced Pediatrics Centre, Post Graduate Institute of Medical Education and Research, Chandigarh, India. meenusingh4@rediffmail.com Several new drugs have resulted from innovative pharmacological and immunomodulatory approaches towards treatment of asthma. Diverse therapeutic targets have provided new agents. The new classes of drugs available are newer "on site activated inhaled corticisteroids" and soft steroids, anti IgE compounds, leukotriene inhibitors and single isomer agents which are available for clinical use. Anti interleukin agents and phosphodiesterase inhibitors are in the stage of clinical trials. Antisense therapy and pharmacogenetics are the on horizon for treatment of asthma. Publication Types: Review

Infect Dis Clin North Am. 2004 Dec;18(4):743-59, vii. Related Articles, Links Community-acquired pneumonia: pathophysiology and host factors with focus on possible new approaches to management of lower respiratory tract infections. Wunderink RG, Waterer GW. Northwestern University Feinberg School of Medicine, 676 North St. Clair, Suite 14-044, Chicago, IL 60611, USA. r-wunderink@northwestern.edu The present understanding of the pathophysiology of community-acquired pneumonia (CAP) explains the mechanism for many specific manifestations, but does not address adequately why only some patients experience complications. Recent advances in under-standing the genetics of complex illnesses offer hope for a more complete insight into the pathogenesis of CAP. This article reviews genetic variation in the molecules involved in the known patho-genic mechanisms of CAP, including cough, bacterial recognition, inflammation and the compensatory anti-inflammatory response,and organ dysfunction. Publication Types: Review

Infection. 2004 Apr;32(2):82-8. Related Articles, Links Safety, efficacy and development of resistance under the new protease inhibitor lopinavir/ritonavir: 48-week results. Voigt E, Wasmuth JC, Vogel M, Mauss S, Schmutz G, Kaiser R, Rockstroh JK. Department of Internal Medicine, University of Bonn, Sigmund Freud Str. 25, D-53105, Bonn, Germany. esther.voigt@uni-bonn.de BACKGROUND: Within this open-label, uncontrolled prospective trial we evaluated safety, efficacy and development of genotypic resistance under the new protease inhibitor lopinavir/ritonavir (LPV/r) in antiretroviral (ARV) HIV patients. PATIENTS AND METHODS: 58 patients with virological failure under their current ARV therapy were started on a LPV/r containing regimen. Median baseline HIV RNA and CD4 count were 4.6 log(10) cps/ml (range 2.1-6.4) and 128 x 10(6)/l (0-767), respectively. CD4 count, HIV RNA and metabolic parameters were assessed at weeks 0, 4, 8, 12, 16, 24, 32, 40, 48. Genotypic resistance testing was performed at baseline and again at weeks 12, 24 and 48 in the event of virological failure. RESULTS: Until week 48, viral load (VL) decreased by a median of 1.9 log(10) cps/ml (-0.8-3.8). A VL below 80 cps/ml was found in 20/58 patients (34.5%) at week 48. In parallel, CD4 cells increased to a median of 332 x 10(6)/l (8-905). Nine patients discontinued study treatment. At 48 weeks, median triglyceride and cholesterol levels increased significantly. While the median number of overall protease mutations at baseline was four in all patients, it was six in patients virologically failing on LPV/r. The average number of mutations increased significantly to eight at week 48. Several mutations were detected considerably more often in the event of failure than in response to treatment, e. g. at amino acid positions 10, 24, 54, 71, 82, 84. CONCLUSION: LPV/r is effective in heavily pretreated patients. Discontinuation due to adverse events is infrequent. No individual mutation can be associated with failure on LPV/r. However, a greater number of protease mutations at baseline is associated with poorer treatment outcome and several mutations seem to be related to treatment failure. Publication Types: Clinical Trial

Inflamm Bowel Dis. 2004 Mar;10(2):148-58. Related Articles, Links Pharmacogenetics and inflammatory bowel disease: progress and prospects. Ho GT, Lees C, Satsangi J. Department of Gastroenterology, Western General Hospital, Edinburgh EH,4 2XU. gho@ed.ac.uk Publication Types: Review

Inflamm Bowel Dis. 2005 Nov;11(11):1013-9. Related Articles, Links Multidrug resistance (MDR1) gene in inflammatory bowel disease: a key player? Ho GT, Gaya DR, Satsangi J. Gastrointestinal Unit, Western General Hospital, Edinburgh, United Kingdom. gho@ed.ac.uk Publication Types: Review

Int Arch Occup Environ Health. 2005 Jun;78(5):343-54. Epub 2005 May 10. Related Articles, Links Mercapturic acids revisited as biomarkers of exposure to reactive chemicals in occupational toxicology: a minireview. Haufroid V, Lison D. Universite catholique de Louvain, Unite de Toxicologie Industrielle et Environnementale, Clos Chapelle-aux-Champs 30 boite 54, 1200 Bruxelles, Belgium. haufroid@toxi.ucl.ac.be A minireview is presented concerning the use of mercapturic acids as biological exposure index for electrophilic chemicals. Besides pure analytical aspects, this minireview considers possible issues in relation to (a) the added value of mercapturic acids as compared to other well validated biomarkers of exposure and (b) the high inter-individual variability in mercapturic acids excretion. Recent field and/or experimental studies confirm the usefulness of mercapturic acids as biological exposure index for electrophilic chemicals and suggest the interest of a toxicogenetic approach for a better interpretation of the results of biological monitoring. Publication Types: Review

Int J Clin Oncol. 2005 Feb;10(1):14-9. Related Articles, Links Cancer pharmacogenomics: achievements in basic research. Nakajima M, Yokoi T. Drug Metabolism and Toxicology, Division of Pharmaceutical Sciences, Graduate School of Medical Science, Kanazawa University, Kakuma-machi, Kanazawa, 920-1192, Japan. nmiki@kenroku.kanazawa-u.ac.jp Pharmacogenomics is the study of how genetic inheritance influences the responses to drugs. Genetic polymorphisms in drug-metabolizing enzymes result in altered pharmacokinetics in therapeutic drugs. In recent years, there has been great progress in our knowledge of the effects of cytochrome P450 (CYP) polymorphisms on the pharmacokinetics of therapeutic drugs. CYP enzymes catalyze the activation or detoxification of several anticancer drugs. Anticancer drugs generally have a narrow therapeutic margin. Therefore, the interindividual variability in their efficacy and toxicity is a major problem in clinical practice. In this review, genetic polymorphisms of CYP enzymes and their clinical relevance in cancer chemotherapy are discussed. Publication Types: Review

Int J Clin Oncol. 2005 Feb;10(1):3-4. Related Articles, Links Cancer pharmacogenomics: progress and obstacles toward the goal. Nishiyama M. Department of Translational Cancer Research, Research Institute for Radiation Biology and Medicine,

Hiroshima University, Hiroshima, 734-8551, Japan. yamacho@hiroshima-u.ac.jp

Int J Clin Oncol. 2005 Feb;10(1):5-13. Related Articles, Links Cancer pharmacogenomics: international trends. Yamayoshi Y, Iida E, Tanigawara Y. Department of Hospital Pharmacy, School of Medicine, Keio University, 35 Shinanomachi, Shinjuku-ku, Tokyo, 160-8582, Japan. It is well known that inter-individual variability exists in the responses to many drugs. Many nongenetic factors, such as age, sex, diet, and organ function, are known to affect the therapeutic effects of drugs. However, recent advances in pharmacogenomics have revealed that genetic polymorphisms also significantly influence both the efficacy and the toxicity of drugs. Mutations in the genes encoding drug-metabolizing enzymes, transporters, and target molecules may alter their expression, activity, or affinity to drugs, thereby influencing the drugs' pharmacokinetics and pharmacodynamics. Numerous studies have reported on the correlations between therapeutic outcomes and polymorphisms in drug-metabolizing enzymes, transporters, target molecules, and DNA repair enzymes. These pharmacogenomic discoveries are expected to be useful for the individualization and optimization of cancer chemotherapy. Publication Types: Review

Int J Clin Pharmacol Ther. 2004 Mar;42(3):133-8. Related Articles, Links Single-step identification of all length polymorphisms in the UGT1A1 gene promoter. Skarke C, Grosch S, Geisslinger G, Lotsch J. Pharmazentrum Frankfurt, Institute of Clinical Pharmacology, Johann Wolfgang Goethe University, Frankfurt, Germany. skarke@em.uni-frankfurt.de AIM: To provide a sensitive genetic screening method for rapid identification of all known length polymorphisms in the promoter region of the uridine 5'-diphosphoglucose glucuronosyltransferase (UGT) 1A1 gene comprising (TA)5, (TA)7 and (TA)8 repeats as opposed to the non-mutated (TA)6 allele. METHODS: The UGT1A1 promoter genotype was assessed in 115 subjects by means of a newly developed pyrosequencing method. PCR-generated DNA templates of heterozygous (TA)5 and (TA)7 carriers were cloned into a TOPO TA vector and verified by sequencing. In addition, a (TA)8 segment was produced by cloning to demonstrate the ability of the method to detect this mutation. RESULTS: All length polymorphisms of the UGT1A1 promoter described in the literature were clearly identified. Fifteen subjects had Gilbert's syndrome with elevated serum bilirubin associated with a homozygous (TA)7TAA/(TA)7TAA genotype. Two subjects with the rare genotypes (TA)5TAA/(TA)6TAA and (TA)5TAA/(TA)7TAA were found, where only the latter one displayed elevated serum bilirubin levels. Allelic frequencies were 0.9%, 66.1% and 33% for the (TA)5TAA, (TA)6TAA and (TA)7TAA allele, respectively. CONCLUSION: Our method enables reliable genetic single-step screening for all known length polymorphisms in the UGT1A1 gene promoter that cause Gilbert's syndrome. This facilitates pharmacogenetic-guided dosing of drugs with known toxicity metabolized by UGT1A1.

Int J Clin Pharmacol Ther. 2005 Dec;43(12):577-8. Related Articles, Links Current pharmacogenetics in colorectal cancer--do they have an impact on our clinical treatment strategies? Goekkurt E, Stoehlmacher J. Department of Internal Medicine I, University Hospital Carl

Gustav Carus, University Dresden, Germany.

Int J Eat Disord. 2005;37 Suppl:S90-4. Related Articles, Links The future of treatment research in anorexia nervosa. Strober M. Eating Disorders Program, Department of Psychiatry and Biobehavioral Sciences, David Geffen School of Medicine, University of California at Los Angeles, Los Angeles, California, USA. mstrober@mednet.ucla.edu In spite of much being written on the treatment of anorexia nervosa (AN), and the well-documented long-term morbidity of this illness, treatment effects have been little investigated. The current article considers the prospects for treatment research, taking note of the formidable challenges that lie ahead for the design, implementation, and interpretation of controlled clinical trials, and highlighting opportunities for effectiveness studies. In the light of increasing evidence of the role played by biologic susceptibility factors in AN, the potential future contribution to treatment research of advances in pharmacogenetics and molecular neuroscience also receives comment. 2005 by Wiley Periodicals, Inc.

Int J Hematol. 2004 Oct;80(3):295-6. Related Articles, Links Genetic polymorphism of the CYP2C9 subfamily of 3 different races in warfarin maintenance dose. Gan GG, Phipps ME, Ku CS, Teh A, Sangkar V. Publication Types: Letter

Int J Neuropsychopharmacol. 2004 Dec;7(4).381-5. Related Articles, Links Comment on: Int J Neuropsychopharmacol. 2004 Dec;7(4):453-60. Int J Neuropsychopharmacol. 2004 Dec;7(4):501-6. Focus on The 5-HT1A receptor: emerging role of a gene regulatory variant in psychopathology and pharmacogenetics. Lesch KP, Gutknecht L. Clinical and Molecular Psychobiology, Department of Psychiatry and Psychotherapy, University of Wurzburg, Wurzburg, Germany. kplesch@mail.uni-wuerzburg.de While multiple lines of evidence implicate the 5-HT1A receptor in the pathophysiology of anxiety and depression as well as in the mechanism of action of anxiolytics/antidepressants, its relevance to the therapeutic effectiveness of these drugs has been a matter of considerable debate (for review see Griebel, 1995; Hensler, 2003; Hjorth et al., 2000; Lesch et al., 2003). In the current issue of the International Journal of Neuropsychopharmacology, however, both Serretti et al. (2004) and Lemonde et al. (2004) make a strong argument for contribution of a functional 5-HT1A receptor gene variant in the pharmacogenetics of antidepressant treatment with prototypic tricyclics and selective serotonin reuptake inhibitors (SSRIs). Furthermore, the third study in this series by Huang and associates (2004) reveals an association of allelic variation of 5-HT1A receptor expression in a wide spectrum of psychopathology including schizophrenia, substance abuse, and panic disorder. Not unexpectedly, the failure to detect a consistent effect of this gene variation on 5-HT1A receptor functionality in the mature brain as indicated by both receptor binding in post-mortem brain and in-vivo receptor responsivity further supports a critical role of the 5-HT1A receptor in engineering neurodevelopmental processes which may have the potential to set the stage for the brain's permissiveness for psychopathology in later life. The availability of an increasing number of functional gene variants within the serotonergic pathway together with integration of emerging concepts of developmental genetics of complex traits will provide the groundwork for the molecular dissection of syndromal dimensions and treatment response. Publication Types: Comment Review

Int J Neurosci. 2005 Nov;115(11):1539-47. Related Articles, Links Dopamine D4 receptor gene exon III polymorphism and interindividual variation in response to clozapine. Zhao AL, Zhao JP, Zhang YH, Xue ZM, Chen JD, Chen XG. Departmernt of Psychiatry, The Second Xiangya Hospital Central South University, Changsha, Hunan, PR China. To investigate the relationship between 48 bp variant number tandem repeat polymorphism in dopamine D4 receptor gene and response to clozapine in schizophrenic patients, the authors included 81 inpatients with a DSM-IV diagnosis of schizophrenia and patients meeting criteria for refractory to treatment were excluded. This study found that the frequencies of five 48 bp repeats homozygous genotype and five 48 bp repeats allele were significantly less in the responders than the nonresponders, which divided by improving total schizophrenic symptom. The results of this study suggest that inherited variants of D4 may explain some of the interindividual variation seen in patient response to clozapine.

Int J Obstet Anesth. 2005 Oct;14(4):316-23. Related Articles, Links Pharmacogenetics: implications for obstetric anesthesia. Landau R. Service d'Anesthesiologie, Hopitaux Universitaires de Geneve, Geneva, Switzerland. ruth.landau@hcuge.ch Publication Types: Review

Int J Toxicol. 2005 May-Jun;24(3):153-5. Related Articles, Links Application of emerging technologies in toxicology and safety assessment: regulatory perspectives. Leighton JK. Division of Oncology Drug Products, Food and Drug Administration, Center for Drug Evaluation and Research, Rockville, Maryland 20852, USA. LEIGHTONJ@cder.fda.gov Emerging technologies applied in the regulatory field encompass a group of technologies that are used in addition to or in replacement of the standard toxicology studies conducted to support an Investigational New Drug Application (IND) or New Drug Application (NDA). The standard package includes general toxicology studies of various duration, safety pharmacology studies, genetic toxicology studies, and reproductive toxicology studies. New and emerging technologies applied to the regulation of new drugs include the use of novel biomarkers, transfected cells and transgenic animals, and the "omics" technologies (toxicogenomics, proteomics, and metabonomics). These technologies are at various stages of regulatory development and acceptance. For example, the use of transgenic animals have gained acceptance by regulatory authorities to replace a 2-year carcinogenicity assay. Alternatively, the "omics" technologies are not sufficiently advanced to achieve regulatory acceptance as replacements, although these assays have a role early in drug development and they may prove useful as supplements to standard studies. Data from these assays have been used to address specific mechanistic questions in combination with standard toxicology assays. Publication Types: Review

Int Rev Psychiatry. 2004 Nov;16(4):311-9. Related Articles, Links Pharmacogenomics--can genetics help in the care of psychiatric patients? Bolonna AA, Arranz MJ, Mancama D, Kerwin RW. Clinical Neuropharmacology, Division of Psychological Medicine, Institute of Psychiatry, KCL, London, UK. Psychiatric patients demonstrate varied responses to treatment. Consequently, treatment strategies are trial-and-error, which has a negative effect on prognosis and compliance. The aim of pharmacogenomic research is to enable customised drug treatment by identifying variations within multiple candidate genes (those encoding drug-targeted neurotransmitter receptors, transporters and metabolic enzymes) that are likely to confer the inter-individual differences in drug response and development of drug-induced side effects. Pharmacogenetic and pharmacogenomic research to date has identified genetic polymorphisms of dopamine (DA) and serotonin (5-HT) receptor subtypes, the serotonin transporter (5-HTT) and metabolic enzymes (cytochrome P450 [CYP] family) as important contributors to the variability in response to psychiatric drugs and the development of drug-induced side effects such as tardive dyskinesia and weight gain. It is anticipated that technological and methodological advances will provide further candidate genes and refine association analyses of existing candidates, enabling pharmacogenomic research to move towards future treatment regimes that are catered to the individual. Publication Types: Review

Internist (Berl). 2005 Aug;46(8):835-6, 838-42, 844-6. Related Articles, Links [Basics of molecular diagnostics and therapy of malignant tumors] [Article in German] Daniel PT, Dorken B. Medizinische Klinik mit Schwerpunkt Hamatologie und Onkologie, Charite-Universitatsmedizin Berlin, Campus Virchow Klinikum, Humboldt Universitat, Berlin, Germany. pdaniel@mdc-berlin.de Recent insights in disease pathogenesis and mechanisms of resistance to therapy of malignant tumors provide a rational basis for the development of novel therapeutic strategies that target genetic defects and deregulated signaling events in malignant tumors. In contrast to conventional therapeutics, small molecule inhibitors or monoclonal antibodies allow for a far more selective, targeted therapy of tumors that carry a corresponding target structure or gene expression profile. Molecular therapeutics therefore necessitate clinical deployment of genetic diagnostics for the identification of those patients who have a chance to benefit from these novel targeted therapies. Publication Types: Review

Internist (Berl). 2005 Nov;46(11):1270-7. Related Articles, Links [Implications of pharmacogenetics in every-day practice.] [Article in German] Gerloff T, Roots I. Institut fur Klinische Pharmakologie, Charite Universitatsmedizin Berlin, . Pharmacogenetics as one of the areas of clinical pharmacology addresses hereditary factors involved in individually different responses to drugs. Clinical trials combined with molecular genetics seek for underlying reasons influencing efficacy and toxicity of drugs. The declared goal of pharmacogenetics is to provide physicians with knowledge and tools to allow an individualized patient-directed pharmacotherapy. This concept is best evolved for clinical practice in the field of drug-metabolizing enzymes, especially for the cytochromes P450 (CYP) 2D6, CYP2C19 and thiopurine S-methyltransferase (TPMT). Patients with inherited enzyme deficiencies are at risk to accumulate excessive drug concentrations when treated with standard doses which may lead to adverse drug reactions or even to life-threatening conditions. Genetic factors are also involved in drug-target interactions (e. g. receptors). Prospective controlled clinical trials are needed to evaluate the benefit of pharmacogenetics for therapy outcome and to define its role in clinical practice.

Invest New Drugs. 2004 Aug;22(3):285-9. Related Articles, Links Pharmacogenetics of tipifarnib (R115777) transport and metabolism in cancer patients. Sparreboom A, Marsh S, Mathijssen RH, Verweij J, McLeod HL. Clinical Pharmacology Research Core, National Cancer Institute, Bethesda, MD, USA. SparrebA@mail.nih.gov The purpose of this study was to perform exploratory relationships between the pharmacokinetics of the farnesyl transferase inhibitor, tipifarnib (R115777, Zarnestra) and allelic variants of genes coding for ATP binding-cassette transporters and drug-metabolizing enzymes. Twenty-eight patients with advanced solid tumors were treated with tipifarnib administered orally at a dose of 200 or 300 mg. Blood samples were collected for pharmacokinetics and genotyping of 10 variants in genes encoding P-glycoprotein (ABCB1), cytochrome P450 isozymes CYP3A4 and CYP3A5, and UDP glucuronosyltransferase isozyme UGT1A1. The homozygous T -allele of ABCB1*8 (1236C > T) was associated with a trend for a higher area under the curve of tipifarnib as compared to patients with only one or no variant alleles [mean (+/-SD), 5,303 +/- 1,620 ng.h/mL vs. 3,619 +/- 1,275 ng.h/mL; P = 0.047). No statistically significant differences were observed with any other genetic variant (P > 0.15). Overall, this study indicates that ABCB1 genotype might be correlated with tipifarnib pharmacokinetics, although considerable overlap in exposure measures between genotype groups was observed. Publication Types: Clinical Trial

Invest New Drugs. 2005 Dec;23(6):513-22. Related Articles, Links Cancer treatment and pharmacogenetics of cytochrome P450 enzymes. van Schaik RH. Department of Clinical Chemistry, Erasmus University Medical Center, Rotterdam, The Netherlands. r.vanschaik@erasmusmc.nl For the treatment of cancer, the window between drug toxicity and suboptimal therapy is often narrow. Interindividual variation in drug metabolism therefore complicates therapy. Genetic polymorphisms in phase I and phase II enzymes may explain part of the observed interindividual variation in pharmacokinetics and pharmacodynamics of anticancer drugs. The cytochrome P450 superfamily is involved in many drug metabolizing reactions. Information on variant alleles for the different isoenzymes of this family, encoding proteins with decreased enzymatic activity, is rapidly growing. The ultimate goal of ongoing research on these enzymes would be to enable pharmacogenetic screening prior to anticancer therapy. At this moment, potential clinically relevant application of CYP450 pharmacogenetics for anticancer therapy may be found for CYP1A2 and flutamide, CYP2A6 and tegafur, CYP2B6 and cyclophosphamide, CYP2C8 and paclitaxel, CYP2D6 and tamoxifen, and CYP3A5. For this latter enzyme, the drugs of interest still need to be identified.

Invest New Drugs. 2005 Dec;23(6):533-7. Related Articles, Links Thymidylate synthase pharmacogenetics. Marsh S. Division of Molecular Oncology, Washington University School of Medicine in St. Louis, 660, South Euclid Avenue, Campus Box 8069, St. Louis, MO 63110, USA. smarsh@im.wustl.edu Thymidylate synthase (TYMS) is an important target for chemotherapy drugs, such as 5-fluorouracil (5FU) and methotrexate. Over-expression of TYMS is linked to resistance to TYMS-targeted chemotherapy drugs. Currently there is no protocol for selecting cancer patients at risk for drug resistance prior to chemotherapy treatment. Three polymorphisms in the 5' and 3' untranslated regions (5'UTR and 3'UTR) of the thymidylate synthase gene have been shown to influence TYMS expression. Preliminary data has suggested a poorer response rate to 5FU or methotrexate is seen in patients with 3 copies of a 28 bp tandem repeat in the 5'UTR enhancer region (TSER polymorphism) and this relationship may be further clarified by the presence of a single nucleotide polymorphism (SNP) with the second repeat of the 3 repeat (TSER(*)3) allele. A 6 bp deletion in the 3'UTR of the TYMS gene has also been shown to affect TYMS RNA expression and has a significant association with poor outcome in 5FU treated patients. Evidence linking all 3 TYMS polymorphisms with TYMS expression and patient response to TYMS-targeted chemotherapy treatment will be highlighted.

Invest New Drugs. 2005 Dec;23(6):539-45. Related Articles, Links Pharmacogenetics of irinotecan: a promoter polymorphism of UGT1A1 gene and severe adverse reactions to irinotecan. Ando M, Hasegawa Y, Ando Y. Department of Medicine, Division of Respiratory Diseases, Nagoya University Graduated School of Medicine, Nagoya, Japan. This review focuses on a pharmacogenetic association between genetic polymorphism of UGT1A1 gene and severe adverse reactions to irinotecan. Although many studies used pharmacokinetic parameters as surrogate measures for predicting clinical outcomes of irinotecan chemotherapy, they have not produced consistent evidence. On the other hand, genotyping results of UGT1A1 gene appear to predict severe adverse reactions more straightforward than the pharmacokinetic parameters or the phenotypes of the enzymatic activity. A case-control study of Japanese cancer patients revealed that those with the variant UGT1A1 alleles were at significantly higher risk of severe adverse reactions to irinotecan, suggesting that the genotyping strategy would be clinically useful. Nevertheless, clinical importance of the pharmacogenetic testing should differ for different patient groups and for different clinical situations. We need to keep this issue in mind in applying the pharmacogenetic evidence in clinical practice.

J Acquir Immune Defic Syndr. 2004 Aug 15;36(5):1034-40. Related Articles, Links Coadministration of lopinavir/ritonavir and phenytoin results in two-way drug interaction through cytochrome P-450 induction. Lim ML, Min SS, Eron JJ, Bertz RJ, Robinson M, Gaedigk A, Kashuba AD. School of Pharmacy, University of North Carolina at Chapel Hill, Chapel Hill, NC 27599, USA. Lopinavir/ritonavir (LPV/RTV) is a CYP3A4 inhibitor and substrate; it also may induce cytochrome P-450 (CYP) isozymes. Phenytoin (PHT) is a CYP3A4 inducer and CYP2C9/CYP2C19 substrate. This study quantified the pharmacokinetic (PK) drug interaction between LPV/RTV and PHT. Open-label, randomized, multiple-dose, PK study in healthy volunteers. Subjects in arm A (n = 12) received LPV/RTV 400/100 mg twice daily (BID) (days 1-10), followed by LPV/RTV 400/100 mg BID + PHT 300 mg once daily (QD) (days 11-22). Arm B (n = 12) received PHT 300 mg QD (days 1-11), followed by PHT 300 mg QD + LPV/RTV 400/100 mg BID (days 12-23). Plasma samples were collected on day 11 and day 22; PK parameters were compared by geometric mean ratio (GMR, day 22:day 11). P values <0.05 were considered significant. Following PHT addition, LPV area under the concentration-time curve (AUC0-12h) decreased from 70.9 +/-37.0 to 49.6 +/-25.1 microg.h/mL (GMR 0.67, P = 0.011) and C0h decreased from 6.0 +/- 3.2 to 3.6 +/- 2.3 microg/mL (GMR 0.54, P = 0.001). Following LPV/RTV addition, PHT AUC0-24h decreased from 191.0+/-89.2 to 147.8+/-104.5 microg.h/mL (GMR 0.69, P = 0.009) and C0h decreased from 7.0+/-4.0 to 5.3+/-4.1 microg/mL (GMR 0.66, P = 0.033). Concomitant LPV/RTV and PHT use results in a 2-way drug interaction. Phenytoin appears to increase LPV clearance via CYP3A4 induction, which is not offset by the presence of low-dose RTV. LPV/RTV may increase PHT clearance via CYP2C9 induction. Management should be individualized to each patient; dosage or medication adjustments may be necessary. Publication Types: Clinical Trial Randomized Controlled Trial

J Allergy Clin Immunol. 2004 Jul;114(1):13-9; quiz 20. Related Articles, Links The biology of Kit in disease and the application of pharmacogenetics. Akin C, Metcalfe DD. Laboratory of Allergic Diseases, National Institute of Allergy and Infectious Disease, National Institutes of Health, Bethesda, MD, USA. cemakin@med.umich.edu C-kit encodes a transmembrane protein with intrinsic tyrosine kinase activity, which functions as the receptor for stem cell factor. It is expressed on a variety of cell types, including mast cells, hematopoietic progenitor cells, melanocytes, germ cells, and gastrointestinal pacemaker cells. Mutations resulting in alteration of Kit function are associated with diseases involving each of these cells. Recent development of tyrosine kinase inhibitors led to their evaluation as novel therapies for diseases associated with Kit activation. This review will discuss the pathobiology of Kit in human disease, with a particular emphasis on implications for potential targeted treatment strategies in mast cell disease. Publication Types: Review

J Allergy Clin Immunol. 2005 Apr;115(4 Suppl):S532-8. Related Articles, Links Genetics and the variability of treatment response in asthma. Israel E. Division of Pulmonary and Critical Care Medicine, Brigham and Women's Hospital, Harvard Medical School, Boston, Mass, USA. Pharmacogenetics is the study of how genetic differences influence the variability in patients' responses to therapy. Using specific examples in asthma, I will define the concepts of variability in response to therapy in asthma. I will then use the relationship between specific genetic polymorphisms and the response to beta-adrenergic agonists and leukotriene modifiers to illustrate pharmacogenetic interactions and to acquaint the reader with the applicability of these findings to clinical practice. Publication Types: Case Reports Review

J Allergy Clin Immunol. 2005 Mar;115(3):470-7. Related Articles, Links Advances in pediatric and adult asthma. Szefler SJ, Apter A. Division of Clinical Pharmacology, Department of Pediatrics, National Jewish Medical and Research Center, Denver, Colo 80206, USA. szeflers@njc.org Last year's review on adult and pediatric asthma highlighted reports related to asthma genetics, the importance of upper airway management, the costs of asthma, and the importance of early recognition and intervention. This year we will organize our discussion to review recent reports related to the origins and persistence of asthma in both adults and children. We highlight Journal publications from 2004, along with recent key publications from other medical journals, to provide a perspective on the rapidly developing areas of genetics, including pharmacogenetics, respiratory infection, biomarker measurements, and asthma pharmacotherapy. This new understanding of the pathogenesis of asthma combined with clinical applications of genetics and biomarkers should lead to new management strategies. Asthma management is likely to change in the coming years from a strategy directed to the best outcome in groups of patients to an individualized approach to assessment and management. Publication Types: Review

J Am Acad Nurse Pract. 2005 Jun;17(6):219-24. Related Articles, Links Genetics of essential hypertension. Coy V. Trauma Services/Austin Medical Education Program, Brackenridge Hospital, Austin, TX 78701, USA. PURPOSE: To inform healthcare providers of the genetics involved in the development of essential hypertension and to illustrate the role the healthcare provider has in the management of patients with essential hypertension. DATA SOURCES: Research-based articles in the medical literature, selected published literature in refereed journals, and Internet sites. CONCLUSIONS: Essential hypertension is a complex chronic disease that affects many people and has grave implications for the patient. Genetics involved in the development of essential hypertension and treatment choices is evolving; therefore, the healthcare provider must be knowledgeable in these areas to effectively care for patients with hypertension. IMPLICATIONS FOR PRACTICE: Essential hypertension is a chronic disease that affects over 50 million people in the United States. Advances in genetics are allowing scientists to discover the genetic basis of hypertension. With knowledge of genetics and environmental factors involved in the development of essential hypertension, healthcare providers will be able to more effectively screen, manage, and treat individuals with hypertension. Publication Types: Case Reports Review

J Am Chem Soc. 2006 Jan 18;128(2):658-62. Related Articles, Links DNA hole transport on an electrode: application to effective photoelectrochemical SNP typing. Okamoto A, Kamei T, Saito I. Department of Synthetic Chemistry and Biological Chemistry, Faculty of Engineering, Kyoto University, Japan. okamoto@sbchem.kyoto-u.ac.jp A useful feature of DNA is that long-range hole transport through DNA is readily achieved. Photostimulated long-range hole transport through DNA has prospective use in the development of a conceptually new electrochemical single-nucleotide polymorphism (SNP) typing method for use as a versatile platform for gene diagnostics and pharmacogenetics. We have applied artificial DNAs designed for photostimulated long-range hole transport through DNA to SNP typing. By hybridizing photosensitizer-equipped DNA probes, immobilized on gold working electrodes, with a target DNA strand containing an SNP site, we observed a cathodic photocurrent, which markedly changed depending on the nature of the base at the specific site. The use of a combination of hole-transporting bases constitutes a very powerful method for a single-step electrochemical assay applicable to SNP typing of all types of sequences.

J Am Coll Cardiol. 2005 Dec 6;46(11):1965-77. Epub 2005 Nov 9. Related Articles, Links New paradigms in cardiovascular medicine: emerging technologies and practices: perioperative genomics. Podgoreanu MV, Schwinn DA. Department of Anesthesiology, Duke University Medical Center, Durham, North Carolina 27710, USA. mihai.podgoreanu@duke.edu Considerable progress has been made in understanding the pathophysiology of perioperative stress responses and their impact on the cardiovascular system; however, researchers are just beginning to unravel genetic and molecular determinants that predispose to increased risk for postoperative cardiovascular adverse events. A new field, coined perioperative genomics, aims to apply functional genomic approaches to uncover the biological reasons why similar patients can have dramatically different clinical outcomes after surgery. For the perioperative physician, such findings may soon translate into prospective risk assessment incorporating genomic profiling of markers important in inflammatory, thrombotic, vascular, and neurologic responses to perioperative stress, with implications ranging from individualized additional pre-operative testing and physiological optimization, to perioperative decision-making, choice of monitoring strategies, and critical care resource utilization. We review current knowledge regarding genomic technologies in perioperative cardiovascular disease characterization and outcome prediction, as well as discuss future trends/challenges for translating integrated "omic" information into daily clinical management of the surgical patient. Publication Types: Review

J Am Coll Cardiol. 2005 May 17;45(10):1611-9. Epub 2005 Apr 21. Related Articles, Links Comment in: J Am Coll Cardiol. 2005 May 17;45(10):1620-1. A common PCSK9 haplotype, encompassing the E670G coding single nucleotide polymorphism, is a novel genetic marker for plasma low-density lipoprotein cholesterol levels and severity of coronary atherosclerosis. Chen SN, Ballantyne CM, Gotto AM Jr, Tan Y, Willerson JT, Marian AJ. Section of Cardiology, Center for Preventive Cardiology, Department of Medicine, Baylor College of Medicine, Houston, Texas 77030, USA. OBJECTIVES: We sought to determine the effects of PCSK9 variants on plasma low-density lipoprotein cholesterol (LDL-C) levels, severity of coronary atherosclerosis, and response to statin therapy in the Lipoprotein Coronary Atherosclerosis Study (LCAS) population. BACKGROUND: Mutations in PCSK9 cause autosomal-dominant hypercholesterolemia. We hypothesized that PCSK9 variants could affect plasma LDL-C in individuals with polygenic hypercholesterolemia. METHODS: We sequenced all 12 exons and boundaries to detect novel polymorphisms, and genotyped 372 subjects in LCAS and 319 subjects in a second independent population for six polymorphisms, including novel leucine repeats, by fluorescently tagged markers. We reconstructed haplotypes using a Bayesian algorithm. RESULTS: Permutation test results showed statistically significant differences in global haplotype distribution among the tertiles of LDL-C (odds ratio [OR]: 2.36, 95% confidence interval [CI]: 1.90 to 4.32, $p = 0.005$) and minimum lumen diameter of coronary lesions (OR: 1.83, 95% CI: 1.01 to 3.55, $p = 0.045$). Regression analysis identified haplotype 3 as an independent determinant of LDL-C levels (adjusted R2 = 2.2%, F = 9.37, p = 0.002). Haplotype structure analysis identified E670G as the determinant variant, exerting a dose effect (GG > EG > EE) and accounting for 3.5% of plasma LDL-C variability (F = 14.6, p < 0.001). Plasma total cholesterol, apolipoprotein B, and lipoprotein (a) levels were also associated with the E670G variant. Distributions of the E670G genotypes in an independent normolipidemic and the hyperlipidemic LCAS populations were significantly different (F = 7.2, p = 0.027). No significant treatment-by-genotype interactions were detected. The false positive report probability was between 2% and 8%. CONCLUSIONS: Haplotype 3 encompassing the E670G variant is an independent determinant of plasma LDL-C levels and the severity of coronary atherosclerosis. Publication Types: Clinical Trial Controlled Clinical Trial

J Am Coll Cardiol. 2005 Nov 1;46(9):1615-27. Epub 2005 Oct 10. Related Articles, Links Prospects for personalized cardiovascular medicine: the impact of genomics. Ginsburg GS, Donahue MP, Newby LK. Division of Cardiovascular Medicine, Department of Medicine, Institute for Genome Sciences and Policy, Center for Genomic Medicine, Duke University, Durham, North Carolina 27708, USA. geoffrey.ginsburg@duke.edu Sequencing of the human genome has ushered in prospects for individualizing cardiovascular health care. There is growing evidence that the practice of cardiovascular medicine might soon have a new toolbox to predict and treat disease more effectively. The Human Genome Project has spawned several important "omic" technologies that allow "whole genome" interrogation of sequence variation (re-sequencing, genotyping, comparative genome hybridization), transcription (expression profiling, tissue arrays), proteins (gas or liquid chromatography and tandem mass spectroscopy [MS]), and metabolites (MS or nuclear magnetic resonance profiling); deoxyribonucleic acid, ribonucleic acid, protein, and metabolic approaches all provide more exacting detail of cardiovascular disease mechanisms and, in some cases, are redefining its taxonomy. Pharmacogenomic approaches are emerging across broad classes of cardiovascular therapeutics to assist practitioners in making more precise decisions about which drugs to give to which patients to optimize the benefit-to-risk ratio. Molecular imaging is developing chemical and biological probes that can sense molecular pathway mechanisms that will allow us to monitor health and disease. Together, these tools will enable a paradigm shift from genetic medicine--on the basis of the study of individual inherited characteristics, most often single genes--to genomic medicine, which by its nature is comprehensive and focuses on the functions and interactions of multiple genes and gene products, among themselves and with their environment. The information gained from such analyses, in combination with clinical data, is now allowing us to assess individual risks and guide clinical management and decision-making, all of which form the basis for cardiovascular genomic medicine. Publication Types: Review

J Am Med Inform Assoc. 2005 Mar-Apr;12(2):121-9. Epub 2004 Nov 23. Related Articles, Links Erratum in: J Am Med Inform Assoc. 2005 May-Jun;12(3):364. A statistical approach to scanning the biomedical literature for pharmacogenetics knowledge. Rubin DL, Thorn CF, Klein TE, Altman RB. Section of Medical Informatics, MSOB X-215,

Stanford, CA 94305, USA. rubin@smi.stanford.edu OBJECTIVE: Biomedical databases summarize current scientific knowledge, but they generally require years of laborious curation effort to build, focusing on identifying pertinent literature and data in the voluminous biomedical literature. It is difficult to manually extract useful information embedded in the large volumes of literature, and automated intelligent text analysis tools are becoming increasingly essential to assist in these curation activities. The goal of the authors was to develop an automated method to identify articles in Medline citations that contain pharmacogenetics data pertaining to gene-drug relationships. DESIGN: The authors built and evaluated several candidate statistical models that characterize pharmacogenetics articles in terms of word usage and the profile of Medical Subject Headings (MeSH) used in those articles. The best-performing model was used to scan the entire Medline article database (11 million articles) to identify candidate pharmacogenetics articles. RESULTS: A sampling of the articles identified from scanning Medline was reviewed by a pharmacologist to assess the precision of the method. The authors' approach identified 4,892 pharmacogenetics articles in the literature with 92% precision. Their automated method took a fraction of the time to acquire these articles compared with the time expected to be taken to accumulate them manually. The authors have built a Web resource (http://pharmdemo.stanford.edu/pharmdb/main.spy) to provide access to their results. CONCLUSION: A statistical classification approach can screen the primary literature to pharmacogenetics articles with high precision. Such methods may assist curators in acquiring pertinent literature in building biomedical databases.

J Anal Toxicol. 2005 Oct;29(7):590-8. Related Articles, Links Pharmacogenomics as molecular autopsy for forensic toxicology: genotyping cytochrome P450 3A4*1B and 3A5*3 for 25 fentanyl cases. Jin M, Gock SB, Jannetto PJ, Jentzen JM, Wong SH. Department of Pathology, Medical College of Wisconsin, Milwaukee 53226, USA. Pharmacogenomics, the study on genetic contributions to drug action may help in certifying fentanyl toxicity. Fentanyl is used clinically as an adjunct to surgical anesthesia and for chronic pain management. Its toxicity may be partially due to cytochrome P450 (CYP) 3A4*1B and 3A5*3 variant alleles, resulting in variable fentanyl metabolism. In this study, we examined 25 fentanyl-related deaths (22 Caucasians, 1 African-American, and 2 Native-Americans) from the Milwaukee County Medical Examiner's Office and referral cases. Fentanyl and norfentanyl in postmortem blood samples were analyzed by radioimmunoassay and liquid chromatography-mass spectrometry-mass spectrometry. The samples were then genotyped for CYP3A4*1B and 3A5*3 using Pyrosequencing. Genotyping showed: 1 CYP3A4*1B homozygous and CYP3A5*3 heterozygous, 1 compound CYP3A4*1B and CYP3A5*3 heterozygous, 22 CYP3A4*1B wild type and CYP3A5*3 homozygous, and 1 CYP3A5*3 and CYP3A4*1B wild type. CYP variant allelic frequencies of the 25 cases were 6% for CYP3A4*1B and 92% for CYP3A5*3, compared with normal Caucasian CYP3A4*1B, 3-8%, and CYP3A5*3, 85-95%. The mean fentanyl concentration and metabolic ratio of fentanyl to norfentanyl of the 2 cases with CYP3A4*1B and CYP3A5*3 variants were 12.8 and 1.4 microg/L, respectively, lower than those of 22 cases with wild type CYP3A4*1B and CYP3A5*3 homozygous variants, 16.7 and 7.3 microg/L, respectively. The postmortem/in vivo data provided the first scientific evidence that CYP3A5 is involved in the fentanyl metabolism, and homozygous CYP3A5 *3 causes impaired metabolism of fentanyl, and genotyping CYP3A4*1B and 3A5*3 variants may help to certify the fentanyl toxicity.

J Appl Genet. 2004;45(4):395-7. Related Articles, Links Molecular biomedicine and the unraveling of complex phenotypes. Pignatti PF. Publication Types: Editorial

J Autoimmun. 2005;25 Suppl:1-5. Related Articles, Links Pharmacogenetics of autoimmune diseases: research issues in the case of Multiple Sclerosis and the role of IFN-beta. Macciardi F, Boneschi FM, Cohen D. Serono Genetics Institute, 5, rue Henri Desbrueres, 91030 Evry Cedex, France. fabio.macciardi@serono.fr Pharmacogenetics of auto-immune diseases is a complex field of application for this relatively new discipline, since we still have a partial knowledge of the biological mechanisms of the disease and of the drugs currently used to treat it. We address a few key issues that emerge when planning a pharmacogenetic investigation in Multiple Sclerosis and that relate to the complexities existing at the biological-genetic level and at the phenotypic characterization. In fact, we think that a clearer characterization of the clinical phenotype representing the end-point of the investigation together with a critical appraisal of the multi-faceted dimension of the genetic component of either the disease and the pharmacogenetic profile of the drug investigated, will help to design more thorough study and to achieve deeper understanding of the practical results. We will primarily focus our research considerations on the role of Interferon Beta (IFN-beta) as a prototypal therapeutic agent in Multiple Sclerosis.

J Biol Chem. 2006 Mar 17;281(11):7364-73. Epub 2006 Jan 6. Related Articles, Links Human arsenic methyltransferase (AS3MT) pharmacogenetics: gene resequencing and functional genomics studies. Wood TC, Salavagionne OE, Mukherjee B, Wang L, Klumpp AF, Thomae BA, Eckloff BW, Schaid DJ, Wieben ED, Weinshilboum RM. Division of Clinical Pharmacology, Department of Molecular Pharmacology and Experimental Therapeutics, Mayo Clinic College of Medicine, 200 First Street SW, Rochester, MN 55905, USA. Arsenic contaminates ground water worldwide. Methylation is an important reaction in the biotransformation of arsenic. We set out to study the pharmacogenetics of human arsenic methyltransferase (AS3MT, previously CYT19). After cloning the human AS3MT cDNA, we annotated the human gene and resequenced its 5'-flanking region, exons, and splice junctions using 60 DNA samples from African-American (AA) and 60 samples from Caucasian-American (CA) subjects. We observed 26 single nucleotide polymorphisms (SNPs), including 3 non-synonymous cSNPs, as well as a variable number of tandem repeats in exon 1 within an area encoding the cDNA 5'-untranslated region. The nonsynonymous cSNPs included T860C (M287T) with frequencies of 10.8 and 10% in AA and CA subjects, respectively, as well as C517T (A173W) in one AA and C917T (T306I) in one CA sample. Haplotype analysis showed that Ile(306) was linked to Thr(287), so this double variant allozyme was also studied functionally. After expression in COS-1 cells and correction for transfection efficiency, the Trp(173) allozyme displayed 31%, Thr(287) 350%, Ile(306)

4.8%, and Thr(287)/Ile(306) 6.2% of the activity of the wild type (WT) allozyme, with 20, 190, 4.4, and 7.9% of the level of WT immunoreactive protein, respectively. Apparent K(m) values for S-adenosyl-l-methionine were 4.6, 3.1, and 11 mum for WT, Trp(173), and Thr(287) allozymes, with K(m) values for sodium arsenite with the same allozymes of 11.8, 8.9, and 4.5mum. The Ile(306) and Thr(287)/Ile(306) allozymes expressed too little activity for inclusion in the substrate kinetic studies. Expression of reporter gene constructs for the 5'-flanking region and the variable number of tandem repeats in the 5'-untranslated region demonstrated cell line-dependent variation in reporter gene expression, with shorter repeats associated with increased transcription in HepG2 cells. These results raise the possibility that inherited variation in AS3MT may contribute to variation in arsenic metabolism and, perhaps, arsenic-dependent carcinogenesis in humans.

J Biolaw Bus. 2004;7(3):16-9. Related Articles, Links How molecular medicine transforms policy (and everything else). Kean MA, Batchelder KF. Feinstein Kean Healthcare, Cambridge, Massachusetts, USA. Molecular medicine (also known as pharmacogenomics, pharmacogenetics, gene-based medicine, personalized medicine), after being heralded prematurely as the next revolution in medicine, is in the process now of becoming the first big change in healthcare of the 21st century. Because its scientific, clinical, ethical, financial, and regulatory implications are so far-reaching, it is important to define who and what will be affected in order to put the right societal systems and policies in place to cope with the change. Leaders of the personalized medicine field will be those organizations that see the wave and prepare to adjust their traditional planning, relationships, attitudes and management approach.

J Biolaw Bus. 2005;8(3):28-36. Related Articles, Links Ethics and policy perspectives on personalized medicine in the post-genomic era. Landon MR. Boston University, USA. The completion of the human genome project and the accompanying biotechnological revolution hold great promise for the creation of pharmaceutical agents to combat not only previously incurable diseases, but also those for which therapeutics exist, yet they either cause severe adverse effects or exhibit no benefit in subsets of the population. In many instances variation in therapy response can be attributed to genetic differences, more particularly single nucleotide polymorphism (SNPs). Detection of the genetic differences which affect drug response, commonly referred to as pharmacogenomics, may result in further classification of diseases, and consequently, the development of 'personalized' therapies. While of potential great benefit, the widespread use of pharmacogenomic data poses social, ethical, and economic risks that need to be addressed by regulatory agencies such as the Food and Drug Administration (FDA). This paper explores some of the common problems associated with the use of pharmacogenomic data including validation of the data, patient confidentiality, social stratification, economic risks faced by pharmaceutical and insurance companies, and offers suggestions for regulatory procedures to ensure the appropriate use of the data in drug development and clinical trials.

J Biomed Sci. 2004 May-Jun;11(3):418-22. Related Articles, Links Medicinal herb extract and a single-compound drug confer similar complex pharmacogenomic activities in mcf-7 cells. Yang NS, Shyur LF, Chen CH, Wang SY, Tzeng CM. Institute of BioAgricultural Sciences, Academia Sinica, Taipei, Taiwan, ROC. nsyang@gate.sinica.edu.tw Metabolite profiling and DNA microarray analysis of global gene expression profiles were employed to characterize the bioactivities of the herbal extract of Anoectochilus formosanus (AF), a popular folk medicine with anticancer activity, in MCF-7 cancer cells. The pharmacogenomic activities of this plant extract as a crude phytocompound mixture were compared to those conferred by the single-compound drug, plumbagin. A similar level of complexity in transcriptional regulation at the genomic level was observed for both AF extract- and plumbagin-treated MCF-7 cells, as revealed by the number of up- or downregulated genes as well as by the specific but distinct patterns found in the gene-clustering analysis. This finding offers evidence to support the search for fractionated medicinal herb extracts or phytocompound mixtures, in addition to single-compound drugs, as defined therapeutic agents. Copyright 2004 National Science Council, ROC and S. Karger AG, Basel

J Biopharm Stat. 2004 Aug;14(3):535-7. Related Articles, Links Microarrays in pharmacogenomics. Chen JJ. Publication Types: Editorial

J Biopharm Stat. 2004 Aug;14(3):539-52. Related Articles, Links Some statistical and regulatory issues in the evaluation of genetic and genomic tests. Campbell G. Division of Biostatistics, Center for Devices and Radiological Health, US Food and Drug Administration, Rockville, Maryland 20850, USA. gxc@cdrh.fda.gov The genomics revolution is reverberating throughout the worlds of pharmaceutical drugs, genetic testing and statistical science. This revolution, which uses single nucleotide polymorphisms (SNPs) and gene expression technology, including cDNA and oligonucleotide microarrays, for a range of tests from home-brews to high-complexity lab kits, can allow the selection or exclusion of patients for therapy (responders or poor metabolizers). The wide variety of US regulatory mechanisms for these tests is discussed. Clinical studies to evaluate the performance of such tests need to follow statistical principles for sound diagnostic test design. Statistical methodology to evaluate such studies can be wide ranging, including receiver operating characteristic (ROC) methodology, logistic regression, discriminant analysis, multiple comparison procedures resampling, Bayesian hierarchical modeling, recursive partitioning, as well as exploratory techniques such as data mining. Recent examples of approved genetic tests are discussed. Publication Types: Review

J Biopharm Stat. 2004 Aug;14(3):553-73. Related Articles, Links A generalized additive model for microarray gene expression data analysis. Tsai CA, Hsueh HM, Chen JJ. Division of Biometry and Risk Assessment, National Center for Toxicological Research, Food and Drug Administration, Jefferson, Arkansas 72079, USA. Microarray technology allows the measurement of expression levels of a large number of genes simultaneously. There are inherent biases in microarray data generated from an experiment. Various statistical methods have been proposed for data normalization and data analysis. This paper proposes a generalized additive model for the analysis of gene expression data. This model consists of two sub-models: a non-linear model and a linear model. We propose a two-step normalization algorithm to fit the two sub-models sequentially. The first step involves a non-parametric regression using lowess fits to adjust for non-linear systematic biases. The second step uses a linear ANOVA model to estimate the remaining effects including the interaction effect of genes and treatments, the effect of interest in a study. The proposed model is a generalization of the ANOVA model for microarray data analysis. We show correspondences between the lowess fit and the ANOVA model methods. The normalization procedure does not assume the majority of genes do not change their expression levels, and neither does it assume two channel intensities from the same spot are independent. The procedure can be applied to either one channel or two channel data from the experiments with multiple treatments or multiple nuisance factors. Two toxicogenomic experiment data sets and a simulated data set are used to contrast the proposed method with the commonly known lowess fit and ANOVA methods.

J Biopharm Stat. 2005;15(2):327-41. Related Articles, Links Class prediction in toxicogenomics. Raghavan N, Amaratunga D, Nie AY, McMillian M. Department of Non-Clinical Biostatistics, Johnson and Johnson Pharmaceutical Research and Development, LLC, Raritan, New Jersey 08869, USA. nraghava@prdus.jnj.com The intent of this article is to discuss some of the complexities of toxicogenomics data and the statistical design and analysis issues that arise in the course of conducting a toxicogenomics study. We also describe a procedure for classifying compounds into various hepatotoxicity classes based on gene expression data. The methodology involves first classifying a compound as toxic or nontoxic and subsequently classifying the toxic compounds into the hepatotoxicity classes, based on votes by binary classifiers. The binary classifiers are constructed by using genes selected to best elicit differences between the two classes. We show that the gene selection strategy improves the misclassification error rates and also delivers gene pathways that exhibit biological relevance.

J Bone Joint Surg Am. 2005 Nov;87(11):2550-64. Related Articles, Links Molecular biology in orthopaedics: the advent of molecular orthopaedics. Evans CH, Rosier RN. Center for Molecular Orthopaedics, Harvard Medical School, 221 Long-wood Avenue, BLI-152, Boston, MA 02115, USA. cevans@rics.bwh.harvard.edu Molecular biology is the study, at the molecular level, of how genetic information is stored, inherited, and expressed and how it influences the structure and function of cells. Although molecular biology approaches have been used for decades in orthopaedic research, they are only now beginning to influence clinical practice. A variety of sophisticated techniques permit rapid and affordable DNA sequencing, gene expression profiling, gene cloning, gene manipulation, gene transfer, recombinant protein production, and other technologies of enormous biomedical importance. Success in genomics has spawned additional ambitious endeavors, including proteomics, pharmacogenetics, and bioinformatics. These techniques are providing new diagnostic, staging, prognostic, and therapeutic opportunities in all areas of medicine, including orthopaedics. With the use of molecular criteria, treatment of the orthopaedic patient may become more individualized, and greater emphasis will be placed on preventative strategies based on the patient's genetic makeup. Both surgical and nonsurgical decisions will increasingly accommodate molecular criteria.

J Cardiothorac Vasc Anesth. 2004 Jun;18(3):353-65. Related Articles, Links Pharmacogenetics as related to the practice of cardiothoracic and vascular anesthesia. Bukaveckas BL, Valdes R Jr, Linder MW. Department of Pathology and Laboratory Medicine, University of Louisville, Louisville, KY, USA. Publication Types: Review

J Cell Physiol. 2005 Sep;204(3):742-9. Related Articles, Links Pharmacogenomics in colorectal carcinomas: future perspectives in personalized therapy. Russo A, Corsale S, Cammareri P, Agnese V, Cascio S, Di Fede G, Macaluso M, Bazan V. Department of Oncology, University of Palermo, Italy. Lab-oncobiologia@usa.net The recent introduction of new drugs such as capecitabine, irinotecan, and oxaliplatinum has greatly improved the clinical outcome of patients with advanced/metastatic colorectal cancer. Nevertheless, some patients may suffer from the adverse drug reactions which will probably be the main cause of chemotherapy failure. The goal of pharmacogenomics is to find correlations between therapeutic responses to drugs and the genetic profiles of patients; the different responses to a particular drug are due, in fact, not only to the specific clinico-pathological features of the patient or to environmental factors, but also to the ethnic origins and the particular individual's genetic profile. Genes which codify for the metabolism enzymes, receptor proteins, or protein targets of chemotherapy agents often present various genetic polymorphisms. The main aim of this review is to provide an overview of the known polymorphisms present in the genes which codify for factors (thymidylate synthase dihydropyrimidine dehydrogenase, uridine diphosphate (UDP)-glucuronosyl-transferase 1A1, enzymes implicated in DNA repair) involved in the action mechanisms of the drugs now utilized in chemotherapeutic treatment of colorectal carcinoma, such as fluoropyrimidines, irinotecan, and platinum agents. Copyright 2005 Wiley-Liss, Inc. Publication Types: Review

J Chemother. 2004 Aug;16(4):337-42. Related Articles, Links Molecular characterization of beta-lactam resistance of Salmonella isolates from pediatric patients in Romania. Filip R, Chihu-Amparan L, Coman G, Velazquez ME, Silva J. Department of Microbiology, Faculty of Medicine, University of Medicine and Pharmacy Gr.T. Popa Iasi, Romania. The molecular characterization of 16 clinical isolates of Salmonella enterica (14 serotype Typhimurium and 2 serotype Kingston) obtained between January and June 1999 from feces of children hospitalized in Iasi, Romania were genotypically compared by pulse field gel electrophoresis of XbaI restricted bacterial DNA. The majority of the clinical isolates (12/16) belonged to cluster A and (4/16) to unrelated strains, correlating to the OMP profile. Two major different patterns of beta-lactamases were identified: the first with pI of 5.4, 8.2 in 6/16 strains and the second with pI of 5.4 in 5/16. The blaTEM beta-lactamase was identified in 14/16 of the clinical isolates and the blaSHV-5 gene in one strain. We concluded that extended spectrum beta-lactamase (ESBL) with pIs of 8.2 was the most frequent enzyme produced by serotype Typhimurium isolates which were related.

J Chemother. 2004 Aug;16(4):347-9. Related Articles, Links The contribution of a novel ribosomal S12 mutation to aminoglycoside resistance of Escherichia coli mutants. Gill AE, Amyes SG. Division of Medical Microbiology, School of Biomedical and Clinical Laboratory Sciences, University of Edinburgh, Medical School, Teviot Place, Edinburgh EH8 9AG, UK. This study characterised the contribution of a novel ribosomal S12 mutation to aminoglycoside resistance in Escherichia coli via step-wise mutation analysis. Mutants of E. coli NCTC 10418 were selected in four separate progressive series (I-IV) on plates containing increasing aminoglycoside (streptomycin, neomycin, gentamicin, tobramycin, and kanamycin) concentrations. Minimum inhibitory concentrations (MICs) of these aminoglycosides were established for the most resistant mutants in each series. There was no cross-resistance between streptomycin and the other aminoglycosides tested; however there was cross-resistance between the neomycin, tobramycin and kanamycin resistant mutants. DNA sequencing of a 423bp region of the rpsL gene encoding S12 revealed a novel Lys87-->Glu mutation in the streptomycin selected resistant mutants, while there were no S12 mutations in resistant mutants resulting from selection with neomycin, gentamicin, and tobramycin and kanamycin.

J Chemother. 2004 Dec;16 Suppl 6:35-48. Related Articles, Links Resistance phenotypes and multi-drug resistance in Streptococcus pneumoniae (PROTEKT years 1-3 [1999-20021). Reinert RR. Institute of Medical Microbiology, National Reference Center for Streptococci, University Hospital, Pauwelsstr. 30, D-52057 Aachen, Germany. Reinert@rwth-aachen.de Publication Types: Multicenter Study

J Chemother. 2004 Nov;16 Suppl 4:22-4. Related Articles, Links Pharmacogenetics and pharmacogenomics as new tools to optimise cancer chemotherapy. Robert J. Universite Victor Segalen Bordeaux 2, Institut Bergonie, 33076 Bordeaux Cedex, France. robert@bergonie.org Pharmacogenetics takes into account the individual variability of the genome and its relationships with drug activity. Numerous gene polymorphisms occurring at the level of drug metabolising enzymes, drug transporters or drug targets have been identified; they may be responsible for an alteration of the phenotype, and of individual changes in drug efficacy and/or toxicity. Pharmacogenomics takes into account the genetic alterations present in tumours and their role in drug activity. It may be possible to establish correlations between the activity of a drug and the level of expression of tumour genes, and thus select the most appropriate drugs to prescribe for the treatment of individual tumours. Pharmacogenetics and pharmacogenomics are acting synergistically for the personalisation of treatments, on the basis of the constitutive singularity of patients and of the molecular characteristics of tumours. Publication Types: Review

J Chemother. 2004 Nov;16 Suppl 4:25-30. Related Articles, Links Prospective clinical trials using a pharmacogenetic/pharmacogenomic approach. Peters GJ, Smorenburg CH, Van Groeningen CJ. Dept Medical Oncology, VU University Medical Center, 1007 MB Amsterdam, The Netherlands. gj.peters@vumc.nl The antitumor activity of most anticancer agents is limited by a number of different factors, such as their cellular targets and activating enzymes, while constitutive genetic polymorphisms may limit drug bioavailability and influence either antitumor efficacy or toxic side effects. An example of a drug for which clear predictive parameters have been identified is 5-fluorouracil (5FU): its antitumor activity is limited by either a high activity of the target enzyme thymidylate synthase (TS) and/or a high activity of its degrading enzyme, dihydropyrimidine dehydrogenase (DPD). Retrospective studies showed a clear correlation between a high expression of TS and a poor response, which was stronger when DPD was included in the evaluation (high DPD, poor response). Therefore we initiated a clinical prospective study in which we treated previously untreated patients with advanced colorectal cancer with tailored chemotherapy: at a low TS-mRNA and low DPD-mRNA patients were stratified to receive a standard weekly 5FU-leucovorin regimen. At a high TS and/or DPD, patients were stratified to receive a combination of oxaliplatin and irinotecan. Up to now this proof-of-principle study demonstrated that selection of patients is possible and can clearly improve the clinical outcome. The next step is to develop algorithms to select patients for combination chemotherapy with 5FU-leucovorin and new compounds, such as oxaliplatin or irinotecan, or novel targeted agents such as bevacizumab or cetuximab. For these combination schedules the optimal combination of predictive factors has to be explored. Publication Types: Review

J Chemother. 2004 Nov;16 Suppl 4:31-5. Related Articles, Links Uridine diphosphoglucuronosyl transferase and methylenetetrahydrofolate reductase polymorphisms as genomic predictors of toxicity and response to irinotecan-, antifolate- and fluoropyrimidine-based chemotherapy. Toffoli G, Cecchin E. Experimental and Clinical Pharmacology, CRO - National Cancer Institute, Via Pedemontana Occidentale 12, 33081 Aviano, Italy. gtoffoli@cro.it Pharmacogenetics could be a useful tool for performing tailored anticancer chemotherapy. Several polymorphisms potentially affecting enzymes responsible for metabolism, transport and mechanism of action of irinotecan, fluoropyrimidines and antifolate agents have been investigated and sometimes associated with toxicity and response. In particular, uridine diphosphoglucuronosyl transferase 1A1 (UGT1A1) enzyme is responsible for detoxification of irinotecan active metabolite, SN38. A polymorphic structure in the promoter region (UGT1A1*28) may affect irinotecan toxicity and SN38 plasma level. Methylenetetrahydrofolate reductase (MTHFR) is a key enzyme in the folate cycle, presenting two common polymorphisms (677C>T and 1298 A>C) which have impact on toxicity and efficacy of methotrexate and 5-fluorouracil. Publication Types: Review

J Chemother. 2004 Nov;16 Suppl 4:7-12. Related Articles, Links Reversing resistance to targeted therapy. Vidal L, Attard G, Kaye S, De Bono J. Institute of Cancer Research and Royal Marsden Hospital, Sutton, UK. The development of molecular targeted anticancer drugs is rapidly changing cancer therapeutics. However, drug resistance to these novel agents remains a real clinical concern. Reports now indicate that resistance to many of these molecular targeted agents--including hormone therapies, trastuzumab, imatinib, and gefitinib--occurs via common resistance mechanisms. These include 1) inadequate target blockade due to sub-optimal drug delivery; 2) altered target expression at the DNA (gene amplification), mRNA or protein level; 3) an altered target such as a mutated kinase domain; 4) modified target regulating proteins (e.g. altered expression of co-activators and/or co-repressors for nuclear steroid hormone receptors); 5) signalling by alternative proteins (functional redundancy) or different signalling pathways. It is envisioned that the molecular evaluation of clinical anticancer drug resistance, which requires the detailed study of pharmacokinetics, pharmacogenetics and pharmacodynamics, will allow the development of rational reversal strategies and improved patient outcome. Publication Types: Review

J Chemother. 2005 Apr;17(2):131-7. Related Articles, Links T serotyping and genomic profile of erythromycin-resistant or -sensitive Streptococcus pyogenes isolated in Campania Region, Italy. Catalanotti P, Catania MR, Lucido M, Martini S, Galle F, Ortega De Luna L, Rossano F. Dipartimento di Medicina Sperimentale, Sezione di Microbiologia e Microbiologia Clinica, Seconda Universita di Napoli, Naples, Italy. piergior.catalanotti@unina2.it Streptococcus pyogenes causes mild infections, such as pharyngitis, and severe infections, such as necrotizing fascitis. In recent years, erythromycin-resistant strains of S. pyogenes have been reported in many countries. In some areas of Italy, increased rates of erythromycin resistance were first observed in the mid-1990s. Here, we report epidemiological T serotyping, invasiveness, erythromycin resistance, and PFGE patterns of 99 S. pyogenes strains isolated at the Laboratory of Clinical Microbiology of the Second University of Naples, Italy. Regarding T serotyping, 26 of 99 strains were W+, 16 strains were U+, 16 were X+, and 14 were agglutinated by anti T serum. A low percentage revealed Y+. Twelve strains were not T serotyped. PFGE patterns showed species polymorphism; however, inside the various serotypes, we demonstrated a fair homogeneity. No correlation among invasiveness and T serotype or PFGE pattern has been shown. Twenty-two of 99 strains were erythromycin-resistant.

J Chemother. 2005 Aug;17(4):385-92. Related Articles, Links Accumulation of azithromycin and roxithromycin in tracheal epithelial fetal cell lines expressing wild type or mutated cystic fibrosis transmembrane conductance regulator protein (CFTR). Labro MT, Babin-Chevaye C, Mergey M. INSERM U479, CHU X. Bichat, Paris, France. labro@bichat.inserm.fr Macrolides are accumulated in phagocytes, partially via an active transport system; the membrane carrier is not identified but many data indicate a link with the P-glycoprotein family which includes the Cystic Fibrosis Transmembrane Conductance Regulator (CFTR) protein. We have used two epithelial cell lines which express either wild-type (N cells) or mutated (homozygous deltaF508) (F cells) CFTR to study the cellular accumulation of two macrolides (azithromycin and roxithromycin). Adherent cells were incubated with the radiolabeled drugs before extensive washings and counting. Azithromycin was better (about 2-fold) accumulated in F cells up to 60 min but then plateaued, whereas accumulation continued without saturation over 3 hours in N cells. Roxithromycin was also better (1.5-fold) accumulated in F cells at 15 and 30 min, but there were no differences at further incubation times. Macrolide efflux from loaded N and F cells, and the susceptibilities of the carrier systems (entry and efflux) to various pharmacologic agents were similar to those previously observed with phagocytes. These data suggest that the macrolide carriers (for entry and efflux) are not strictly specific for phagocytes and that the CFTR protein plays a role in macrolide uptake.

J Child Neurol. 2004 Mar;19(3):155-64. Related Articles, Links Pharmacologic treatment of autism. Palermo MT, Curatolo P. Research Center for Autism, Associazione Anni Verdi, Via Silvio Sbricoli 8, 00148 Rome, Italy. marktpalermo@virgilio.it Autism is a chronic and lifelong pervasive developmental disorder for which there is yet no effective cure, and medical management remains a major challenge for clinicians. In spite of the possible similarities with conditions that have an established pharmacotherapy, and despite improvements in some associated "problematic behaviors" following the use of available medications, effective medical treatment for the core symptoms involving language and social cognition remains elusive. The purpose of the present article is to review current biologic knowledge about autism in an attempt to correlate clinical trials with known mechanisms of disease. In addition, the need for controlled studies and for the creation of homogeneous subgroups of patients based on clinical and genetic characteristics is emphasized. The application of molecular genetic investigations and pharmacogenetics in the diagnostic work-up of autistic patients can lead to more effective individualized medical care. Publication Types: Review

J Chromatogr B Analyt Technol Biomed Life Sci. 2004 May 25;804(2):263-7. Related Articles, Links Simple and rapid docetaxel assay in plasma by protein precipitation and high-performance liquid chromatography-tandem mass spectrometry. Hou W, Watters JW, McLeod HL. Department of Medicine, Washington University School of Medicine, 660 S. Euclid Avenue, Campus Box 8069, St. Louis, MO 63110, USA. A simple, rapid and low cost sample preparation method was developed for quantification of docetaxel in mouse plasma by high-performance liquid chromatography/tandem mass spectrometry with paclitaxel as the internal standard. A small volume of plasma (40 microl) and one-step protein precipitation using methanol and acetonitrile (1:1 (v/v)) were used for sample preparation. The calibration curve for docetaxel in mouse plasma was linear over the range 25-2500 nM. The detection limit was 8 nM. The lower limit of quantitation is 25 nM. The intra- and inter-day precisions (CV) of analysis were 9.5 and 9.7% for the low quality control (LQC), 5.5 and 4.9% for the medium quality control (MQC) and 3.9 and 6.3% for the high quality control (HQC), respectively. The accuracy was 102.5% for LQC, 97.9% for MQC and 108.8% for HQC. This assay has now been applied to evaluation of mouse pharmacogenetics and other clinical pharmacology applications.

J Clin Endocrinol Metab. 2004 Dec;89(12):6208-17. Related Articles, Links X-chromosome inactivation patterns and androgen receptor functionality influence phenotype and social characteristics as well as pharmacogenetics of testosterone therapy in Klinefelter patients. Zitzmann M, Depenbusch M, Gromoll J, Nieschlag E. Institute of Reproductive Medicine, University of Munster, D-48129 Munster, Germany. Klinefelter syndrome is characterized by a vast range of phenotypes related to androgen effects. Testosterone (T) acts via the X-linked androgen receptor gene carrying the CAG repeat (CAGn) polymorphism, the length of which is inversely associated with androgen action and might account for the marked variation in phenotypes. In 77 newly diagnosed and untreated Klinefelter patients with a 47,XXY karyotype we assessed phenotype and social traits in relation to X-weighted biallelic CAGn length using X-chromosome inactivation analysis after digestion of leukocyte DNA with methylation-sensitive HpaII. Forty-eight men were hypogonadal and received T substitution therapy; in these, pharmacogenetic effects were investigated. The shorter CAGn allele was preferentially inactive. CAGn length was positively associated with body height. Bone density and the relation of arm span to body height were inversely related to CAGn length. The presence of long CAGn was predictive for gynecomastia and smaller testes, whereas short CAGn were associated with a stable partnership and professions requiring higher standards of education also when corrected for family background. There was a trend for men with longer CAGn to be diagnosed earlier in life. Under T substitution, men with shorter CAGn exhibited a more profound suppression of LH levels, augmented prostate growth, and higher hemoglobin concentrations. A significant genotype-phenotype association exists in Klinefelter patients: androgen effects on appearance and social characteristics are modulated by the androgen receptor CAGn polymorphism. The effects of T substitution are pharmacogenetically modified. This finding is magnified by preferential inactivation of the more functional short CAGn allele.

J Clin Endocrinol Metab. 2006 Mar;91(3):1076-80. Epub 2005 Nov 15. Related Articles, Links Growth hormone (GH) pharmacogenetics: influence of GH receptor exon 3 retention or deletion on first-year growth response and final height in patients with severe GH deficiency. Jorge AA, Marchisotti FG, Montenegro LR, Carvalho LR, Mendonca BB, Arnhold IJ. Hospital das Clinicas, Laboratorio de Hormonios, Avenida Dr Eneas de Carvalho Aguiar 155 PAMB, 2 andar Bloco 6, 05403-900, Sao Paulo, Brazil. alexj@usp.br CONTEXT: A polymorphism in GHR gene, the presence or absence of exon 3, has been shown to influence the 1- and 2-yr growth responses to human recombinant GH (hGH) therapy in children without GH deficiency (GHD). OBJECTIVE: The objective of this study was to assess the influence of GHR-exon-3 genotype on the short and long-term response to hGH therapy in children with GHD. SETTING: The study was conducted in the university hospital. DESIGN AND PATIENTS: Genotype and retrospective analysis was performed on data of 75 children with GHD. Intervention: Intervention consisted of hGH treatment at a mean dose of 33 mug/kg.d and GHR-exon-3 genotype by multiplex PCR. MAIN OUTCOME MEASURES: The main outcome measures were GHR genotype: full-length (fl) and exon 3-deleted (d3) alleles, growth velocity in 58 children who remained prepubertal during the first year, and adult height in 44 patients with GHD after 7.5 +/- 3.0 yr of treatment. RESULTS: Clinical and laboratory data at the start of treatment and hGH doses were indistinguishable among patients with different GHR-exon-3 genotypes (fl/fl vs. fl/d3 or d3/d3). Patients carrying at least one GHRd3 allele had a significantly better growth velocity in the first year of hGH replacement (12.3 +/- 2.6 vs. 10.6 +/- 2.3 cm/yr; $P < 0.05$) and achieved a taller adult height (final height sd score, -0.8 +/- 1.1 vs. -1.7 +/- 1.2; $P < 0.05$) when compared with patients homozygous for GHRfl alleles. CONCLUSIONS: Patients with GHD who are homozygous for GHR exon 3 fl were less responsive to short- and long-term hGH therapy. Approximately half of the population is homozygous for GHRfl, and future studies adjusting hGH therapy to genotype may improve outcome.

J Clin Epidemiol. 2005 Jul;58(7):651-4. Epub 2005 Apr 18. Related Articles, Links A review on the design and reporting of studies on drug-gene interaction. Smits KM, Schouten JS, Smits LJ, Stelma FF, Nelemans P, Prins MH. Department of Epidemiology, University of Maastricht, P.O. Box 616, 6200 MD Maastricht, The Netherlands. kim.smits@epid.unimaas.nl OBJECTIVE: Methodological standards for clinical pharmacogenetic studies should be developed to improve reporting of studies and facilitate their inclusion in systematic reviews. The essence of these studies lies within the concept of effect modification. STUDY DESIGN AND SETTING: A narrative review discussing methodological issues in the design and reporting of pharmacogenetic studies. RESULTS: Studying effect modification within a trial leads to the comparison of subgroups based on genotype. Differences in effect based on genotype should preferably be expressed in absolute terms (risk differences) to facilitate clinical decisions on treatment. Information on the distribution of potential effect modifiers or prognostic factors should be available to prevent a biased comparison of differences in effect between genotypes. The distribution of genotypes should also be presented and compared to Hardy-Weinberg equilibrium to check for selection bias. Additional points of interest include the possibility of selective nonavailability of biomaterial and the choice of a statistical model to study effect modification. CONCLUSION: Additional methodological issues should be taken into account when designing and reporting pharmacogenetic studies, to ensure high study quality. We present several important issues for future studies investigating drug-gene interactions that can serve as a basis for further discussion on methodology in pharmacogenetics. Publication Types: Review

J Clin Gastroenterol. 2005 May-Jun;39(4 Suppl 3):S251-6. Related Articles, Links What does the future hold for irritable bowel syndrome and the functional gastrointestinal disorders? Drossman DA. Department of Medicine, University of North Carolina at Chapel Hill, Chapel Hill, NC 27599-7080, USA. Our understanding of irritable bowel syndrome and the functional GI disorders has grown considerably over the last 15 years. In part this relates changes in their classification and definition from being due solely to motility disturbances, to being symptom based (eg, Rome criteria). This opened the door to the study of many other factors that contribute to the clinical expression of these disorders, including visceral hypersensitivity, sensitization, altered mucosal immunity, and dysfunction in brain-gut regulatory processes. New knowledge has been gained in areas of genetics, central nervous system and enteric nervous system neurotransmitters of motility, sensitivity and secretion, the effect of altered mucosal inflammation on cytokine and paracrine activation, and neural sensitization, postinfectious disorders, the influence of psychologic stress on gut functioning via alterations in regulatory pathways (eg, hypothalamic-pituitary adrenal axis, or pain regulatory system like the cingulate cortex), improved accuracy of diagnosis using Rome II criteria plus "red flags" the institution of behavioral treatments, and the use of new pharmacologic treatments both at the gut and brain level. Future research will improve upon this new knowledge via basic and translational studies of neuropeptide signaling with new neurotransmitters, new knowledge on the mechanisms for central nervous system-enteric nervous system communication and dysfunction, and more advanced clinical research on education, communication skills and their effects on outcome, genetics, pharmacogenetics and genetic epidemiology, better understanding as to how certain psychosocial domains (eg, catastrophizing, abuse) affect symptom behavior and outcome, newer pharmacologic treatments, and the use of combined pharmacologic and behavioral treatment packages. I am pleased to have the opportunity to provide a personal perspective on what the future will be for irritable bowel syndrome and the other functional GI disorders. Having been involved in this field for almost 30 years, I have been fortunate to witness tremendous changes. The focus of this presentation is to address the advances that have recently occurred that set the stage for proposing future research to help move the field along and ultimately to help our patients. Publication Types: Review

J Clin Gastroenterol. 2005 May-Jun;39(5 Suppl):S251-6. Related Articles, Links What does the future hold for irritable bowel syndrome and the functional gastrointestinal disorders? Drossman DA. From the Department of Medicine and Psychiatry and UNC Center for Functional GI and Motility Disorders, University of North Carolina at Chapel Hill, Chapel Hill, NC. Our understanding of irritable bowel syndrome and the functional GI disorders has grown considerably over the last 15 years. In part this relates changes in their classification and definition from being due solely to motility disturbances, to being symptom based (eg, Rome criteria). This opened the door to the study of many other factors that contribute to the clinical expression of these disorders, including visceral hypersensitivity, sensitization, altered mucosal immunity, and dysfunction in brain-gut regulatory processes. New knowledge has been gained in areas of genetics, central nervous system and enteric nervous system neurotransmitters of motility, sensitivity and secretion, the effect of altered mucosal inflammation on cytokine and paracrine activation, and neural sensitization, postinfectious disorders, the influence of psychologic stress on gut functioning via alterations in regulatory pathways (eg, hypothalamic-pituitary adrenal axis, or pain regulatory system like the cingulate cortex), improved accuracy of diagnosis using Rome II criteria plus "red flags" the institution of behavioral treatments, and the use of new pharmacologic treatments both at the gut and brain level. Future research will improve upon this new knowledge via basic and translational studies of neuropeptide signaling with new neurotransmitters, new knowledge on the mechanisms for central nervous system-enteric nervous system communication and dysfunction, and more advanced clinical research on education, communication skills and their effects on outcome, genetics, pharmacogenetics and genetic epidemiology, better understanding as to how certain psychosocial domains (eg, catastrophizing, abuse) affect symptom behavior and outcome, newer pharmacologic treatments, and the use of combined pharmacologic and behavioral treatment packages. I am pleased to have the opportunity to provide a personal perspective on what the future will be for irritable bowel syndrome and the other functional GI disorders. Having been involved in this field for almost 30 years, I have been fortunate to witness tremendous changes. The focus of this presentation is to address the advances that have recently occurred that set the stage for proposing future research to help move the field along and ultimately to help our patients.

J Clin Oncol. 2005 Dec 20;23(36):9312-8. Related Articles, Links Pharmacogenetics of tamoxifen biotransformation is associated with clinical outcomes of efficacy and hot flashes. Goetz MP, Rae JM, Suman VJ, Safgren SL, Ames MM, Visscher DW, Reynolds C, Couch FJ, Lingle WL, Flockhart DA, Desta Z, Perez EA, Ingle JN. Department of Oncology, Mayo Clinic College of Medicine, Rochester, MN 55905, USA. goetz.matthew@mayo.edu PURPOSE: Polymorphisms in tamoxifen metabolizing genes affect the plasma concentration of tamoxifen metabolites, but their effect on clinical outcome is unknown. METHODS: We determined cytochrome P450 (CYP)2D6 (*4 and *6) and CYP3A5 (*3) genotype from paraffin-embedded tumor samples and buccal cells (living patients) in tamoxifen-treated women enrolled onto a North Central Cancer Treatment Group adjuvant breast cancer trial. The relationship between genotype and disease outcome was determined using the log-rank test and Cox proportional hazards modeling. RESULTS: Paraffin blocks were obtained from 223 of 256 eligible patients, and buccal cells were obtained from 17 living women. CYP2D6 (*4 and *6) and CYP3A5 (*3) genotypes were determined from 190, 194, and 205 patient samples and in 17 living women. The concordance rate between buccal and tumor genotype was 100%. Women with the CYP2D6 *4/*4 genotype had worse relapse-free time (RF-time; P = .023) and disease-free survival (DFS; P = .012), but not overall survival (P = .169) and did not experience moderate to severe hot flashes relative to women heterozygous or homozygous for the wild-type allele. In the multivariate analysis, women with the CYP2D6 *4/*4 genotype still tended to have worse RFS (hazard ratio [HR], 1.85; P = .176) and DFS (HR, 1.86; P = .089). The CYP3A5*3 variant was not associated with any of these clinical outcomes. CONCLUSION: In tamoxifen-treated patients, women with the CYP2D6 *4/*4 genotype tend to have a higher risk of disease relapse and a lower incidence of hot flashes, which is consistent with our previous observation that CYP2D6 is responsible for the metabolic activation of tamoxifen to endoxifen.

J Clin Oncol. 2005 Jan 10;23(2):267-75. Related Articles, Links Integrative epidemiology: from risk assessment to outcome prediction. Spitz MR, Wu X, Mills G. Department of Epidemiology, The University of Texas M. D. Anderson Cancer Center, 1515 Holcombe Blvd., Box 189, Houston, TX 77030, USA. mspitz@mdanderson.org In this paper, we advance the concept of integrative epidemiology. Our unifying premise is that the same genes that are implicated in cancer risk may also be involved in a person's propensity to carcinogenic exposure and/or to modulation of therapeutic outcome. In the coming years, molecular epidemiology will play an increasingly prominent role in early detection of cancer and in identifying genetically high-risk subgroups that might benefit disproportionately from more intensive screening or chemoprevention interventions. Molecular epidemiology is also integral to pharmacogenetic research, by constructing genetic profiles that could be used to individualize therapy and to understand the functional consequences of chemoprevention, chemotherapy, or radiotherapy response. At the level of risk assessment, the focus might be on germline polymorphisms in candidate genes; for early detection, epigenetic events in these same or other genes may be relevant; and tumor tissue expression levels, loss of heterozygosity, genomic amplification, rearrangements, or somatic mutations in the same classes of genes may determine outcome. We will provide examples of how changes in the function of a single gene can contribute to susceptibility to carcinogenic exposure, predisposition to cancer development, patient prognosis, and prediction of outcome. Publication Types: Review

J Clin Oncol. 2005 Jan 10;23(2):311-23. Related Articles, Links Treating tobacco dependence: state of the science and new directions. Lerman C, Patterson F, Berrettini W. Tobacco Use Research Center, 3535 Market St, Suite 4100, Philadelphia, PA 19104, USA. clerman@mail.med.upenn.edu Despite almost two decades of intensive tobacco control efforts, nearly one quarter of Americans continue to smoke. The two United States Food and Drug Administration-approved medications used to treat tobacco dependence, bupropion and nicotine replacement therapy, are effective for only a fraction of smokers. Investigations of medications approved for affective disorders and other forms of substance abuse, such as fluoxetine and naltrexone, have yielded mixed results as tobacco dependence treatments. A particular challenge in tobacco dependence treatment is the development of effective approaches for smokers with unique needs, such as cancer patients and pregnant women. Despite new developments in these areas, significant gaps in knowledge and practice remain. Basic research in the neurobiologic and genetic basis of nicotine dependence offers promise for the development of novel and more effective treatment approaches. For example, emerging research in pharmacogenetics explores how genetic variation in drug-metabolizing enzymes and drug targets modifies response to pharmacotherapy. These discoveries could someday help practitioners to individualize the type, dosage, and duration of tobacco dependence treatment based on genotype, and maximize the efficacy. Publication Types: Review

J Clin Oncol. 2005 May 20;23(15):3517-25. Related Articles, Links Clinical value of mitochondrial mutations in colorectal cancer. Lievre A, Chapusot C, Bouvier AM, Zinzindohoue F, Piard F, Roignot P, Arnould L, Beaune P, Faivre J, Laurent-Puig P. INSERM U490 Laboratoire de Toxicologie Moleculaire, 45 Rue des Saints Peres, 75006 Paris, France. PURPOSE: Prognostic factors that could select high-risk recurrence colorectal cancer patients and predict chemosensitivity are needed. Since mutations of mitochondrial DNA (mtDNA) have been described in different types of cancers and since they may play a role in response to anticancer agents, we investigated in a population-based series of colorectal cancer patients the clinical value of mtDNA mutations. PATIENTS AND METHODS: The displacement loop (D-loop) region of mtDNA was sequenced on a series of 365 patients recorded in the Digestive Cancer Registry of Cote-d'Or (France) between 1998 and 2000. Clinicopathologic characteristics were correlated to the presence of a D-loop mutation. Survival rates were compared with the log-rank test. A multivariate survival analysis was performed.

RESULTS: D-loop mutations were found in 38.3% of the tumors. The 3-year survival rate was 53.5% in patients with D-loop mutation versus 62.1% in patients without (P = .05). After adjustment for age, stage, and microsatellite instability status, the relative risk of death in patients with D-loop mutation was 1.40 (95% CI, 1.02 to 1.93; P = .034) as compared with those without. In stage III colon cancers, adjuvant chemotherapy was beneficial only for patients without D-loop mutation (3-year survival, 78.3% v 45.4%, P < .02). In those with D-loop mutation who received adjuvant chemotherapy, the relative risk of death was 4.30 (95% CI, 1.23 to 15.00; P < .02). CONCLUSION: The D-loop region is a hotspot for somatic mutations in colorectal tumors. Moreover, presence of tumor D-loop mutation appears to be a factor of poor prognosis in colorectal patients and a factor of resistance to fluorouracil-based adjuvant chemotherapy in stage III colon cancers.

J Clin Oncol. 2005 Oct 1;23(28):7230-1; author reply 7231. Related Articles, Links Comment on: J Clin Oncol. 2005 Mar 1;23(7):1365-9. Studying the predictive/prognostic role of thymidylate synthase genotypes in patients with colorectal cancer: Is one polymorphism enough? Graziano F, Kawakami K. Publication Types: Comment Letter

J Clin Oncol. 2005 Oct 10;23(29):7342-9. Epub 2005 Sep 6. Related Articles, Links Comment in: J Clin Oncol. 2005 Oct 10;23(29):7253-6. Pharmacogenomic discovery approaches: will the real genes please stand up? Walgren RA, Meucci MA, McLeod HL. Department of Medicine, Washington University School of Medicine, 660 S Euclid Ave, Campus Box 8069, St Louis, MO 63110, USA. Genetic inheritance plays a significant role in the interindividual variability of drug response. The field of pharmacogenomics seeks to identify genetic factors that influence drug response, including both those that are inherited and those that arise within tumors, and use this information to improve drug therapy. Candidate gene approaches have led to clinical tests for toxicity avoidance (eg, TPMT, UGT1A1) and efficacy prediction (eg, epidermal growth factor receptor-activating mutations). However, the "right" genes are not known for most anticancer drugs. Strategies for uncovering pharmacogenomic associations vary widely from monogenic candidate gene approaches to polygenic genome-wide approaches. This review will place in context clinically relevant pharmacogenomic discovery approaches, including the relative strengths and weaknesses and the challenges inherent with achieving the goal of individualized therapy. Publication Types: Review

J Clin Pharm Ther. 2005 Apr;30(2):185-8. Related Articles, Links A study of the in vitro interaction between lidocaine and premedications using human liver microsomes. Nagashima A, Tanaka E, Inomata S, Honda K, Misawa S. Institute of Community Medicine, University of Tsukuba, Ibaraki-ken, Japan. OBJECTIVE: To investigate potential interactions between lidocaine (lignocaine) metabolism and premedication drugs, i.e. psychotropic and antianxiety agents (diazepam, midazolam), hypnotics (pentobarbital, thiamylal), depolarizing neuromuscular blocking agents (vecuronium, pancuronium and suxamethonium), an antihypertensive agent (clonidine) and an H2-receptor blocking agent (cimetidine) using human liver microsomes in vitro. METHODS: The interaction effects between lidocaine and premedication were examined using human liver microsomal preparations and monitored for enzyme activity. The lidocaine and its main metabolite (monoethylglycinexylide) were measured by HPLC/UV. RESULTS: Lidocaine metabolism was non-competitively inhibited by midazolam (Ki = 77.6 microM). Thiamylal was a competitive inhibitor of lidocaine metabolism (Ki = 885 microM). Cimethidine, pancuronium and vecuronium weakly inhibited lidocaine metabolism in a concentration-depend manner over the therapeutic range in human liver microsomes. On the contrary, suxamethonium, pentobarbital and clonidine did not inhibit lidocaine metabolism over the therapeutic range in human liver microsomes. CONCLUSION: These results show that the interactions between lidocaine and midazolam and thiamylal are of potential toxicological and clinical significance.

J Clin Pharm Ther. 2005 Aug;30(4):305-12. Related Articles, Links A second (non-genomic) steroid mechanism of action: possible opportunity for novel pharmacotherapy? Craig MA, Beppler GA, Santos C, Raffa RB. Department of Pharmaceutical Sciences, Temple University School of Pharmacy, Philadelphia, PA 19140, USA. Publication Types: Editorial

J Clin Pharm Ther. 2005 Feb;30(1):1-4. Related Articles, Links Drug evaluation, drug development and pharmacogenetics: celebrating 30 years of progress. Li Wan Po A. Publication Types: Editorial Historical Article

J Clin Pharmacol. 2004 Jun;44(6):559-69. Related Articles, Links Drug-drug, drug-dietary supplement, and drug-citrus fruit and other food interactions: what have we learned? Huang SM, Lesko LJ. Office of Clinical Pharmacology and Biopharmaceutics, HFD-850, Center for Drug Evaluation and Research, Food and Drug Administration, 5600 Fishers Lane, PKLN 6A/19, Rockville, MD 20850, USA. Serious drug-drug interactions have contributed to recent U.S. market withdrawals and also recent nonapprovals of a few new molecular entities. Many of these interactions involved the inhibition or induction of metabolizing enzymes and efflux transporters, resulting in altered systemic exposure and adverse drug reactions or loss of efficacy. In addition to drug-drug interactions, drug-dietary supplement and drug-citrus fruit interactions, among others, could also cause adverse drug reactions or loss of efficacy and are important issues to consider in the evaluation of new drug candidates. This commentary reviews (1). the current understanding of the mechanistic basis of these interactions, (2). issues to consider in the interpretation of study results, and (3). recent labeling examples to illustrate the translation of study results to information useful for patients and health care providers. Publication Types: Review

J Clin Pharmacol. 2005 Jun;45(6):649-58. Related Articles, Links A single administration of recombinant human interleukin-12 is associated with increased expression levels of interferon-gamma and signal transducer and activator of transcription in healthy subjects. Trudeau C, Cotreau MM, Stonis L, Dykstra KH, Oestreicher JL, Strahs A, Dorner AJ, Van Cleave VH, Trepicchio WL, Schwertschlag US. Experimental Medicine, Wyeth Research, 35 Cambridge Park Drive, Cambridge, MA 02140, USA. The objectives of this study were to assess the safety and tolerability of single doses of 1, 4, and 8 mug of recombinant human interleukin-12 (rhIL-12) administered subcutaneously to healthy subjects. The pharmacokinetics, pharmacodynamics, and pharmacogenomics of rhIL-12 were evaluated. Recombinant human IL-12 was well tolerated in these healthy male and female subjects. The most frequently reported adverse events were flu-like symptoms, which exhibited a dose-response relationship. Pharmacokinetic analysis suggested that serum IL-12 levels increased with dose. Analysis of serum levels indicated that interferon-gamma increased with the dose of rhIL-12, whereas IL-6 levels showed no changes with rhIL-12 treatment. The messenger ribonucleic acid expression of signal transducer and activator of transcription was significantly increased 24 hours after the administration of rhIL-12 for all dose groups versus placebo, and results indicated that the magnitude of increase may be dose dependent. This study suggests that interferon-gamma and signal transducer and activator of transcription are biomarkers of rhIL-12 activity.

J Clin Psychiatry. 2004 Sep;65(9):1228-34. Related Articles, Links Breastfeeding during maternal antidepressant treatment with serotonin reuptake inhibitors: infant exposure, clinical symptoms, and cytochrome p450 genotypes. Berle JO, Steen VM, Aamo TO, Breilid H, Zahlsen K, Spigset O. Centre for Child and Adolescent Mental Health, University of Bergen, Bergen, Norway. jean.berle@psyk.uib.no BACKGROUND: The aims of the study were to quantify the drug exposure in breastfed infants of antidepressant-treated mothers, to identify possible adverse events, and to correlate these variables to maternal and infant drug metabolism-relevant genotypes and milk triglyceride content. METHOD: The study included 25 lactating women treated with citalopram (N = 9), sertraline (N = 6), paroxetine (N = 6), fluoxetine (N = 1), or venlafaxine (N = 3) and their 26 breastfed infants. Drug concentrations in maternal and infant serum and milk were analyzed using liquid chromotography mass spectrometry methods; milk triglyceride levels were measured with a commercial kit. Cytochrome P450 (CYP) 2D6 and CYP2C19 activity was determined by polymerase chain reaction-based genotyping of the mothers and infants. An infant adverse event questionnaire was completed by the medication-treated mothers as well as by a control group of medication-free breastfeeding mothers of 68 infants. RESULTS: Sertraline and paroxetine were not detected in any of the drug-exposed infants. The infant serum level of citalopram was either undetectable (N = 4) or low (N = 6). All venlafaxine-exposed infants had measurable drug concentrations. We identified a paroxetine-treated mother and her infant who were both CYP2D6 poor metabolizers, as well as a citalopram-treated mother with CYP2C19 poor metabolizer status, but the serum drug levels of their infants were still either undetectable (paroxetine) or low (citalopram). There was no evidence of adverse events in the drug-exposed infants. CONCLUSION: Serum drug levels in breastfed infants of antidepressant-treated mothers were undetectable or low. This study adds further evidence to previously published data indicating that breastfeeding should not be generally discouraged in women using serotonin reuptake inhibitor anti-depressants.

J Clin Psychiatry. 2005 Jan;66(1):15-27. Related Articles, Links The CYP2D6 poor metabolizer phenotype may be associated with risperidone adverse drug reactions and discontinuation. de Leon J, Susce MT, Pan RM, Fairchild M, Koch WH, Wedlund

PJ. University of Kentucky Mental Health Research Center at Eastern State Hospital, Lexington, KY 40508, USA. jdeleon@uky.edu OBJECTIVE: The cytochrome P450 2D6 (CYP2D6) enzyme metabolizes risperidone. CYP2D6 poor metabolizers have no CYP2D6 activity (7% of whites and 1%-2% of other races). This study tested whether the CYP2D6 poor metabolizer phenotype was associated with adverse drug reactions (ADRs) and discontinuation due to ADRs. METHOD: Adult inpatients and outpatients were recruited from July 2000 to March 2003 including (1) 325 who were stabilized on risperidone therapy and classified as either expressing moderate-to-marked ADRs (22%, 73/325) or not (78%, 252/325) and (2) 212 who discontinued risperidone and were classified as discontinued due to ADRs (38%, 81/212) or for other reasons (62%, 131/212). Genetic tests were performed by allele-specific polymerase chain reaction and/or by the AmpliChip CYP450 microarray system for up to 34 separate CYP2D6 alleles. Two logistic regression models with dependent variables (moderate-to-marked ADRs while taking risperidone and risperidone discontinuation due to ADRs) were evaluated with respect to the CYP2D6 phenotype. RESULTS: The odds ratios (ORs) and 95% confidence intervals (CIs) for the CYP2D6 poor metabolizer phenotype in the univariate analyses and after correcting for clinical variables were (1) OR = 3.1 (CI = 1.4 to 7.0) and 3.4 (CI = 1.5 to 8.0) for moderate-to-marked ADRs on risperidone and (2) OR = 3.0 (CI = 0.85 to 10.6) and 6.0 (CI = 1.4 to 25.4) for discontinuation due to ADRs. CONCLUSIONS: The CYP2D6 poor metabolizer phenotype appears to be associated with risperidone ADRs and discontinuation due to ADRs; however, this finding requires further study in larger patient populations. The CYP3A5 and p-glycoprotein exon 21 and 26 genotypes were not significantly associated with risperidone response.

J Clin Psychiatry. 2005 Jun;66(6):799. Related Articles, Links Cultural competence in clinical psychopharmacology. Thompson JW. The Association of American Indian Physicians.

J Clin Psychiatry. 2005 Jun;66(6):800. Related Articles, Links Comment in: J Clin Psychiatry. 2005 Nov;66(11):1491; author reply 1491-2. An African patient with ziprasidone intolerance. Hein J, Gregor A, Bartholoma A, Heinz A, Juckel G. Publication Types: Case Reports Letter

J Clin Psychiatry. 2005 Nov;66(11):1491; author reply 1491-2. Related Articles, Links Comment on: J Clin Psychiatry. 2005 Jun;66(6):800. Applying parsimony to "An African patient with ziprasidone intolerance". Anders JL. Publication Types: Comment Letter

J Clin Psychopharmacol. 2005 Oct;25(5):427-34. Related Articles, Links Pharmacogenetic testing in the clinical management of schizophrenia: a decision-analytic model. Perlis RH, Ganz DA, Avorn J, Schneeweiss S, Glynn RJ, Smoller JW, Wang PS. Pharmacogenomics Research Program, Department of Psychiatry, Massachusetts General Hospital and Harvard Medical School, Boston, MA 02114, USA. rperlis@partners.org Clinical application of pharmacogenetic testing has been proposed as a means of improving treatment outcomes in psychiatry. The identification of a putative genetic test for better clozapine response in schizophrenia offers an opportunity to evaluate the cost-effectiveness of such testing. The authors performed a cost-effectiveness analysis of a genetic test that may identify individuals with greater likelihood of responding to clozapine treatment. We modeled a target population of schizophrenia patients in an acute psychotic episode, using a lifetime time horizon and societal perspective. Outcome measures included life expectancy, quality-adjusted life expectancy, costs, and incremental cost-effectiveness. Effects of variations in testing parameters were also examined. For a 30-year-old with schizophrenia, applying the pharmacogenetic test and treating those predicted to respond to clozapine with clozapine-first cost US $47,705 per additional quality-adjusted life-year, compared with treating all patients with conventional agents and reserving clozapine for treatment-resistant patients. In 1-way sensitivity analyses, test sensitivity and cost had the greatest impact on the incremental cost-effectiveness. We conclude that pharmacogenetic tests may achieve utility in clinical psychiatry, although their cost-effectiveness depends on several clinical parameters. More consistent reporting of test parameters such as sensitivity and specificity would greatly facilitate assessment of future pharmacogenetic studies.

J Clin Psychopharmacol. 2005 Oct;25(5):448-56. Related Articles, Links Polymorphic variations in GSTM1, GSTT1, PgP, CYP2D6, CYP3A5, and dopamine D2 and D3 receptors and their association with tardive dyskinesia in severe mental illness. de Leon J, Susce MT, Pan RM, Koch WH, Wedlund PJ. University of Kentucky Mental Health Research Center at Eastern State Hospital, Lexington, KY 40508, USA. jdeleon@uky.edu This study tested the association between tardive dyskinesia (TD) and polymorphic variations in (a) 2 cytochrome P450 (CYP) genes (CYP2D6 or CYP3A5), (b) 2 DRD2 variants (Ser311Cys and -141C Ins/del) and the Ser9Gly DRD3 variants, (c) 2 glutathione S-transferases (GSTT1 and GSTM1), and (d) variations in the PgP gene, MDR1. The study sample included 516 severely mentally ill patients from Central Kentucky facilities. Logistic regression models that included clinical variables associated with TD were developed. Gene variants were added to these clinical models. The total sample included 31% (162/516) with TD where 30% (49/162) of those had severe TD. Polymorphisms in DRD2, MDR1, and GSTT1 were never significant. Two gene variants appeared to be significant after adding them to the clinical regression models: (1) Ser9Gly DRD3 polymorphism was associated with severe TD (odds ratio for patients with 1 mutant allele when compared with individuals with 2 wild types was 2.5, 95% confidence interval 1.1-5.6, whereas the odds ratio for patients with 2 mutant alleles when compared with individuals with 1 mutant was 2.8, 95% confidence interval 1.0-7.4), and (2) GSTM1 absence was associated with TD (odds ratio 1.7, 95% confidence interval 1.2-2.4) particularly in white women. The CYP2D6 and CYP3A5 absence showed potential for significant associations in larger samples, particularly in white men. New studies need to replicate whether these or other genes could be used conjointly with clinical variables to identify subjects at risk for TD in clinical settings.

J Comput Biol. 2004;11(4):714-26. Related Articles, Links Sample size for identifying differentially expressed genes in microarray experiments. Wang SJ, Chen JJ. Division of Biometrics II, Office of Biostatistics, Center for Drug Evaluation and Research, Food and Drug Administration, 5600 Fishers Lane, Rockville, Maryland 20857, USA.

wangs@cder.fda.gov Microarray technology allows simultaneous comparison of expression levels of thousands of genes under each condition. This paper concerns sample size calculation in the identification of differentially expressed genes between a control and a treated sample. In a typical experiment, only a fraction of genes (altered genes) is expected to be differentially expressed between two samples. Sample size determination depends on a number of factors including the specified significance level (alpha), the desired statistical power (1-beta), the fraction (eta) of truly altered genes out of the total g genes studied, and the effect sizes (Delta) for the altered genes. This paper proposes a method to calculate the number of arrays required to detect at least 100lambda % (where 0 < lambda < or = 1) of the truly altered genes under the model of an equal effect size for all altered genes. The required numbers of arrays are tabulated for various values of alpha, beta, Delta, eta, and lambda for the one-sample and two-sample t-tests for g = 10,000. Based on the proposed approach, to identify up to 90% of truly altered genes among the unknown number of truly altered genes, the estimated numbers of arrays needed appear to be manageable. For instance, when the standardized effect size is at least 2.0, the number of arrays needed is less than or equal to 14 for the two-sample t-test and is less than or equal to 10 for the one-sample t-test. As the cost per array declines, such array numbers become practical. The proposed method offers a simple, intuitive, and practical way to determine the number of arrays needed in microarray experiments in which the true correlation structure among the genes under investigation cannot be reasonably assumed. An example dataset is used to illustrate the use of the proposed approach to plan microarray experiments.

J Control Release. 2005 Jan 3;101(1-3):259-71. Related Articles, Links Polymer genomics: shifting the gene and drug delivery paradigms. Kabanov AV, Batrakova EV, Sriadibhatla S, Yang Z, Kelly DL, Alakov VY. Pharmaceutical Sciences Department, College of Pharmacy and Eppley, University of Nebraska Institute for Research in Cancer and Allied Diseases, Nebraska Medical Center, Omaha, NE 68198-5830, USA. akabanov@unmc.edu Pluronic, the A-B-A amphiphilic block copolymers of poly(ethylene oxide) and poly(propylene oxide), can up-regulate the expression of selected genes in cells and alter genetic responses to antineoplastic agents in cancer. Two key new findings are discussed in relation to current drug and gene delivery strategies. First, these block copolymers alone and in combination with a polycation, polyethyleneimine, can up-regulate the expression of reporter genes in stably transfected cells. This underscores the ability of selected synthetic polymers to enhance transgene expression through a mechanism that augments improved DNA delivery into a cell. Second, although, when used alone, Pluronic is "genetically benign," when combined with an antineoplastic agent, doxorubicin, it drastically alters pharmacogenomic responses to this agent and prevents the development of multidrug resistance in breast cancer cells. Collectively, these studies propose the need for a thorough assessment of pharmacogenomic effects of polymer therapeutics to maximize the clinical outcomes and understand the pharmacological and toxicological effects of polymer-based drugs and delivery systems. Publication Types: Review

J Cyst Fibros. 2004 Mar;3(1):37-44. Related Articles, Links Genotyping of Pseudomonas aeruginosa in cystic fibrosis suggests need for segregation. Edenborough FP, Stone HR, Kelly SJ, Zadik P, Doherty CJ, Govan JR. Adult Cystic Fibrosis Unit, Northern General Hospital, Herries Road, Sheffield, S5 7AU, UK. fedenborough@yahoo.com BACKGROUND: Emerging resistance of Pseudomonas aeruginosa within cystic fibrosis (CF) populations is attributed to antibiotic pressure and spread of transmissible strains. We describe increasing resistance of P. aeruginosa isolates, resulting in the identification of two multiresistant strains and their impact on morbidity. METHODS: Susceptibility reports of all P. aeruginosa isolates since 1998 in our unit were reviewed. Isolates were submitted for genomic finger-printing by pulsed-field gel electrophoresis. Clinical measures and the consumption of treatment resources were compared between those harbouring resistant organisms and those with sensitive strains. RESULTS: Analysis of 407 reports from 43 patients revealed isolation of multiresistant (MR) organisms increased during 1999. Those harbouring MR strains consumed more resources than non-MR. Strain typing showed a new 'Sheffield' strain in seven patients (100% MR), and the 'Liverpool' strain in 10 patients (40% MR). Individuals in these groups consumed significantly more resources than 23 patients with unique, susceptible strains (4% MR). DISCUSSION: Increasing resistance in isolates of P. aeruginosa may herald the arrival of a transmissible strain in CF Units which though sometimes sensitive, may become multiply resistant and require more intensive treatment. We now segregate those with transmissible strains from each other and from those with unique strains.

J Drug Target. 2005 Aug;13(7):431-43. Related Articles, Links Polypropylenimine dendrimer-induced gene expression changes: the effect of complexation with DNA, dendrimer generation and cell type. Omidi Y, Hollins AJ, Drayton RM, Akhtar S. Tabriz University of Medical Sciences, Department of Pharmaceutics, Tabriz, Iran. Polypropylenimine (PPI) dendrimers appear attractive non-viral vectors for the delivery of genes, antisense oligonucleotides, and small interfering RNA (siRNA). However, the effects of these synthetic gene delivery vectors on global gene expression are poorly understood. Here we have examined the toxicogenomics of generation 2 (DAB-8) and generation 3 (DAB-16) PPI dendrimers in two human cell lines. At concentrations and treatment protocols routinely used for gene and oligonucleotide transfection, PPI dendrimers alone elicited marked changes in endogenous gene expression in A431 epithelial cells. The extent of PPI-induced gene changes appeared to be dependent on the dendrimer generation as the number of genes affected was greater with G3 compared to G2 PPI dendrimers in A431 cells. The signature of DAB16-induced gene changes in A549 cells was different to those elicited in A431 cells implying a strong dependence on cell type. The DAB-16 polymer complexed with DNA (dendriplexes) also elicited marked gene expression changes in A549 cells but with a signature that was different from the polymer alone implying that dendriplexes are "recognised" by cells as chemical entities that are distinct from the polymer alone. Alterations in expression of a variety of gene ontologies were observed including those involved in defence responses, cell proliferation and apoptosis. Although there was a tendency for increased DNA damage in cells treated with DAB16 alone or its DNA dendriplexes as detected by the COMET assay, these differences were not statistically significant. These data show for the first time that PPI-dendrimers, separate from their capability as transfection reagents, can intrinsically alter the expression of many endogenous genes that could potentially lead to them exerting multiple biological effects in cells. The impact and consequences of polymer-induced gene changes should guide their rational use as delivery systems for gene-based therapeutics.

J Dtsch Dermatol Ges. 2005 Mar;3(3):214-21; quiz 222, 224. Related Articles, Links [Pharmacogenomics in dermatology] [Article in German] Harr T, Itin PH. Publication Types: Review

J Endocrinol Invest. 2005;28(10 Suppl):2-7. Related Articles, Links Genetics and pharmacogenetics of osteoporosis. Carbonell Sala S, Masi L, Marini F, Del Monte F, Falchetti A, Franceschelli F, Brandi ML. Department of Internal Medicine, University of Florence, and DEGENE Srl, Florence, Italy. Osteoporosis is a skeletal chronic multifactorial disease characterised by abnormal low bone mass and microarchitectural deterioration of bone tissue. This disorder, present in both sexes, related to environmental and genetic factors, is becoming a major public health problem in developed countries. It has a polygenic pattern of inheritance that complicates identification of disease genes [cytokines, calciotropic hormones, sex hormones pathway synthesis and their receptors, bone matrix proteins synthesis genes involved on estrogenic metabolism (CYP19) and LDL receptor-related protein 5 (LRP5) gene]. It is possible to identify associations between candidate genes polymorphisms and disease phenotype in population-based and case-control studies. This could give us promising data for earlier identification of osteoporosis susceptibility and fracture risk. Preventive therapy could be targeted to patients at risk of osteoporosis before fractures occur. Genetic polymorphisms are also starting to be used to predict drug response. A new era of pharmacogenetics represents an interesting prospective to identify the potential individuals to receive customised treatments.

J Exp Ther Oncol. 2004 Oct;4(3):253-7. Related Articles, Links The 24th International Symposium of Sapporo Cancer Seminar "Pharmacogenomics in Cancer Chemotherapy: Recent Advances in ABC Transporters and Genome Analyses". Hokkaido University Conference Hall, Sapporo, Japan, June 20-22, 2004. Ishikawa T. Department of Biomolecular Engineering, Graduate School of Bioscience and Biotechnology, Tokyo Institute of Technology, 4259-B-60 Nagatsuta, Midori-ku, Yokohama 226-8501, Japan. tishikaw@bio.titech.ac.jp Publication Types: Congresses

J Formos Med Assoc. 2004 Feb;103(2):85-95. Related Articles, Links Recent advances in childhood acute lymphoblastic leukemia. Pui CH. Department of Hematology-Oncology, St. Jude Children's Research Hospital, 332 North Lauderdale St., Memphis, TN 38105-2794, USA. Contemporary risk-directed therapy has advanced the cure rate for childhood acute lymphoblastic leukemia to near 80%. Molecular genetic analyses of leukemic cells, pharmacodynamic studies of antileukemic agents, and pharmacogenetic studies of the host's drug-metabolizing enzymes, drug transporters, and drug targets are providing a rational base for further improvement of treatment efficacy and the reduction of complications. Early treatment response, as defined by the measurement of minimal residual disease, which reflects both the drug responsiveness of leukemic cells and host pharmacodynamics/pharmacogenomics, is the most reliable prognostic indicator for gauging the intensity of treatment. Recent advances in high-throughput biotechnology, including gene expression profiling, proteomics and gene silencing promise to identify molecular targets for specific treatment. The ultimate goal is to elucidate central mechanisms of leukemogenesis so that preventive measures can be devised. Publication Types: Review

J Gastroenterol Hepatol. 2005 Aug;20(8):1149-57. Related Articles, Links Azathioprine and 6-mercaptopurine pharmacogenetics and metabolite monitoring in inflammatory bowel disease. Gearry RB, Barclay ML. Department of Gastroenterology, Christchurch Hospital, Christchurch School of Medicine and Health Sciences, New Zealand. Richard.Gearry@cdhb.govt.nz The thiopurine drugs azathioprine and 6-mercaptopurine (6-MP) are well-established in the treatment of inflammatory bowel disease (IBD). However, there is a wide inter- and intra-patient variation in the concentrations of active and toxic metabolites due to their complex metabolism and genetic polymorphisms in metabolizing enzymes. Serious drug toxicity leads to cessation of therapy in 9-25% of patients, and there is failure to achieve efficacy in approximately 15% of cases. Advances in the understanding of thiopurine drug metabolism have led to new genetic and metabolite tests to help clinicians optimize thiopurine use. Thiopurine methyltransferase (TPMT) enzyme activity can predict life-threatening myelotoxicity in the one in 300 patients who are TPMT-deficient. However, myelotoxicity can also occur in the presence of normal TPMT activity so blood count monitoring should remain standard practice. TPMT testing may also aid in dose individualization. 6-Thioguanine nucleotides (6-TGN) are thought to be the predominant active metabolites of the thiopurines. 6-thioguanine nucleotide concentration is correlated with bone marrow toxicity and may also correlate with efficacy in IBD. Measurement of 6-TGN and 6-methylmercaptopurine (6-MMP) concentration is most useful in determining why a patient is not responding to a standard dose of a thiopurine drug and may help in avoiding myelosuppression. The ratio of these metabolites can help distinguish non-compliance, under-dosing, thiopurine-resistant and thiopurine-refractory disease. Some of these investigations are entering routine clinical practice but more research is required to determine their optimal use in patients with IBD. Publication Types: Review

J Geriatr Psychiatry Neurol. 2004 Sep;17(3):172-80. Related Articles, Links Neuropsychiatric complications of medical and surgical therapies for Parkinson's disease. Burn DJ, Troster AI. Department of Neurology, Regional Neurosciences Centre, Newcastle General Hospital, Westgate Road, Newcastle upon Tyne NE4 6BE. d.j.burn@ncl.ac.uk This review deals with the range of neuropsychiatric problems that may arise from the use of medical and surgical therapies in the treatment of Parkinson's disease. As new approaches emerge, these problems are diversifying. Well-recognized drug-related complications include hallucinations and psychosis and the so-called dopamine-dysregulation syndrome. The etiology of these problems has not been fully established and is not clearly dose related, while the management can be difficult and needs to be tailored to the individual patient. Cholinergic and dopaminergic drugs may both influence cognitive function. The development of pharmacogenetics could improve the therapeutic ratio of medical approaches to PD in the future. The literature relating to the neuropsychiatric issues complicating the surgical treatment of Parkinson's disease is more recent and frequently suffers from methodological problems, lack of a systematic approach, and adequate patient follow-up. The emergence of neuropsychiatric problems in association with surgery has shed new light upon the pathophysiological mechanisms underpinning these symptoms. Depression, hypomania, euphoria, mirth, and hypersexuality have all been described following deep brain stimulation procedures, although most studies have concentrated upon the depressive features. Anxiety has been described only rarely to date. Fortunately, permanent cognitive complications appear to be rare. The optimal management approach for surgically related neuropsychiatric problems is unknown at present. Prospective multicenter studies would contribute significantly to resolving this therapeutic uncertainty. Publication Types: Review

J Health Commun. 2004 Nov-Dec;9(6):541-59. Related Articles, Links Comment in: J Health Commun. 2004 Nov-Dec;9(6):561-2. Evaluating direct-to-consumer marketing of race-based pharmacogenomics: a focus group study of public understandings of applied genomic medication. Bates BR, Poirot K, Harris TM, Condit CM, Achter PJ. School of Communication Studies, Ohio University, Athens, Ohio 45710, USA. batesb@ohio.edu Some medical providers have advocated applied genomics, including the use of genetically linked racial phenotypes in medical practice, raising fear that race-based medication will become justified. As with other emerging medical genetic technologies, pharmaceutical companies may advertise these treatments. Researchers fear that consumers will uncritically accept pharmaceutical messages and demand the product. In this exploratory study, we examined public reactions to advertisements for applied genomic medications. A focus group methodology was employed. Participants tended to resist the message and generated warrants for doing so, indicating critical reception of the messages. Message accepters also provided warrants. Warrants for resistance and acceptance differ between self-identified racial groups. Consumers, health care providers, and pharmaceutical corporations will benefit from a better understanding of direct-to-consumer advertisements as medical communication. Our study concludes that both advocates and opponents of direct-to-consumer advertisements should recognize that potential consumers of pharmacogenomics act as critical consumers of health advertising discourse.

J Health Serv Res Policy. 2005 Jan;10(1):40-4. Related Articles, Links Pharmacogenetics: policy needs for personal prescribing. Melzer D, Raven A, Ling T, Detmer D, Zimmern R. Department of Public Health and Primary Care, University of Cambridge, Cambridge CB2 2SR, UK. Pharmacogenetics involves genetic testing of individual patients to guide drug treatment. Proponents argue that pharmacogenetics will achieve major gains in drug safety and efficacy, and revolutionise marketing. Pharmacogenetics also raises several policy concerns, including the need for sound information for clinical decision-making on drug-genetic test combinations. Currently, the pharmacogenetics science base and the rate of emergence of clinical applications are uncertain. Most commentary on pharmacogenetics focuses on new compounds, yet older drugs cause most adverse events. Test regulation in the USA appears fundamentally different from Europe, where evidence of safety or efficacy may not be required. Genetics research is needed as part of post-marketing surveillance systems. In routine clinical practice, computer-based health records with relevant decision support systems will also be needed. Without health policy action, pharmacogenetics could produce a new generation of poorly evaluated tests and drugs, with medicine becoming significantly less evidence-based, leading to rising costs, patient hazard and exclusions of drug-related 'genetic minorities' from evaluated treatments.

J HIV Ther. 2004 Nov;9(4):73-4. Related Articles, Links The challenge of once a day HIV treatment. Pozniak AL. Publication Types: Editorial

J Hum Genet. 2004;49(10):558-72. Epub 2004 Sep 11. Related Articles, Links Inference from the relationships between linkage disequilibrium and allele frequency distributions of 240 candidate SNPs in 109 drug-related genes in four Asian populations. Cha PC, Yamada R, Sekine A, Nakamura Y, Koh CL. Institute of Biological Sciences (Genetics and Molecular Biology), Faculty of Science, University of Malaya, 50603, Lembah Pantai, Kuala Lumpur, Malaysia. genescha@yahoo.com. The extensive nucleotide diversity in drug-related genes predisposes individuals to different drug responses and is a major problem in current clinical practice and drug development. Striking allelic frequency differences exist in these genes between populations. In this study, we genotyped 240 sites known to be polymorphic in the Japanese population in each of 270 unrelated healthy individuals comprising 90 each of Malaysian Malays, Indians, and Chinese. These sites are distributed in 109 genes that are drug related, such as genes encoding drug-metabolizing enzymes and drug transporters. Allele frequency and linkage disequilibrium distributions of these sites were determined and compared. They were also compared with similar data of 752 Japanese. Extensive similarities in allele frequency and linkage disequilibrium distributions were observed among Japanese, Malaysian Chinese, and Malays. However, significant differences were observed between Japanese and Malaysian Chinese with Malaysian Indians. These four populations were grouped into two genetic clusters of different ancestries. However, a higher correlation was found between Malaysian Malays and Indians, indicating the existence of extensive admixture between them. The results also imply the possible and rational use of existing single nucleotide polymorphism databases as references to assist future pharmacogenetic studies involving populations of similar ancestry.

J Hum Genet. 2004;49(7):355-9. Epub 2004 Jun 18. Related Articles, Links Apolipoprotein E polymorphism is associated with age of onset in schizophrenia. Kampman O, Anttila S, Illi A, Mattila KM, Rontu R, Leinonen E, Lehtimaki T. Medical School, University of Tampere, 33014 Tampere, Finland.

olli.kampman@uta.fi The aims of the study were to investigate the relationship between Apolipoprotein E (APOE) polymorphism, risk of schizophrenia, treatment response to conventional anti-psychotics, and age of onset in schizophrenia. The sample comprised 94 Finnish patients with a DSM-IV diagnosis of schizophrenia. Forty-three of the patients were good responders to conventional anti-psychotics and 51 were classified as non-responders. The control group consisted of 98 healthy blood donors. The APOE allele frequencies (epsilon 2, epsilon 3, and epsilon 4) were 4.8, 72.3, and 22.9% in patients and 7.1, 75.0, and 17.9 in controls. None of the differences between groups were statistically significant. No association between treatment response and APOE genotype was found. Patients with APOE epsilon 4/epsilon 4 genotype had a markedly lower age of onset compared with rest of the sample (p=0.0015), which remained significant when controlling for gender (p=0.02). There was an increasing linear trend between the number of epsilon 3 alleles (0, 1, or 2) and age of onset in schizophrenia (p=0.08). An inverse trend was found between the number of epsilon 4 alleles and age of onset (p=0.07). No relationship between APOE polymorphism and risk for schizophrenia was found. APOE epsilon 4/epsilon 4 genotype may be associated with early onset schizophrenia. APOE epsilon 3 allele may function protectively in later onset in this disease.

J Hum Genet. 2005;50(7):321-8. Epub 2005 Jul 23. Related Articles, Links Genetic diversity and new therapeutic concepts. Shastry BS. Department of Biological Sciences, Oakland University, Rochester, MI 48309, USA. shastry@oakland.edu The differences in medicinal drug responses among individuals had been known for quite some time. Some patients exhibit a life-threatening adverse reaction while others fail to show an expected therapeutic effect. Intermediate responses between the above two extreme cases are also known. In fact, it has been recently reported that approximately 100,000 deaths and more than 2 million hospitalizations annually in the United States are due to properly prescribed medications. This interindividual variability could be due in part to genetically determined characteristics of target genes or drug metabolizing enzymes. This has now been substantiated by a variety of studies. We know that "one size fits all" is not correct. Therefore, the application of pharmacogenetic concepts to clinical practice is an excellent goal in the postgenomic era. The successful completion of the human genome project provided necessary molecular tools, such as high-throughput SNP genotyping, HapMap, and microarray, that can be applied to develop proper therapeutic options for individuals. Recently, there have been considerable scientific, corporate, and policy interest in pharmacotherapy. However, identification of causal variations in a target gene is only a starting point, and the progress in this rapidly developing field is slower than expected. One major drawback could be due to the multigene determinant of drug response that requires a genome-wide screening. Additionally, application of pharmacogenetic knowledge into clinical practice requires a high level of accuracy, precision (risk/benefit ratio), and strict regulations. This is because the pharmacogenetic approach raises several ethical, moral, and legal questions. It is also necessary that both health professionals and the general public must be urgently educated. Despite these limitations, translation of pharmacogenomic data into clinical practice would certainly provide better opportunities to increase the safety and efficacy of medicine in the future. Publication Types: Review

J Hypertens. 2004 Dec;22(12):2273-5. Related Articles, Links Comment on: J Hypertens. 2004 Dec;22(12):2321-8. Pharmacogenomics of left ventricular hypertrophy reversal: beyond the 'one size fits all' approach to antihypertensive therapy. Schillaci G. Publication Types: Comment Editorial Review

J Hypertens. 2004 Dec;22(12):2321-8. Related Articles, Links Comment in: J Hypertens. 2004 Dec;22(12):2273-5. Single nucleotide polymorphisms predict the change in left ventricular mass in response to antihypertensive treatment. Liljedahl U, Kahan T, Malmqvist K, Melhus H, Syvanen AC, Lind L, Kurland L. Department of Medical Sciences, Uppsala University, Sweden. BACKGROUND: Our aim was to determine whether the change in left ventricular (LV) mass in response to antihypertensive treatment could be predicted by multivariate analysis of single nucleotide polymorphisms (SNPs) in candidate genes reflecting pathways likely to be involved in blood pressure control. METHODS: Patients with mild to moderate primary hypertension and LV hypertrophy were randomized in a double-blind fashion to treatment with either the angiotensin II type 1 receptor antagonist irbesartan (n = 48) or the beta1 adrenoreceptor blocker atenolol (n = 49). A microarray-based minisequencing system was used for genotyping 74 SNPs in 25 genes. These genotypes were related to the change in LV mass index by echocardiography, after 12 weeks treatment as monotherapy, using stepwise multiple regression analysis. RESULTS: The blood pressure reductions were similar and significant in both treatment groups. Two SNPs in two separate genes (the angiotensinogen T1198C polymorphism, corresponding to the M235T variant and the apolipoprotein B G10108A polymorphism) for those treated with irbesartan, and the adrenoreceptor alpha2A A1817G for those treated with atenolol, significantly predicted the change in LV mass. The predictive power of these SNPs was independent of the degree of blood pressure reduction. CONCLUSION: SNPs in the angiotensinogen, apolipoprotein B, and the alpha2 adrenoreceptor gene predicted the change in LV mass during antihypertensive therapy. These results illustrate the potential of using microarray-based technology for SNP genotyping in predicting individual drug responses. Publication Types: Clinical Trial Multicenter Study Randomized Controlled Trial

J Hypertens. 2005 Dec;23(12):2127-43. Related Articles, Links Genetic determinants of blood pressure regulation. Marteau JB, Zaiou M, Siest G, Visvikis-Siest S. INSERM U525, Equipe 4, Faculte de Pharmacie, Universite Henri Poincare, Nancy, France. Hypertension is a multifactorial disorder that probably results from the inheritance of a number of susceptibility genes and involves multiple environmental determinants. Existing evidence suggests that the genetic contribution to blood pressure variation is about 30-50%. Although a number of candidate genes have been studied in different ethnic populations, results from genetic analysis are still inconsistent and specific causes of hypertension remain unclear. Furthermore, the abundance of data in the literature makes it difficult to piece together the puzzle of hypertension and to define candidate genes involved in the dynamic of blood pressure regulation. In this review, we attempt to highlight the genetic basis of hypertension pathogenesis, focusing on the most important existing genetic variations of candidate genes and their potential role in the development of this disease. Our objective is to review current knowledge and discuss limitations to clinical applications of genotypic information in the diagnosis, evaluation and treatment of hypertension. Finally, some principles of pharmacogenomics are presented here along with future perspectives of hypertension. Publication Types: Review

J Hypertens. 2005 Jul;23(7):1311-25. Related Articles, Links Comment in: J Hypertens. 2005 Jul;23(7):1327-9. Pharmacogenomics of blood pressure response to antihypertensive treatment. Mellen PB, Herrington DM. Department of Internal Medicine/Cardiology, Wake Forest University School of Medicine, Winston-Salem, North Carolina 27157, USA. PURPOSE IDENTIFICATION: Inter-individual variability in blood pressure response to treatment is well documented, but a clinically useful means to distinguish responders from non-responders has been elusive. With the advent of new technologies and genomic knowledge, more investigators are seeking to identify genetic determinants of blood pressure response to therapy. STUDY SELECTION: We identified studies of candidate polymorphisms from an initial PubMed search using the MESH terms 'Hypertension: Drug Therapy' and 'Genetics' or 'Pharmacogenetics', limiting results to English-language publications on studies in human adults. We further identified specific polymorphisms of interest noted in earlier reviews and performed additional PubMed searches based on these candidate genes. Pertinent studies were further extracted from the references of studies already identified. We focused on clinical trials that measured blood pressure response to a medication or class of medications over a minimum of 4 weeks. DATA EXTRACTION: We evaluated studies looking at blood pressure response to commonly used classes of antihypertensive medications by major genetic variants. RESULTS OF ANALYSIS: Although many studies show that blood pressure response to a given class of antihypertensive medications varies by genotype for different polymorphisms, none of the genotypes identified consistently predicted blood pressure response. CONCLUSIONS: Common variants may influence response to diuretics, beta-blockers, angiotensin-converting enzyme inhibitors, and angiotensin receptor blockers, but studies of polymorphisms have generally yielded conflicting results. The inclusion of pharmacogenomic studies in large clinical trials and other more innovative investigative methods may provide greater clarity of the potential role for genotyping in the treatment of patients with hypertension. Publication Types: Review

J Hypertens. 2005 Jul;23(7):1327-9. Related Articles, Links Comment on: J Hypertens. 2005 Jul;23(7):1311-25. Pharmacogenomics in hypertension: present practicalities and future potential. Brain N Jr, Dominiczak AF. Publication Types: Comment Editorial

J Hypertens. 2005 May;23(5):929-32. Related Articles, Links Comment in: J Hypertens. 2005 Nov;23(11):2109-10; author reply 2110-1. Comment on: J Hypertens. 2005 Mar;23(3):543-9. J Hypertens. 2005 May;23(5):961-9. Studies on genes and hypertension: a daunting task. Saavedra JM. Publication Types: Comment Editorial

J Infect Dis. 2005 Dec 1;192(11):1931-42. Epub 2005 Nov 1. Related Articles, Links Pharmacogenetics of long-term responses to antiretroviral regimens containing Efavirenz and/or Nelfinavir: an Adult Aids Clinical Trials Group Study. Haas DW, Smeaton LM, Shafer RW, Robbins GK, Morse GD, Labbe L, Wilkinson GR, Clifford DB, D'Aquila RT, De Gruttola V, Pollard RB, Merigan TC, Hirsch MS, George AL Jr, Donahue JP, Kim RB. Vanderbilt University School of Medicine, Nashville, TN 37203, USA. david.w.haas@vanderbilt.edu BACKGROUND: Efavirenz and nelfinavir are metabolized by cytochrome P-450 (CYP) 2B6 and CYP2C19, respectively, with some involvement by CYP3A. Nelfinavir is a substrate for P-glycoprotein, which is encoded by MDR1. The present study examined associations between genetic variants and long-term responses to treatment. METHODS: Adult AIDS Clinical Trials Group study 384 randomized antiretroviral-naive subjects to receive efavirenz and/or nelfinavir plus 2 nucleoside analogues, with follow-up lasting up to 3 years. Population pharmacokinetics were estimated from a nonlinear mixed-effects model. Polymorphisms in CYP2B6, CYP2C19, CYP3A4, CYP3A5, and MDR1 were characterized. RESULTS: The 504 participants in the genetic study included 340 efavirenz recipients and 348 nelfinavir recipients (184 of the 504 participants received both efavirenz and nelfinavir). Of the participants, 49% were white, 31% were black, and 19% were Hispanic. Plasma exposure to efavirenz and nelfinavir in each population was significantly associated with the polymorphisms CYP2B6 516G-->T and CYP2C19 681G-->A, respectively. Among efavirenz recipients, the MDR1 position 3435 TT genotype was associated with decreased likelihood of virologic failure and decreased emergence of efavirenz-resistant virus but not with plasma efavirenz exposure. Among nelfinavir recipients, a trend toward decreased virologic failure was associated with the polymorphism CYP2C19 681G-->A. CONCLUSIONS: Genetic variants predict plasma exposure to efavirenz and nelfinavir, and they may predict virologic failure and/or emergence of drug-resistant virus. These associations with treatment responses must be validated in other studies. Publication Types: Randomized Controlled Trial

J Infect Dis. 2005 May 1;191(9):1397-400. Epub 2005 Mar 22. Related Articles, Links Comment on: J Infect Dis. 2005 May 1;191(9):1419-26. Pharmacogenomics and HIV therapeutics. Haas DW. Publication Types: Comment Editorial

J Invest Dermatol. 2006 Jan;126(1):229-31. Related Articles, Links Aminoglycosides as potential pharmacogenetic agents in the treatment of Hailey-Hailey disease. Kellermayer R, Szigeti R, Keeling KM, Bedekovics T, Bedwell DM. Publication Types: Letter

J Lipid Res. 2004 Oct;45(10):1885-91. Epub 2004 Aug 1. Related Articles, Links Polymorphisms in the gene encoding lipoprotein lipase in men with low HDL-C and coronary heart disease: the Veterans Affairs HDL Intervention Trial. Brousseau ME, Goldkamp AL, Collins D, Demissie S, Connolly AC, Cupples LA, Ordovas JM, Bloomfield HE, Robins SJ, Schaefer EJ. Lipid Metabolism Laboratory, Jean Mayer-United States Department of Agriculture Human Nutrition Research Center on Aging at Tufts University, and

Department of Medicine, New England Medical Center, Boston, MA, USA. margaret.brousseau@tufts.edu Our goal was to further define the role of LPL gene polymorphisms in coronary heart disease (CHD) risk. We determined the frequencies of three LPL polymorphisms (D9N, N291S, and S447X) in 899 men from the Veterans Affairs HDL Intervention Trial (VA-HIT), a study that examined the potential benefits of increasing HDL with gemfibrozil in men with established CHD and low high density lipoprotein cholesterol (HDL-C; < or =40 mg/dl), and compared them with those of men without CHD from the Framingham Offspring Study (FOS). In VA-HIT, genotype frequencies for LPL D9N, N291S, and S447X were 5.3, 4.5, and 13.0%, respectively. These values differed from those for men in FOS having an HDL-C of >40, who had corresponding values of 3.2% (P = 0.06), 1.5% (P < 0.01), and 18.2% (P < 0.01). On gemfibrozil, carriers of the LPL N9 allele in VA-HIT had lower levels of large LDL (-32%; P < 0.01) but higher levels of small, dense LDL (+59%; P < 0.003) than did noncarriers. Consequently, mean LDL particle diameter was smaller in LPL N9 carriers than in noncarriers (20.14 +/- 0.87 vs. 20.63 +/- 0.80 nm; P < 0.003). In men with low HDL-C and CHD: 1) the LPL N9 and S291 alleles are more frequent than in CHD-free men with normal HDL-C, whereas the X447 allele is less frequent, and 2) the LPL N9 allele is associated with the LDL subclass response to gemfibrozil. Publication Types: Clinical Trial

J Med Ethics. 2005 Mar;31(3):144-8. Related Articles, Links Pharmacogenetics, ethical issues: review of the Nuffield Council on Bioethics Report. Corrigan OP. Centre for Family Research and Cambridge Genetics Knowledge Park, Faculty of Social and Political Sciences, University of Cambridge, Free School Lane, Cambridge, B2 3RF, UK. opc22@cam.ac.uk In September this year the Nuffield Council on Bioethics held a meeting to disclose and discuss the main findings of their newly published report on the ethical issues associated with developments in pharmacogenetics research. The basics of pharmacogenetics science is briefly outlined, and then the extent to which the report was successful in addressing (or at least highlighting) the attendant social, ethical, and policy implications of pharmacogenetics research is evaluated.

J Med Genet. 2005 Jul;42(7):583-7. Related Articles, Links Melanocortin-1 receptor gene variants affect pain and mu-opioid analgesia in mice and humans. Mogil JS, Ritchie J, Smith SB, Strasburg K, Kaplan L, Wallace MR, Romberg RR, Bijl H, Sarton EY, Fillingim RB, Dahan A. Department of Psychology and Centre for Research on Pain, McGill University, Montreal, Canada. jeffrey.mogil@mcgill.ca BACKGROUND: A recent genetic study in mice and humans revealed the modulatory effect of MC1R (melanocortin-1 receptor) gene variants on kappa-opioid receptor mediated analgesia. It is unclear whether this gene affects basal pain sensitivity or the efficacy of analgesics acting at the more clinically relevant mu-opioid receptor. OBJECTIVE: To characterise sensitivity to pain and mu-opioid analgesia in mice and humans with non-functional melanocortin-1 receptors. METHODS: Comparisons of spontaneous mutant C57BL/6-Mc1r(e/e) mice to C57BL/6 wildtype mice, followed by a gene dosage study of pain and morphine-6-glucuronide (M6G) analgesia in humans with MC1R variants. RESULTS: C57BL/6-Mc1r(e/e) mutant mice and human redheads--both with non-functional MC1Rs--display reduced sensitivity to noxious stimuli and increased analgesic responsiveness to the mu-opioid selective morphine metabolite, M6G. In both species the differential analgesia is likely due to pharmacodynamic factors, as plasma levels of M6G are similar across genotype. CONCLUSIONS: Genotype at MC1R similarly affects pain sensitivity and M6G analgesia in mice and humans. These findings confirm the utility of cross species translational strategies in pharmacogenetics.

J Mol Endocrinol. 2005 Jun;34(3):617-23. Related Articles, Links Pharmacogenetic analysis of human steroid 5 alpha reductase type II: comparison of finasteride and dutasteride. Makridakis N, Reichardt JK. Department of Biochemistry and Molecular Biology and Institute for Genetic Medicine, Keck School of Medicine of the University of Southern California, 2250 Alcazar Street, IGM240, Los Angeles, California 90089-9075, USA. Human steroid 5 alpha-reductase type II is a prostate-specific, membrane-associated enzyme that catalyzes the conversion of testosterone to dihydrotestosterone, the most potent androgen in the prostate gland. Genetic variants of this enzyme have been associated with both the development and the progression of prostate cancer. Both finasteride and dutasteride are competitive inhibitors of the type II steroid 5 alpha-reductase that have been effectively used for the treatment of benign prostatic hyperplasia. Finasteride has also been successfully utilized for prostate cancer chemoprevention. We here investigate 5 alpha-reductase inhibition assays in vitro to measure the effect of incubation time on the apparent inhibition constant (Ki) for both constitutional and somatic (prostate cancer) enzyme variants. Our systematic pharmacogenetic analysis shows that both finasteride and dutasteride are slow, time-dependent inhibitors of steroid 5 alpha-reductase type II, and that the inhibition kinetics depend on the 5 alpha-reductase genotype. We also show that, overall, dutasteride is a more efficient steroid 5 alpha-reductase inhibitor than finasteride. Based on our data, we are able to map areas of the enzyme that are responsible for this time-dependent inhibition for either (or both) enzyme inhibitor(s). This comprehensive pharmacogenetic analysis of steroid 5 alpha-reductase variants unveiled significant pharmacogenetic variation for both finasteride and dutasteride and thus should be taken into account when designing protocols for treatment and/or chemoprevention of prostatic diseases with either one of these 5 alpha-reductase inhibitors since there is considerable pharmacogenetic variation for both drugs.

J Natl Cancer Inst. 2005 Mar 16;97(6):412-3. Related Articles, Links Erratum in: J Natl Cancer Inst. 2005 Apr 6;97(7):480. Tamoxifen pharmacogenetics moves closer to reality. Garber K. Publication Types: News

J Natl Med Assoc. 2004 Apr;96(4):556-7. Related Articles, Links Comment on: J Natl Med Assoc. 2003 Dec;95(12):1201-3. J Natl Med Assoc. 2004 Feb;96(2):196-9. JNMA points to the need of more drug metabolism studies on black patients. Floyd MD. Publication Types: Comment Letter

J Neurol. 2004 Jun;251(6):651-7. Related Articles, Links The future prospects in the classification, diagnosis and therapies of inflammatory myopathies: a view to the future from the "bench-to-bedside". Dalakas MC. Neuromuscular Diseases

Section, National Institue of Neurological Disorders and Stroke, National Institues of Health, Building 10, Room 4N248, 10 Center Dr. MSC 1382, Bethesda, MD 20892-1382, USA. Publication Types: Review

J Neurol. 2004 Oct;251(10):1169-72. Related Articles, Links Genetic approaches to solving common diseases. Abou-Sleiman PM, Healy DG, Wood NW. Department of Molecular Neuroscience, Institute of Neurology, Queen Square, London WC1N 3BG, UK. The pathway to solving simple Mendelian inherited neurological disease is now well established. Barely a month goes by without new linkage data or mutations in a novel gene being reported. These developments are giving insights into a range of neurological conditions from the cortex to the muscle. However, most of these diseases are individually rare, and one of the major challenges facing neuroscience is to devise methods to find the genetic variants that confer risk of common diseases and differential response to treatment. This latter area is an important emerging field known as pharmacogenomics.Unlike Mendelian genetics where effective strategies are well established, the strategies for detecting moderate genetic effects in populations have been problematic. It is likely that a combination of techniques will be used, involving both linkage analysis and linkage disequilibrium mapping. In this review we consider some of the approaches that can be taken to resolve the common genetic variation underlying common disease. Publication Types: Review

J Neurol. 2005 Sep;252 Suppl 3:iii21-iii27. Related Articles, Links Genomics and proteomics: role in the management of multiple sclerosis. Kappos L, Achtnichts L, Dahlke F, Kuhle J, Naegelin Y, Sandbrink R, Lindberg RL. Outpatient Clinic Neurology-Neurosurgery, University Hospital, Petersgraben 4, 4031 Basel, Switzerland. lkappos@uhbs.ch Epidemiological studies and neuro-imaging have provided important insights into the natural course and prognostic factors of multiple sclerosis (MS), but our ability to predict different courses of the disease, and especially its response to treatment, is still very limited. Pharmacogenetic, pharmacogenomic and proteomic studies aim to assess gene and protein function in disease and promise to help to fill this important gap in our knowledge. Such studies may increase our understanding of disease mechanisms and responses to therapeutic compounds. Large-scale transcriptional expression profiling can be performed using gene chip microarrays; this technology allows screening for differentially expressed genes without having well-defined underlying hypotheses ("discovery-driven research"). To complement the technique, real time reverse transcription and polymerase chain reaction (RT-PCR) can be used for more targeted profiling and provides quantitative data on pre-selected genes. However, to maximise their clinical utility, expression profiling results need to be combined with well-documented clinical and imaging data.Two forthcoming studies will investigate the long-term effects of early treatment with interferon beta-1b (IFNbeta) on the course of MS. The BENEFIT (BEtaseron/Betaferon in Newly Emerging MS for Initial Treatment) study will incorporate pharmacogenetic and pharmacogenomic analyses to determine the genetic elements controlling treatment response. BEST-PGx (Betaferon/Betaseron in Early relapsing-remitting MS Surveillance Trial-Pharmacogenomics) is an exploratory 2-

year study that will investigate the value of RNA expression profiling and pharmacogenetics in predicting treatment response to IFNbeta in patients with early relapsing MS. The main goal of BEST-PGx is the identification of differences in gene expression profiles of patients showing differential treatment responses. In addition, this study may reveal new information relevant to the mechanism of action of interferon treatment in MS and also to differences in the underlying pathology of the immune system. These data may help us approach the goal of a really "individualised therapy" with increased efficacy, reduced adverse drug reactions and more efficient use of health care resources. Publication Types: Review

J Nutr. 2004 Jun;134(6 Suppl):1600S-1604S; discussion 1630S-1632S, 1667S-1672S. Related Articles, Links Pharmacogenetics and individual variation in the range of amino acid adequacy: the biological aspects. Caldwell J. The University of Liverpool, Liverpool L69 3GA, UK. jcc@liv.ac.uk There have been major developments in our understanding of the ways in which genetic variation among individuals in a population can affect responses to drugs, and use of such information can improve the safety and efficacy of medicines. The brief review summarizes the emergence of modern pharmacogenetics, illustrating the importance of the field using the CYP 2D6 polymorphism as a paradigm. These pharmacogenetic polymorphisms are compared and contrasted with the long-established inborn errors of amino acid biochemistry, exemplified by phenylketonuria, suggesting ways in which the approaches of pharmacogenetics might inform the safe and effective use of amino acids as food additives and supplements. Publication Types: Review

J Nutr. 2005 Nov;135(11):2698-702. Related Articles, Links Nutrigenetics in cancer research--folate metabolism and colorectal cancer. Ulrich CM. Cancer Prevention Program, Fred Hutchinson Cancer Research Center, Seattle, WA, USA. nulrich@fhcrc.org The B vitamin folate is essential for one-carbon transfer reactions, including those related to the methylation of DNA or other substrates and nucleotide synthesis. Epidemiologic and experimental studies implicate low-folate intakes in elevated risk of colorectal neoplasia and suggest that biologic mechanisms underlying this relation include disturbances in DNA methylation patterns or adverse effects on DNA synthesis and repair. With the completion of the Human Genome Project, a vast amount of data on inherited genetic variability has become available. This genetic information can be used in studies of molecular epidemiology to provide information on multiple aspects of folate metabolism. First, studies linking polymorphisms in folate metabolism to an altered risk of cancer provide evidence for a causal link between this pathway and colorectal carcinogenesis. Second, studies on genetic characteristics can help clarify whether certain individuals may benefit from higher or lower intakes of folate or nutrients relevant to folate metabolism. Third, studies on genetic polymorphisms can generate hypotheses regarding possible biologic mechanisms that connect this pathway to carcinogenesis. Last, genetic variability in folate metabolism may predict survival after a cancer diagnosis, possibly via pharmacogenetic effects. To solve the puzzle of the folate-cancer relation, a transdisciplinary approach is needed that integrates knowledge from epidemiology, clinical studies, experimental nutrition, and mathematical modeling. This review illustrates knowledge that can be gained from molecular epidemiology in the context of nutrigenetics, and the questions that this approach can answer or raise.

J Pharmacokinet Pharmacodyn. 2005 Aug;32(3-4):377-400. Related Articles, Links Unified pharmacogenetics-based parent-metabolite pharmacokinetic model incorporating acetylation polymorphism for talampanel in humans. Buchwald P, Juhasz A, Bell C, Patfalusi M, Howes J, Bodor N. IVAX Research, Inc., 4400 Biscayne Boulevard, Miami, FL 33137, USA. Peter_Buchwald@ivax.com The N-acetylation of the noncompetitive AMPA antagonist talampanel (TLP) represents a route of varying significance in various species. For a detailed analysis in humans, plasma concentrations of TLP and its N-acetyl metabolite (NAc-TLP) were measured for up to 48 h after administration of a single oral dose of 75 mg in 28 healthy volunteers following genotyping for the N-acetyltansferase NAT2 isozymes (alleles NAT2*4, *5, *6, and *7). Unified parent-metabolite pharmacokinetic (PK) models that allowed three different rates of acetylation were used to simultaneously fit plasma levels for both the parent drug and its metabolite following genotype-based classification as slow, intermediate, or fast acetylator. A perfect correspondence was found between the phenotype inferred from genotyping and the phenotype determined by using plasma metabolite-to-parent molar ratios indicating that this route of metabolism is indeed mediated by NAT2. Linear parent-metabolite PK models (first-order input, first-order elimination through two parallel routes one of which is through a metabolite with polymorphic rate of formation) gave adequate and sufficiently consistent fit. Parameters obtained suggest that for TLP in humans, N-acetylation represents only about 1/4th of the total elimination even in true (*4/*4 homozygous) fast acetylators, acetylation is about 8-12 times faster in fast and 3-6 times faster in intermediate acetylators than in slow acetylators, and the N-acetyl metabolite is eliminated faster than the parent drug. Such PK models can provide quantitative estimates of relative in vivo metabolism rates for routes catalyzed by functionally polymorphic enzymes.

J Pharmacol Exp Ther. 2004 Aug;310(2):656-65. Epub 2004 Mar 25. Related Articles, Links UDP-glucuronosyltransferase (UGT) 2B15 pharmacogenetics: UGT2B15 D85Y genotype and gender are major determinants of oxazepam glucuronidation by human liver. Court MH, Hao Q, Krishnaswamy S, Bekaii-Saab T, Al-Rohaimi A, von Moltke LL, Greenblatt DJ. Comparative and Molecular Pharmacogenetics Laboratory, Department of Pharmacology and Experimental Therapeutics, Tufts University School of Medicine, Boston, Massachusetts, USA. michael.court@tufts.edu Oxazepam is a commonly used 1,4-benzodiazepine anxiolytic drug that is polymorphically metabolized in humans. However, the molecular basis for this phenomenon is currently unknown. We have previously shown that S-oxazepam glucuronide, the major oxazepam metabolite, is selectively formed by UDP-glucuronosyltransferase (UGT) 2B15, whereas the minor R-oxazepam glucuronide is produced by multiple UGTs other than UGT2B15. Phenotype-genotype studies were conducted using microsomes and DNA prepared from the same set of 54 human livers. Sequencing of the UGT2B15 gene revealed three nonsynonymous polymorphisms, D85Y, T352I, and K523T, with variant allele frequencies of 0.56, 0.02, and 0.40, respectively. D85Y genotype showed a significant effect ($p = 0.012$) on S-oxazepam glucuronidation with lower median activities in 85Y/Y livers (49 pmol/min/mg protein) compared with 85D/D livers (131 pmol/min/mg), whereas 85D/Y livers were intermediate in activity (65 pmol/min/mg). There was also a significant trend (p = 0.049) for higher S-oxazepam activities in the two 352T/I livers (135 and 210 pmol/min/mg) compared with the remaining 352T/T livers (median, 64 pmol/min/mg). Conversely, K523T genotype had no apparent effect on oxazepam glucuronidation (p > 0.05). Donor gender also significantly influenced S-oxazepam glucuronidation with higher median activities in male (65 pmol/min/mg) compared with female (39 pmol/min/ mg) livers (p = 0.042). R-Oxazepam glucuronidation was not affected by either genotype or gender (p > 0.05). In conclusion, gender and D85Y genotype are identified as major determinants of S-oxazepam glucuronidation by human liver and may explain in part polymorphic oxazepam glucuronidation by human subjects.

J Pharmacol Exp Ther. 2005 Jun;313(3):1331-9. Epub 2005 Mar 10. Related Articles, Links UDP glucuronosyltransferase (UGT) 1A6 pharmacogenetics: I. Identification of polymorphisms in the 5'-regulatory and exon 1 regions, and association with human liver UGT1A6 gene expression and glucuronidation. Krishnaswamy S, Hao Q, Al-Rohaimi A, Hesse LM, von Moltke LL, Greenblatt DJ, Court MH. Molecular Pharmacogenetics Laboratory, Department of Pharmacology and Experimental Therapeutics, Tufts University, Boston, MA 02111, USA. UDP glucuronosyltransferase (UGT) 1A6 is a major isoform in human liver that glucuronidates numerous drugs, toxins, and endogenous substrates with high interindividual variability. The molecular basis for this variability remains unknown, although it likely involves genetic and environmental factors. Phenotype-genotype studies were conducted using a well characterized human liver bank (n = 54) and serotonin glucuronidation as a UGT1A6-specific phenotype marker. A positive moderate-to-heavy alcohol use history (>14 drinks per week) was the only demographic factor examined that correlated with phenotype and was associated with 2-fold higher serotonin glucuronidation (p < 0.001), UGT1A6 protein content (p = 0.004), and UGT1A6 mRNA content (p = 0.025). UGT1A6 gene resequencing identified three nonsynonymous polymorphisms (S7A, T181A, and R184S) in exon 1 and eight novel polymorphisms in the 5'-regulatory region (to -2052 base pairs). S7A was in complete linkage disequilibrium with three 5'-regulatory region polymorphisms (-1710c-->g, -1310del5, and -652g-->a). Initial univariate analyses did not identify any significant phenotype-genotype associations. However, in livers without substantial alcohol exposure, 50% lower UGT1A6 mRNA levels (p = 0.026) were found in carriers of the linked S7A-enhancer polymorphisms compared with noncarriers but without significant effect on UGT1A6 protein content or glucuronidation activities. Three major haplotypes, including (*)1A (reference), (*)1B (-1535g-->a and -427g-->c), and (*)2 (-1710c-->g, -1310del5, -652g-->a, S7A, T181A, and R184S), were identified, accounting for 90% of alleles. No association of haplotype with any of the phenotype measures could be discerned. In conclusion, although the identified UGT1A6 polymorphisms did not explain the observed glucuronidation variability, there does seem to be a significant role for environmental factors associated with alcohol consumption.

J Pharmacol Exp Ther. 2005 Jun;313(3):1340-6. Epub 2005 Mar 10. Related Articles, Links UDP glucuronosyltransferase (UGT) 1A6 pharmacogenetics: II. Functional impact of the three most common nonsynonymous UGT1A6 polymorphisms (S7A, T181A, and R184S). Krishnaswamy S, Hao Q, Al-Rohaimi A, Hesse LM, von Moltke LL, Greenblatt DJ, Court MH. Molecular Pharmacogenetics Laboratory, Department of Pharmacology and Experimental Therapeutics, Tufts University, Boston, MA 02111, USA. The objective of this study was to use recombinant enzymes and human liver microsomes (HLMs) to comprehensively evaluate the functional impact of the three most common nonsynonymous polymorphisms (S7A, T181A, and R184S) identified in the human UDP glucuronosyltransferase (UGT) 1A6 gene. In addition to the known allozymes, other possible amino acid variants were expressed in human embryonic kidney (HEK)293 cells to enable structure-function analysis. Initial studies using different substrates (serotonin, 5-hydroxytryptophol, 4-nitrophenol, acetaminophen, and valproic acid) showed similar results with 2-fold higher glucuronidation by UGT1A6(*)2 (S7A/T181A/R184S) compared with UGT1A6(*)1 (reference), and intermediate activities for other variants. Enzyme kinetic analyses with the UGT1A6-specific substrate (serotonin) showed 50% lower K(m) values for all R184S variants and 2-fold higher V(max) values for both S7A/T181A variants compared with UGT1A6(*)1. Furthermore, intrinsic clearance (V(max)/K(m)) values were highest for the UGT1A6(*)2 allozyme (2.3-fold over UGT1A6(*)1), resulting from additive effects of higher enzyme affinity and activity. As expected, K(m) values of (*)1/(*)1 genotyped HLMs (5.4 +/- 0.2 mM) were similar to recombinant UGT1A6(*)1 (5.8 +/- 0.6 mM). Conversely, (*)2/(*)2 HLMs showed higher K(m) values (7.0 +/- 0.3 mM) rather than the lower K(m) values displayed by recombinant UGT1A6(*)2 (3.6 +/- 0.3 mM), suggesting that this allozyme may display different enzyme kinetic behavior in HLMs compared with HEK293 cells. At best, these polymorphisms were predicted to account for 15 to 20% of the observed 13-fold variability in glucuronidation of UGT1A6 substrates by HLMs, indicating that there are likely other genetic or environmental factors responsible for the majority of this variation.

J Pharmacol Sci. 2005 Jan;97(1):83-90. Epub 2005 Jan 15. Related Articles, Links Utilization of human liver microsomes to explain individual differences in paclitaxel metabolism by CYP2C8 and CYP3A4. Taniguchi R, Kumai T, Matsumoto N, Watanabe M, Kamio K, Suzuki S, Kobayashi S. Department of Pharmacology, St. Marianna University School of Medicine, Kawasaki, Japan. yakuri@marianna-u.ac.jp Paclitaxel is widely used for treatment of malignant tumors. Paclitaxel is metabolized by CYP2C8 and CYP3A4, and these enzymes are known to differ between individuals, although the details have not been clarified. Recent progress in pharmacogenetics has shown that genetic polymorphisms of metabolic enzymes are related to these individual differences. We investigated the effect of the polymorphisms on paclitaxel metabolism by analyzing metabolic activities of CYP2C8 and CYP3A4 and expressions of mRNA and protein. Production of 6alpha-hydroxypaclitaxel, a metabolite of CYP2C8, was 2.3-fold larger than 3'-p-hydroxypaclitaxel, a metabolite of CYP3A4. Significant inter-individual differences between these two enzyme activities were shown. The expressions of mRNA and protein levels correlated well with the enzyme activities, especially with CYP3A4. Although it was previously reported that CYP2C8*3 showed lower activity than the wild type, two subjects that had the CYP2C8*3 allele did not show lower activities in our study. Inter-individual differences in paclitaxel metabolism may be related to CYP2C8 and CYP3A4 mRNA expression. CYP2C8 is the primary metabolic pathway of paclitaxel, but there is a "shifting phenomenon" in the metabolic pathway of paclitaxel in the liver of some human subjects.

J Pharmacol Toxicol Methods. 2004 May-Jun;49(3):183-6. Related Articles, Links Identification and measurement of genomic biomarkers of nephrotoxicity. Goodsaid FM. Department of Genetic and Molecular Toxicology, Schering-Plough Research Institute, 144 Route 94, Lafayette, NJ 07871, USA. federico.goodsaid@fluidigm.com An accelerated pace for drug discovery and development requires the application of measurements of novel parameters for drug-induced toxicity. Genomic biomarkers can contribute to this process as indicators or predictors of toxicity. Transcript levels for genes such as the kidney injury molecule have been identified and evaluated as genomic biomarkers of nephrotoxicity. Publication Types: Review

J Pharmacol Toxicol Methods. 2006 Jan-Feb;53(1):31-7. Epub 2005 Oct 19. Related Articles, Links Toxicogenomic analysis methods for predictive toxicology. Maggioli J, Hoover A, Weng L. Rosetta Biosoftware, 401 Terry Avenue, North Seattle, WA 98109, USA. myra_ozeta@rosettabio.com Toxicogenomics, the application of genomic data to elucidate or predict an organism's response to a toxicant, can inform the drug development process in important ways. It is apparent that standardized approaches to many types of toxicogenomic questions are still being formulated. Specifically, a significant body of proof of principle studies has emerged that demonstrates a range of statistical methodologies applied to predictive toxicology. These studies rely on class prediction methods--mathematical models generated using the gene expression profiles of known toxins from representative toxicological classes--to predict the toxicological effect of a compound based on the similarities between its gene expression profile and the profiles of a given toxicological class. Class prediction methods hold promise for increasing the rate at which compounds can be evaluated for toxicity early in the drug discovery process, while at the same time reducing the length of toxicological studies and their associated costs. Class prediction methods are informed by class comparison and class discovery steps, which inform, respectively, the selection of genes whose response can be used to distinguish among the toxicological classes and the number of classes distinguishable using the response of these genes. Together these steps use a variety of complementary statistical techniques to achieve a successful class prediction model. This report attempts to review some of the themes that appear to be emerging in the application of these techniques to predictive toxicology methods over toxicogenomics' short history. Publication Types: Review

J Pharmacol Toxicol Methods. 2006 Jan-Feb;53(1):38-66. Epub 2005 Jul 27.

Related Articles, Links Systems-ADME/Tox: resources and network approaches. Ekins S. GeneGo, 500 Renaissance Drive, Suite 106, St. Joseph, MI 49085, USA. sean@genego.com The increasing cost of drug development is partially due to our failure to identify undesirable compounds at an early enough stage of development. The application of higher throughput screening methods have resulted in the generation of very large datasets from cells in vitro or from in vivo experiments following the treatment with drugs or known toxins. In recent years the development of systems biology, databases and pathway software has enabled the analysis of the high-throughput data in the context of the whole cell. One of the latest technology paradigms to be applied alongside the existing in vitro and computational models for absorption, distribution, metabolism, excretion and toxicology (ADME/Tox) involves the integration of complex multidimensional datasets, termed toxicogenomics. The goal is to provide a more complete understanding of the effects a molecule might have on the entire biological system. However, due to the sheer complexity of this data it may be necessary to apply one or more different types of computational approaches that have as yet not been fully utilized in this field. The present review describes the data generated currently and introduces computational approaches as a component of ADME/Tox. These methods include network algorithms and manually curated databases of interactions that have been separately classified under systems biology methods. The integration of these disparate tools will result in systems-ADME/Tox and it is important to understand exactly what data resources and technologies are available and applicable. Examples of networks derived with important drug transporters and drug metabolizing enzymes are provided to demonstrate the network technologies. Publication Types: Review

J Prof Nurs. 2004 Jul-Aug;20(4):222-9. Related Articles, Links Genetic discoveries and nursing implications for complex disease prevention and management. Frazier L, Meininger J, Halsey Lea D, Boerwinkle E. School of Nursing, University of Texas Health Science Center at Houston, 1100 Holcombe, Houston, TX 77030, USA. lorraine.frazier@uth.tmc.edu The purpose of this article is to examine the management of patients with complex diseases, in light of recent genetic discoveries, and to explore how these genetic discoveries will impact nursing practice and nursing research. The nursing science processes discussed are not comprehensive of all nursing practice but, instead, are concentrated in areas where genetics will have the greatest influence. Advances in genetic science will revolutionize our approach to patients and to health care in the prevention, diagnosis, and treatment of disease, raising many issues for nursing research and practice. As the scope of genetics expands to encompass multifactorial disease processes, a continuing reexamination of the knowledge base is required for nursing practice, with incorporation of genetic knowledge into the repertoire of every nurse, and with advanced knowledge for nurses who select specialty roles in the genetics area. This article explores the impact of this revolution on nursing science and practice as well as the opportunities for nursing science and practice to participate fully in this revolution. Because of the high proportion of the population at risk for complex diseases and because nurses are occupied every day in the prevention, assessment, treatment, and therapeutic intervention of patients with such diseases in practice and research, there is great opportunity for nurses to improve health care through the application (nursing practice) and discovery (nursing research) of genetic knowledge. Publication Types: Review

J Proteome Res. 2004 Jul-Aug;3(4):697-711. Related Articles, Links Clinical and pharmacogenomic data mining: 2. A simple method for the combination of information from associations and multivariances to facilitate analysis, decision, and design in clinical research and practice. Robson B, Mushlin R. T. J. Watson Research Center, Yorktown Heights, New York 10598, USA. The physician and researcher must ultimately be able to combine qualitative and quantitative features from a variety of combinations of observations on data of many component items (i.e., many dimensions), and hence reach simple conclusions about interpretation, rational courses of action, and design. In the first paper of this series, it was noted that such needs are challenging the classical means of using statistics. Hence, the paper proposed the use of a Generalized Theory of Expected Information or "Zeta Theory". The conjoint event [a,b,c,..] is seen as a rule of association for a,b,c,.. associated with a rule strength I(a;b;c;...) = xi(s,o[a,b,c,..]) - xi (s,e[a,b,c,...]), where xi is the incomplete Zeta Function. Here, o[a,b,c,...] is the observed, and e[a,b,c,..] the expected, frequency of occurrence of conjoint event [a,b,c,...]. The present paper explores how output from this approach might be assembled in a form better suited for decision support. Related to this is the difficulty that the treatment of covariance and multivariance was previously rendered as a "fuzzy association" so that the output would fall into a similar form as the true associations, but this was a somewhat ad hoc approach in which only the final I( ) had any meaning. Users at clinical research sites had subsequently requested an alternative approach in which "effective frequencies" o[ ] and e[ ] calculated from the above variances and used to evaluate I( ) give some intuitive feeling analogous to the association treatment, and this is explored here. Though the present paper is theoretical, real examples are used to illustrate application. One clinical-genomic example illustrates experimental design by identifying data which is, or is not, statistically germane to the study. We also report on some impressions based on applying these techniques in studies of real, extensive patient record data which are now emerging, as well as on molecular design data originally studied in part to test the ability to deduce the effects of simple natural patient sequence variations ("SNPs") on patient protein activity. On the basis of these study experiences, methods of rationalizing and condensing the rules implied by associations and variances between data, as well as discussion of the difficulty of what is meant by "condensed", are presented in the Appendix.

J Proteome Res. 2004 Mar-Apr;3(2):218-27. Related Articles, Links Mining disease susceptibility genes through SNP analyses and expression profiling using MALDI-TOF mass spectrometry. Tang K, Oeth P, Kammerer S, Denissenko MF, Ekblom J, Jurinke C, van den Boom D, Braun A, Cantor CR. Sequenom Inc., 3595 John Hopkins Court, San Diego, California 92121, USA. To find genes that underlie disease susceptibilities, genome-wide single nucleotide polymorphisms (SNPs) have been analyzed using high-throughput matrix assisted laser desorption/ionization (MALDI) time-of-flight (TOF) mass spectrometry (MS). As a proof-of-concept for this approach, gene regions have been identified that were previously associated by others with certain diseases or traits. On the same technology platform, accurate and absolute transcriptional profiling can be performed and applied to allele expression analysis. Here, we provide a brief review of the technology and its applications to disease gene discovery.

J Proteome Res. 2005 Mar-Apr;4(2):445-55. Related Articles, Links Clinical and pharmacogenomic data mining: 3. Zeta theory as a general tactic for clinical bioinformatics. Robson B. T. J. Watson Research Center (IBM), 1101 Kitchawan Road, Yorktown Heights, New York 10598, USA. A new approach, a Zeta Theory of observations, data, and data mining, is being forged from a theory of expected information into an even more cohesive and comprehensive form by the challenge of general genomic, pharmacogenomic, and proteomic data. In this paper, the focus is not on studies using the specific tool FANO (CliniMiner) but on extensions to a new broader theoretical approach, aspects of which can easily be implemented into, or otherwise support, excellent existing methods, such as forms of multivariate analysis and IBM's product Intelligent Miner. The theory should perhaps be distinguished from an existing purely number-theoretic area sometimes also known as Zeta Theory, which focuses on the Riemann Zeta Function and the ways in which it governs the distribution of prime numbers. However, Zeta Theory as used here overlaps heavily with it and actually makes use of these same matters. The distinction is that it enters from a Bayesian information theory and data representation perspective. It could thus be considered an application of the 'mathematician's version'. The application is by no means confined to areas of modern biomedicine, and indeed its generality, even merging into quantum mechanics, is a key feature. Other areas with some similar challenges as modern biology, and which have inspired data mining methods such as IBM's Intelligent Miner, include commerce. But for several reasons discussed, modern molecular biology and medicine seem particularly challenging, and this relates to the often irreducible high dimensionality of the data. This thus remains our main target.

J Psychosoc Nurs Ment Health Serv. 2006 Feb;44(2):13-6. Related Articles, Links Personalized drug therapy with pharmacogenetics--part 2: pharmacodynamics. Howland RH. University of Pittsburgh School of Medicine, Western Psychiatric Institute and Clinic, Pennsylvania 15213, USA. HowlandRH@upmc.edu

J Psychosoc Nurs Ment Health Serv. 2006 Jan;44(1):13-6. Related Articles, Links Personalized drug therapy with pharmacogenetics. Part 1: Pharmacokinetics. Howland RH. University of Pittsburgh, School of Medicine, Western Psychiatric Institute and Clinic, Pittsburgh, Pennsylvania 15213, USA. HowlandRH@upmc.edu Publication Types: Review

J Rheumatol. 2005 Jan;32(1):11-16. Related Articles, Links Comment in: J Rheumatol. 2005 Jan;32(1):6-10. Factors influencing response to disease modifying antirheumatic drugs in patients with rheumatoid arthritis. Hider SL, Buckley C, Silman AJ, Symmons DP, Bruce IN. Publication Types: Editorial

J Stud Alcohol Suppl. 2005 Jul;(15):56-64; discussion 33. Related Articles, Links COMBINE genetics study: the pharmacogenetics of alcoholism treatment response: genes and mechanisms. Goldman D, Oroszi G, O'Malley S, Anton R. Laboratory of Neurogenetics, NIAAA, NIH, 5625 Fishers Lane, Room 3S32, MSC9412, Rockville, Maryland 20852, USA. dgneuro@box-d.nih.gov OBJECTIVE: Partial efficacy of treatment and differences in adverse events across individuals are a challenge and an opportunity in the treatment of alcoholism. Individuation of therapy and understanding origins of differential treatment response may require identification of inherited functional variants of genes. The neurobiology of reward, executive cognitive function, anxiety and dysphoria have been identified as critical domains that may have a genetic basis that could predict treatment response. METHOD: The COMBINE Study presents a unique opportunity to evaluate specific genetic loci (markers) that affect neurobiology central to addiction and extended withdrawal. The study also addresses variation in drug metabolism and action. Candidate genetic markers are selected for study based on functionality and abundance. RESULTS: COMT Vall58Met is a common (minor allele frequency 0.42), functional, catecholamine-metabolizing enzyme polymorphism with threefold relevance. Vall58Met alters executive cognitive function, stress and anxiety responses and brain endogenous opioid function. OPRM1 Asn40Asp is a common (minor allele frequency 0.10), functional polymorphism of the mu-opioid receptor, which may serve as a gatekeeper molecule in naltrexone's actions and was recently reported to affect naltrexone response. HTTLPR (minor allele frequency 0.40) alters serotonin transporter function to affect anxiety, dysphoria and obsessional behavior, which are assessed in COMBINE and may be related to relapse and addictive behavior. CONCLUSIONS: All genetic testing is consented through a separate human research protocol, and the testing is conducted nonclinically, confidentially and apart from the clinical record to protect human research participants who have volunteered for this aspect of COMBINE. Publication Types: Review

J Surg Oncol. 2004 Dec 1;88(3):182-8. Related Articles, Links Medication errors in pediatrics--the octopus evading defeat. Sullivan JE, Buchino JJ. Department of Pediatrics, University of Louisville, Louisville, Kentucky 40202, USA. sully@louisville.edu Medication errors have come to the forefront in healthcare and oversight organizations as well as to the public over the past several years. There has been an increasing focus on this area of patient care requiring more intensive evaluation and intervention to prevent these errors. Although it is difficult to ascertain the true occurrence of medication errors, they may occur as frequently as once in every 20 orders. Children are at higher risk for medication errors and adverse drug events for numerous reasons. Not only is there great variability in weight and body surface area in this population, there is also significant differences in the pharmacokinetics and pharmacodynamics of many medications when compared to adults. In addition, our knowledge of pharmacogenetics and phenotypic ontogeny must be applied. Sources of medication errors are identified, and specific examples and solutions to improve medication use in children are provided. It is critical to have 1) personnel trained in pediatrics to prescribe, prepare, dispense and administer medications, 2) a quality review system in place to review drug use and medication errors, and 3) to implement computerized physician order entry with decision support and other tools in the next decade to improve pharmacologic therapy for pediatric patients. Publication Types: Review

J Thromb Haemost. 2005 Aug;3(8):1655-62. Related Articles, Links Aspirin resistance. Szczeklik A, Musial J, Undas A, Sanak M. Department of Medicine, Jagiellonian University School of Medicine, Cracow, Poland. mmszczek@cyf-kr.edu.pl Treatment failures occur with any drug and aspirin is no exception. Evidence is growing to indicate that there are subpopulations that do not respond to antithrombotic action of aspirin. The term 'aspirin resistance' has been used to describe a number of different phenomena, including inability of aspirin to: (i) protect against cardiovascular events despite its regular intake; (ii) to affect various laboratory tests, reflecting platelet activity. Research on aspirin resistance yielded interesting results in clinical pharmacology and pharmacogenetics. Future studies will show whether genotyping for polymorphisms might be of value in everyday clinical use of aspirin. Present data indicate that in survivors of recent myocardial infarction or unstable angina, patients receiving coronary artery bypass grafts, as well as in subjects with hypercholesterolemia, aspirin resistance has to be considered when implementing antithrombotic therapy. However, in individual patients the available laboratory tests are of no particular use to predict reliably the clinical outcome or to guide in making therapeutic decision. Prospective clinical trials seem necessary to reach such conclusions. Publication Types: Review

J Thromb Haemost. 2005 Feb;3(2):287-91. Related Articles, Links A potential pharmacogenomic strategy for anticoagulant treatment in non-ST elevation acute coronary syndromes: the role of interleukin-1 receptor antagonist genotype. Ray KK, Francis S, Crossman DC. Cardiovascular Research Unit, Clinical Sciences Centre North, Northern General Hospital, Sheffield, UK. kkray@partners.org OBJECTIVES: Our aim was to determine a pharmacogenomic approach to heparin use in non-ST elevation acute coronary syndromes, specifically the impact of interleukin (IL)-1 receptor antagonist polymorphisms upon von Willebrand factor (vWF) responses to unfractionated heparin (UFH) and low molecular weight heparin (LMWH). BACKGROUND: In acute coronary syndromes (ACS), identification of specific biological or genetic targets to direct pharmacological treatment remains a challenge. vWF has been shown to predict future cardiovascular risk and the response to anticoagulant treatments during non-ST elevation ACS. IL-1 receptor antagonist (IL-1RN) polymorphisms predict the change in vWF between 24 and 48 h (Delta vWF) during non-ST elevation ACS. METHODS: We genotyped at the IL-1 locus, 67 patients with non-ST elevation ACS who received either LMWH or UFH, and measured vWF levels at 24 and 48 h. RESULTS: LMWH was superior to UFH in reducing the rise in vWF between 24 and 48 h in the cohort as a whole. However, when patients were stratified by IL-1RN genotype, LMWH was superior to UFH in reducing Delta vWF only in allele *2 carriers (0.51 iU mL(-1) vs. 1.37, $P < 0.01$), but not in non-carriers (- 0.03 iU mL(-1) vs. 0.15, P = NS). CONCLUSION: IL-1RN genotype may be a useful marker to identify patients that benefit from LMWH in non-ST elevation ACS.

J Thromb Haemost. 2005 Oct;3(10):2340-5. Epub 2005 Sep 9. Related Articles, Links Cyclooxygenase-1 haplotype modulates platelet response to aspirin. Maree AO, Curtin RJ, Chubb A, Dolan C, Cox D, O'Brien J, Crean P, Shields DC, Fitzgerald DJ. Department of Clinical Pharmacology, Royal College of Surgeons, Ireland. amaree@partners.org BACKGROUND: Aspirin (acetylsalicylic acid) irreversibly inhibits platelet cyclooxygenase (COX)-1, the enzyme that converts arachidonic acid (AA) to the potent platelet agonist thromboxane (TX) A2. Despite clear benefit from aspirin in patients with cardiovascular disease (CAD), evidence of heterogeneity in the way individuals respond has given rise to the concept of 'aspirin resistance.'AIMS: To evaluate the hypothesis that incomplete suppression of platelet COX as a consequence of variation in the COX-1 gene may affect aspirin response and thus contribute to aspirin resistance. PATIENTS AND METHODS: Aspirin response, determined by serum TXB2 levels and AA-induced platelet aggregation, was prospectively studied in patients (n = 144) with stable CAD taking aspirin (75-300 mg). Patients were genotyped for five single nucleotide polymorphisms in COX-1 [A-842G, C22T (R8W), G128A (Q41Q), C644A (G213G) and C714A (L237M)]. Haplotype frequencies and effect of haplotype on two platelet phenotypes were estimated by maximum likelihood. The four most common haplotypes were considered separately and less common haplotypes pooled. RESULTS: COX-1 haplotype was significantly associated with aspirin response determined by AA-induced platelet aggregation (P = 0.004; 4 d.f.). Serum TXB2 generation was also related to genotype (P = 0.02; 4 d.f.). CONCLUSION: Genetic variability in COX-1 appears to modulate both AA-induced platelet aggregation and thromboxane generation. Heterogeneity in the way patients respond to aspirin may in part reflect variation in COX-1 genotype.

J Toxicol Environ Health A. 2004 Sep 24;67(18):1423-41. Related Articles, Links Gene expression profiling in spleens of deoxynivalenol-exposed mice: immediate early genes as primary targets. Kinser S, Jia Q, Li M, Laughter A, Cornwell P, Corton JC, Pestka J. Department of Food Science and Human Nutrition, Center for Integrative Toxicology, Michigan State University, East Lansing, Michigan 48824, USA. Exposure to the trichothecene mycotoxin deoxynivalenol (DON) alters immune functions in vitro and in vivo. To gain further insight into DON's immunotoxic effects, microarrays were used to determine how acute exposure to this mycotoxin modulates gene expression profiles in murine spleen. B6C3F1 mice were treated orally with 25mg/kg body weight DON, and 2h later spleens were collected for macroarray analysis. Following normalization using a local linear regression model, expression of 116 out of 1176 genes was significantly altered compared to average expression levels in all treatment groups. When genes were arranged into an ontology tree to facilitate comparison of expression profiles between treatment groups, DON was found primarily to modulate genes associated with immunity, inflammation, and chemotaxis. Real-time polymerase chain reaction was used to confirm modulation for selected genes. DON was found to induce the cytokines interleukin (IL)-1alpha, IL-1beta, IL-6 and IL-11. In analogous fashion, DON upregulated expression of the chemokines macrophage inhibitory protein-2 (MIP-2), cytokine-induced chemoattractant protein-1 (CINC-1), monocyte chemoattractant protein (MCP)-1, MCP-3, and cytokine-responsive gene-2 (CRG-2). c-Fos, Fra-, c-Jun, and

JunB, components of the activator protein-1 (AP-1) transcription factor complex, were induced by DON as well as another transcription factor, NR4A1. Four hydrolases were found to be upregulated by DON, including mitogen-activated protein kinase phosphatase 1 (MKP1), catalytic subunit beta isoform (CnAbeta), protein tyrosine phosphatase receptor type J (Ptprj), and protein tyrosine phosphatase nonreceptor type 8 (Ptpn8), whereas three other hydrolases, microsomal epoxide hydrolase (Eph) 1, histidine triad nucleotide binding protein (Hint), and proteosome subunit beta type 8 (Psmb8) were significantly decreased by the toxin. Finally, cysteine-rich protein 61 (CRP61) and heat-shock protein 40 (Hsp40), genes associated with signaling, were increased, while Jun kinase 2 (JNK2) was decreased. Taken together, data suggest that DON upregulated the expression of multiple immediate early genes, many of which are likely to contribute to the complex immunological effects reported for this and other trichothecenes. Copyright Taylor and Francis Inc.

J Vet Med Sci. 2004 Nov;66(11):1335-8. Related Articles, Links The intelligent data management system for toxicogenomics. Lee WS, Lee GJ, Lee GJ, Yeo CD, Kang JS, Kim YH, Kim SJ, Kim JS, Hwang SY, Park JS, Hwang JW, Kang KS, Lee YS, Jeon KS, Um CH, Hong SI, Kim YS. Bioinformatics Unit, ISTECH Inc., Goyang, Gyeonggi-do, South Korea. Toxicogenomics is now emerging as one of the most important genomic application because the toxicity test based on gene expression profiles is expected to be more precise and efficient than current histopathological approaches in a pre-clinical phase. One of the challenging issues in toxicogenomics is the construction of intelligent database management system which can deal with heterogeneous and complex data from many different experimental and information sources. TEST(Toxicogenomics for Efficient Safety Test) database is especially focused on the connectivity of heterogeneous data and the intelligent query system which enable users to obtain relevant useful information from the complex data sets. The database deals with four kinds of information; compound, histopathology, gene expression, and annotation information. Currently, TEST database maintains toxicogenomics information for 16 compounds, 45 microarrays, 190 animal experiments, and customized 4.8 K rat clone set. Our presented system is expected to be a good information source for studying of toxicology mechanism in the genome-wide level and can also be applied to the designing toxicity test chip.

J Vet Med Sci. 2004 Nov;66(11):1339-45. Related Articles, Links cDNA microarray gene expression analysis and toxicological phenotype for anticancer drug. Lee GJ, Lee WS, Jeon KS, Um CH, Kim YS, Kim SJ, Lee CH, Yoon HK, Hwang SY, Park JS, Hwang JW, Kang KS, Lee YS, Kim MS, Chon KJ, Yeo CD, Kang JS. Research Institute, Shin-Won Scientific Co., Ltd. Gyeonggi-do, South Korea. Toxicogenomics, the subdiscipline that merges genomics with toxicology, hold the promise to contributing toward the goal of elucidating mechanism by studying genomic profiling related with various drugs. The application of gene expression profiling technology to examine multiple genes and signaling pathways promises a significant advance in understanding the toxic mechanisms of various drugs and prediction of new drug candidate. Toxicogenomics is emerging field combining genomics and bioinformatics to identify and characterize mechanisms of toxicity of drug and various compounds. The principal hypothesis underlying on this field is that chemical-specific pattern of altered gene expression is related with each chemicals properties, especially toxicological property, and it will be revealed using high-density microarray analysis of sample from exposed organisms. So, in this study we compare the gene expression pattern of two anticancer drugs paclitaxel and orally absorbable paclitaxel, using the cDNA microarray. And from the result of this study, it is possible to provide the new possibility for genome-wide insight into mechanism of their anticancer activity and toxicological phenotype.

J Viral Hepat. 2005 May;12(3):251-61. Related Articles, Links Characteristic sequence changes of hepatitis C virus genotype 2b associated with sustained biochemical response to IFN therapy. Tanabe Y, Nagayama K, Enomoto N, Izumi N, Tazawa J, Kurosaki M, Sakamoto N, Sato C, Watanabe M. Department of Gastroenterology and Hepatology, Faculty of Medicine, Tokyo Medical and Dental University, Tokyo 113-8519, Japan. In hepatitis C virus (HCV) genotype 2b infection, viral eradication (sustained viral response; sVR) is obtained in about 40% by interferon monotherapy, whereas a considerable proportion of non-sVR patients exhibit sustained biochemical response (sBR) showing normal biochemical values despite persistent viraemia. However, the mechanism of sBR has not yet been established. In this study, we analysed serial changes in full-length sequences of HCV genotype 2b before and after interferon (IFN) therapy in five patients with sBR and five with no response (NR; persistent viraemia and abnormal biochemical values after IFN therapy). The overall substitution rate of amino acids in the full-length HCV genome was higher in the sBR group than in the NR group [2.22 +/- 0.48 (10(-3) changes/site/year) vs 1.04 +/- 0.30: P = 0.002]. When the genetic changes were analysed for individual HCV proteins, the sBR group had significantly higher substitution rates of amino acid in NS4A [8.82 +/- 2.80 (10(-3) changes/site/year) vs 0: P = 0.001]. These amino acid changes in sBR were mainly located in the binding motifs of HLA class I molecules including those frequently found in the Japanese population. These results demonstrated that the greater amino acid changes of HCV arising during interferon therapy are associated with the establishment of sBR. Although functional significance of these changes awaits further investigation, the finding that amino acid changes in NS4A in sBR patients are mainly located in the HLA class I binding motifs illustrated the potential roles of the escape mutations of HCV genome from CTLs in the decreasing activities of hepatitis in sBR.

J Womens Health (Larchmt). 2005 Jan-Feb;14(1):19-29. Related Articles, Links Sex and racial differences in pharmacological response: where is the evidence? Pharmacogenetics, pharmacokinetics, and pharmacodynamics. Anderson GD. Department of Pharmacy, University of Washington, Seattle, Washington, USA. gaila@u.washington.edu The Food and Drug Administration (FDA) reviewed 300 new drug applications between 1995 and 2000. Of the 163 that included a sex analysis, 11 drugs showed a >40% difference in pharmacokinetics between males and females, which was listed on the product label, yet no dosing recommendations were made based on sex. Female sex has been shown to be a risk factor for clinically relevant adverse drug reactions. Would simply dosing females based on their different pharmacokinetics decrease the incidence of adverse events? The answer is not known. Sex-dependent pharmacodynamic effects have been identified. The role of pharmacokinetics vs. pharmacodynamics is unclear, as is the impact of pharmacogenetics on both. This review highlights a few specific examples in each area in which sex differences in pharmacokinetics and pharmacodynamics are important and provides recommendations for additional needed research. Publication Types: Review

J Zhejiang Univ Sci B. 2006 Feb;7(2):169-70. Related Articles, Links Pharmacogenetics, pharmacogenomics and ecogenetics. Motulsky AG, Qi M. Department of Medicine Medical Genetics and Genome Sciences, University of Washington, Seattle, WA 98195, USA. agmot@u.washington.edu Pharmacogenetics and pharmacogenomics deal with the role of genetic factors in drug effectiveness and adverse drug reactions. The promise of a personalized medicine is beginning to be explored but requires much more clinical and translational research. Specific DNA abnormalities in some cancers already have led to effective targeted treatments. Racially determined frequency differences in pharmacogenetic traits may affect choice of treatment requiring specific testing rather than basing treatments according to racial designation. The role of genes in variable responses to foreign chemicals (xenobiotics) has been termed ecogenetics or toxicogenetics raising problems in public health and occupational medicine. Nutrigenetics refers to genetic variation in response to nutrients and may affect nutritional requirements and predisposition to chronic disease.

JAAPA. 2004 Jul;17(7):31-2, 47. Related Articles, Links The role of pharmacogenetics in future practice. Carey L. Philadelphia University, Philadelphia, PA, USA.

JAMA. 2004 Jun 16;291(23):2869-71. Related Articles, Links Comment on: JAMA. 2004 Jun 16;291(23):2821-7. Using pharmacogenetics to improve drug safety and efficacy. Haga SB, Burke W. The Center for the Advancement of Genomics, Rockville, Md, USA. Publication Types: Comment

JAMA. 2005 May 11;293(18):2199. Related Articles, Links Gene variants explain patient differences in antiepileptic drug responses. Hampton T. Publication Types: News

Jurimetrics. 2000 Fall;41(1):23-52. Related Articles, Links Separating predictive genetic testing from snake oil: regulation, liabilities, and lost opportunities. Malinowski MJ. Widener University School of Law, USA. This article explores the extent to which completion of maps of the human genome, coupled with the introduction of technology that will accelerate the identification of gene and protein function, have introduced immeasurable potential to advance life science and health care through genetic profiling. In light of definitional uncertainty, the regulatory and legal environment surrounding predictive genetic testing threatens to impede clinical utilization of genetic profiling technologies that could significantly improve human health. Especially given that genetic testing technologies have been stigmatized in the public and medical community, they must enter the marketplace with a regulatory framework that assures safety, efficacy, and market responsibility.

Kardiol Pol. 2004 Mar;60(3):304-8. Related Articles, Links [Pharmacogenetics--new perspectives in the treatment of cardiovascular diseases] [Article in Polish] Dzida G. Katedra i Klinika Chorob Wewnetrznych, Akademia Medyczna, Lublin, Poland. Publication Types: Review

Kobe J Med Sci. 2003;49(5-6):143-51. Related Articles, Links Effects of mefloquine usage on genetic polymorphism of Plasmodium falciparum in Thai-Myanmarese border. Matsuo T, Shirakawa T, Singhasivanon P, Looareesuwan S, Kawabata M. International Center for Medical Research, Kobe University School of Medicine, 7-5-1 Kusunoki-cho, Chuo-ku, Kobe 650-0017, Japan. We studied the polymorphism of msp-1, which encodes a major surface protein on the merozoite, isolated from blood samples from western Thailand in 1999. Our study area was a low-transmission area for malaria, where mefloquine has been used as an antimalarial drug since 1994. Forty-nine patients were confirmed to have contracted falciparum malaria twice within 24 weeks. The number of detected haplotypes in 49 patients was 89 at the first diagnosis and 68 at the second diagnosis. The mean number of haplotypes per patient significantly decreased from 1.82 to 1.39 but the frequency distributions of msp-1 haplotypes did not change significantly with the use of mefloquine. Our study strongly suggests that the antigenic diversity of Plasmodium falciparum is retained during mefloquine therapy in low-transmission areas.

Lancet Infect Dis. 2005 Jan;5(1):10. Related Articles, Links Live smallpox experiments may go ahead. Senior K. Publication Types: News

Lancet Neurol. 2006 Feb;5(2):189-96. Related Articles, Links Update on pharmacogenetics in epilepsy: a brief review. Szoeke CE, Newton M, Wood JM, Goldstein D, Berkovic SF, OBrien TJ, Sheffield LJ. Department of Medicine, University of Melbourne, Melbourne, Australia. cassandra.szoeke@mh.org.au Recent developments in the pharmacogenetics of antiepileptic drugs provide new prospects for predicting the efficacy of treatment and potential side-effects. Epilepsy is a common, serious, and treatable neurological disorder, yet current treatment is limited by high rates of adverse drug reactions and lack of complete seizure control in a significant proportion of patients. The disorder is especially suitable for pharmacogenetic investigation because treatment response can be quantified and side-effects can be assessed with validated measures. Additionally, there is substantial knowledge of the pharmacodynamics and kinetics of antiepileptic drugs, and some candidate genes implicated in the disorder have been identified. However, recent studies of the association of particular genes and their genetic variants with seizure control and adverse drug reactions have not provided unifying conclusions. This article reviews the published work and summarises the state of research in this area. Future directions for research and the application of this technology to the clinical practice of individualising treatment for epilepsy are discussed. Publication Types: Review

Lancet Oncol. 2006 Jan;7(1):61-8. Related Articles, Links Comparative pharmacogenomics of antiretroviral and cytotoxic treatments. Stebbing J, Bower M. Chelsea and Westminster Hospital, 369 Fulham Road, London SW10 9NH, UK. Few genetic markers are used routinely to predict clinical effectiveness and toxic effects despite the fact that physicians and their patients are consistently confronted with this balance. Because one of the goals of pharmacogenomics is to identify individuals and target populations that might have adverse outcomes, pharmaceutical companies have been reluctant to use a strategy that might identify patients who are not eligible for a particular treatment. This view is changing because drug-discovery programmes and treatments that target specific pathways, are showing improvements in surrogate and survival endpoints. HIV and cancer are now regarded as chronic diseases, which commonly need life-long systemic treatment from the time of diagnosis. HIV and cancer medicine have used pharmacogenomics to some extent in clinical care. Common and classic features of pharmacogenomics that are related to both antiretroviral treatment and to cytotoxic treatment are discussed in this review, providing a framework for individual treatment of these diseases. Publication Types: Review

Leuk Lymphoma. 2003;44 Suppl 3:S115-22. Related Articles, Links Pharmacogenetics and proteomics of anticancer drugs in non-Hodgkin's lymphoma. Loni L, De Braud F, Zinzani PL, Danesi R. Division of Pharmacology and Chemotherapy, Department of Oncology, Transplants and Advanced Technologies in Medicine, via Roma 55, University of Pisa, Pisa 56126 Italy. The variability of tumor responses to chemotherapeutic agents is a topic of major interest in current cancer research. Advances in the knowledge of dysregulation of key molecular pathways in cancer cells have enabled techniques to be developed that can profile tumor cells for their genetic background, allowing selection of anticancer agents on an individual basis. The next generation of anticancer treatments might therefore be tailored according to the molecular alterations identified in tumor cells of individual patients. However, before these alterations can be exploited from a therapeutic point of view, it is necessary to understand how such alterations influence the cellular pathways that control sensitivity to chemotherapeutic agents. Pharmacogenetics and pharmacoproteomics, novel disciplines that investigate the relationship between gene and protein expression in tumor cells and the response to anticancer agents, will be instrumental in developing optimal chemotherapeutic regimens for patients with non-Hodgkin's lymphoma. Publication Types: Review

Liver Transpl. 2005 Jul;11(7):826-33. Related Articles, Links Erratum in: Liver Transpl. 2005 Sep;11(9):1150. Comment in: Liver Transpl. 2005 Oct;11(10):1300-1. Pharmacogenetic association with adverse drug reactions to azathioprine immunosuppressive therapy following liver transplantation. Breen DP, Marinaki AM, Arenas M, Hayes PC. College of Medicine and Veterinary Medicine, University of Edinburgh, Edinburgh, Scotland, UK. davebreen@lycos.com Azathioprine (AZA) is a thiopurine prodrug commonly used in triple-immunosuppressive therapy following liver transplantation. Approximately 1 in 10 patients suffers side effects in response to the drug, the most problematic being bone marrow toxicity. There is evidence that polymorphisms in the genes encoding thiopurine methyltransferase (TPMT) and inosine triphosphate pyrophosphatase (ITPase) predict adverse drug reactions to AZA therapy. Furthermore, common genetic polymorphisms in the gene encoding methylenetetrahydrofolate reductase (MTHFR) may have an indirect impact on thiopurine drug methylation by influencing levels of the methyl donor S-adenosylmethionine (SAM). The aim of this study was to determine whether polymorphisms in these candidate pharmacogenetic loci predict adverse drug reactions to AZA immunosuppressive therapy in liver transplant patients. A series of 65 liver transplant recipients were recruited to the study from the Liver Transplant Out-Patient clinic at The Royal Infirmary of Edinburgh. Clinical response to AZA was retrospectively correlated against TPMT activity, TPMT*2, *3A, and *3A genotypes, inosine triphosphatase (ITPA) 94C>A and IVS2+21A>C genotypes, and MTHFR 677C>T and 1298A>C genotypes. Variant TPMT, ITPA, and MTHFR genotypes were not significantly associated with adverse drug reactions to AZA, including bone marrow suppression. However, the 2 patients who suffered nodular regenerative hyperplasia (NRH) were both heterozygous for the TPMT*3A mutation. In conclusion, our findings suggest that TPMT, ITPA, and MTHFR genotypes do not predict adverse drug reactions, including bone marrow suppression, in liver transplant patients. However, the possible association between NRH and a heterozygous TPMT genotype should be investigated further.

Lung Cancer. 2005 Oct;50 Suppl 1:S13-4. Related Articles, Links Using translational research to tailor the use of chemotherapy in the treatment of NSCLC. Bepler G. H. Lee Moffitt Cancer Center and Research Institute, Tampa, FL 33612-9497, USA. BeplerG@moffitt.usf.edu The treatment of advanced non-small-cell lung cancer (NSCLC) has improved over the past two decades with the availability of new agents such as gemcitabine, the taxanes and vinorelbine. Despite these advances, survival prospects remain disappointingly low for most patients. Further improvements in response rate and survival requires the development of new agents with novel mechanisms of action, such as molecularly targeted therapies, which are currently being tested in clinical trials. The conventional treatment approach to NSCLC is beginning to shift towards the application of specific strategies and techniques, such as pharmacogenomics, to tailor treatment to individual patients. Many efforts are in progress to identify the clinical predictors of outcome. The discovery of prognostic molecular markers, such as the putative suppressor gene (RRM1), represents a novel and potential parameter to help guide clinical treatment decisions.

Lymphat Res Biol. 2005 Summer;3(2):81-6. Related Articles, Links Pharmacogenomics: its role in re-establishing coumarin as treatment for lymphedema. Farinola N, Piller N. Lymphedema Assessment Clinic, Department of Surgery, School of Medicine, Flinders University and Flinders Medical Centre, Adelaide, South Australia. Although there remains some significant controversy regarding the use and benefits of coumarin (5,6-benzo-alpha pyrone), it would seem that targeted appropriate and monitored use of the drug does have a significant role in the treatment of lymphedemas. The particular benefits are its cost and ease of administration. Given today's demands for high level investigative clinical trials, it would be virtually impossible to conduct a study large enough to make any significant conclusions about hepatotoxic effects. However, it seems without doubt that the majority of studies conducted thus far suggest that coumarin (and other benzopyrones, i.e., the ruto-sides, which do not have hepatotoxic effects and which are often discussed in aggregate with coumarin) is effective in treating lymphedema, particularly when used in conjunction with complex physical therapy. The use of pharmacogenomics could significantly lower the risk of coumarin-associated hepatotoxicity, by targeting the use of coumarin to those with functional CYP2A6. Further research in this area will be required to re-evaluate the cost- benefit ratio and to determine the potential for the reintroduction of coumarin as a potent treatment for lymphedema. The perceived negative image of coumarin should not be allowed to carry across to the other benzopyrones, as they still confer a significant benefit in the management of lymphedemas. Publication Types: Review

Manag Care. 2004 Nov;13(11):54-5. Related Articles, Links Pharmacogenetic, pharmacogenomic testing rapidly gaining acceptance. Morrow T. National Association of Managed Care Physicians, USA.

Math Biosci. 2005 Jan;193(1):79-100. Epub 2004 Dec 28. Related Articles, Links Multi-class clustering and prediction in the analysis of microarray data. Tsai CA, Lee TC, Ho IC, Yang UC, Chen CH, Chen JJ. Division of Biometry and Risk Assessment, National Center for Toxicological Research, Food and Drug Administration NCTR/FDA/HFT-20 Jefferson, AR 72079, USA. DNA microarray technology provides tools for studying the expression profiles of a large number of distinct genes simultaneously. This technology has been applied to sample clustering and sample prediction. Because of a large number of genes measured, many of the genes in the original data set are irrelevant to the analysis. Selection of discriminatory genes is critical to the accuracy of clustering and prediction. This paper considers statistical significance testing approach to selecting discriminatory gene sets for multi-class clustering and prediction of experimental samples. A toxicogenomic data set with nine treatments (a control and eight metals, As, Cd, Ni, Cr, Sb, Pb, Cu, and AsV with a total of 55 samples) is used to illustrate a general framework of the approach. Among four selected gene sets, a gene set omega(I) formed by the intersection of the F-test and the set of the union of one-versus-all t-tests performs the best in terms of clustering as well as prediction. Hierarchical and two modified partition (k-means) methods all show that the set omega(I) is able to group the 55 samples into seven clusters reasonably well, in which the As and AsV samples are considered as one cluster (the same group) as are the Cd and Cu samples. With respect to prediction, the overall accuracy for the gene set omega(I) using the nearest neighbors algorithm to predict 55 samples into one of the nine treatments is 85%.

Med Clin North Am. 2006 Jan;90(1):39-60. Related Articles, Links Asthma: diagnosis and management. Mathur SK, Busse WW. Section of Allergy, Pulmonary, and Critical Care, Department of Medicine, University of Wisconsin Medical School, Madison, WI 53792, USA. The diagnosis and management of asthma continue to be of critical importance, as recent trends have demonstrated its increasing prevalence, morbidity, and perhaps mortality. Because current treatments for asthma are effective and safe, it is important to diagnose asthma early and to use treatments effectively, particularly those directed toward airway inflammation. The diagnostic measures and array of medications, both those currently available and on the horizon, provide an armamentarium for effective diagnosis, management, and monitoring of asthma. In the coming years, it is expected that additional testing modalities will be available for more precise monitoring of asthma control, and an increased understanding of pharmacogenetics will enable the tailoring of asthma medications to specific patients, providing customized therapy to maximize asthma control. Publication Types: Review

Med Etika Bioet. 2001 Spring-Summer;8(1-2):3-5. Related Articles, Links Ethical perspectives on life sciences research after mapping the human genome. Magill G. Center for Health Care Ethics, Health Sciences, St. Louis University, 3525 Caroline Mall, St. Louis, MO 63104, USA. The essay discusses ethical perspectives of life sciences research that can help us navigate a path across the genetic landscape that opens before us with the map of the human genome that was announced recently. We can rightly anticipate many drug discoveries and genetic therapies to cure, prevent, or alleviate devastating conditions. But we must also pause with appropriate apprehension about the possible dangers and difficulties we may encounter.

Med J Aust. 2005 Jan 17;182(2):78-81. Related Articles, Links Advances in childhood leukaemia: successful clinical-trials research leads to individualised therapy. Ziegler DS, Dalla Pozza L, Waters KD, Marshall GM. Centre for Children's Cancer and Blood Disorders, Sydney Children's Hospital, Randwick, NSW, Australia. In most cases, childhood leukaemia has a fetal origin, but multiple molecular events are required after birth for pre-leukaemic cells to progress to leukaemia. Cure rates for acute lymphoblastic leukaemia (ALL) now approach 80%. A high level of minimal residual disease detected by polymerase chain reaction in patients with ALL in remission has profound prognostic importance and is the focus of a major Australian study attempting to prevent relapse in these children. Greater awareness of the late effects of chemotherapy has led to changes in the treatment protocols for ALL, with improvement in neurocognitive outcomes and reduced rates of second malignancies. Pharmacogenetics is a new field of research that aims to enhance treatment efficacy by assessing the individual's metabolism of and response to chemotherapeutic agents. Targeted therapies currently being developed show some promise of being able to further improve cure rates. Adolescents with ALL have a better prognosis if treated with paediatric rather than adult protocols. Publication Types: Review

Med J Aust. 2005 Jun 20;182(12):607-8. Related Articles, Links Tailoring access to high cost, genetically targeted drugs. Assessment of real cost effectiveness, with data linked to individual health outcomes while protecting patient privacy, is an essential challenge we need to meet. Hall WD, Ward R, Liauw WS, Lu CY, Brien JA. Publication Types: Editorial

Med Law. 2005 Jun;24(2):343-54. Related Articles, Links Reprogenetics and pharmacogenetics: in whose best interests? Mackenzie R. University of Kent, Kent Law School, Eliot College, University of Kent, Canterbury, United Kingdom. Reprogenetics involves embryonic pre-implantation genetic diagnosis, provoking controversy over the creation of saviour siblings, eugenics and genetic enhancement. It will soon ascertain pharmacogenetic susceptibilities. Pharmacogenetics impacts upon public health initiatives underpinned by resource allocation constraints in that genetic epidemiological studies assist in administering health care resources and public health strategies. Knowing how likely sections of the population are to develop specific medical conditions so that lifestyle and environmental factors influencing these conditions can be targeted has the potential to save public money and improve public health. Aligning population groups with genetic susceptibilities with specific medications would enable cost-effective prescribing. Reprogenetics and pharmacogenetics also possess great commercial potential for nation states and biotechnology companies. Hence ethical legal safeguards for members of the public whose reproductive or genetic tissue is a research or health care resource are essential. Both legal measures such as informed consent and mechanisms for including the public in policy decisions over reprogenetics and pharmacogenetics must be rethought to ensure that they provide protection rather than function as rubber stamps which preclude deeper inquiry into justifications of projects.

Med Pr. 2004;55(2):193-202. Related Articles, Links [Toxicogenomics. New perspectives for the molecular toxicology] [Article in Polish] Lutz W, Kur B. Zakladu Immunotoksykologii, Instytutu Medycyny Pracy im. prof. I. Nofera w Lodzi. lutz@imp.lodz.pl Gene expression in the cellular genome is subject to changes caused by internal and external factors. Due to different expression of gene sets (polymorphism), cells show different morphological and functional characteristics. Environmental and occupational toxic agents may influence cells at the level of transcription and translation. The functional toxicogenomics attempts to explain those influences. Due to recent developments in molecular biology and bioinformatics, it has become possible to analyze protein transcript (toxicogenomics) and profile (toxicoproteomics). This work reports new opportunities to study gene sequencing and expression by means of the DNA chip technique (rapid analysis of the genetic polymorphism) and the microarrays technique (simultaneous analysis of hundreds or thousands of genes). The authors report examples of some practical applications of toxicogenomics in the assessment of the effects of pathological exposures to environmental and occupational toxic (carcinogenic, hepatotoxic and/or neurotoxic) agents, due to the development of new groups of biomarkers, such as biomarkers of individual susceptibility, biomarkers of toxic effects combined with the assay of the relationship between a toxic agent and its dose, and the effect measured at the level of the cellular genome and results of histopathological and biochemical tests. Publication Types: Review

Med Princ Pract. 2005;14 Suppl 1:35-48. Related Articles, Links Mechanisms of drug resistance in cancer chemotherapy. Luqmani YA. Department of Pharmaceutical Chemistry, Faculty of Pharmacy, Kuwait University, Kuwait. yunus@hsc.edu.kw The management of cancer involves procedures, which include surgery, radiotherapy and chemotherapy. Development of chemoresistance is a persistent problem during the treatment of local and disseminated disease. A plethora of cytotoxic drugs that selectively, but not exclusively, target actively proliferating cells include such diverse groups as DNA alkylating agents, antimetabolites, intercalating agents and mitotic inhibitors. Resistance constitutes a lack of response to drug-induced tumour growth inhibition; it may be inherent in a subpopulation of heterogeneous cancer cells or be acquired as a cellular response to drug exposure. Resistance varies. Although regulatory approval may require efficacy in as few as 20% of trial cohorts, a drug may subsequently be used in unselected patients displaying resistance to the treatment. Principal mechanisms may include altered membrane transport involving the P-glycoprotein product of the multidrug resistance (MDR) gene as well as other associated proteins, altered target enzyme (e.g. mutated topoisomerase II), decreased drug activation, increased drug degradation due to altered expression of drug-metabolising enzymes, drug inactivation due to conjugation with increased glutathione, subcellular redistribution, drug interaction, enhanced DNA repair and failure to apoptose as a result of mutated cell cycle proteins such as p53. Attempts to overcome resistance mainly involve the use of combination drug therapy using different classes of drugs with minimally overlapping toxicities to allow maximal dosages and with narrowest cycle intervals, necessary for bone marrow recovery. Adjuvant therapy with P-glycoprotein inhibitors and, in specific instances, the use of growth factor and protein kinase C inhibitors are newer experimental approaches that may also prove effective in abrogating or delaying onset of resistance. Gene knockout using antisense molecules may be another effective way of blocking drug resistance genes. Conversely, drug resistance may also be used to good purpose by transplanting retrovirally transformed CD34 cells expressing the MDR gene to protect the bone marrow during high-dose chemotherapy. Copyright 2005 S. Karger AG, Basel Publication Types: Review

Med Sci (Paris). 2004 Jun-Jul;20(6-7):634-6. Related Articles, Links [Pharmacogenomics: the link between genes and response to drugs] [Article in French] Loriot MA, Beaune P. Publication Types: News

Med Sci (Paris). 2004 Nov;20(11):964-5. Related Articles, Links [Pharmacogenomics of the growth hormone: polymorphism of the receptor in the front line] [Article in French] Bougneres P. Publication Types: News

Med Sci Monit. 2004 May;10(5):RA111-23. Epub 2004 Apr 28. Related Articles, Links Challenge of personalized health care: to what extent is medicine already individualized and what are the future trends? Fierz W. Institute for Clinical Microbiology and Immunology, St. Gallen, Switzerland. walter.fierz@logolab.ch Personalized medicine: is it hype or revolution? In any case, there is not only real demand for it, but it also has a history. As it is, the personal aspects of health care have been partly neglected in the current era of evidence-based, scientific medicine. We now know that a 'one fits all' type of treatment has its limits. Medicine needs to be (re-)personalized. The time is right: the post-genomic era provides the necessary molecular tools, but does it provide for the risks involved? Privacy, protection of minorities, and prevention of discrimination are at stake. Regulations are required. The health-care process needs redesigning to render personalized medicine effective. Information and communication management is challenged to handle the wealth of personal information and link to global medical knowledge. But the goal is magnificent: personal health planning, early diagnosis, the right drug for the right patient, and predictable side effects. Publication Types: Review

Med Wieku Rozwoj. 2003 Oct-Dec;7(4 Pt 2):531-46. Related Articles, Links [I. Single nucleotide polymorphism in human genetic analyses] [Article in Polish] Czerska K, Nawara M, Bal J. Pracownia Genetyki Molekularnej, Zaklad Genetyki Medycznej, Instytut Matki i Dziecka, Kasprzaka 17a, 01-211 Warszawa, Poland. czerska@imid.med.pl The new era of human genetic analyses has been began by finishing of The Human Genome Project. Discovery of the almost complete sequence of human DNA showed surprisingly small differences between the genetic materials of randomly chosen people. Genetists pay intensive attention to the very small part of nucleotide sequence - 0.1% - which contains polymorphic changes. The most frequent type of these changes is polymorphism of a single nucleotide (SNP). It makes up about 90% of all molecular differences in human DNA sequence. There are about 3 mln positions in DNA sequence containing SNPs. Polymorphic changes serve as genetic markers and they enable to map genes or to follow their inheritance. Changes of this kind seem also to be the possible cause of the remarkable variety of susceptibility to many common diseases e.g.: diabetes, cancer and cardiovascular disorders. SNPs are also the object of interest of intensively developing scientific domain - pharmacogenetics. Scientists working on this interdisciplinary field - connecting pharmacology and genetics - try to find out the reason of great variety of response to medicines and their side effects in case of patients belonging to the same therapeutical groups. Progress in this kind of research in near future will enable a significant improvement of pharmacological therapy, which will be based on matching the drug to genetically determined traits of patients. Publication Types: Review

Med Wieku Rozwoj. 2004 Oct-Dec;8(4 Pt 1):967-91. Related Articles, Links [II. Pharmacogenetics--the future of modern pharmacology and genetics] [Article in Polish] Czerska K, Bal J. Zaklad Genetyki Medycznej, Instytut Matki i Dziecka, ul. Kasprzaka 17a, 01-211 Warszawa. czerska@imid.med.pl Pharmacogenetics is a scientific discipline connecting pharmacology and genetics. Its point of interest is an analysis of the variable, genetically determined patient's response to drugs. The basic discovery in this field was the elucidation of the heterogenic response of patients to the tuberculostatic drug -- isoniazid. The new era of searching for the molecular background of the variable drugs metabolism has begun after identification, in the 50's, of the polymorphic variants of NAT2 gene. It encodes for N-acetyltransferase 2, an isoniazid metabolizing enzyme. The key catalysts of the biotransformation reactions are cytochrome P450 isoenzymes. Identification of the polymorphic variants of genes encoding these enzymes enabled an explanation of the heterogenic drugs tolerance. The current knowledge shows that the genetic defects that are responsible for variable pharmacological response concern not only genes encoding the metabolising enzymes but also transporter proteins and drug receptors. Due to achievements of the molecular genetics and putting into practice the modern bioinformatic technics new pharmacological opportunities have been created. It becomes possible to predict the patient's individual reactions and needs, without the necessity of treatment by "trial and error". Pharmacogenetics will allow to implement personalized therapy leading to safer and more effective drugs usage. Identification of the individual metabolising paths will reduce patient's exposition to the side effects of many drugs. In spite of many financial and logistic limitations there are chances of introducing the pharmacogenetic analysis -- as an obligatory step -- to the phases II and III of clinical trials by 2020. Publication Types: Review

Medicina (B Aires). 2004;64(6):563-7. Related Articles, Links [Pharmacogenetics/pharmacogenomics in clinical practice] [Article in Spanish] Sookoian S, Pirola CJ. Publication Types: Editorial

Medinfo. 2004;11(Pt 2):793-7. Related Articles, Links A resource to acquire and summarize pharmacogenetics knowledge in the literature. Rubin DL, Carrillo M, Woon M, Conroy J, Klein TE, Altman RB. Department of Genetics, Stanford University, Stanford, CA 94305-5210, USA. To determine how genetic variations contribute the variations in drug response, we need to know the genes that are related to drugs of interest. But there are no publicly available data-bases of known gene-drug relationships, and it is time-consuming to search the literature for this information. We have developed a resource to support the storage, summarization, and dissemination of key gene-drug interactions of relevance to pharmacogenetics. Extracting all gene-drug relationships from the literature is a daunting task, so we distributed a tool to acquire this knowledge from the scientific community. We also developed a categorization scheme to classify gene-drug relationships according to the type of pharmacogenetic evidence that supports them. Our resource (http://www.pharmgkb.org/home/project-community.jsp) can be queried by gene or drug, and it summarizes gene-drug relationships, categories of evidence, and supporting literature. This resource is growing, containing entries for 138 genes and 215 drugs of pharmacogenetics significance, and is a core component of PharmGKB, a pharmacogenetics knowledge base (http://www.pharmgkb.org).

Methods Enzymol. 2004;382:115-44. Related Articles, Links NAD(P)H:quinone oxidoreductase 1 (NQO1, DT-diaphorase), functions and pharmacogenetics. Ross D, Siegel D. Department of Pharmaceutical Sciences, School of Pharmacy, University of Colorado, Denver 80262, USA. Publication Types: Review

Methods Enzymol. 2005;400:485-510. Related Articles, Links High-speed screening of human ATP-binding cassette transporter function and genetic polymorphisms: new strategies in pharmacogenomics. Ishikawa T, Sakurai A, Kanamori Y, Nagakura M, Hirano H, Takarada Y, Yamada K, Fukushima K, Kitajima M. Department of Biomolecular Engineering, Tokyo Institute of Technology, Graduate School of Bioscience and Biotechnology, Midoriku, Yokohama, Japan. Drug transporters represent an important mechanism in cellular uptake and efflux of drugs and their metabolites. Hitherto a variety of drug transporter genes have been cloned and classified into either solute carriers or ATP-binding cassette (ABC) transporters. Such drug transporters are expressed in various tissues such as the intestine, brain, liver, kidney, and, importantly, cancer cells, where they play critical roles in the absorption, distribution, and excretion of drugs. We developed high-speed functional screening and quantitative structure-activity relationship analysis methods to study the substrate specificity of ABC transporters and to evaluate the effect of genetic polymorphisms on their function. These methods would provide powerful and practical tools for screening synthetic and natural compounds, and the deduced data can be applied to the molecular design of new drugs. Furthermore, we demonstrate a new "SNP array" method to detect genetic polymorphisms of ABC transporters in human samples.

Methods Inf Med. 2005;44(2):257-61. Related Articles, Links An OGSA-based integration of life-scientific resources for drug discovery. Kosaka T, Tohsato Y, Date S, Matsuda H, Shimojo S. Graduate School of Information Science and Technology, Osaka University, 5-1 Mihogaoka, Ibaraki, Osaka 567-0047, Japan. tak-k@ais.cmc.osaka-u.ac.jp OBJECTIVES: The rapid progress of life-scientific research has the potential to dramatically change the paradigm of drug discovery. Efficient utilization of life-scientific resources, i.e., databases and analytic software tools, poses a challenging issue with regard to the reduction of time and cost in the drug discovery process. In this paper, a variety of heterogeneous Web-based life-scientific resources are integrated toward the improvement of drug discovery performance. METHODS: For the integration of heterogeneous life-scientific resources, a database federation technique based on three-layer architecture has been utilized. With the federation technique, life-scientific resources are integrated step by step through database layers, database integration layers and analysis layers to encapsulate complexity and heterogeneity. In this study, we have taken advantage of the latest Grid technology based on OGSA (Open Grid Services Architecture) for the implementation of our approach. RESULTS: The actual case of life-scientific resources for drug discovery demonstrates that our prototype system developed with the proposed technique works well for the identification process of candidate compounds to a target protein. In other words, the prototype system allows a researcher to retrieve candidate compounds with less effort than before. CONCLUSIONS: The usefulness of the prototypic system represents the ability of our approach to integrate heterogeneous life-scientific resources, which have the potential to dramatically improve efficiency in drug discovery, resulting in the shortening of drug development. On the other hand, the system requires further consideration from the aspect of practical use. Dynamic aggregation of the resources is one example of such a consideration.

Methods Mol Biol. 2005;291:399-414. Related Articles, Links Genotyping technologies: application to biotransformation enzyme genetic polymorphism screening. Romkes M, Buch SC. Center for Clinical Pharmacology, University of Pittsburgh, PA, USA. Pharmacogenomics encompasses several major areas: the study of polymorphic variations in drug response and disease susceptibility, identification of the effects of drugs/xenobiotics at the genomic level, and genotype/phenotype associations. The most common type of human genetic variations is single-nucleotide polymorphisms (SNPs). Several novel approaches to detection of SNPs are currently available. The range of new methods includes modifications of several conventional techniques, such as PCR, mass spectrometry (ms), and sequencing, as well as more innovative technologies such as fluorescence resonance energy transfer (FRET) and microarrays. The application of each of these techniques is largely dependent on the number of SNPs to be screened and sample size. The current chapter presents an overview of the general concepts of a variety of genotyping technologies, with an emphasis on the recently developed methodologies, including a comparison of the advantages, applicability, cost efficiency, and limitations of these methods. Publication Types: Review

Methods Mol Biol. 2005;297:243-52. Related Articles, Links SNaPshot for pharmacogenetics by minisequencing. Bender K. Institut fur Rechtsmedizin, Mainz, Germany. Genetic polymorphisms of genes coding for metabolic enzymes are helpful to predict how an individual may respond to medication or drugs. The described approach for the identification of genetic variations for the cytochrome P450 enzymes CYP2D6 and CYP2C19 has been designed for the rapid genotyping of relevant alleles (CYP2D6*1, -*3, -*4, -*6, -*7, and -*8 and CYP2C19*1, -*2, -*3, -*4, and -*5) by performing polymerase chain reaction amplifications of genomic regions containing the SNP followed by a single-tube multiplex single base extension (minisquencing) reaction. This multiplex assay can easily be expanded for additional genes and single nucleotide polymorphisms (SNPs). Minisequencing is a sensitive, reproducible, and time-saving method for SNP typing that can be performed using ordinary laboratory equipment.

Methods Mol Biol. 2005;311:179-91. Related Articles, Links PharmGKB: the pharmacogenetics and pharmacogenomics knowledge base. Thorn CF, Klein TE, Altman RB. Department of Genetics, Stanford University School of Medicine, Stanford, CA, USA. The Pharmacogenetics and Pharmacogenomics Knowledge Base (PharmGKB) is an interactive tool for researchers investigating how genetic variation effects drug response. The PharmGKB web site, www.pharmgkb.org, displays genotype, molecular, and clinical primary data integrated with literature, pathway representations, protocol information, and links to additional external resources. Users can search and browse the knowledge base by genes, drugs, diseases, and pathways. Registration is free to the entire research community but subject to an agreement to respect the rights and privacy of the individuals whose information is contained within the database. Registered users can access and download primary data to aid in the design of future pharmacogenetics and pharmacogenomics studies. Publication Types: Review

Methods Mol Biol. 2005;311:193-208. Related Articles, Links Systems for the management of pharmacogenomic information. Sturn A, Maurer M, Molidor R, Trajanoski Z. Institute for Genomics and Bioinformatics, Graz University of Technology, Graz, Austria. Recent breakthroughs in biological research have been made possible by remarkable advances in high-performance computing and the establishment of a highly sophisticated information technology infrastructure. This chapter gives an overview of the main and most important technologies needed for the management of pharmacogenomic information, namely database management systems and software and hardware architectures. Because pharmacogenomics deals with a great many of public and/or proprietary data, the most prominent ways for easy storage, retrieval, analysis, and exchange are presented. Processing these data requires the use of sophisticated software architectures. Several most recent practices useful for a pharmacogenomic environment are explained. Multitiered application design and web services are discussed and described independent of the major enterprise development platforms. Because life sciences are becoming increasingly quantitative and because state-of-the-art software architectures use many system resources, this chapter presents the most recent and powerful systems for parallel data processing and data storage. Finally, shared and distributed memory systems and combinations of them as well as different storage architectures such as directly attached storage, network-attached storage, and storage-area network are explained in detail. Publication Types: Review

Methods Mol Biol. 2005;311:3-15. Related Articles, Links Pharmacogenomics: historical perspective and current status. Kalow W. Department of Pharmacology, University of Toronto, Toronto, Canada. Pharmacogenomics is an extension of pharmacogenetics, a science described here in terms of five stages of development: 1) some clinical observations predicted genetic alterations of drug response; 2) additional case discoveries led to the term "pharmacogenetics," a concept broadened by 3) many systemic case studies, and the realization of its wide applicability; 4) came the recognition of systematic pharmacogenetic differences between human populations. Then it became clear that 5) most human drug-response differences were multifactorial, caused by many genetic alterations plus environmental factors. The recognition of these complexities, and the advance of genetics into genomics led to the broader science of pharmacogenomics. This led to plans to create "personalized medicine," that is, making drug use more effective and safer by giving drugs that fit a person's genes. Much of the science of genetics, dealing with gene structure, was changed by the realization that gene expression and thereby gene function was variable; this leads to systematic studies of drug action on genes, reversing the traditional studies of genes affecting drug action. Finally, the realization that gene-protein variations contribute to most common diseases leads to efforts of creating new drugs that act on these variants. Publication Types: Historical Article Review

Methods Mol Biol. 2005;311:63-72. Related Articles, Links Aspects influencing genotyping method selection. Imle P. Hartwell Center for Bioinformatics and Biotechnology, St. Jude Children's Research Hospital, Memphis, TN, USA. The variety of genotyping methods currently available and the evolution of their capabilities have facilitated an expansion of the field of pharmacogenomics. Traditionally, limited genotyping capabilities have restricted the generation and application of genotyping data for pharmacogenomic studies. With the variety of platforms and chemistries available for flexible, high-throughput genotyping, it is important to keep in mind the limitations imposed by both the polymorphisms that are to be interrogated and the type of pharmacogenomics study for which the data are being generated. This chapter is an overview of the constraints these factors impose on different genotyping methods and describes aspects important to the integration of genotyping into a pharmacogenomics study. Publication Types: Review

Methods Mol Med. 2004;108:235-60. Related Articles, Links Pharmacogenetics and pharmacogenomics. Lindpaintner K. The advances made over the last 30 yr in molecular biology, molecular genetics, and genomics, and the development of associated methods and technologies, have had a major impact on our understanding of biology, including the action of drugs and other biologically active xenobiotics. The tools that have been developed and the knowledge of the fundamental principles underlying cellular function have become indispensable for almost any field of biological research, including biomedicine and health care. It is important to realize that, with regard to pharmacology and drug discovery, these accomplishments have in the last 30 yr led gradually to a rather fundamental shift from the "chemical paradigm" to a "biological paradigm." Where previously medicinal chemistry drove new developments in drug discovery, with biology almost an ancillary service that examined new molecules for biological function, biology, based on a new-found understanding of physiological effects of biomolecules and pathways, has now taken the lead. Biology is now requesting from the chemist compounds that modulate the function of these biomolecules or pathways, with (at least theoretically) a predictable functional impact in the setting of integrated physiology. One particular aspect of the progress in biology, namely, our understanding of genetics and especially the cataloging of genome sequences, has uniquely captured the imagination of both scientists and the public. The austere beauty of Mendel's laws, the compeling esthetics of the double-helix structure, and the awe-inspiring accomplishment coupled with an unprecedented public relations campaign of the Human Genome Project have combined to generate public excitement and almost certainly unrealistically high expectations regarding the impact that genetics/genomics will have on the practice of health care. The interface between genetics/genomics and pharmacology, pharmacogenetics, and pharmacogenomics (usually in the most loosely defined terms) is commonly touted as heralding a "revolution" in medicine, yet as soon as one begins to probe more carefully, little substance is yet to be found to support these enthusiastic claims.

Methods Mol Med. 2005;108:235-60. Related Articles, Links Pharmacogenetics and pharmacogenomics. Lindpaintner K. Roche Genetics, F. Hoffmann-La Roche, Ltd, Basel, Switzerland. Pharmacogenetics, in the different scenarios included in this term, will represent an important new avenue toward understanding disease pathology and drug action, and will offer new opportunities of stratifying patients to achieve optimal treatment success. As such, it represents a logical, consequent step in the history of medicine-evolution, rather than revolution. Its implementation will take time, and will not apply to all diseases and all treatments equally. If society finds ways to sanction the proper use of this information, thus allowing and protecting its unencumbered use for the patient's benefit, important progress in health care will be made.

Methods Mol Med. 2005;108:459-86. Related Articles, Links Biomedical informatics methods in pharmacogenomics. Yan Q. MedImmune Inc, Mountain View, CA, USA. Pharmacogenomics is the study of the genetic basis of individual variation in response to therapeutic agents. Pharmacogenomics may potentially affect on every step of health care and every drug treatment protocol. The optimal approach to pharmacogenomics in hypertension requires the integration of different disciplines, in which biomedical informatics plays an essential role. This chapter describes biomedical informatics methods used in dealing with key issues in pharmacogenomics. These key issues include the association between structure and function, the interaction between gene and drug, and the correlation between genotype and phenotype. Heterogeneous resources, including web sites, databases, and software analysis tools, are selected, organized, and integrated in practical methods to support these studies. Bioinformatics methods described in this chapter include genetic sequence searching, comparison, structural modeling, functional analysis, and systems biology studies, with emphasis on single-nucleotide polymorphism (SNP) analysis. Medical informatics methods such as disease and drug information and clinical terminology are also embraced in this chapter. This combination of both biological and medical informatics provides comprehensive methodologies to resolve complex problems in pharmacogenomics.

Methods Mol Med. 2005;111:197-231. Related Articles, Links Gene expression profiling to characterize anticancer drug sensitivity. Breaux JK, Los G. Rebecca and John Moores UCSD Cancer Center, University of California-San Diego, La Jolla, USA. This chapter presents a protocol for using cDNA microarrays to acquire gene expression profiles that characterize anticancer drug sensitivity. The protocol includes steps for drug exposure, RNA isolation, preparation of fluorescently labeled samples, microarray hybridization, data processing, and data analysis. In addition to the detailed protocol, important experimental design issues are discussed, and some preliminary experiments are recommended.

Methods. 2005 Nov;37(3):274-9. Related Articles, Links Convergent functional genomics: a Bayesian candidate gene identification approach for complex disorders. Bertsch B, Ogden CA, Sidhu K, Le-Niculescu H, Kuczenski R, Niculescu AB. Laboratory of Neurophenomics, Institute of Psychiatric Research, Indiana University School of Medicine, Indianapolis, IN 46202, USA. Identifying genes involved in complex neuropsychiatric disorders through classic human genetic approaches has proven difficult. To overcome that barrier, we have developed a translational approach called Convergent Functional Genomics (CFG), which cross-matches animal model microarray gene expression data with human genetic linkage data as well as human postmortem brain data and biological role data, as a Bayesian way of cross-validating findings and reducing uncertainty. Our approach produces a short list of high probability candidate genes out of the hundreds of genes changed in microarray datasets and the hundreds of genes present in a linkage peak chromosomal area. These genes can then be prioritized, pursued, and validated in an individual fashion using: (1) human candidate gene association studies and (2) cell culture and mouse transgenic models. Further bioinformatics analysis of groups of genes identified through CFG leads to insights into pathways and mechanisms that may be involved in the pathophysiology of the illness studied. This simple but powerful approach is likely generalizable to other complex, non-neuropsychiatric disorders, for which good animal models, as well as good human genetic linkage datasets and human target tissue gene expression datasets exist.

Mini Rev Med Chem. 2005 Jan;5(1):13-20. Related Articles, Links Medicinal chemistry, metabolic profiling and drug target discovery: a role for metabolic profiling in reverse pharmacology and chemical genetics. Harrigan GG, Brackett DJ, Boros LG. Global High Throughput

Screening, Pfizer Corporation, Chesterfield, MO 63198, USA. george.g.harrigan@pfizer.com Comprehensive analysis of the metabolome can contribute to mechanism of action studies for small molecules discovered in phenotypic screens. Examples are presented in this overview of the rapidly developing field of "metabolic profiling." These examples include the use of NMR in gene function analysis, GC-based studies on the identification of metabolic pathways affected by PPAR-gamma agonists, applications of Fourier-transform MS and the use of stable isotope-based metabolic profiling (SIDMAP) to investigate metabolic adaptive changes induced by effective anticancer agents. Publication Types: Review

MLO Med Lab Obs. 2005 Mar;37(3):20-7. Related Articles, Links Erratum in: MLO Med Lab Obs. 2005 May;37(5):28. Pharmacogenomics and its applications. White RM Sr, Wong SH. DSI Laboratories in Fort Myers, FL, USA.

MMW Fortschr Med. 2004 Nov 18;146(47):39-40. Related Articles, Links [Present day hypertension research is determined by cell biology and genetics. Modern therapies protect the organs] [Article in German] Haller H, Schrader J. Zentrum Innere Medzin, Medizinische Hochschule Hannover. Publication Types: Editorial

Mol Biol (Mosk). 2005 May-Jun;39(3):403-12. Related Articles, Links [Biochip development for polymorphism analysis in biotransformation system genes] [Article in Russian] Glotov S, Nasedkina TV, Ivashchenko TE, Iurasov RA, Surzhikov SA, Pan'kov SV, Chudinov AV, Baranov VS, Zasedatelev AS. Large-scale population researches, diagnostics of genetic predisposition to multifactorial diseases, screening of the polymorphic loci associated with individual sensitivity to pharmaceutical preparations, require the development of effective, exact and rapid methods of analysis for detection of many mutations simultaneously. One of the most perspective methods to solve these problems is a method of allele-specific hybridization with biochips. Taking the analysis of mutations in genes CYP1A1, CYP2D6, GSTM1, GSTT1, NAT2, CYP2C9, CYP2C19 and MTHFR as an example we showed the efficiency of using the approach for identification of individual genetic polymorphism. We believe that the biochips can be also a convenient tool in pharmacogenetics researches.

Mol Cancer Res. 2006 Mar;4(3):135-50. Related Articles, Links Pharmacogenetics and Regulation of Human Cytochrome P450 1B1: Implications in Hormone-Mediated Tumor Metabolism and a Novel Target for Therapeutic Intervention. Sissung TM, Price DK, Sparreboom A, Figg WD. Medical Oncology Clinical Research Unit, Clinical Pharmacology Research Core, National Cancer Institute, 9000 Rockville Pike, Building 10, Room 5A01, Bethesda, MD 20892. wdfigg@helix.nih.gov. Several of the hormone-mediated cancers (breast, endometrial, ovarian, and prostate) represent major cancers in both incidence and mortality rates. The etiology of these cancers is in large part modulated by the hormones estrogen and testosterone. As advanced disease develops, the common treatment for these cancers is chemotherapy. Thus, genes that can alter tissue response to hormones and alter clinical response to chemotherapy are of major interest. The cytochrome P450 1B1 (CYP1B1) may be involved in disease progression and modulate the treatment in the above hormone-mediated cancers. This review will focus on the pharmacogenetics of CYP1B1 in relation to hormone-mediated cancers and provide an assessment of cancer risk based on CYP1B1 polymorphisms and expression. In addition, it will provide a summary of CYP1B1 gene regulation and expression in normal and neoplastic tissue. (Mol Cancer Res 2006;4(3):1-16). n process]

Mol Cancer Ther. 2005 May;4(5):843-54. Related Articles, Links Irinotecan pharmacokinetic and pharmacogenomic alterations induced by methylselenocysteine in human head and neck xenograft tumors. Azrak RG, Yu J, Pendyala L, Smith PF, Cao S, Li X, Shannon WD, Durrani FA, McLeod HL, Rustum YM. Department of Cancer Biology, Roswell Park Cancer Institute, Elm and Carlton Streets, Buffalo, NY 14263, USA. The combination of methylselenocysteine and irinotecan (CPT-11) is synergistic against FaDu and A253 xenografts. Methylselenocysteine/CPT-11 increased tumor cure rate to 100% in FaDu and to 60% in A253. In this study, the effect of methylselenocysteine on pharmacokinetic and pharmacogenetic profiles of genes relevant to CPT-11 metabolic pathway was evaluated to identify possible mechanisms associated with the observed combinational synergy. Nude mice bearing tumors (FaDu and A253) were treated with methylselenocysteine, CPT-11, and a combination of methylselenocysteine/CPT-11. Samples were collected and analyzed for plasma and intratumor concentration of CPT-11 and 7-ethyl-10-hydroxyl-camptothecin (SN-38) by high-performance liquid chromatography. The intratumor relative expression of genes related to the CPT-11 metabolic pathway was measured by real-time PCR. After methylselenocysteine treatment, the intratumor area under the concentration-time curve of SN-38 increased to a significantly higher level in A253 than in FaDu and was associated with increased expression of CES1 in both tumors. Methylselenocysteine/CPT-11 treatment, compared with CPT-11 alone, resulted in a significant decrease in levels of ABCC1 and DRG1 in FaDu tumors and an increase in levels of CYP3A5 and TNFSF6 in A253 tumors. No statistically significant changes induced by methylselenocysteine/CPT-11 were observed in the levels of other investigated variables. In conclusion, the significant increase in the cure rate after methylselenocysteine/CPT-11 could be related to increased drug delivery into both tumors (CES1), reduced resistance to SN-38 (ABCC1 and DRG1) in FaDu, and induced Fas ligand apoptosis (TNFSF6) in A253. No correlation was observed between cure rate and other investigated variables (transporters, degradation enzymes, DNA repair, and cell survival/death genes) in either tumor.

Mol Diagn. 2005;9(3):119-27. Related Articles, Links Applications of AmpliChip CYP450. Jain KK. Jain PharmaBiotech, Basel, Switzerland. jain@pharmabiotech.ch Pharmacogenetics has assumed increasing importance with the developing concepts of personalized medicine. There is a need to determine the metabolic status of an individual when using drugs, the actions of which are influenced by drug-metabolizing enzymes. Cytochrome P450 (CYP) and its variants, particularly CYP2D6 and CYP2C19, play a role in the metabolism of approximately 25% of all prescription drugs.This review covers the role of the CYP system not only in the metabolism of drugs but also in the pathophysiology of disease. Various technologies for the assessment of CYP status are described, with the focus on AmpliChip CYP450 (Roche Molecular Diagnostics, Alameda, CA, USA), the first approved microarray molecular diagnostic test for the analysis of 29 polymorphisms and mutations of the CYP2D6 gene, and two polymorphisms of the CYP2C19 gene. It combines Roche's PCR technology with the GeneChip microarray system (Affymetrix, Santa Clara, CA, USA). Examples of numerous drugs that are metabolized by the CYP system are listed, and categories of antidepressants, antipsychotics, immunosuppressive and anticancer drugs are described to illustrate the role of testing for CYP polymorphisms in the therapeutic use of these drugs. CYP testing has applications in toxicology and absorption, distribution, metabolism and excretion (ADME) profiling as a guide to drug development.AmpliChip CYP450 may be used in conjunction with pharmacotherapy to guide decision making about selection of drugs and dosage. The test is not a solitary tool to determine optimum drug dosage, but is meant for use along with clinical evaluation and other methods for the selection of the treatment that is best suited for an individual patient. AmpliChip CYP450 is the first DNA microarray test to be cleared by the US FDA, and its clearance paves the way for similar microarray-based diagnostic tests to be developed in the future. This will facilitate the development of personalized medicine.

Mol Interv. 2004 Apr;4(2):109-23. Related Articles, Links Serotonin transporter: gene, genetic disorders, and pharmacogenetics. Murphy DL, Lerner A, Rudnick G, Lesch KP. Laboratory of Clinical Science, Building 10, Room 3D41, 10 Center Drive, MSC 1264, NIMH, NIH, Bethesda, MD 20892. The highly evolutionarily conserved serotonin transporter (SERT) regulates the entire serotoninergic system and its receptors via mod-ulation of extracellular fluid serotonin concentrations. Differences in SERT expression and function produced by three SERT genes and their variants show associations with multiple human disorders. Screens of DNA from patients with autism, ADHD, bipolar disorder, and Tourette's syndrome have detected signals in the chromosome 17q region where SERT is locat-ed. Parallel investigations of SERT knockout mice have uncovered multiple phenotypes that identify SERT as a candidate gene for additional human disorders ranging from irritable bowel syndrome to obesity. Replicated studies have demonstrated that the SERT 5'-flanking region polymorphism SS genotype is associated with poorer therapeutic responses and more frequent serious side effects during treatment with antidepressant SERT antagonists, namely, the serotonin reuptake inhibitors (SRIs).

Mol Pharmacol. 2005 Apr;67(4):1360-8. Epub 2005 Jan 20. Related Articles, Links EDGE: a centralized resource for the comparison, analysis, and distribution of toxicogenomic information. Hayes KR, Vollrath AL, Zastrow GM, McMillan BJ, Craven M, Jovanovich S, Rank DR, Penn S, Walisser JA, Reddy JK, Thomas RS, Bradfield CA. McArdle Laboratory for Cancer Research, 1400 University Avenue, Madison, WI 53706, USA. Transcriptional profiling via microarrays holds great promise for toxicant classification and hazard prediction. Unfortunately, the use of different microarray platforms, protocols, and informatics often hinders the meaningful comparison of transcriptional profiling data across laboratories. One solution to this problem is to provide a low-cost and centralized resource that enables researchers to share toxicogenomic data that has been generated on a common platform. In an effort to create such a resource, we developed a standardized set of microarray reagents and reproducible protocols to simplify the analysis of liver gene expression in the mouse model. This resource, referred to as EDGE, was then used to generate a training set of 117 publicly accessible transcriptional profiles that can be accessed at http://edge.oncology.wisc.edu/. The Web-accessible database was also linked to an informatics suite that allows on-line clustering and K-means analyses as well as Boolean and sequence-based searches of the data. We propose that EDGE can serve as a prototype resource for the sharing of toxicogenomics information and be used to develop algorithms for efficient chemical classification and hazard prediction.

Mol Pharmacol. 2005 Jul;68(1):110-8. Epub 2005 Mar 28. Related Articles, Links Cellular and pharmacogenetics foundation of synergistic interaction of pemetrexed and gemcitabine in human non-small-cell lung cancer cells. Giovannetti E, Mey V, Nannizzi S, Pasqualetti G, Marini L, Del Tacca M, Danesi R. Division of Pharmacology and Chemotherapy, Department of Oncology, Transplants and Advanced Technologies in Medicine, 55, Via Roma, 56126 Pisa, Italy. elisagio@tiscalinet.it Gemcitabine and pemetrexed are effective agents in the treatment of non-small-cell lung cancer (NSCLC), and the present study investigates cellular and genetic aspects of their interaction against A549, Calu-1, and Calu-6 cells. Cells were treated with pemetrexed and gemcitabine, and their interaction was assessed using the combination index. The role of drug metabolism in gemcitabine cytotoxicity was examined with inhibitors of deoxycytidine kinase (dCK), 5'-nucleotidase, and cytidine deaminase, whereas the role of pemetrexed targets, thymidylate synthase (TS), dihydrofolate reductase (DHFR), and glycinamide ribonucleotide formyltransferase (GARFT) in drug chemosensitivity was analyzed in cytotoxicity rescue studies. The effect of gemcitabine and pemetrexed on Akt phosphorylation was investigated with enzyme-linked immunosorbent assay, whereas quantitative polymerase chain reaction (PCR) was used to study target gene-expression profiles and its modulation by each drug. Synergistic cytotoxicity was demonstrated, and pemetrexed significantly decreased the amount of phosphorylated Akt, enhanced apoptosis, and increased the expression of dCK in A549 and Calu-6 cells, as well as the expression of the human nucleoside equilibrative transporter 1 (hENT1) in all cell lines. PCR demonstrated a correlation between dCK expression and gemcitabine sensitivity, whereas expression of TS, DHFR, and GARFT was predictive of pemetrexed chemosensitivity. These data demonstrated that 1) gemcitabine and pemetrexed synergistically interact against NSCLC cells through the suppression of Akt phosphorylation and induction of apoptosis; 2) the gene expression profile of critical genes may predict for drug chemosensitivity; and 3) pemetrexed enhances dCK and hENT1 expression, thus suggesting the role of gene-expression modulation for rational development of chemotherapy combinations.

Mol Psychiatry. 2004 Nov;9(11):1007-29. Related Articles, Links Candidate genes, pathways and mechanisms for bipolar (manic-depressive) and related disorders: an expanded convergent functional genomics approach. Ogden CA, Rich ME,

Schork NJ, Paulus MP, Geyer MA, Lohr JB, Kuczenski R, Niculescu AB. Laboratory of Neurophenomics, University of California, San Diego, CA, USA. Identifying genes for bipolar mood disorders through classic genetics has proven difficult. Here, we present a comprehensive convergent approach that translationally integrates brain gene expression data from a relevant pharmacogenomic mouse model (involving treatments with a stimulant--methamphetamine, and a mood stabilizer--valproate), with human data (linkage loci from human genetic studies, changes in postmortem brains from patients), as a bayesian strategy of crossvalidating findings. Topping the list of candidate genes, we have DARPP-32 (dopamine- and cAMP-regulated phosphoprotein of 32 kDa) located at 17q12, PENK (preproenkephalin) located at 8q12.1, and TAC1 (tachykinin 1, substance P) located at 7q21.3. These data suggest that more primitive molecular mechanisms involved in pleasure and pain may have been recruited by evolution to play a role in higher mental functions such as mood. The analysis also revealed other high-probability candidates genes (neurogenesis, neurotrophic, neurotransmitter, signal transduction, circadian, synaptic, and myelin related), pathways and mechanisms of likely importance in pathophysiology.

Mol Psychiatry. 2004 Sep;9(9):879-89. Related Articles, Links Investigation of serotonin-related genes in antidepressant response. Peters EJ, Slager SL, McGrath PJ, Knowles JA, Hamilton SP. Department of Psychiatry, University of California, San Francisco, CA 94143-0984, USA. In this study, we sought out to test the hypothesis that genetic factors may influence antidepressant response to fluoxetine. The investigation focused on seven candidate genes in the serotonergic pathway involved in the synthesis, transport, recognition, and degradation of serotonin. Our clinical sample consisted of 96 subjects with unipolar major depression treated with fluoxetine with response variables assessed after a 12-week trial. Patient data were also collected to investigate the pattern of drug response. Using a high-throughput single-nucleotide polymorphism (SNP) genotyping platform and capillary electrophoresis, we genotyped patients at 110 SNPs and four repeat polymorphisms located in seven candidate genes (HTR1A, HTR2A, HTR2C, MAOA, SLC6A4, TPH1, and TPH2). Statistical tests performed included single-locus and haplotype association tests, and linkage disequilibrium (LD) estimation. Little evidence of population stratification was observed in the sample with 20 random SNPs using a genomic control procedure. Our most intriguing result involved three SNPs in the TPH1 gene and one SNP in the SLC6A4 gene, which show significant single-locus association when response to fluoxetine is compared to nonresponse (P=0.02-0.04). All odds ratios indicated an increased risk of not responding to fluoxetine. In the specific response vs nonspecific and nonresponse comparison, three SNPs in the TPH2 gene (P=0.02-0.04) were positively associated and one SNP in the HTR2A gene (P=0.02) was negatively associated. When comparing specific response to nonspecific response, we found significant negative associations in three SNPs in the HTR2A gene (P=0.001-0.03) and two SNPs in the MAOA gene (P=0.03-0.05). We observed variable, although strong LD, in each gene and unexpectedly low numbers of estimated haplotypes, formed from tagged SNPs. Significant haplotype associations were found in all but the HTR1A and

HTR2C genes. Although these data should be interpreted cautiously due to the small sample size, these results implicate TPH1 and SLC6A4 in general response, and HTR2A, TPH2, and MAOA in the specificity of response to fluoxetine. Intriguingly, we observe that a number of the less frequent alleles of many of the SNP markers were associated with the nonresponse and nonspecific phenotypes.

Mol Psychiatry. 2005 Aug;10(8):713. Related Articles, Links Pharmacogenomics in psychiatry: genomic considerations. Licinio J, Wong ML. Publication Types: Editorial

Mol Psychiatry. 2005 Jul;10(7):615. Related Articles, Links Pharmacogenomics in psychiatry: clinical issues to be considered. Licinio J, Wong ML. Publication Types: Editorial

Monash Bioeth Rev. 2004 Apr;23(2):9-20. Related Articles, Links The ethics of pharmacogenomics. Neil D, Craigie J. Centre for Human Bioethics, School of Philosophy and Bioethics, Monash University, Australia. Of the future technologies arising from the Human Genome Project, pharmacogenomics will probably be the first to have a widespread impact on the everyday practice of medicine. This technology offers great benefits but also presents some difficult ethical challenges. This paper explains what pharmacogenomics is and examines three of the issues that it raises: orphan populations, the use of ethnicity in drug trials, and potential obstacles to informed consent for genetic testing.

Mov Disord. 2005 Jun;20(6):734-9. Related Articles, Links Genetic polymorphism of catechol-O-methyltransferase and levodopa pharmacokinetic-pharmacodynamic pattern in patients with Parkinson's disease. Contin M, Martinelli P, Mochi M, Riva R, Albani F, Baruzzi A. Neurology Clinic, Department of Neurological Sciences, University of Bologna, Via Foscolo 7, 40123 Bologna, Italy. manuela.contin@unibo.it We explored the potential effect of catechol-O-methyltransferase (COMT) genetic polymorphism on the pharmacokinetics and pharmacodynamics of a standard oral dose of levodopa in patients with Parkinson's disease (PD). We prospectively collected blood samples for COMT genotyping from a population of 104 PD patients. Each patient was examined by a standard oral levodopa/benserazide test, based on simultaneous serial measurements of plasma levodopa concentrations, finger-tapping motor effects and dyskinesia ratings, up to 4 hours after dosing. The main levodopa pharmacokinetic outcome variables were time to peak and peak plasma concentration, plasma elimination half-life, and the area under the plasma concentration-time curve. The main outcome levodopa pharmacodynamic variables were latency, duration, and magnitude of the motor effect elicited by the levodopa test dose, the area under the tapping effect-time curve, and the presence of dyskinesias. Nineteen patients (18%) harbored the low-activity homozygous COMT genotype (A/A), 63 patients (61%) carried the intermediate-activity heterozygous COMT genotype (A/G) and 22 patients (21%) had the high-activity homozygous COMT genotype (G/G). The three groups were comparable for vital and clinical characteristics. No significant difference was found in levodopa main pharmacokinetic-pharmacodynamic variables and dyskinesia incidence among the three subgroups of patients. We failed to identify clinically relevant levodopa pharmacokinetic-pharmacodynamic response patterns associated with the COMT polymorphism in PD patients. (c) 2005 Movement Disorder Society. Publication Types: Clinical Trial

Mutat Res. 2004 Apr 14;548(1-2):97-105. Related Articles, Links Microarray-based method for genotyping of functional single nucleotide polymorphisms using dual-color fluorescence hybridization. Ji M, Hou P, Li S, He N, Lu Z. Chien-Shiung Wu Laboratory, Department of Biological Science and Medical Engineering, Southeast University, Nanjing 210096, China. Screening disease-related single nucleotide polymorphism (SNP) markers in the whole genome has great potential in complex disease genetics and pharmacogenetics researches. It has led to a requirement for high-throughput genotyping platforms that can maximize the efficient screening functional SNPs with respect to accuracy, speed and cost. In this study, we attempted to develop a microarray-based method for scoring a number of genomic DNA in parallel for one or more molecular markers on a glass slide. Two SNP markers localized to the methylenetetrahydrofolate reductase gene (MTHFR) were selected as the investigated targets. Amplified PCR products from nine genomic DNA specimens were spotted and immobilized onto a poly-l-lysine coated glass slide to fabricate a microarray, then interrogated by hybridization with dual-color probes to determine the SNP genotype of each sample. The results indicated that the microarray-based method could determine the genotype of 677 and 1298 MTHFR polymorphisms. Sequencing was performed to validate these results. Our experiments successfully demonstrate that PCR products subjected to dual-color hybridization on a microarray could be applied as a useful and a high-throughput tool to analyze molecular markers.

Mutat Res. 2005 Aug 4;575(1-2):102-15. Epub 2005 Apr 25. Related Articles, Links Toxicogenomics in the pharmaceutical industry: hollow promises or real benefit? Luhe A, Suter L, Ruepp S, Singer T, Weiser T, Albertini S. F. Hoffmann-La Roche Ltd., Non-Clinical Drug Safety, 4070 Basel, Switzerland. anke.luehe@roche.com Almost 10 years ago, microarray technology was established as a new powerful tool for large-scale analysis of gene expression. Soon thereafter the new technology was discovered by toxicologists for the purpose of deciphering the molecular events underlying toxicity, and the term "Toxicogenomics" appeared in scientific literature. Ever since, the toxicology community was fascinated by the multiplicity of sophisticated possibilities toxicogenomics seems to offer: genome-wide analysis of toxicant-induced expression profiles may provide a means for prediction of toxicity prior to classical toxicological endpoints such as histopathology or clinical chemistry. Some researchers even speculated of the classical methods being superfluous before long. It was assumed that by using toxicogenomics it would be possible to classify compounds early in drug development and consequently save animals, time, and money in pre-clinical toxicity studies. Moreover, it seemed within reach to unravel the molecular mechanisms underlying toxicity. The feasibility of bridging data derived from in vitro and in vivo systems, identifying new biomarkers, and comparing toxicological responses "across-species" was also excessively praised. After several years of intensive application of microarray technology in the field of toxicology, not only by the pharmaceutical industry, it is now time to survey its achievements and to question how many of these wishes and promises have really come true. Publication Types: Review

Mutat Res. 2005 Aug 4;575(1-2):116-7. Related Articles, Links Toxicogenomics in genetic toxicology and hazard determination--concluding remarks. Sarrif A, van Delft JH, Gant TW, Kleinjans JC, van Vliet E. European Centre for Ecotoxicology and Toxicology of Chemicals, Avenue E. Van Nieuwenhuyse 4, Box 6, 1160 Brussels, Belgium. henk.vrijhof@ecetoc.org

Mutat Res. 2005 Aug 4;575(1-2):1-3. Epub 2005 Apr 25. Related Articles, Links Toxicogenomics in genetic toxicology and hazard determination: introduction and overview. Sarrif A, van Delft JH, van Schooten FJ, Gant TW, Elliott BM, van Ravenzwaay B, van Steeg H, Vrijhof H. Publication Types: Editorial

Mutat Res. 2005 Aug 4;575(1-2):4-16. Related Articles, Links In pursuit of effective toxicogenomics. Gant TW, Zhang SD. MRC Toxicology Unit, University of Leicester, P.O. Box 138, Lancaster Road, Leicester LE1 9HN, UK. twg1@le.ac.uk Biological systems exhibit complex responses to xenobiotics varying from generic stress responses to very specific changes closely associated with the mechanism of toxicity. Until recently our view of this complexity was obscured by the simplicity of available analysis tools which allowed determination of only a few genes in any one study. Then genome sequencing and high throughput library screening projects delivered data on the genome sequence of many organisms, and clones were collected and made available to researchers in a previously unparalleled quantity. To exploit this new resource the microarray was developed from its predecessor the dot blot. Further development has expanded the number of clones contained on any one microarray to a point where the expression of many tens of thousands of genes in a biological system can be determined in a short period of time. What these data are revealing is the full complexity of the gene expression response to stimuli such as xenobiotic exposure. Toxicogenomics seeks to use the complexity of this response as a fingerprint or signature characteristic of that xenobiotic exposure. There are though two major experimental challenges that need to be dealt with for toxicogenomics to be successful. The first is technical and relates to the intrinsic difficulties associated with the accurate measurement of gene expression. For microarrays, this problem is multiplied by the number of genes on the microarray itself. To overcome this technical variability correct experimental design is critical. The second challenge concerns the biological system used. What genetic background, time point and dose of xenobiotic should be chosen? For in vitro systems should cell lines or primary cells be used? These factors, and more, could affect the gene expression profile obtained in response to the same xenobiotic exposure. Using both our data and data from public databases these issues are explored in this paper. Publication Types: Review

Mutat Res. 2005 Jun 3;573(1-2):111-35. Related Articles, Links Assessment of two flexible and compatible SNP genotyping platforms: TaqMan SNP Genotyping Assays and the SNPlex Genotyping System. De la Vega FM, Lazaruk KD, Rhodes MD, Wenz MH. Applied Biosystems, 850 Lincoln Centre Dr., Foster City, CA 94404, USA. delavefm@appliedbiosystems.com In this review we describe the principles, protocols, and applications of two commercially available SNP genotyping platforms, the TaqMan SNP Genotyping Assays and the SNPlex Genotyping System. Combined, these two technologies meet the requirements of multiple SNP applications in genetics research and pharmacogenetics. We also describe a set of SNP selection tools and validated assay resources which we developed to accelerate the cycle of experimentation on these platforms. Criteria for selecting the more appropriate of these two genotyping technologies are presented: the genetic architecture of the trait of interest, the throughput required, and the number of SNPs and samples needed for a successful study. Overall, the TaqMan assay format is suitable for low- to mid-throughput applications in which a high assay conversion rate, simple assay workflow, and low cost of automation are desirable. The SNPlex Genotyping System, on the other hand, is well suited for SNP applications in which throughput and cost-efficiency are essential, e.g., applications requiring either the testing of large numbers of SNPs and samples, or the flexibility to select various SNP subsets.

Mutat Res. 2005 Jun 3;573(1-2):180-94. Related Articles, Links Pharmacogenetic testing: proofs of principle and pharmacoeconomic implications. Dervieux T, Meshkin B, Neri B. Prometheus Laboratories, 5739 Pacific Center Boulevard, San Diego, 92121 CA, USA. tdervieux@prometheuslabs.com Several proofs of principle have established that pharmacogenetic testing for mutations altering expression and functions of genes associated with drug disposition and response can decrease the "trial-and-error" dosing and reduce the risk of adverse drug reactions. These proofs of principle include thiopurine methyltransferase and thiopurine therapy, dihydropyrimidine dehydrogenase/thymidylate synthase and 5-fluorouracil therapy, folate enzyme MTHFR and methotrexate therapy, UGT1A1 and irinotecan therapy and CYP450 2C9 and S-warfarin therapy. These evidences advocate for the prospective identification of mutations associated with drug response, serious adverse reactions and treatment failure. More recent evidence with the HLA basis of hypersensitivity to the retroviral agent abacavir demonstrates the potential of pharmacogenetic testing and its pharmacoeconomic implications. With the convergence of rising drug costs and evidence supporting the clinical benefits of pharmacogenetic testing, it will be important to demonstrate the improved net health outcomes attributed to the additional costs for this testing. Publication Types: Review

N Engl J Med. 2004 Apr 8;350(15):1535-48. Related Articles, Links Comment in: N Engl J Med. 2004 Jul 1;351(1):102; author reply 102. Acute lymphoblastic leukemia. Pui CH, Relling MV, Downing JR. Department of Hematology/Oncology, St. Jude Children's Research Hospital, Memphis, TN 38105, USA. ching-hon.pui@stjude.org Publication Types: Review

N Engl J Med. 2004 Nov 11;351(20):2035-7. Epub 2004 Nov 8. Related Articles, Links Comment on: N Engl J Med. 2004 Nov 11;351(20):2049-57. Race-based therapeutics. Bloche MG. Georgetown University Law Center, Washington, DC, USA. Publication Types: Comment

N Engl J Med. 2005 Jun 2;352(22):2285-93. Related Articles, Links Effect of VKORC1 haplotypes on transcriptional regulation and warfarin dose. Rieder MJ, Reiner AP, Gage BF, Nickerson DA, Eby CS, McLeod HL, Blough DK, Thummel KE, Veenstra DL, Rettie AE. Department of Genome

Sciences, University of Washington, Seattle, USA. BACKGROUND: The management of warfarin therapy is complicated by a wide variation among patients in drug response. Variants in the gene encoding vitamin K epoxide reductase complex 1 (VKORC1) may affect the response to warfarin. METHODS: We conducted a retrospective study of European-American patients receiving long-term warfarin maintenance therapy. Multiple linear-regression analysis was used to determine the effect of VKORC1 haplotypes on the warfarin dose. We determined VKORC1 haplotype frequencies in African-American, European-American, and Asian-American populations and VKORC1 messenger RNA (mRNA) expression in human liver samples. RESULTS: We identified 10 common noncoding VKORC1 single-nucleotide polymorphisms and inferred five major haplotypes. We identified a low-dose haplotype group (A) and a high-dose haplotype group (B). The mean (+/-SE) maintenance dose of warfarin differed significantly among the three haplotype group combinations, at 2.7+/-0.2 mg per day for A/A, 4.9+/-0.2 mg per day for A/B, and 6.2+/-0.3 mg per day for B/B (P<0.001). VKORC1 haplotype groups A and B explained approximately 25 percent of the variance in dose. Asian Americans had a higher proportion of group A haplotypes and African Americans a higher proportion of group B haplotypes. VKORC1 mRNA levels varied according to the haplotype combination. CONCLUSIONS: VKORC1 haplotypes can be used to stratify patients into low-, intermediate-, and high-dose warfarin groups and may explain differences in dose requirements among patients of different ancestries. The molecular mechanism of this warfarin dose response appears to be regulated at the transcriptional level. Copyright 2005 Massachusetts Medical Society.

N Engl J Med. 2005 May 26;352(21):2211-21. Related Articles, Links Comment in: N Engl J Med. 2005 Sep 1;353(9):955-6; author reply 955-6. Drug metabolism and variability among patients in drug response. Wilkinson GR. Department of Pharmacology, Vanderbilt University, Nashville, TN 37232-6600, USA. grant.wilkinson@vanderbilt.edu Publication Types: Review

N Engl J Med. 2006 Jan 26;354(4):421-2. Related Articles, Links Comment in: N Engl J Med. 2006 Jan 26;354(4):408-11. Comment on: N Engl J Med. 2003 Mar 20;348(12):1166-70. N Engl J Med. 2003 Mar 20;348(12):1170-5. Self-reported race and genetic admixture. Sinha M, Larkin EK, Elston RC, Redline S. Publication Types: Comment Letter

N Z Bioeth J. 2002 Jun;3(2):29-30. Related Articles, Links In that case. A multi-national pharmaceutical company wishes to recruit some of your patients to a pharmaco-genetic study. Response. Holloway JW. Asthma Genetics Research Group, Human Genetics Division, University of Southampton, UK.

N Z Bioeth J. 2002 Jun;3(2):31-2. Related Articles, Links In that case. A multi-national pharmaceutical company wishes to recruit some of your patients to a pharmaco-genetic study. Response. Wee R. weer@paradise.net.nz

Nagoya J Med Sci. 2004 May;67(1-2):1-7. Related Articles, Links Pharmacogenetics of antipsychoatics. Ozaki N. Department of Psychiatry, Nagoya University Graduate School of Medicine, Aichi, Japan. ozaki-n@med.nagoya-u.ac.jp Although a number of antipsychotics have been introduced for the treatment of schizophrenia, inter-individual differences of in antipsychotic response and the number of refractory schizophrenic patients have become two of the most challenging problems in clinical psychiatry. Thus, the pharmacogenetics of antipsychotics have been aimed at providing genetic components of this inter-individual variability in antipsychotic response in order to establish an individually-based pharmacotherapy for schizophrenia and to elucidate the mechanism of antipsychotic response so as to solve the refractoriness of schizophrenia. Pharmacogenetics, which is defined as the science of pharmacological response and its modification by hereditary influence can be divided into two categories: the genetic background of pharmacokinetics, i.e. the absorption, distribution, tissue localization, biotransformation and excretion of drugs, and pharmacodynamics, i.e. the biochemical and physiological consequences of a drug and its mechanism of action. Pharmacokinetics of antipsychotics has been focused mainly on the association between genetic polymorphisms in CYP genes, including CYP2D6, and the metabolism of these drugs. Polymorphism in CYP2D6 enables a division of individuals within a given population into at least two groups, i.e. poor metabolizers (PMs), extensive metabolizers (EMs), and ultrarapid metabolizers (UMs) of certain drugs. PMs have higher plasma concentrations of and more adverse effects from antipsychotics. UMs could be one of the important factors that induce treatment-refractoriness to antipsychotics. Genetic polymorphisms in serotonin and dopamine receptors that have a high affinity for antipsychotics have so far been extensively investigated in the pharmacodynamics of this type of drug. Not just one gene but multiple genes play a role in complex phenotypes, including the clinical response to medication. Thus, a multiple candidate genes approach has recently been adopted in the pharmacogenetics of antipsychotics. The new field of pharmacogenomics using DNA microarray analysis, which focuses on the genetic determinants of drug response at the level of the entire human genome, is important for development and prescription of safer and more effective individually-tailored antipsychotics. Publication Types: Review Items 1001 - 1239 of 1239 Previous of 3 1001: Eur J Clin Microbiol Infect Dis. 2004 Aug;23(8):653-5. Epub 2004 Jul 23. Related Articles, Links Prevalence of mutations in dihydrofolate reductase and dihydropteroate synthetase genes of Plasmodium falciparum: analysis of imported cases of malaria in Italy. De Fatima M, Ligozzi M, Bonora MG, Bisoffi Z, Fontana R. Dipartimento di Patologia, Sezione di Microbiologia, Universita di Verona, Strada Le Grazie 8, 37100 Verona, Italy.

Nat Biotechnol. 2004 Jul;22(7):813. Related Articles, Links Bargains in the basement. Jacobs T. Complete Growth Investor, USA. tom@completegrowth.com

Nat Biotechnol. 2005 May;23(5):510. Related Articles, Links Cautious welcome for FDA pharmacogenomics guidance. Katsnelson A; United States Food And Drug Administration. Publication Types: News

Nat Biotechnol. 2005 Oct;23(10):1317-8. Related Articles, Links An individual approach. Lewis R.

Nat Biotechnol. 2005 Sep;23(9):1036. Related Articles, Links RandD deals boom in 2004. Lawrence S.

Nat Biotechnol. 2005 Sep;23(9):1089-91. Related Articles, Links Protozoan genomics for drug discovery. Chaudhary K, Roos DS. Publication Types: News

Nat Clin Pract Cardiovasc Med. 2005 Jan;2(1):2-3. Related Articles, Links Pharmacogenetics: the outlook for genetic testing in statin therapy. Chasman DI, Ridker PM. Brigham and Women's Hospital and Harvard Medical School, Boston, MA 02215, USA. dchasman@rics.bwh.harvard.edu

Nat Clin Pract Cardiovasc Med. 2005 Sep;2(9):475-83. Related Articles, Links Mechanisms of disease: beta-adrenergic receptors--alterations in signal transduction and pharmacogenomics in heart failure. Feldman DS, Carnes CA, Abraham WT, Bristow MR. Davis Heart and Lung Research Institute, Division of Cardiology/Medicine, Ohio State University, Columbus, OH 43210, USA. feldman-1@medctr.osu.edu Beta-adrenergic signaling is an important regulator of myocardial function. During the progression of heart failure (HF), a reproducible series of biochemical events occurs that affects beta-adrenergic receptor (beta-AR) signaling and cardiac function. Furthermore, there are pathophysiologic alterations in the expression and regulation of proteins that are regulated by beta-ARs during HF. Analyses of these complex signaling pathways have led to a better understanding of HF mechanisms and the use of beta-adrenergic antagonists, which have notably altered HF-related morbidity and mortality. Despite therapeutic advances that have affected beta-AR signaling, HF remains a leading cause of hospitalization and a principal cause of death in industrialized nations. In this review, we summarize current insights into beta-adrenergic signal-transduction pathways, the best-described beta-AR polymorphisms, and therapies that target the beta-AR pathway in HF. Publication Types: Review

Nat Genet. 2004 Jul;36(7):720-4. Epub 2004 Jun 20. Related Articles, Links Comment in: Nat Genet. 2004 Jul;36(7):661. A common polymorphism of the growth hormone receptor is associated with increased responsiveness to growth hormone. Dos Santos C, Essioux L, Teinturier C, Tauber M, Goffin V, Bougneres P. U561 INSERM, Saint Vincent de Paul Hospital, Paris V University, 82 Avenue Denfert-Rochereau, 75014 Paris, France. Growth hormone is used to increase height in short children who are not deficient in growth hormone, but its efficacy varies largely across individuals. The genetic factors responsible for this variation are entirely unknown. In two cohorts of short children treated with growth hormone, we found that an isoform of the growth hormone receptor gene that lacks exon 3 (d3-GHR) was associated with 1.7 to 2 times more growth acceleration induced by growth hormone than the full-length isoform ($P < 0.0001$). In transfection experiments, the transduction of growth hormone signaling through d3-GHR homo- or heterodimers was approximately 30% higher than through full-length GHR homodimers ($P < 0.0001$). One-half of Europeans are hetero- or homozygous with respect to the allele encoding the d3-GHR isoform, which is dominant over the full-length isoform. These observations suggest that the polymorphism in exon 3 of GHR is important in growth hormone pharmacogenetics.

Nat Genet. 2004 Nov;36(11 Suppl):S34-42. Related Articles, Links Will tomorrow's medicines work for everyone? Tate SK,

Goldstein DB. Department of Biology, University College London, Darwin Building, Gower Street, London, WC1E 6BT, UK. Throughout much of the world, 'race' and 'ethnicity' are key determinants of health. For example, African Americans have, by some estimates, a twofold higher incidence of fatal heart attacks and a 10% higher incidence of cancer than European Americans, and South Asian- or Caribbean-born British are approximately 3.5 times as likely to die as a direct result of diabetes than are British of European ancestry. The health care that people receive also depends on 'race' and 'ethnicity'. African Americans are less likely to receive cancer-screening services and more likely to have late-stage cancer when diagnosed than European Americans. Health disparities such as these are one of the greatest social injustices in the developed world and one of the most important scientific and political challenges. Publication Types: Review

Nat Genet. 2005 Aug;37(8):794-5. Related Articles, Links Comment on: Nat Genet. 2005 Aug;37(8):878-82. Pharmacogenetics goes 3D. McLeod HL, Marsh S. Publication Types: Comment News

Nat Genet. 2005 Jan;37(1):84-9. Epub 2004 Dec 19. Related Articles, Links Comment in: Nat Genet. 2005 Sep;37(9):915-6; author reply 916. A single-nucleotide polymorphism tagging set for human drug metabolism and transport. Ahmadi KR, Weale ME, Xue ZY, Soranzo N, Yarnall DP, Briley JD, Maruyama Y, Kobayashi M, Wood NW, Spurr NK, Burns DK, Roses AD, Saunders AM, Goldstein DB. Department of Biology (Galton Lab), University College London, The Darwin Building, Gower Street, London WC1E 6BT, UK. Interindividual variability in drug response, ranging from no therapeutic benefit to life-threatening adverse reactions, is influenced by variation in genes that control the absorption, distribution, metabolism and excretion of drugs. We genotyped 904 single-nucleotide polymorphisms (SNPs) from 55 such genes in two population samples (European and Japanese) and identified a set of tagging SNPs that represents the common variation in these genes, both known and unknown. Extensive empirical evaluations, including a direct assessment of association with candidate functional SNPs in a new, larger population sample, validated the performance of these tagging SNPs and confirmed their utility for linkage-disequilibrium mapping in pharmacogenetics. The analyses also suggest that rare variation is not amenable to tagging strategies.

Nat Genet. 2005 Jul;37(7):671-81. Related Articles, Links Priorities and standards in pharmacogenetic research. Need AC, Motulsky AG, Goldstein DB. Institute for Genome Sciences and Policy, Center for Population Genomics and Pharmacogenetics, Duke University, 103 Research Drive, DUMC Box 3471, Durham, North Carolina 27710, USA. The current enthusiasm for pharmacogenetics draws much of its inspiration from the relatively few examples of polymorphisms that have marked and seemingly clinically relevant effects on drug response. In this regard, pharmacogenetic research has paralleled the study of human disease, which has enjoyed success in identifying mutations underlying mendelian conditions. Progress in deciphering the genetics of complex diseases, involving the interaction of multiple genes with each other and with the environment has been considerably less successful. In most instances, drug responses will probably also prove to be complex, influenced by both the environment and multiple genetic factors. For pharmacogenetics to deliver on its potential, this complexity will need to be recognized and accommodated, both in basic research and in clinical application of pharmacogenetics. As the attention of researchers begins to shift toward more systematic pharmacogenetic investigations, we suggest some priorities and standards for pharmacogenetic research. Publication Types: Review

Nat Med. 2004 Dec;10(12):1289-91. Related Articles, Links Creating incentives for genomic research to improve targeting of therapies. Evans BJ, Flockhart DA, Meslin EM. Pharmacogenomics, Ethics, and Public Policy Program, Indiana University Center for Bioethics, Indianapolis, USA.

Nat Med. 2005 May;11(5):462. Related Articles, Links Personalized medicine prompts push to redesign clinical trials. Singer E. Publication Types: News

Nat Rev Cancer. 2006 Feb;6(2):117-29. Related Articles, Links Erratum in: Nat Rev Cancer. 2006 Mar;6(3):249. Acute lymphoblastic leukaemia: a model for the pharmacogenomics of cancer therapy. Cheok MH, Evans WE. St. Jude Children's Research Hospital, Department of Pharmaceutical Sciences, 332 North Lauderdale Street, Memphis, Tennessee 38105, USA. The use of combination chemotherapy to cure acute lymphoblastic leukaemia (ALL) in children emerged in the 1980s as a paradigm for curing any disseminated cancer, and many of the therapeutic principles were subsequently applied to the treatment of other disseminated human cancers. Similarly, elucidation of the pharmacogenomics of ALL and its translation into new chemotherapeutic approaches might serve as a model for optimizing the treatment of other human cancers. Germline polymorphisms and gene-expression patterns in ALL cells have been linked to the toxicity and efficacy of chemotherapy for ALL and are beginning to emerge as useful clinical diagnostics. Publication Types: Review

Nat Rev Cancer. 2006 Feb;6(2):130-40. Related Articles, Links Non-steroidal anti-inflammatory drugs for cancer prevention: promise, perils and pharmacogenetics. Ulrich CM, Bigler J, Potter JD. Fred Hutchinson Cancer Research Center, 1100 Fairview Avenue North, Seattle, Washington 98109, USA. nulrich@fhcrc.org Aspirin and other non-steroidal anti-inflammatory drugs (NSAIDs) show indisputable promise as chemopreventive agents. Possible targets include cancers of the colon, stomach, breast and lung. However, recent studies raise concern about potential cardiovascular toxicity associated with the use of NSAIDs that specifically target the enzyme cyclooxygenase 2. These findings, and others that show that inherited genetic characteristics might determine preventive success, argue for new strategies that are tailored to individual medical history and genetic make-up. Publication Types: Review

Nat Rev Drug Discov. 2004 Feb;3(2):136-51. Related Articles, Links From monoamines to genomic targets: a paradigm shift for drug discovery in depression. Wong ML, Licinio J. Center for Pharmacogenomics, Neuropsychiatric Institute and David Geffen School of Medicine at UCLA, 695 Charles Young Drive South, Los Angeles, California 90095-1761, USA. mali@ucla.edu Depression, a complex psychiatric disorder that affects approximately 15% of the population, has an enormous social cost. Although the disorder is thought to be the outcome of gene-environmental interactions, the causative genes and environmental factors underlying depression remain to be identified. All the antidepressant drugs now in use--the forerunner of which was discovered serendipitously 50 years ago--modulate monoamine neurotransmission, and take six to eight weeks to exert their effects, but each drug is efficacious in only 60-70% of patients. A conceptually novel antidepressant that acted rapidly and safely in a high proportion of patients would almost certainly become the world's bestselling drug. Yet such a drug is not on the horizon. Here, we cover the different phases of antidepressant drug discovery in the past, present and future, and comment on the challenges and opportunities for antidepressant research. Publication Types: Review

Nat Rev Drug Discov. 2004 Feb;3(2):160-70. Related Articles, Links Cytokine-receptor pairing: accelerating discovery of cytokine function. Foster D, Parrish-Novak J, Fox B, Xu W. Cytokine Biology Program, ZymoGenetics, Inc. 1201 Eastlake Avenue, East Seattle, Washington 98102, USA. fosterd@zgi.com Over the past decade, advances in both gene discovery and ligand-receptor pairing techniques have led to the recognition that systematic pairing of 'orphan' database-derived cytokines and/or cytokine receptors with their cognate partners can lead to a marked acceleration in the elucidation of biological function. The sometimes-restricted tissue distribution of the receptor, coupled with the highly specific bioactivity of the corresponding ligand, can direct investigators rapidly towards regulatory function and site-of-action studies. The power of cytokine-receptor pairing to accelerate the understanding of function will be illustrated, citing several examples of candidate drug discoveries. Several of these discoveries, resulting from cytokine-receptor pairings, are at present advancing towards human clinical evaluation. Publication Types: Review

Nat Rev Drug Discov. 2004 May;3(5):382. Related Articles, Links Allen D. Rose. Rose AD. Publication Types: Interview

Nat Rev Drug Discov. 2004 Oct;3(10):822. Related Articles, Links Jonathan K. C. Knowles discusses the impact of pharmacogenomics on market segmentation. Knowles JK. Publication Types: News

Nat Rev Drug Discov. 2004 Sep;3(9):723. Related Articles, Links Plotting the trajectories of tomorrow's magic bullets. [No authors listed] Publication Types: Editorial

Nat Rev Drug Discov. 2004 Sep;3(9):725. Related Articles, Links Lack of data privacy could hamper pharmacogenomics studies. Howard K. Publication Types: News

Nat Rev Drug Discov. 2004 Sep;3(9):739-48. Related Articles, Links Pharmacogenomics: bench to bedside. Weinshilboum R, Wang L. Mayo Medical School-Mayo Graduate School, Mayo Clinic College of Medicine, Department of Molecular Pharmacology and Experimental Therapeutics, Rochester, Minnesota 55905, USA. weinshilboum.richard@mayo.edu Pharmacogenetics is the study of the role of inheritance in inter-individual variation in drug response. Since its origins in the mid-twentieth century, a major driving force in pharmacogenetics research has been the promise of individualized drug therapy to maximize drug efficacy and minimize drug toxicity. In recent years, the convergence of advances in pharmacogenetics with rapid developments in human genomics has resulted in the evolution of pharmacogenetics into pharmacogenomics, and led to increasing enthusiasm for the 'translation' of this evolving discipline into clinical practice. Here, we briefly summarize the development of pharmacogenetics and pharmacogenomics, and then discuss the key factors that have had an influence on - and will continue to affect - the translation of pharmacogenomics from the research bench to the bedside, highlighting the challenges that need to be addressed to achieve this goal. Publication Types: Review

Nat Rev Drug Discov. 2004 Sep;3(9):749-61. Related Articles, Links Technology platforms for pharmacogenomic diagnostic assays. Koch WH. Roche Molecular Systems, Pharmacogenetics Department, 4300 Hacienda Drive, Pleasanton, California 94588, USA. walter_h.koch@roche.com Rapid advances in the understanding of genomic variation affecting drug responses, and the development of multiplex assay technologies, are converging to form the basis for new in vitro diagnostic assays. These molecular diagnostic assays are expected to guide the therapeutic treatment of many diseases, by informing physicians about molecular subtypes of disease that require differential treatment, which drug has the greatest probability of effectively managing the disease, and which individual patients are at the highest risk of experiencing adverse reactions to a given drug therapy. This article reviews some of the relative strengths and limitations of the most widely used technologies and platforms for such assays. Publication Types: Review

Nat Rev Drug Discov. 2004 Sep;3(9):763-9. Related Articles, Links Translation of pharmacogenomics and pharmacogenetics: a regulatory perspective. Lesko LJ, Woodcock J. Office of Clinical Pharmacology and Biopharmaceutics, Center for Drug Evaluation and Research, Food and Drug Administration, Rockville, Maryland 20857, USA. leskol@cder.fda.gov Pharmacogenomics and pharmacogenetics provide methodologies that can lead to DNA-based tests to improve drug selection, identify optimal dosing, maximize drug efficacy or minimize the risk of toxicity. Rapid advances in basic research have identified many opportunities for the development of 'personalized' treatments for individuals and/or subsets of patients defined by genetic and/or genomic tests. However, the integration of these tests into routine clinical practice remains a major multidisciplinary challenge, and even for well-established biomarkers there has been little progress. Here, we consider this challenge from a regulatory perspective, highlighting recent initiatives from the FDA that aim to facilitate the integration of pharmacogenetics and pharmacogenomics into drug development and clinical practice. Publication Types: Review

Nat Rev Drug Discov. 2004 Sep;3(9):811. Related Articles, Links Desperately seeking biostatisticians. Gimalac A. Serono Genetics Institute, Route Nationale 7, 91030 Evry Cedex, France. anne.gimalac@serono.com

Nat Rev Drug Discov. 2005 Apr;4(4):345-50. Related Articles, Links How molecular profiling could revolutionize drug discovery. Stoughton RB, Friend SH. GHC Technologies, Inc., 505 Coast Boulevard South, Suite 309, La Jolla, California 92037, USA.

roland_stoughton@ghctechnologies.com Information from genomic, proteomic and metabolomic measurements has already benefited target discovery and validation, assessment of efficacy and toxicity of compounds, identification of disease subgroups and the prediction of responses of individual patients. Greater benefits can be expected from the application of these technologies on a significantly larger scale; by simultaneously collecting diverse measurements from the same subjects or cell cultures; by exploiting the steadily improving quantitative accuracy of the technologies; and by interpreting the emerging data in the context of underlying biological models of increasing sophistication. The benefits of applying molecular profiling to drug discovery and development will include much lower failure rates at all stages of the drug development pipeline, faster progression from discovery through to clinical trials and more successful therapies for patient subgroups. Upheavals in existing organizational structures in the current 'conveyor belt' models of drug discovery might be required to take full advantage of these methods. Publication Types: Review

Nat Rev Drug Discov. 2005 Aug;4(8):639-47. Related Articles, Links Pharmacogenetics-based therapeutic recommendations--ready for clinical practice? Kirchheiner J, Fuhr U, Brockmoller J. Department of Pharmacology, University of Cologne, Gleueler Strasse 24, 50931, Koln, Germany. julia.kirchheiner@uk-koeln.de Although considerable progress has been made in basic pharmacogenetic research, less has been demonstrated in the application of pharmacogenetics (PGx)-based diagnostics to drug development and in clinical practice. There are drugs that are currently used in the clinic for which individualized therapy could be beneficial based on PGx data. However, specific, actionable recommendations on how to implement individualized therapy--particularly with respect to dosage--still have to be developed. Moreover, to apply PGx efficiently in clinical drug development, and later in drug therapy, study designs and the generation and handling of PGx data need to become more standardized. Here, we argue for the development of concise guidelines for implementation of PGx analyses in drug development and therapy. Publication Types: Editorial

Nat Rev Drug Discov. 2005 Dec;4(12):947. Related Articles, Links First phase of HapMap project already helping drug discovery. Andrawiss M. Publication Types: News

Nat Rev Drug Discov. 2005 Jun;4(6):500-9. Related Articles, Links Measuring the value of pharmacogenomics. Phillips KA, Van Bebber SL. School of Pharmacy and Institute for Health Policy Studies, University of California, San Francisco, 3333 California Street, Box 0613, San Francisco, California 94143, USA. Pharmacogenetics and pharmacogenomics offer the potential of developing DNA-based tests to help maximize drug efficacy and enhance drug safety. Major scientific advances in this field have brought us to the point where such tests are poised to enter more widespread clinical use. However, many questions have been raised about whether such tests will be of significant value, and how to assess this. Here, we review the application of economics-based resource-allocation frameworks to assess the value of pharmacogenomics, and the findings so far. We then develop a resource-allocation framework for assessing the potential value of pharmacogenomic testing from a population perspective, and apply this framework to the example of testing for variant alleles of CYP2D6, an important drug-metabolizing enzyme. This review provides a framework for analysing the value of pharmacogenomic interventions, and suggests where further research and development could be most beneficial. Publication Types: Review

Nat Rev Drug Discov. 2005 May;4(5):359. Related Articles, Links FDA pharmacogenomics guidance sends clear message to industry. Ratner M. Publication Types: News

Nat Rev Drug Discov. 2005 Nov;4(11):872-3. Related Articles, Links Royal Society puts personalized medicine in perspective. Branca MA. Publication Types: News

Nat Rev Drug Discov. 2005 Nov;4(11):911-8. Related Articles, Links Combinatorial pharmacogenetics. Wilke RA, Reif DM, Moore JH. Center for Human Genetics, Marshfield Clinic Research Foundation, Marshfield, Wisconsin, USA. Combinatorial pharmacogenetics seeks to characterize genetic variations that affect reactions to potentially toxic agents within the complex metabolic networks of the human body. Polymorphic drug-metabolizing enzymes are likely to represent some of the most common inheritable risk factors associated with common 'disease' phenotypes, such as adverse drug reactions. The relatively high concordance between polymorphisms in drug-metabolizing enzymes and clinical phenotypes indicates that research into this class of polymorphisms could benefit patients in the near future. Characterization of other genes affecting drug disposition (absorption, distribution, metabolism and elimination) will further enhance this process. As with most questions concerning biological systems, the complexity arises out of the combinatorial magnitude of all the possible interactions and pathways. The high-dimensionality of the resulting analysis problem will often overwhelm traditional analysis methods. Novel analysis techniques, such as multifactor dimensionality reduction, offer viable options for evaluating such data. Publication Types: Review

Nat Rev Drug Discov. 2006 Jan;5(1):23-6. Related Articles, Links A call for the creation of personalized medicine databases. Gurwitz D, Lunshof JE, Altman RB. Department of Human Genetics and Molecular Medicine, Sackler Faculty of Medicine, Tel-Aviv University, Israel. gurwitz@post.tau.ac.il The success of the Human Genome Project raised expectations that the knowledge gained would lead to improved insight into human health and disease, identification of new drug targets and, eventually, a breakthrough in healthcare management. However, the realization of these expectations has been hampered by the lack of essential data on genotype--drug-response phenotype associations. We therefore propose a follow-up to the Human Genome Project: forming global consortia devoted to archiving and analysing group and individual patient data on associations between genotypes and drug-response phenotypes. Here, we discuss the rationale for such personalized medicine databases, and the key practical and ethical issues that need to be addressed in their establishment.

Nat Rev Genet. 2004 Apr;5(4):262-75. Related Articles, Links Chemogenomics: an emerging strategy for rapid target and drug discovery. Bredel M, Jacoby E. Division of Oncology, Stanford University School of Medicine, 269 Campus Drive, CCSR-1110, Stanford, California 94305-5151,

USA. mbredel@stanford.edu Publication Types: Review

Nat Rev Genet. 2004 Dec;5(12):936-48. Related Articles, Links Toxicogenomics and systems toxicology: aims and prospects. Waters MD, Fostel JM. National Center for Toxicogenomics, National Institute of Environmental Health Sciences, PO Box 12233, MD F1-05, 111 Alexander Drive, Research Triangle Park, North Carolina 27709-2233, USA. waters2@niehs.nih.gov Toxicogenomics combines transcript, protein and metabolite profiling with conventional toxicology to investigate the interaction between genes and environmental stress in disease causation. The patterns of altered molecular expression that are caused by specific exposures or disease outcomes have revealed how several toxicants act and cause disease. Despite these success stories, the field faces noteworthy challenges in discriminating the molecular basis of toxicity. We argue that toxicology is gradually evolving into a systems toxicology that will eventually allow us to describe all the toxicological interactions that occur within a living system under stress and use our knowledge of toxicogenomic responses in one species to predict the modes-of-action of similar agents in other species. Publication Types: Review

Nat Rev Genet. 2004 Sep;5(9):645-56. Related Articles, Links Pharmacogenetics and drug development: the path to safer and more effective drugs. Roses AD. Genetics Research, GlaxoSmithKline, Five Moore Drive, Research Triangle Park, North Carolina 27709, USA. allen.d.roses@gsk.com Pharmacogenetics provides opportunities for informed decision-making along the pharmaceutical pipeline. There is a growing literature of retrospective studies of marketed medicines that describe efficacy or safety on the basis of patient genotypes. These studies emphasize the potential prospective use of genome information to enhance success in finding new medicines. An example of a prospective efficacy pharmacogenetic Phase-IIA proof-of-concept study is described. Inserting a rapidly performed efficacy pharmacogenetic step after initial clinical data are obtained can provide confidence for a commitment to full drug development. The rapid identification of adverse events during and after drug development using genomic mapping tools is also reviewed. Publication Types: Review

Nat Rev Genet. 2004 Sep;5(9):657-63. Related Articles, Links Genetically modified mouse models for pharmacogenomic research. Liggett SB. University of Cincinnati College of Medicine, 231 Albert Sabin Way, Room G062, Cincinnati, Ohio 45267-0564, USA. stephen.liggett@uc.edu It is now evident that differences in the DNA sequence of genes involved with drug action can lead to interindividual differences in effectiveness and adverse reactions to therapeutic drugs. Pharmacogenomics raises the possibility that drug discovery and patient management could move from a 'one drug fits all' approach to one in which therapy is tailored to patients' genomes. Genetically modified mice that mimic human variation in drug response can provide one of the tools to move the field towards these goals. Publication Types: Review

Nat Rev Genet. 2004 Sep;5(9):663-9. Related Articles, Links Integrating pharmacogenetics into society: in search of a model. Webster A, Martin P, Lewis G,

Smart A. Science and Technology Studies Unit, University of York, York YO10 5DD, United Kingdom. There has been considerable scientific, corporate and policy interest in the more effective use of genetics in both drug development and delivery. Pharmacogenetics - the study of the relationship between an individual's genetic makeup and response to medicinal drugs - has attracted global interest, but will it live up to its promise? Looking beyond the hype that has accompanied much of the commentary in the area, the future of pharmacogenetics will depend on how competing interests and options are resolved. Publication Types: Review

Nat Rev Genet. 2004 Sep;5(9):669-76. Related Articles, Links Pharmacogenetics - five decades of therapeutic lessons from genetic diversity. Meyer UA. Biozentrum, University of Basel, CH-4056 Basel, Switzerland. Urs-A.Meyer@unibas.ch Physicians have long been aware of the subtle differences in the responses of patients to medication. The recognition that a part of this variation is inherited, and therefore predictable, created the field of pharmacogenetics fifty years ago. Knowing the gene variants that cause differences among patients has the potential to allow 'personalized' drug therapy and to avoid therapeutic failure and serious side effects. Publication Types: Historical Article Review

Nat Rev Genet. 2004 Sep;5(9):676-80. Related Articles, Links Pharmacogenetics: ethical problems and solutions. Breckenridge A, Lindpaintner K, Lipton P, McLeod H, Rothstein M, Wallace H. UK Medicines and Healthcare products Regulatory Agency. Regulators, drug companies, academic scientists, bioethicists, clinicians and, increasingly, the general public are starting to realize that pharmacogenetics (PGx) will probably have a huge impact on the way in which we treat both common and rare diseases. But how much thought has gone into the ethical issues that the incorporation of phamacogenetic testing into drug discovery, prescription and use will entail? It seems that "quite a bit" is the answer, as the diverse viewpoints of representatives of all of these groups presented here illustrate. However, these views also highlight that now is the time to start formulating and implementing solutions to these potential problems. Publication Types: Review

Nat Rev Genet. 2005 Mar;6(3):241-6. Related Articles, Links Pharmacogenetics and geographical ancestry: implications for drug development and global health. Daar AS, Singer PA. Canadian Program on Genomics and Global Health, University of Toronto Joint Centre for Bioethics, 88 College Street, Toronto, Ontario M5G 1L4, Canada. a.daar@utoronto.ca Understanding and harnessing genomic variation will contribute significantly to improving the health of people in developing countries. We need to explore the nexus between pharmacogenetics, genotyping projects in developing countries, and the evolution of the pharmaceutical industry in both the developed and developing worlds. Here, we argue that, for the foreseeable future, we should focus not on boutique 'personalized' medicine, but on carefully defined differences between populations and ethical ways of using emerging genomics knowledge to develop drugs and improve health.

Nature. 2004 Jul 1;430(6995):30. Related Articles, Links Cancer: understanding the target. Stratton MR, Futreal PA. Publication Types: News

Nature. 2004 Jul 8;430(6996):276. Related Articles, Links Recruiters and industry. Building biostatistics. Gimalac A. Serono Genetics Institute, Evry, France.

Nature. 2004 Jun 17;429(6993):696-8. Related Articles, Links Comment in: Nature. 2004 Aug 5;430(7000):611. Mental health: Asia's tigers get the blues. Dennis C. Publication Types: News

Nature. 2004 Mar 25;428(6981):379-82. Related Articles, Links Medicine: profile of a tumour. Kallioniemi O. Publication Types: Letter

Nature. 2004 May 27;429(6990):453-6. Related Articles, Links Predicting disease using genomics. Bell J. University of Oxford, Academic Centre, John Radcliffe Hospital, Headington, Oxford OX3 9DU, UK. regius@medsci.ox.ac.uk Information from the human genome sequence will eventually alter many aspects of clinical practice. It will increase through our understanding of disease mechanisms, and guide the development of new drugs and therapeutic procedures. In the short term, however, knowledge of the genome will have a profound clinical impact on the diagnostic capability of clinical genetics laboratories. Molecular phenotyping using genetic and genomic information will allow early and more accurate prediction and diagnosis of disease and of disease progression. Medicine will become oriented towards disease prevention rather than efforts to cure people at late stages of illness. Publication Types: Review

Nature. 2004 May 27;429(6990):464-8. Related Articles, Links Moving towards individualized medicine with pharmacogenomics. Evans WE, Relling MV. Department of Pharmaceutical Sciences, St Jude Children's Research Hospital, Memphis, Tennessee 38105, USA. william.evans@stjude.org Individuals respond differently to drugs and sometimes the effects are unpredictable. Differences in DNA that alter the expression or function of proteins that are targeted by drugs can contribute significantly to variation in the responses of individuals. Many of the genes examined in early studies were linked to highly penetrant, single-gene traits, but future advances hinge on the more difficult challenge of elucidating multi-gene determinants of drug response. This intersection of genomics and medicine has the potential to yield a new set of molecular diagnostic tools that can be used to individualize and optimize drug therapy. Publication Types: Review

Nature. 2004 Nov 25;432(7016):426. Related Articles, Links Summit calls for clear view of deposits in all biobanks. Pearson H. Publication Types: News

Nature. 2005 Aug 4;436(7051):746-7. Related Articles, Links An individual approach. Lewis R.

Nature. 2005 Jul 28;436(7050):492-3. Related Articles, Links Strength in numbers. Padma TV.

Nature. 2005 Jun 23;435(7045):1008-9. Related Articles, Links Drug targeting: is race enough? Wadman M. Publication Types: News

Nature. 2005 Oct 6;437(7060):796. Related Articles, Links Erratum in: Nature. 2005 Oct 20;437(7062):1079. Japan jumps towards personalized medicine. Cyranoski D. Publication Types: News

Nature. 2006 Jan 19;439(7074):274-5. Related Articles, Links Comment on: Nature. 2006 Jan 19;439(7074):353-7. Nature. 2006 Jan 19;439(7074):358-62. Cancer biology:

signatures guide drug choice. Downward J. Publication Types: Comment News

Nefrologia. 2005;25(4):381-6. Related Articles, Links [Pharmacogenetics of angiotensin system in non diabetic nephropathy] [Article in Spanish] Coto E, Marin R, Alvarez V, Praga M, Fernandez Andrade C, Arias M, Poveda R, Valles M, Galceran JM, Luno J, Rivera F, Campistol JM. Genetica Molecular, Hospital Central de Asturias e Instituto Reina Sofia de Investigacion Nefrologica, eliecer.coto@sespa.princast.es BACKGROUND: Genetic variability could contribute to the response to pharmacological treatment in patients with nephropathy. In albuminuric diabetic patients the renoprotective effect of angiotensin I-converting enzyme (ACE) inhibition should be lower among homozygotes for the deletion allele (DD) compared to II-homozygotes. METHODS: A total of 71 non-diabetic chronic nephropathy patients were treated with losartan (n = 37) or amlodipine (n = 34). Blood pressure and proteinuria were determined before and after the treatment, and changes in the mean values were statistically compared. Patients were genotyped for the ACE-I/D, angiotensin I receptor type 1 (AGTR1)-1166 A/C, and angiotensinogen (AGT)-M235T polymorphims, and the reduction of blood pressure and proteinuria between the different genotypes were compared. RESULTS: The reduction in systolic or diastolic blood pressure was not found to be different between the ACE-I/D or AGT-M/T genotypes in patients treated with losartan or amlodipine. In patients treated with losartan, we found a significantly higher reduction of diastolic blood pressure in AGTR1-AA patients compared to AC patients (p = 0,0024). We did not find differences in proteinuria-reduction between the different genotypes in patients treated with losartan or amlodipine. CONCLUSIONS: Our data show that the effects of losartan and amlodipine on the absolute mean reduction of blood pressure and proteinuria in non-diabetic nephropathy patients are similar between the different ACE or AGT genotypes. Although based on a small number of patients, the AGTR1-AA genotype was associated with a significantly higher reduction in diastolic blood pressure among losartan-treated patients. Additional studies are necessary to refute or confirm this association.

Neurology. 2004 Nov 23;63(10 Suppl 4):S3-8. Related Articles, Links Pharmacogenetics and enzyme induction/inhibition properties of antiepileptic drugs. Anderson GD. Department of Pharmacy, Box 357630,University of Washington, Seattle, WA 98195, USA. gaila@u.washington.edu One of the major differences between the older antiepileptic drugs (AEDs) and the newer AEDs is the potential of the older AEDs for significant interactions with other medications. Many of the drug-drug interactions involving the older AEDs are reciprocal, i.e., both drugs affect each other. In contrast, the newer AEDs have either no or limited drug interaction potential. Despite our extensive understanding of and our ability to predict drug-drug interactions, serious drug interactions still occur. More than 30% of all new seizures occur in the elderly, and because this population may be taking a variety of other medications the addition of an AED can have profound impact on these other therapies. In women, the use of enzyme-inducing AEDs can cause significant alterations of sex hormones and can decrease the efficacy of oral contraceptives. In children and adults, the use of enzyme inducers may result in long-term endocrine effects, including bone loss and lipid, thyroid, and sex hormone abnormalities. Phenytoin and phenobarbital are metabolized by cytochrome P450 isozymes, with activity dependent on genetic polymorphism (CYP2C9, CYP2C19). The dosing of the newer AEDs is not affected by genetic polymorphism. The decreased induction and inhibition effects and the lack of significant genetic polymorphism of the newer AEDs allow increased ease of use and perhaps greater safety, especially for patients taking multiple medications. Publication Types: Review

Neuropsychopharmacol Hung. 2004 Sep;6 Suppl 1:15-47. Related Articles, Links [Abstracts of the VII Magyar Neuropsychopharmacology Congress. Tihany, Hungary, September 30-October 2, 2004] [Article in Hungarian] [No authors listed] Publication Types: Congresses Overall

Neuropsychopharmacology. 2006 Jan;31(1):231-42. Related Articles, Links Role of Functional Genetic Variation in the Dopamine D2 Receptor (DRD2) in Response to Bupropion and Nicotine Replacement Therapy for Tobacco Dependence: Results of Two Randomized Clinical Trials. Lerman C, Jepson C, Wileyto EP, Epstein LH, Rukstalis M, Patterson F, Kaufmann V, Restine S, Hawk L, Niaura R, Berrettini W. 1Department of Psychiatry and Abramson Cancer Center, Tobacco Use Research Center, University of Pennsylvania, Philadelphia, PA, USA. Although bupropion and nicotine replacement therapy (NRT) are efficacious tobacco dependence treatments, there is substantial interindividual variability in therapeutic response and most smokers relapse. Pharmacogenetics research may improve treatment outcomes by identifying genetic variants predictive of therapeutic response. We investigated the roles of two functional genetic variants in the dopamine D2 receptor (DRD2) gene in response to pharmacotherapy for tobacco dependence among participants in two randomized clinical trials with a 6-month follow-up period: a double-blind placebo-controlled trial of bupropion (n=414) and an open label trial of transdermal nicotine vs nicotine nasal spray (n=368). At the end of the treatment phase, a statistically significant (p=0.01) interaction between the DRD2 - 141C Ins/Del genotype and treatment indicated a more favorable response to bupropion among smokers homozygous for the Ins C allele compared to those carrying a Del C allele. By contrast, smokers carrying the Del C allele had statistically significantly (p=0.006) higher quit rates on NRT compared to those homozygous for the Ins C allele, independent of NRT type. The C957T variant was also associated (p=0.03) with abstinence following NRT. These results suggest that bupropion may be the preferred pharmacologic treatment for smokers homozygous for the DRD2 - 141 Ins C allele, while NRT may be more beneficial for those who carry the Del C allele. Study findings require confirmation in additional larger samples before they are applied in practice.Neuropsychopharmacology (2006) 31, 231-242. doi:10.1038/sj.npp.1300861; published online 10 August 2005.

NeuroRx. 2005 Oct;2(4):683-95. Related Articles, Links Central nervous system drug development: an integrative biomarker approach toward individualized medicine. Gomez-Mancilla B, Marrer E, Kehren J, Kinnunen A, Imbert G, Hillebrand R, Bergstrom M, Schmidt ME. Neuroscience-Biomarker Development,

Novartis Pharma, CH-4002 Basel, Switzerland. baltazar.gomezmancilla@novartis.com Drug development for CNS disorders faces the same formidable hurdles as other therapeutic areas: escalating development costs; novel drug targets with unproven therapeutic potential; and health care systems and regulatory agencies demanding more compelling demonstrations of the value of new drug products. Extensive clinical testing remains the core of registration of new compounds; however, traditional clinical trial methods are falling short in overcoming these development hurdles. The most common CNS disorders targeted for drug treatment are chronic, slowly vitiating processes manifested by highly subjective and context dependent signs and symptoms. With the exception of a few rare familial degenerative disorders, they have ill-defined or undefined pathophysiology. Samples selected for treatment trials using clinical criteria are inevitably heterogeneous, and dependence on traditional endpoints results in early proof-of-concept trials being long and large, with very poor signal to noise. It is no wonder that pharmaceutical and biotechnology companies are looking to biomarkers as an integral part of decision-making process supported by new technologies such as genetics, genomics, proteomics, and imaging as a mean of rationalizing CNS drug development. The present review represent an effort to illustrate the integration of such technologies in drug development supporting the path of individualized medicine. Publication Types: Review

NeuroRx. 2006 Jan;3(1):117-30. Related Articles, Links Imaging genomics and response to treatment with antipsychotics in schizophrenia. Blasi G, Bertolino A. Psychiatric Neuroscience Group, Department of Neurological and Psychiatric Sciences, University of Bari, Bari, Italy 70125. Recent important advancements in genomic research have opened the way to new strategies for public health management. One of these questions pertains to how individual genetic variation may be associated with individual variability in response to drug treatment. The field of pharmacogenetics may have a profound impact on treatment of complex psychiatric disorders like schizophrenia. However, pharmacogenetic studies in schizophrenia have produced conflicting results. The first studies examined potential associations between clinical response and drug receptor genes. Subsequent studies have tried to use more objective phenotypes still in association with drug receptor genes. More recently, other studies have sought the association between putative causative or modifier genes and intermediate phenotypes. Thus, conflicting results may be at least in part explained by variability and choice of the phenotype, by choice of candidate genes, or by the relatively little knowledge about the neurobiology of this disorder. We propose that choosing intermediate phenotypes that allow in vivo measurement of specific neuronal functions may be of great help in reducing several of the potential confounds intrinsic to clinical measurements. Functional neuroimaging is ideally suited to address several of these potential confounds, and it may represent a powerful strategy to investigate the relationship between behavior, brain function, genes, and individual variability in the response to treatment with antipsychotic drugs in schizophrenia. Preliminary evidence with potential susceptilibity genes such as COMT, DISC1, and GRM3 support these assumptions.

Neurosci Lett. 2005 Mar 7;376(1):51-5. Epub 2004 Dec 10. Related Articles, Links Long-term response to lithium salts in bipolar illness is influenced by the glycogen synthase kinase 3-beta -50 T/C SNP. Benedetti F, Serretti A, Pontiggia A, Bernasconi A, Lorenzi C, Colombo C, Smeraldi E. Istituto Scientifico Universitario Ospedale San Raffaele, Department of Neuropsychiatric Sciences, San Raffaele Turro, 20127 Milano, Italy. benedetti.francesco@hsr.it The molecular mechanisms driving the biological clock in the suprachiasmatic nucleus of the hypothalamus may play a role in mood disorders. A single nucleotide polymorphism (SNP) (-50 T/C) falling into the effective promoter region (nt -171 to +29) of the gene coding for glycogen synthase kinase 3-beta (GSK3-beta) has been linked with different age at onset of bipolar illness and with different antidepressant effects of total sleep deprivation. GSK3-beta codes for an enzyme which is a target for the action of lithium and possibly of valproic acid. We studied the effect of this polymorphism on the therapeutic response to lithium salts of 88 bipolar type I patients. Data about recurrence rate of mood episodes were collected for at least 2 years before lithium and 2 years on lithium. Results showed that homozygotes for the wild variant did not change their recurrence index while carriers of the mutant allele improved, thus supporting the hypothesis that GSK is a target for the therapeutic action of lithium. Results warrant interest for the variants of genes pertaining to the molecular clock as possible endophenotypes of bipolar disorder, but caution ought to be taken in interpreting these preliminary results and future replication studies must be awaited because of the low frequency of the GSK3-beta*C/C genotype in the studied populations. Publication Types: Clinical Trial

New Genet Soc. 2004 Apr;23(1):89-103. Related Articles, Links Human genetic banking: altruism, benefit and consent. Williams G, Schroeder D. Institute for Environment, Philosophy and Public Policy (IEPPP), Furness College, Lancaster University, Lancaster LA1 4YG, UK. g.d.williams@lancaster.ac.uk This article considers how we should frame the ethical issues raised by current proposals for large-scale genebanks with on-going links to medical and lifestyle data, such as the Wellcome Trust and Medical Research Council's 'UK Biobank'. As recent scandals such as Alder Hey have emphasised, there are complex issues concerning the informed consent of donors that need to be carefully considered. However, we believe that a preoccupation with informed consent obscures important questions about the purposes to which such collections are put, not least that they may be only haphazardly used for research (especially that of commercial interest)--an end that would not fairly reflect the original altruistic motivation of donors, and the trust they must invest. We therefore argue that custodians of such databases take on a weighty pro-active duty, to encourage public debate about the ends of such collections and to sponsor research that reflects publicly agreed priorities and provides public benefits.

New Sci. 2004 Feb 21-27;181(2435):16-7. Related Articles, Links The moral imperative for human cloning. Wilmut I. Roslin Institute, Edinburgh, UK.

New Sci. 2005 Jun 11-17;186(2503):3. Related Articles, Links Not black and white: BiDil may work best for African Americans--but do we know why? [No authors listed] Publication Types: Editorial

New Sci. 2005 Jun 11-17;186(2503):42-7. Related Articles, Links Colour-coded cures. Kingsland J.

Newsweek. 2003 May 19;141(20):44-6, 48, 51-2. Related Articles, Links Taking a new look at pain. Kalb C. Publication Types: News

Nicotine Tob Res. 2005 Apr;7(2):181-97. Related Articles, Links Nicotine addiction through a neurogenomic prism: ethics, public health, and smoking. Caron L, Karkazis K, Raffin TA, Swan G, Koenig BA. Agence d'evaluation des technologies et des modes d'intervention en sante, Montreal, Canada. Studies are under way to examine the neurogenetic factors contributing to smoking behaviors. The combined approaches of genomics, molecular biology, neuroscience, and pharmacology are expected to fuel developments in pharmacogenetics, to create new genetic tests, and ultimately to provide the basis for innovative strategies for smoking cessation and prevention. The emergence of a neurogenomic understanding of nicotine addiction is likely to induce fundamental changes in popular, clinical, and public health views of smoking, which could significantly shape existing practices and policies to reduce tobacco use. Still a nascent area of research, nicotine addiction provides an excellent case study through which to anticipate key ethical and policy issues in both behavioral genetics and the neurogenomics of addictive behaviors. Publication Types: Review

Nihon Shinkei Seishin Yakurigaku Zasshi. 2005 Jun;25(3):129-35. Related Articles, Links [Clinical pharmacogenetics in the treatment of schizophrenia] [Article in Japanese] Saito M, Yasui-Furukori N, Kaneko S. Department of Neuropsychiatry, Hirosaki University, School of Medicine, Japan. smanabu@mama.plala.or.jp Numerous investigations on metabolic enzymes, cytochrome P450 (CYP), have been conducted since 1990. In the psychiatric field, the focus has been on CYP2D6, which is a major enzyme involved in metabolism of antidepressants and antipsychotics. Poor metabolizers (deficit metabolizers) for CYP2D6 represent 7% among Caucasians, while they accouut for less than 1% of Asians. The frequency of a mutated allele for CYP2D6*10, which leads to the decrease in CYP2D6 activity, is 40% in Asians. It has been reported that steady-state plasma concentration of haloperidol in subjects with mutated alleles for CYP2D6 is significantly higher than that in subjects without mutated alleles. At the same time, steady-state plasma concentration of risperidone is very different between CYP2D6 genotypes. In addition, several studies suggest that better efficacy or higher scores of side effects are observed in the subjects with mutated alleles for CYP2D6. Recently receptor polymorphism has become a concern and association between clinical response and polymorphism of dopamine and serotonin has been reported. In the dopamine D2, subjects with -141C Ins allele in -141C Ins/Del polymorphism and subjects with A1 allele in Taq1A have a better response to dopamine antagonists. Association between Ser allele and typical antipsychotics and between Gly allele and atypical antipsychotics has been investigated. There are still no data indicating significant association between dopamine D1 and clinical response to antipsychotics. Clinical pharmacogenetical studies from both a pharmacokinetical and a pharmacogynamical point of view are required in order to introduce and practice individualized medicine in psychiatric field easily. Publication Types: Review

Nihon Shinkei Seishin Yakurigaku Zasshi. 2005 Jun;25(3):137-41. Related Articles, Links [In vivo evaluation of expressed protein function by PET] [Article in Japanese] Matsumoto R, Suhara T. Brain Imaging Project, National Institute of Radiological Sciences, Chiba, Japan. rmat@nirs.go.jp Positron Emission Tomography (PET) allows in vivo visualization of the expression and function of protein using a radioligand. Quantitative analysis of serotonin transporter, receptors, and the function of P-Glycoprotein has been performed in living human brains. Furthermore, the relationship between the phenotype of those proteins and their genetic polymorphism has also been investigated. Regarding the effect of antipsychotics on dopamine D2 receptor, occupancy and its time-course have been measured in a living body using PET. This approach can provide in vivo pharmacological evidences of antipsychotics and establish a rational therapeutic strategy. PET is a powerful tool not only in the field of brain research but also drug discovery and individual medicine. Publication Types: Review

Nippon Naika Gakkai Zasshi. 2004 Mar 10;93(3):574-9. Related Articles, Links [Recent progress in diagnosis of and therapy for patients with leukemia] [Article in Japanese] Ueda T. Publication Types: Review

Nippon Naika Gakkai Zasshi. 2005 Dec 10;94(12):2486-94. Related Articles, Links [Present status and future prospects in genetic tests] [Article in Japanese] Miyachi H. Publication Types: Review

Nippon Rinsho. 2004 Dec;62 Suppl 12:351-5. Related Articles, Links [Clinical evaluation of therapeutic drug monitoring] [Article in Japanese] Kohno H. Division of Pharmacy, National Hospital Organization Disaster Medical Center. Publication Types: Review

Nippon Rinsho. 2004 Jul;62 Suppl 7(Pt 1):441-7. Related Articles, Links [Therapeutic strategies for hepatitis C] [Article in Japanese] Tsubota A, Kumada H. Institute of Clinical Medicine and Research, Jikei University School of Medicine. Publication Types: Review

Nippon Rinsho. 2004 Mar;62 Suppl 3:104-7. Related Articles, Links [ACE gene polymorphism as a risk factor in the development of hypertensive organ damage] [Article in Japanese] Yamasaki E, Nakura J. Department of Geriatric Medicine, Ehime University School of Medicine. Publication Types: Review

Nippon Rinsho. 2004 Mar;62 Suppl 3:116-21. Related Articles, Links [Gene polymorphisms of angiotensin II-type 1 receptor in hypertension] [Article in Japanese] Katsuya T, Ogihara T. Department of Geriatric Medicine, Osaka University Graduate School of Medicine. Publication Types: Review

Nippon Rinsho. 2004 Mar;62 Suppl 3:126-30. Related Articles, Links [Polymorphism in guanine nucleotide-binding protein (G-protein) beta 3 subunit (GNB3) gene as a risk factor in the development of hypertensive organ damage] [Article in Japanese] Ogimoto A. Second Department of Internal Medicine, Ehime University School of Medicine. Publication Types: Review

Nippon Rinsho. 2005 Dec;63 Suppl 12:212-6. Related Articles, Links [Gene-based testing for respiratory disease] [Article in Japanese] Saijo Y. Department of Molecular Medicine, Tohoku University Graduate School of Medicine. Publication Types: Review

Nippon Rinsho. 2005 Dec;63 Suppl 12:301-7. Related Articles, Links [Genetic testing and gene-based testing for hyperlipidemia and lipid metabolism disorders] [Article in Japanese] Kajinami K, Okabayashi M, Sato R. Department of Cardiology, Kanazawa Medical University. Publication Types: Review

Nippon Rinsho. 2005 Dec;63 Suppl 12:35-41. Related Articles, Links [BioBank Japan project] [Article in Japanese] Ohnishi Y, Nakamura Y. Laboratory of Molecular Medicine, Institute of Medical Science, University of Tokyo. Publication Types: Review

Nippon Rinsho. 2005 Dec;63 Suppl 12:450-3. Related Articles, Links [Cytochrome P450 2C19 genotype -based second line therapy with amoxicillin and lansoprazole after failure of initial helicobacter pylori eradication therapy] [Article in Japanese] Asano M, Taniwaki H, Tsuji D, Sato Y, Shimizu T. General Research Center, Seirei Hamamatsu General Hospital. Publication Types: Review

Nippon Rinsho. 2005 Dec;63 Suppl 12:463-6. Related Articles, Links [Genetic analyses of morphine sensitivity] [Article in Japanese] Ikeda K, Ogai Y, Nishizawa D, Ide S, Sora I. Division of Psychobiology, Tokyo Institute of Psychiatry. Publication Types: Review

Nippon Rinsho. 2005 Dec;63 Suppl 12:50-6. Related Articles, Links [Pharmacogenomics: current status and future prospectives] [Article in Japanese] Ishikawa T. Department of Biomolecular Engineering, Graduate School of Bioscience and Biotechnology, Tokyo Institute of Technology. Publication Types: Review

Nippon Rinsho. 2005 Feb;63 Suppl 2:166-70. Related Articles, Links [PPARgamma gene Pro12Ala polymorphism in diabetes mellitus] [Article in Japanese] Yasuda K. Department of Metabolic Disorder, Research Institute, International Medical Center of Japan. Publication Types: Review

Nippon Rinsho. 2005 Jan;63 Suppl 1:686-90. Related Articles, Links [Tailor-made medicine and genomic drug discovery in rheumatoid arthritis] [Article in Japanese] Taniguchi A, Kamatani N. Institute of Rheumatology, Tokyo Women's Medical University. Publication Types: Review

Nippon Rinsho. 2005 Jun;63 Suppl 6:458-63. Related Articles, Links [Recent advances in searching the gene(s) conferring susceptibility to diabetic nephropathy] [Article in Japanese] Maeda S. Laboratory for Diabetic Nephropathy, SNP Research Center, The Institute of Physical and Chemical Research. Publication Types: Review

Nippon Rinsho. 2005 Jun;63(6):1067-70. Related Articles, Links [Future medicine for hypertension in the elderly] [Article in Japanese] Higaki J. Second Department of Internal Medicine, Ehime University School of Medicine. The number of the aged patients with hypertension is now explosively increasing. In near future, progress of new and tailor-made prescribed antihypertensive drugs and curable-gene therapy for hypertension will improve new era of hypertension in the elderly. And finally, resolusion of the aging mechanism and anti-aging medicine may open our future. Publication Types: Review

Nippon Rinsho. 2005 Jun;63(6):926-30. Related Articles, Links [Polymorphism in elderly hypertension] [Article in Japanese] Katsuya T, Ogihara T. Department of

Geriatric Medicine, Osaka University Graduate School of Medicine. Publication Types: Review

Nippon Rinsho. 2005 Nov;63 Suppl 11:426-33. Related Articles, Links [Susceptibility to antibiotics and drug metabolism in patients with H. pylori infection refractory to the initial treatment--therapeutic strategy based on susceptibility to CAM and CYP2C19 polymorphism] [Article in Japanese] Furuta T, Sugimoto M, Nakamura A, Shirai N. First Department of Medicine, Hamamatsu University School of Medicine. Publication Types: Review

Nippon Rinsho. 2005 Nov;63 Suppl 11:569-72. Related Articles, Links [Influence of cytochrome P450 2C19 genetic polymorphism on H. pylori eradication therapy] [Article in Japanese] Hikichi T, Irisawa A, Abe C, Obara K, Sato Y. Department of Internal Medicine II, Fukushima Medical University School of Medicine. Publication Types: Review

Nippon Rinsho. 2005 Sep;63 Suppl 9:288-92. Related Articles, Links [Individualized therapy for glioma] [Article in Japanese] Okada Y, Ueki K. Department of Neurosurgery, Dokkyo University School of Medicine. Publication Types: Review

Nippon Rinsho. 2005 Sep;63 Suppl 9:30-4. Related Articles, Links [Molecular biology of brain tumors] [Article in Japanese] Tamiya T, Morisaki K, Miyake K, Matsumoto Y, Nagao S, Daido S, Ichikawa T. Department of Neurological Surgery, Kagawa University School of Medicine. Publication Types: Review

Nippon Rinsho. 2005 Sep;63 Suppl 9:460-71. Related Articles, Links [Chemoresistance-related genes and individualized adjuvant therapies for brain gliomas] [Article in Japanese] Nagane M. Department of Neurosurgery, Kyorin University School of Medicine. Publication Types: Review

Nippon Rinsho. 2005 Sep;63 Suppl 9:49-54. Related Articles, Links [Analysis of gene expression profiles in malignant brain tumors with respect to sensitivity to therapies] [Article in Japanese] Yamanaka R, Morii K, Takahashi H, Tanaka R, Nishio K. Department of Neurosurgery, Brain Reseach Instiute, Niigata University. Publication Types: Review

Nippon Rinsho. 2006 Jan;64(1):27-33. Related Articles, Links [Tailored medicine for diabetes in the elderly] [Article in Japanese] Ikegami H. Department of Geriatric Medicine, Osaka University Graduate School of Medicine. To establish tailored medicine in the elderly, detailed information on clinical as well as genetic characteristics of each patient is essential. Although current age is all in the elderly, clinical characteristics of elderly patients with diabetes are very heterogeneous, making this category of patients good target for tailored medicine. Several genes conferring susceptibility to diabetic complications, such as insertion/deletion polymorphism of angiotensin--converting enzyme(ACE) gene for diabetic nephropathy, have been identified. Detailed information on genetic factor as well as current status of diabetes-related as well as unrelated complications will contribute a lot in establishing tailored medicine in elderly patients with diabetes. Publication Types: Review

Nippon Shokakibyo Gakkai Zasshi. 2004 Mar;101(3):255-63. Related Articles, Links [Tailored therapy in gastrointestinal and hepatic cancer--toward ideal medicine through genomic science] [Article in Japanese] Imai K, Yoshida Y. First Department of Internal Medicine, Sapporo

Medical University School of Medicine. Publication Types: Review

Nippon Yakurigaku Zasshi. 2005 Apr;125(4):178-84. Related Articles, Links [Overview: molecular variation, specific tissue localization and genetic polymorphisms of drug transporters] [Article in Japanese] Sugiyama Y, Maeda K. sugiyama@mol.f.u-tokyo.ac.jp Publication Types: Review

Nippon Yakurigaku Zasshi. 2005 Dec;126(6):432-5. Related Articles, Links [Tasks and expectations for drug design based on pharmacogenomics] [Article in Japanese] Uyama Y. uyama-yoshiaki@pmda.go.jp Publication Types: Review

Nippon Yakurigaku Zasshi. 2005 Jul;126(1):60-5. Related Articles, Links [Tailor-made medicine] [Article in Japanese] Kamataki T. SNC78123@nifty.com Publication Types: Review

Nippon Yakurigaku Zasshi. 2005 Jul;126(1):66-9. Related Articles, Links [Pharmacogenomics] [Article in Japanese] Azuma J, Imagawa K. Publication Types: Review

Nippon Yakurigaku Zasshi. 2005 Jun;125(6):365-71. Related Articles, Links [Chemogenomics] [Article in Japanese] Eguchi Y. eguchi-y@mki.co.jp Publication Types: Review

Nippon Yakurigaku Zasshi. 2005 Mar;125(3):148-52. Related Articles, Links [Genome-wide analysis of single nucleotide polymorphisms] [Article in Japanese] Ogimoto A, Higaki J. aogimoto@m.ehime-u.ac.jp Publication Types: Review

Nitric Oxide. 2004 Feb;10(1):36-41. Related Articles, Links Dexamethasone lacks effect on blood pressure in mice with a disrupted endothelial NO synthase gene. Wallerath T, Godecke A, Molojavyi A, Li H, Schrader J, Forstermann U. Department of Pharmacology, Johannes Gutenberg University, D-55101 Mainz, Germany. Cushing's syndrome and systemic administration of glucocorticoids are associated with hypertension, but the underlying molecular mechanism is only partially understood. We have shown previously that dexamethasone downregulates the expression of the endothelial NO synthase (eNOS) gene in human endothelial cells and in the rat and that this may contribute to the blood pressure-raising effect of the steroid [Proc. Natl. Acad. Sci. USA 96 (1999) 13357]. In the current communication, we demonstrated that dexamethasone increased mean arterial blood pressure in wild-type C-57 Bl6 mice (eNOS+/+ mice), but had no effect on blood pressure in mice with a disrupted eNOS gene (eNOS-/- mice) derived from the same strain. The NOS inhibitor ethylisothiourea, used for control purposes, showed a hypertensive effect in eNOS+/+ mice, but no such effect in eNOS-/- mice. Serum NO2-/NO3- levels, an indicator of total body NO synthesis, decreased significantly when eNOS+/+ mice were treated with dexamethasone. eNOS-/- mice had lower serum NO2-/NO3- levels per se, which were not changed significantly by dexamethasone. Dexamethasone decreased the expression of eNOS in three major organs of the mouse investigated, namely the heart, the liver, and the kidney. We conclude that the expressional downregulation of eNOS and the ensuing reduction in vascular NO production contributes to the hypertension caused by glucocorticoids.

Novartis Found Symp. 2004;263:41-53; discussion 53-6, 211-8. Related Articles, Links Pharmacogenetics of inflammatory bowel disease. Kelleher D, Farrell R, McManus R. Department of Clinical Medicine and Dublin Molecular Medicine Centre, Trinity College Dublin, Ireland. Therapeutic outcome in inflammatory bowel disease has traditionally been related to disease activity. Recent data suggest that individual differences in drug disposition and metabolism, some of which are genetically determined, may play a significant role in the outcome of therapy for inflammatory diseases. Polymorphisms in the thiopurine methyl transferase gene (TPMT) are known to influence the outcome of therapy with azathioprine although pharmacogenetic analysis of outcome has not entered routine clinical use. The outcome of therapy with drugs such as steroids may be influenced by a wide range of genetic factors including polymorphisms in the multi-drug resistance 1 gene (MDR1), polymorphisms in glucocorticoid receptor genes and potentially other as yet undefined polymorphisms regulating the inflammatory process. Multiple polymorphisms have been identified in MDR1 but their direct contribution to changes in expression and function have not as yet been defined. Lastly, as novel biological agents such as infliximab become established in clinical practice, it is clear that their therapeutic efficacy will likely be modified by polymorphisms downstream of their target molecules. New diagnostic and therapeutic algorithms are needed to directly determine the functional importance of the influence of host genetic factors on choice and dosage scheduling of therapy. Publication Types: Review

Novartis Found Symp. 2005;267:14-9; discussion 19-30. Related Articles, Links Haplotype tagging in pharmacogenetics. Goldstein DB. Department of Biology, Darwin Building, University College London, Gower Street, London WC1E 6BT, UK. Analyses of variation in human populations have become central to understanding how gene variants predispose to disease and influence treatment response. Here I first describe an emerging framework for linkage disequilbrium-(haplotype) based gene mapping focusing on the analysis of patterns of genetic variation in 56 genes that metabolize or transport prescription medicines. Detailed analyses of 754 single nucleotide polymorphisms (SNPs) genotyped in two population samples (European and Japanese) provide a set of haplotype tagging SNPs that economically represent variation in most of the major enzymes that act on prescription drugs. I use these analyses to address a number of outstanding questions relating to haplotype mapping. Following this, I provide a number of applications of haplotype mapping emphasizing the work that needs to be done to translate genotype-phenotype correlations into clinically useful diagnostics, and clinically useful leads concerning new therapeutic targets.

Nurs Clin North Am. 2005 Mar;40(1):33-49. Related Articles, Links Use of prescription drugs: rising or declining? Crockett AB. School of Nursing, Box 81, Middle Tennessee State University, Murfreesboro, TN 37132, USA. acrocket@mtsu.edu Prescribing practices are a reflection of health professionals' abilities to discriminate among the various choices of drugs and determine the ones that will most benefit their patients. As selective as practitioners must be, they cannot limit themselves to knowing only those drugs that fit within the dominant paradigm of acute care. They must broaden their exposure to incorporate knowledge of drugs that permeate clients' lives through media and self-administration. Health promotion drug use is just emerging as a prescriptive activity, but it will become more significant in the future. Primary and secondary prevention drug uses are in flux, and tertiary prevention drug use is likely to overwhelm our system, particularly with the baby boom generation, until our society can switch its focus to more health promotion and disease prevention. It is imperative that health professionals develop shared decision-making capabilities for client education and appropriate prescribing. Only when the health care system exhibits a true client-provider partnership will the "five rights"-right drug, right dose, right route, right time, right client-be accurately applied. With the increasing and overwhelming costs of prescription drugs, health practitioners cannot afford to sit idle; as professionals and stakeholders, they must engage health policy makers and persuade these entities to share their concerns and views, and help their clients, the profession, and themselves. Publication Types: Review

Nursing. 2005 Apr;35(4):22-3. Related Articles, Links Tailoring drug therapy with pharmacogenetics. Lea DH.

Nutr Rev. 2005 Nov;63(11):398-407. Related Articles, Links 5,10-Methylenetetrahydrofolate reductase polymorphisms and pharmacogenetics: a new role of single nucleotide polymorphisms in the folate metabolic pathway in human health and disease. Kim YI. Department of Medicine, University of Toronto, Division of Gastroenterology, St. Michael's Hospital, Room 7258, Medical Sciences Building, 1 King's College Circle, Toronto, Ontario, Canada M5S 1A8. youngin.kim@utoronto.ca Knowledge about the role of folate, a water-soluble B vitamin, and single nucleotide polymorphisms (SNPs) in the folate metabolic pathway in human health and disease has been rapidly expanding. Recently, functionally significant SNPs in 5,10-methylenetetrahydrofolate reductase (MTHFR), a critical enzyme for intracellular folate homeostasis and metabolism, have been identified and characterized. An emerging body of in vitro and clinical evidence suggests that these MTHFR SNPs may be an important pharmacogenetic determinant of predicting response to and toxicity of methotrexate and 5-fluorouracil-based cancer and anti-inflammatory treatments because of their well-defined and highly relevant biochemical effects on intracellular folate composition and one-carbon transfer reactions. Publication Types: Review

NY Times (Print). 2005 Jun 13;:A1, A15. Related Articles, Links U.S. to review drug intended for one race. Saul S. Publication Types: Newspaper Article

Obstet Gynecol Clin North Am. 2006 Mar;33(1):199-224. Related Articles, Links Future directions in myoma research. Brahma PK, Martel KM, Christman GM. Department of Obstetrics and Gynecology, University of Michigan Health System, University of Michigan Medical School, 6422 Medical Science I, 1150 West Medical Center Drive, Ann Arbor, MI 48105, USA. This article highlight our current knowledge of fibroids and addresses future directions for fibroid research and treatment over the next decade. The available data on cytogenetics are discussed, in addition to discoveries into signaling pathways and second messenger molecules in leiomyomas. Current medical management, surgical trends and the barriers to transition to minimally invasive procedures are summarized. Innovations in genetic diagnosis and interventional radiologic-aided therapies may revolutionize therapy for certain populations of patients who have fibroids. From tissue-specific medical management, to minimally invasive surgical techniques, to pharmacogenetics, the current directions of fibroid research are leading us to an exciting new frontier.

Oncogene. 2006 Mar 13;25(11):1629-38. Related Articles, Links Thiopurine S-methyltransferase pharmacogenetics: insights, challenges and future directions. Wang L, Weinshilboum R. Division of Clinical Pharmacology, Department of Molecular Pharmacology and Experimental Therapeutics, Mayo Clinic College of Medicine, Rochester, MN 55905, USA. wang.liewei@mayo.edu The thiopurine S-methyltransferase (TPMT) genetic polymorphism is one of the most 'mature' examples in pharmacogenetics. That is true because of its importance clinically for the individualization of thiopurine drug therapy and also because TPMT has provided novel insights into molecular mechanisms responsible for the functional effects of common genetic polymorphisms. This review will summarize the development of our understanding of the role of inheritance in the regulation of TPMT as well as the clinical implications of that genetic regulation. It will also summarize recent studies in which TPMT pharmacogenetics has enhanced our understanding of molecular mechanisms by which common polymorphisms influence or alter function. TPMT pharmacogenetics highlights the potential clinical importance of the translation of pharmacogenetics from bench to bedside, the potential for basic pharmacogenetic research to provide insight into mechanisms by which genetic polymorphisms can alter function, and the challenges associated with the achievement of both of those goals.

Oncogene. 2006 Mar 13;25(11):1659-72. Related Articles, Links Uridine diphosphoglucuronosyltransferase pharmacogenetics and cancer. Nagar S, Remmel RP. Department of Pharmaceutical Sciences, Temple University School of Pharmacy, Philadelphia, PA 19140, USA. swati.nagar@temple.edu The uridine diphosphoglucuronosyltransferases (UGTs) belong to a superfamily of enzymes that catalyse the glucuronidation of numerous endobiotics and xenobiotics. Several human hepatic and extrahepatic UGT isozymes have been characterized with respect to their substrate specificity, tissue expression and gene structure. Genetic polymorphisms have been identified for almost all the UGT family members. A wide variety of anticancer drugs, dietary chemopreventives and carcinogens are known to be conjugated by members of both UGT1A and UGT2B subfamilies. This review examines in detail each UGT isozyme known to be associated with cancer and carcinogenesis. The cancer-related substrates for several UGTs are summarized, and the functionally relevant genetic polymorphisms of UGTs are reviewed. A number of genotype-phenotype association studies have been carried out to characterize the role of UGT pharmacogenetics in several types of cancer, and these examples are discussed here. In summary, this review focuses on the role of the human UGT genetic polymorphisms in carcinogenesis, chemoprevention and cancer risk.

Oncogene. 2006 Mar 13;25(11):1673-8. Related Articles, Links Pharmacogenetics of human cytosolic sulfotransferases. Nowell S, Falany CN. University of Arkansas for Medical Sciences, Little Rock, AR 72205, USA. sanowell@uams.edu Cytosolic sulfotransferases (SULTs) are phase II detoxification enzymes that are involved in the biotransformation of a wide variety of structurally diverse endo- and xenobiotics, including many therapeutic agents and endogenous steroids. Single-nucleotide polymorphisms (SNPs) in SULTs have functional consequences on the translated protein. For the most part, these SNPs are fairly uncommon in the population, but some, most notably for SULT isoform 1A1, are commonly found and have been associated with cancer risk for a variety of tumor sites and also with response to therapeutic agents. SNPs in the hydroxysteroid sulfotransferase, SULT2A1, have been identified in African-American subjects and influence the ratio of plasma DHEA:DHEA-S. This modification could potentially influence cancer risk in steroidogenic tissues. SNPs in many SULTs are ethnically distributed, another factor that could influence SULT pharmacogenetics. Finally, genetic variation has also been identified in 3'-phosphoadenoside 5'-phosphosulfate synthetase (PAPPS), the enzymes responsible for producing the obligatory cosubstrate for all sulfotransferases. Taken together, this variability could substantially influence the disposition of drugs metabolized by SULTs. Elucidation of the basis and effect of variability in sulfation could greatly impact individualized therapy in the future.

Oncogene. 2006 Mar 13;25(11):1679-91. Related Articles, Links Cytochrome P450 pharmacogenetics and cancer. Rodriguez-Antona C, Ingelman-Sundberg M. Endocrine Cancer Group, Human Cancer Genetics Programme, Spanish National Cancer Center (CNIO), Madrid, Spain. The cytochromes P450 (CYPs) are key enzymes in cancer formation and cancer treatment: They mediate the metabolic activation of numerous precarcinogens and participate in the inactivation and activation of anticancer drugs. Since all CYPs that metabolize xenobiotics are polymorphic, much emphasis has been put on the investigation of a relationship between the distribution of specific variant CYP alleles and risk for different types of cancer, but a consistent view does not yet exist. This is to a great extent explained by the fact that the CYPs involved in activation of precarcinogens are in general not functionally polymorphic. This is in contrast to CYPs that are active in drug biotransformation where large interindividual differences in the capacity to metabolize therapeutic drugs are seen as a consequence of polymorphic alleles with altered function. This includes also some anticancer drugs like tamoxifen and cyclophosphamide metabolized by CYP2D6, CYP2C19 and CYP2B6. Some P450 forms are also selectively expressed in tumours, and this could provide a mechanism for drug resistance, but also future therapies using these enzymes as drug targets can be envisioned. This review gives an up-to-date description of our current knowledge in these areas.

Oncol Rep. 2005 Nov;14(5):1381-4. Related Articles, Links Comparative genomics on ROR1 and ROR2 orthologs. Katoh M, Katoh M. MandM Medical BioInformatics, Hongo 113-0033, Japan. Transmembrane proteins with extracellular Frizzled domain, such as ROR1, ROR2, MUSK, MFRP, FZD1, FZD2, FZD3, FZD4, FZD5, FZD6, FZD7, FZD8, FZD9 and FZD10, are key molecules for WNT signaling network. Here, comparative integromics analyses on ROR1 and ROR2 orthologs were performed by using bioinformatics. Zebrafish ror2 gene, consisting of nine exons, was identified within CR-450684.3 genome sequence. CV490605.1 EST corresponded to the 5'-end of zebrafish ror2 mRNA, and BM533602.1 EST corresponded to the 3'-end. Zebrafish ror2 gene was found to encode a 939-aa transmembrane protein, showing 71.7% and 56.2% total amino-acid identity with human ROR2 and ROR1, respectively. Immunoglobulin-like domain, Frizzled domain, Kringle domain within the extracellular region, tyrosine kinase domain, Ror homology C-terminal (RORHC) domain and juxta-C-terminal LLGD motif within the cytoplasmic region were conserved among vertebrate ROR1 and ROR2 orthologs. SH2 binding site within the RORHC domain was conserved among vertebrate ROR2 orthologs, but not among vertebrate ROR1 orthologs. ROR1 mRNA was expressed in embryonic stem (ES) cells, infant brain, renal cancer, and colon cancer. ROR2 mRNA was expressed in parathyroid, testis, uterus, and also in diffuse type gastric cancer with signet ring cell features. ROR2 promoter rather than ROR1 promoter was more evolutionarily conserved. WNT5A and ROR family receptors, co-expressed in ES cells and gastric cancer, are implicated in the planar cell polarity (PCP) pathway. ROR1 and ROR2 are the pharmacogenomics targets in the fields of stem cell biology and oncology.

Oncol Rep. 2005 Oct;14(4):1083-6. Related Articles, Links Comparative genomics on SNAI1, SNAI2, and SNAI3 orthologs. Katoh M, Katoh M. MandM Medical BioInformatics, Hongo 113-0033, Japan. SNAI1, SNAI2, and SNAI3 genes, encoding transcriptional repressors implicated in epithelial mesenchymal transition (EMT), are human homologs of Drosophila snail (sna) and slug genes. SNAI1 represses transcription of CDH1 (E-cadherin) gene. SNAI2 induces the first phase of EMT, including desmosome dissociation, cell spreading, and initiation of cell separation. Because SNAI family proteins are implicated in EMT during embryogenesis and carcinogenesis, SNAI family genes are potent targets of pharmacogenomics. Here, comparative genomics analyses and comparative proteomics analyses on SNAI family orthologs were performed. Rat Snai3 gene, consisting of three exons, was identified within rat genome sequence AC111791.4. Zebrafish snai1a (NM_131066.1) was identified as SNAI1 ortholog. Chicken ChEST362I17 (CR407272.1), Xenopus slug (AF368041.1), and zebrafish zgc92564 (NM_001008581.1) were identified as SNAI2 orthologs. Chicken snail (NM_ 205142.1), Xenopus snail (BC056857.1), and zebrafish snai1b (NM_130989.1) were identified as SNAI3 orthologs. SNAI1 orthologs consisted of SNAG domain and four zinc finger (ZNF) domains, while SNAI2 and SNAI3 orthologs consisted of SNAG domain and five ZNF domains. Based on the integromics analyses, SNAI2 orthologs were found to be more conserved than SNAI1 and SNAI3 orthologs. SNAI1 mRNA was expressed in placenta, neuroblastoma, and diffuse type gastric cancer. SNAI2 mRNA was expressed in placenta, melanocyte, embryonic stem (ES) cells, leiomyosarcoma, neuroblastoma, and glioblastoma. SNAI3 mRNA was expressed in B cells. Expression of SNAI3 mRNA was repressed due to the existence of anti-sense single-exon transcript. SNAI1, functioning as E-cadherin repressor, is implicated in the malignant infiltrating phenotype of diffuse type gastric cancer through the induction of EMT or fibroblastoid transformation.

Oncologist. 2005 Feb;10(2):104-11. Related Articles, Links Cancer pharmacogenomics: powerful tools in cancer chemotherapy and drug development. Lee W, Lockhart AC, Kim RB, Rothenberg ML. Department of Medicine, Division of Medical Oncology, Vanderbilt University Medical Center, Nashville, Tennessee, USA. wooin.lee@vanderbilt.edu Interindividual differences in tumor response and normal tissue toxicities are consistently observed with most chemotherapeutic agents or regimens. While many clinical variables have been associated with drug responses (e.g., age, gender, diet, drug-drug interactions), inherited variations in drug disposition (metabolism and transport) genes and drug target genes also likely contribute to the observed variability in cancer treatment outcome. Pharmacogenomic studies aim to elucidate the genetic bases for interindividual differences and to use such genetic information to predict the safety, toxicity, and/or efficacy of drugs. There exist several clinically relevant examples of the utility of pharmacogenomics that associate specific genetic polymorphisms in drug metabolizing enzymes (e.g., TPMT, UGT1A1, DPD), drug transporters (MDR1), and drug target enzymes (TS) with clinical outcomes in patients treated with commonly prescribed chemotherapy drugs, such as 5-fluorouracil and irinotecan (Camptosar; Pfizer Pharmaceuticals; New York, NY http://www.pfizer.com). Techniques to discover and evaluate the functional significance of these polymorphisms have evolved in recent years and may soon be applied to clinical practice and clinical trials of currently prescribed anticancer drugs as well as new therapeutic agents. This review discusses the current and future applications of pharmacogenomics in clinical cancer therapy and cancer drug development. Publication Types: Review

Oncology (Williston Park). 2004 Nov;18(13 Suppl 8):70-6. Related Articles, Links The promise of pharmacogenomics: gemcitabine and pemetrexed. Rosell R, Taron M, Sanchez JM, Moran T, Reguart N, Besse B, Isla D, Massuti B, Alberola V, Sanchez JJ. Medical Oncology Service, Hospital Germans Trias i Pujol, Badalona, Spain. rrosell@ns.hugtip.scs.es Although no overall differences in survival have been observed between the many chemotherapy combinations in non-small-cell lung cancer, the clinical application of mRNA expression levels of amplified genes may disclose many genetic influences on cytotoxic drug sensitivity and enable clinicians to tailor chemotherapy according to each individual's gene profile. Specifically, the assessment of ribonucleotide reductase subunit M1 and thymidylate synthase mRNA expression levels might select patients who benefit from gemcitabine (Gemzar) or pemetrexed (Alimta) combinations. Until recently, clinical prognostic factors such as performance status, weight loss, and lactate dehydrogenase were the only parameters used to predict chemotherapy response and survival. However, accumulated data indicate that overexpression of genes involved in cancer glycolysis pathways plays an important role, and might be an independent mechanism of chemoresistance. The dysregulation of glycolytic genes is affected by growth signals involving the PI3K/Akt pathway and downstream genes such as hypoxia-inducible factor-1-alpha. One can thus envision that substantial improvements in therapeutic outcome could benefit from the integration of tailored ribonucleotide reductase-dependent chemotherapy, ribonucleotide reductase antisense therapy, and targeted therapy. Publication Types: Review

Onkologie. 2005 Aug;28(8-9):435-40. Epub 2005 Aug 29. Related Articles, Links Pharmacogenetics in gastrointestinal tumors. Stohlmacher J. Klinik und Polikinik fur Innere Medizin I, Universitatsklinikum Carl Gustav Carus, TU Dresden, Deutschland. jan.stoehlmacher@uniklinikum-dresden.de Treatment of gastrointestinal cancers has significantly advanced over the last few years with the introduction of effective chemotherapeutic and targeted drugs. To provide individual treatment with low toxicity on the one hand but maximum benefit on the other hand is still an unsolved problem. Interindividual variation of drug toxicity and efficacy is determined by genetic polymorphisms. The genetic approach based on single-gene (pharmacogenetics) or multi-gene (pharmacogenomics) analyses is developing as a valuable tool to design tailored therapy. This review focuses on clinically significant polymorphisms in genes involved in the metabolism of the major players in the chemotherapy of gastrointestinal cancer: fluoropyrimidines, irinotecan and platinum. In addition, first results of pharmacogenetics in targeted therapy including cetuximab and bevacizumab are discussed. The pharmacogenetic approach to individualize therapy in gastrointestinal cancers is promising, but additional larger and controlled studies are needed to justify changes of treatment strategies. Publication Types: Review

Onkologie. 2005 Nov;28(11):589-92. Related Articles, Links Pharmacogenetics of extraordinary responses to 5-FU/cisplatin chemotherapy in advanced gastric cancer -- report of 2 cases. Wolschke C, Goekkurt E, Al-Batran SE, Hossfeld DK, Stoehlmacher J. Medizinische Klinik II, Onkologie, Hamatologie und Knochenmarkstransplantation, Universitatsklinikum Hamburg-Eppendorf, Germany. BACKGROUND: Gastric cancer is often diagnosed in the metastatic stage, and only 10% of patients survive for as long as 2 years. Current chemotherapy regimens show significant treatment-related toxicities. It is crucial to identify the patients that will benefit most from certain chemotherapy regimens in order to avoid unnecessary side effects. PATIENTS AND METHODS: 2 patients with advanced gastric cancer repeatedly received 5-FU/cisplatin combination chemotherapy. Genomic DNA was extracted from tumor tissue and mononuclear blood cells. Genotype analysis of genes of metabolizing and DNA repair enzymes was carried out using a PCR-RFLP technique. Direct sequencing was used to identify mutations of the gene dihydropyrimidine dehydrogenase (DPD). RESULTS: Prolonged survival of 51 and 29 months, respectively were observed in our 2 patients. Both patients were positive for genotypes of thymidylate synthase -- the target enzyme of 5-FU -- that are associated with improved drug response. DPD variants connected with increased toxicity were not observed. However, both patients also showed genotypes in cisplatin metabolizing enzymes which enhance the effect of the drug. CONCLUSION: Genotype analysis in drug metabolizing enzymes of 5-FU and cisplatin provide a possible explanation for extraordinary therapy effects observed in 2 patients with advanced gastric cancer. Publication Types: Case Reports

Ophthalmology. 2005 Dec;112(12):2131-6. Related Articles, Links Beta1-adrenergic receptor polymorphisms and clinical efficacy of betaxolol hydrochloride in normal volunteers. Schwartz SG, Puckett BJ, Allen RC, Castillo IG, Leffler CT. Bascom Palmer Eye Institute, University of Miami Miller School of Medicine, Miami, Florida 34102, USA. sschwartz2@med.miami.edu OBJECTIVE: To evaluate the relationship between polymorphisms in the gene encoding the beta1-adrenergic receptor (beta1-AR) and clinical response to betaxolol hydrochloride 0.25% in a small pilot study of normal volunteers. DESIGN: Prospective nonrandomized comparative trial. PARTICIPANTS: Forty-eight consecutive normal volunteers who met all eligibility requirements for inclusion into this study. METHODS: Baseline intraocular pressure (IOP) was recorded. Subjects began treatment with betaxolol (1 drop both eyes twice daily) and underwent follow-up IOP recordings at 3 and 6 weeks. Peripheral blood was obtained for genetic analysis. MAIN OUTCOME MEASURES: Response to betaxolol was calculated as the change in mean IOP from baseline (averaged between both eyes and averaged between both follow-up visits). The beta1-AR genotype was determined by polymerase chain reaction with restriction fragment length polymorphisms at codons 49 (serine [Ser] or glycine [Gly]) and 389 (arginine [Arg] or Gly). RESULTS: There were 32 Ser49 homozygotes and 16 Gly49 carriers. There were no statistically significant differences between the Ser49 homozygotes and the Gly49 carriers with respect to baseline IOP or response to betaxolol therapy. There were 25 Arg389 homozygotes and 23 Gly389 carriers (22 heterozygotes and 1 Gly389 homozygote). As compared with Gly389 carriers, the Arg389 homozygotes had a higher baseline IOP (15.8 mmHg vs. 13.7 mmHg; P = 0.009) and a greater magnitude of response to betaxolol therapy (-3.4 mmHg vs. -1.5 mmHg; P = 0.0009). The Ser49 homozygote genotype was not independently associated with baseline IOP (P = 0.47) or with a response to betaxolol (P = 0.99). The Arg389 homozygote genotype was independently associated with a higher baseline IOP (P = 0.03) and a greater response to betaxolol (P = 0.03), even after adjusting for baseline IOP. CONCLUSIONS: In this small pilot series, a single nucleotide polymorphism at codon 389 in the beta1-AR seems to correlate with a response to betaxolol therapy in normal, nonglaucomatous volunteers. There was no such correlation at codon 49. The polymorphism at codon 389 may predict short-term response to betaxolol and may serve as a determinant of response to betaxolol and other adrenergic agents in glaucomatous eyes requiring treatment. Publication Types: Clinical Trial

Orthopedics. 2005 Oct;28(10):1157-9. Related Articles, Links Pharmacogenomics-Potential applications to orthopedic practice. Sutphin SD, Smith KM. University of Kentucky Chandler Medical Center, Lexington, KY 40536-0293, USA. Pharmacogenomics is developing at a rapid pace. Though ethical and financial considerations still exist, physicians should familiarize themselves with this evolving science. Publication Types: Review

Orv Hetil. 2005 May 15;146(20):995-1001. Related Articles, Links [Multidrug resistance: diagnostic approaches and difficulties] [Article in Hungarian] Rideg O, Csutora P, Magyarlaki T, Teibert A, Nagy T, Kovacs LG, Miseta A. Pecsi Tudomanyegyetem, Altalanos Orvostudomanyi Kar, Laboratoriumi

Medicina Intezet, Pecs. During the mid sixties scientists recognized that tumour cells can be resistant to a variety of chemotherapeutical drugs of different chemical structure simultaneously. They named this phenomenon multidrug resistance (MDR). Following this observation, number of in vitro and in vivo experiments proved that transmembrane proteins of the cell membrane are responsible for the mechanism. Many details of the underlying biochemical mechanisms were explored during the past decade. Nowadays the importance of MDR is well appreciated in different walks of medical science. MDR is an important problem during the treatment of many haematological conditions and solid organ tumors. Also, MDR is an important factor during immunosuppressant therapy of the transplanted patients. In spite of extensive research there are many uncertainties around MDR. This brief review describes the present options in the investigation of MDR. Based upon the MDR genotyping and expression level the likelihood of drug resistance may be predicted with reasonable accuracy. Additional information may be obtained by measuring the P-glycoprotein expression on the cell surface and the outward transport of test molecules from the cells. Although the tests described above provide significant help in predicting MDR or in the confirmation of existing MDR there is no consensus about the laboratory diagnosis. Publication Types: Review

Orv Hetil. 2005 May 22;146(21):1143-50. Related Articles, Links [Pharmacogenetics of inflammatory bowel disease] [Article in Hungarian] Hagymasi Krisztina, Tulassay Z. Semmelweis Egyetem, Altalanos Orvostudomanyi Kar, II. Belgyogyaszati Klinika, Budapest. hkriszti@bel2.sote.hu There are interindividual variations with regard to efficacy and toxicity of many commonly employed drugs. Major causes of interindividual differences of drug effects include genetic variations of drug-metabolizing enzymes, transporters and targets. Pharmacogenetics studies the genetic background of the interindividual variations of drug response. By means of preliminary genetic screening personalized treatment can be achieved, drugs with low efficacy and many side-effects can be avoided. The pharmacogenetically best studied medications of inflammatory bowel disease are azathioprine/6-mercaptopurine. It is obvious that there is a genetic background of the efficacy and toxicity of corticosteroids, 5-ASA drugs, infliximab and other immunosuppressors as well, but further studies now require to confirm the functional significance of it. Therefore, at present, the application and clinical usefulness of pharmacogenetics in the management of inflammatory bowel disease is limited. The aims of future investigations are understanding of the mechanism of drug action, identification of new drug targets and acquainting with genetic factors that determine drug response. Publication Types: Review

Osteoporos Int. 2005 Aug;16(8):857-60. Epub 2005 Feb 1. Related Articles, Links Comment on: Osteoporos Int. 2005 Aug;16(8):943-52. Pharmacogenetics of anti-resorptive therapy efficacy: a Bayesian interpretation. Nguyen TV. Publication Types: Comment Editorial

Pac Symp Biocomput. 2005;:245-7. Related Articles, Links Computational approaches for pharmacogenomics. Ritchie MD, Carillo MW, Wilke RA. Center for Human Genetics Research, Department of Molecular Physiology and Biophysics, Vanderbilt University, Nashville, TN 37232, USA.

Pac Symp Biocomput. 2005;:260-71. Related Articles, Links Enhancing data sharing in collaborative research projects with DASH. Ferrin TE, Huang CC, Greenblatt DM, Stryke D, Giacomini KM, Morris JH. Departments of Pharmaceutical Chemistry and Biopharmaceutical Sciences, University of California San Francisco, San Francisco, CA 94143, USA. We describe a software framework, called DASH, that enables the facile access, maintenance, curation and sharing of computational biology data among collaborating research scientists. The DASH event-based framework enables members of team-based research projects to describe the multistep computational processing pipelines frequently required to generate data for sharing, monitors multiple distributed data stores for changes, and will then automatically invoke the appropriate processing pipeline(s). These pipelines can be used to communicate the results of data analyses to collaborators using mechanisms such as Web Services. We describe the overall design of the DASH system and the application of a simple DASH prototype to a collaborative pharmacogenomics research project involving several dozen researchers located at several different sites--the UCSF Pharmacogenetics of Membrane Transporters project.

Pac Symp Biocomput. 2005;:272-83. Related Articles, Links Threshold gradient descent method for censored data regression with applications in pharmacogenomics. Gui J, Li H. Department of Statistics and Rowe Program in Genetics, University of California, Davis, CA 95616, USA. jgui@ucdavis.edu An important area of research in pharmacogenomics is to relate high-dimensional genetic or genomic data to various clinical phenotypes of patients. Due to large variability in time to certain clinical event among patients, studying possibly censored survival phenotypes can be more informative than treating the phenotypes as categorical variables. In this paper, we develop a threshold gradient descent (TGD) method for the Cox model to select genes that are relevant to patients' survival and to build a predictive model for the risk of a future patient. The computational difficulty associated with the estimation in the high-dimensional and low-sample size settings can be efficiently solved by the gradient descent iterations. Results from application to real data set on predicting survival after chemotherapy for patients with diffuse large B-cell lymphoma demonstrate that the proposed method can be used for identifying important genes that are related to time to death due to cancer and for building a parsimonious model for predicting the survival of future patients. The TGD based Cox regression gives better predictive performance than the L2 penalized regression and can select more relevant genes than the L1 penalized regression.

Pac Symp Biocomput. 2005;:296-307. Related Articles, Links Exploratory visual analysis of pharmacogenomic results. Reif DM, Dudek SM, Shaffer CM, Wang J, Moore JH. Computational Genetics Laboratory, Department of Genetics, Dartmouth Medical School, Lebanon, NH 03756, USA. reif@chgr.mc.vanderbilt.edu Comprehensive analysis of expansive pharmacogenomic datasets is a daunting challenge. A thorough exploration of experimental results requires both statistical and annotative information. Therefore, appropriate analysis tools must bring a readily-accessible, flexible combination of statistics and biological annotation to the user's desktop. We present the Exploratory Visual Analysis (EVA) software and database as such a tool and demonstrate its utility in replicating the findings of an earlier pharmacogenomic study as well as elucidating novel biologically plausible hypotheses. EVA brings all of the often disparate pieces of analysis together in an infinitely flexible visual display that is amenable to any type of statistical result and biological question. Here, we describe the motivations for developing EVA, detail the database and custom graphical user interface (GUI), provide an example of its application to a publicly available pharmacogenomic dataset, and discuss the broad utility of the EVA tool for the pharmacogenomics community.

Paediatr Nurs. 2004 Jul-Aug;16(6):32-5. Related Articles, Links Comment in: Paediatr Nurs. 2004 Jul-Aug;16(6):3. Adverse drug reactions (ADRs) in children: Part 1. Kanneh AB. City University, London. Publication Types: Review

Pain. 2005 Jul;116(1-2):73-8. Related Articles, Links The Val158Met polymorphism of the human catechol-O-methyltransferase (COMT) gene may influence morphine requirements in cancer pain patients. Rakvag TT, Klepstad P, Baar C, Kvam TM, Dale O, Kaasa S, Krokan HE, Skorpen F. Department of Cancer Research and Molecular Medicine, Faculty of Medicine, Norwegian University of Science and Technology (NTNU), N-7489 Trondheim, Norway. Catechol-O-methyltransferase (COMT) inactivates dopamine, epinephrine and norepinephrine in the nervous system. A common functional polymorphism (Val158Met) leads to a three- to-four-fold variation in the COMT enzyme activity, the Met form displaying lower enzymatic activity. The Val158Met polymorphism affects pain perception, and subjects with the Met/Met genotype have the most pronounced response to experimental pain. Based on this information we analyzed the influence from the COMT Val158Met polymorphism on the efficacy of morphine in a cohort of patients suffering from cancer pain. We genotyped 207 Caucasian cancer patients on morphine treatment with respect to the Val158Met polymorphism and compared the morphine doses, serum concentrations of morphine and morphine metabolites between the genotype groups. Patients with the Val/Val genotype (n=44) needed more morphine (155+/-160 mg/24 h) when compared to the Val/Met (117+/-100 mg/24 h; n=96) and the Met/Met genotype (95+/-99 mg/24 h; n=67) groups (P=0.025). This difference was not explained by other factors such as duration of morphine treatment, performance status, time since diagnosis, perceived pain intensity, adverse symptoms, or time until death. These results suggest that genetic variation in the COMT gene may contribute to variability in the efficacy of morphine in cancer pain treatment. Items 501 - 1000 of 1239 Previous of 3 Next 501: Neurol Sci. 2005 May;26 Suppl 2:s143-7. Related Articles, Links Pharmacogenetics of headache treatment. Montagna P, Pierangeli G, Cevoli S, Mochi M, Cortelli P. Department of Clinical Neurology, University of Bologna Medical School, Via Ugo Foscolo 7, I-40123, Bologna, Italy. pmontagn@neuro.unibo.it Headaches and migraines are widely prevalent diseases causing relevant disability and worsened quality of life. Several pharmacological options are available for headache therapy, mostly however without firm rationales and all having high rates of non-responders and often serious side effects. Variability of therapeutic effect and adverse events depend at least in part upon genetic variability, but the genetic factors involved are mostly unknown. Pharmacogenetics, i. e., the application of the knowledge of genomic diversity to the analysis of the phenotypic traits involved in therapeutic response and adverse events, is still in its infancy, but represents a promising approach to therapy in migraine. The extant evidence is summarised here, with special attention to pain therapy and the pharmacogenetics of the serotonergic and the dopaminergic systems.

Pathol Biol (Paris). 2004 Jul;52(6):332-7. Related Articles, Links [Pharmacogenetics and pharmacogenomics of cancers] [Article in French] Robert J. Institut Bergonie et universite Victor-Segalen, 229, cours de l'Argonne, 33076 Bordeaux, France. robert@bergonie.org Sequencing the human genome brings new tools for the individualisation of cancer chemotherapy, firstly thanks to the identification of polymorphisms of genes involved in anticancer drug metabolism or activity (Pharmacogenetics), and secondly thanks to the determination of tumour gene expression profiles and their relationship to chemosensitivity and chemoresistance (Pharmacogenomics). A few functional polymorphisms have been known for a long time (thiopurine methyltransferase, glutathion S-transferases), but several new ones have been identified recently, at the level of the genes encoding drug targets (thymidylate synthase), at the level of DNA repair enzymes (XPD) or at the level of transport proteins (MDR1). On the other hand, the research of correlations between gene expression profiles and chemosensitivity has been performed on the in vitro models of the National Cancer Institute and may allow crucial improvements in the identification of patients who would best take advantage of a specific chemotherapy. Clinical trials, first on a retrospective basis, then on a prospective one, are implemented to validate this approach. Publication Types: Review

Pathol Biol (Paris). 2005 Mar;53(2):116-24. Related Articles, Links [Pharmacogenetics of anticancer drugs.] [Article in French] de Chaisemartin L, Loriot MA. Service de biochimie generale, oncologie moleculaire et pharmacogenetique, hopital europeen Georges-Pompidou, Paris-XV, France. Much progress has been made in treating human malignancies and there are now multiple treatment options with similar efficacy for nearly every type of cancer. However, the narrow therapeutic index of most chemotherapeutic agents and the severe consequences of undertreatment or overdosing have led to research molecular predictive factors of the toxicity and efficacy of cancer treatments. Genetic factors affecting drug metabolism and transport partly explain interindividual variability in drug response. Pharmacogenetic focuses on the molecular mechanisms involved in drug response, and its ultimate goal is the optimisation of the treatments, that combines the optimal efficacy and the minimal risk of severe side effects. Polymorphisms in genes encoding specific drug-metabolising enzymes can result in individuals in the general population being characterised as low, rapid or even ultra-rapid metabolisers. Phenotyping and genotyping tests are now available that determine or predict the metabolic status of an individual and, thus, enable the evaluation of risk of drug failure or toxicity. Some clinical applications of pharmacogenetics (5-FU, irinotecan, thiopurines) have already been developed in routine medicine resulting in significant improvement in patient treatment. The clinical validation of an increasing number of pharmacogenetic tests, as well as the development of new highly efficient technologies for genotyping (real-time PCR, DNA chips...) should further promote pharmacogenetics in clinical practice and lead to the development of a patient-tailored drug therapy. Publication Types: Review

Pediatr Blood Cancer. 2004 Oct;43(5):536-8. Related Articles, Links Comment on: Pediatr Blood Cancer. 2004 Oct;43(5):552-9. Susceptibility to cancer: why did this happen to my child? Davies SM. Cincinnati Children's Hospital and Medical Center, Cincinnati, Ohio, USA. stella.davies@cchmc.org Publication Types: Comment

Pediatr Infect Dis J. 2004 Nov;23(11):1057-9. Related Articles, Links Alternative, age- and viral load-related routes of nelfinavir resistance in human immunodeficiency virus type 1-infected children receiving highly active antiretroviral therapy. Machado ES, Lambert JS, Afonso AO, Cunha SM, Oliveira RH, Tanuri A, Sill AM, Costa AJ, Soares MA. Servico de Doencas Infecciosas e Parasitarias, Hospital Universitario Clementino Fraga Filho, Universidade Federal do Rio de Janeiro, RJ, Brazil. emachado@biologia.ufrj.br To assess prevalence of nelfinavir resistance mutations in children receiving highly active antiretroviral therapy, sequencing of protease gene from plasma of 53 human immunodeficiency virus-infected children was performed. The prevalence of L90M was similar to that of D30N. There was a significant correlation with a higher viral load and lower age and the occurrence of L90M. These findings suggest differential molecular age- and viral load-related routes for nelfinavir resistance.

Pediatr Transplant. 2004 Dec;8(6):551-7. Related Articles, Links The impact of pharmacogenomic factors on steroid dependency in pediatric heart transplant patients using logistic regression analysis. Zheng HX, Webber SA, Zeevi A, Schuetz E, Zhang J, Lamba J, Boyle GJ, Wilson JW, Burckart GJ. School of Pharmacy, University of Southern California, Los Angeles, CA 90033, USA. Many pharmacogenomic predictors of drug response are now available, and include both drug metabolism-disposition factors and drug targets. Information on statistical approaches to analyzing large clinical data sets in relation to genetic polymorphisms is limited. The objective of this study was to evaluate whether logistic regression could identify pharmacogenomic predictors of outcome in a large data set in a complex transplant patient population. Seventy pediatric heart transplant patients were studied. Patients were followed for at least 1 yr post-transplantation as outpatients, and weaned from corticosteroids if clinically appropriate. Logistic regression analysis was used to identify the predictors of steroid dependency. The dependent variable was the presence or absence of steroid therapy at 1 yr post-transplantation. The independent variables were the patients' transplant age, gender, MDR1 C3435T and G2677T, CYP3A53B and cytokine polymorphisms. By chi-square test for the MDR1 C3435T polymorphism, 12 of 18 (67%) patients in the CC group were still on prednisone, whereas only 18 of 47 (38%) of the CT/TT group were still receiving prednisone ($p = 0.04$). For the IL-10 groups, two of 15 patients with the high producer genotype (13.3%) remained on prednisone, in comparison with 16 of 28 patients with the intermediate producer genotype (57.1%) and 15 of 26 patients with the low producer genotype (57.7%, $p = 0.01$). Logistic regression analysis confirmed MDR1 C3435T ($p = 0.021$), and IL-10 polymorphisms (intermediate producer genotype $p = 0.015$; low producer genotype p = 0.013) as independent risk factors for steroid dependency at 1 yr after transplantation. This approach identifies pharmacogenomic factors, which can be studied more extensively in larger data sets, and used in prospective studies to individualize immunosuppressive therapy following solid organ transplantation.

Pharm Res. 2004 Apr;21(4):555-66. Related Articles, Links Neonatal exposure to drugs in breast milk. McNamara PJ, Abbassi M. College of Pharmacy, University of Kentucky, Lexington, Kentucky 40536, USA. pmcnamar@email.uky.edu There are many benefits of breast-feeding both for the infant and for the mother. Nursing mothers who are also taking medications or exposed to environmental hazards may be confronted with a difficult choice to discontinue nursing or maternal medication or risk potential harm to the infant. Frequently, these decisions are made without sufficient information or understanding of the factors influencing exposure. The current review explores two indices of exposure, together with their pharmacokinetic determinants. Both of the indices include the milk to serum (M/S) concentration ratio for a given drug and the volume of milk consumed. The first exposure term, EI(Dose), expresses neonatal dose as a percentage of maternal dose and is inversely related to the maternal systemic clearance. By contrast, the second exposure term, EI(Conc), expresses infant concentration as a percentage of maternal concentration and is inversely related to the infant systemic clearance. Issues related to intersubject variation in M/S (e.g., colostrum vs. mature milk, fore vs. hind milk) and infant clearance (e.g., ontogeny of elimination pathways, pharmacogenetics) and their role in modulating exposure are also discussed. Publication Types: Review

Pharm Res. 2004 May;21(5):777-80. Related Articles, Links Analysis of pharmacokinetics, pharmacodynamics, and pharmacogenomics data sets using VizStruct, a novel multidimensional visualization technique. Bhasi K, Zhang L, Zhang A, Ramanathan M. Department of Pharmaceutical Sciences, State University of New York at Buffalo, Buffalo, New York 14260, USA. PURPOSE: Data visualization techniques for the pharmaceutical sciences have not been extensively investigated. The purpose of this study was to evaluate the usefulness of VizStruct, a multidimensional visualization tool, for applications in pharmacokinetics, pharmacodynamics, and pharmacogenomics. METHODS: The VizStruct tool uses the first harmonic of the discrete Fourier transform to map multidimensional data to two dimensions for visualization. The mapping was used to visualize several published pharmacokinetic, pharmacodynamic, and pharmacogenomic data sets. The VizStruct approach was evaluated using simulated population pharmacokinetics data sets, the data from Dalen and colleagues (Clin. PharmacoL Ther. 63:444-452, 1998) on the kinetics of nortriptyline and its 10-hydroxynortriptyline metabolite in subjects with differing number of copies of the CYP2D6, and the gene expression profiling data of Bohen and colleagues (Proc. Natl. Acad. Sci. USA 100:1926-1930, 2003) on follicular lymphoma patients responsive and nonresponsive to rituximab. RESULTS: The VizStruct mapping preserves the key characteristics of multidimensional data in two dimensions in a manner that facilitates visualization. The mapping is computationally efficient and can be used for cluster detection and class prediction in pharmaceutical data sets. The VizStruct visualization succinctly summarized the salient similarities and differences in the nortriptyline and 10-hydroxynortriptyline pharmacokinetic profiles in subjects with increasing number of CYP2D6 gene copies. In the simulated population pharmacokinetic data sets, it was capable of discriminating the subtle differences between pharmacokinetic profiles derived from 1- and 2-compartment models with the same area under the curve. The two-dimensional VizStruct mapping computed from a subset of 102 informative genes from the Bohen and colleagues data set effectively separated the rituximab responder, rituximab nonresponder, and control subject groups. CONCLUSIONS: The VizStruct approach is a computationally efficient and effective approach for visualizing complex, multidimensional data sets. It could have many useful applications in the pharmaceutical sciences. Publication Types: Review

Pharm Res. 2005 Oct;22(10):1597-613. Epub 2005 Sep 22. Related Articles, Links VeloceGenomics: an accelerated in vivo drug discovery approach to rapidly predict the biologic, drug-like activity of compounds, proteins, or genes. Papoian R, Scherer A, Saulnier M, Staedtler F, Cordier A, Legay F, Maurer G, Staeheli J, Vonderscher J, Chibout SD. Department of Exploratory Development, Biomarker Development, Novartis Pharma A.G., Postfach, 4002, Basel, Switzerland. PURPOSE: The aim of this study is to test the predictive power of in vivo multiorgan RNA expression profiling in identifying the biologic activity of molecules. METHODS: Animals were treated with compound A or B. At the end of the treatment period, in vivo multiorgan microarray-based gene expression data were collected. Investigators masked to the identity of the compounds analyzed the transcriptome signatures to define the molecular pathways affected by treatment and to hypothesize the biologic activity and potential therapeutic indications of the blinded compounds. RESULTS: For compound A, G-protein-coupled receptors and factors associated with cell growth were affected-growth hormone/insulin-like growth factor-1, glucagon/insulin axes, and general somatomedin-like activity. Deblinding showed the compound to be a somatostatin analog, SOM230, confirming the accuracy of the predicted biologic activity. For compound B, components of the inflammatory cascade potentially mediated by lipopolysaccharide, tumor necrosis factor, or proinflammatory cytokines were affected. The gene expression signatures were most consistent with an interleukin-6 family activity. Deblinding revealed that compound B was leukemia inhibitory factor. CONCLUSIONS: VeloceGenomics is a strategy of coupling in vivo compound testing with genomic technologies. The process enables prediction of the mechanism of action and, coupled with other relevant data, prediction of the suitability of compounds for advancement in the drug development process.

Pharm World Sci. 2004 Oct;26(5):253-5. Related Articles, Links Pharmacogenetics in health-care practice. Maitland-van ZA, Klungel OH, de Boer A. Department of Pharmacoepidemiology and Pharmacotherapy, Utrecht Institute of Pharmaceutical Sciences, Utrecht University, Utrecht, The Netherlands. amaitland@sph.uth.tmc.edu Publication Types: Review

Pharm World Sci. 2005 Feb;27(1):20-30. Related Articles, Links Erratum in: Pharm World Sci. 2005 Jun;27(3):267.

Pharmacogenetics as a tool in the therapy of schizophrenia. Wilffert B, Zaal R, Brouwers JR. Department of Social Pharmacy, Pharmacoepidemiology and Pharmacotherapy, Groningen University Institute for Drug Exploration (GUIDE), Groningen, The Netherlands [corrected] B.Wilffert@znb.nl AIM: This review summarises the present knowledge of associations between pharmacogenetics and therapeutic efficacy and side effects of antipsychotics to enable pharmacists to judge the applicability for a more tailor made therapy in patients with schizophrenia. Polymorphisms of Cytochrome P450 isoenzymes and neurotransmitter receptors involved in the efficacy and side effects of antipsychotics are highlighted in this review. METHOD: A search was performed in Medline and EMBASE for the period 1995-August 2002. Also relevant references from the selected papers were incorporated. RESULTS: Poor metabolism with respect to CYP2D6 seems to be related with more pronounced extrapyramidal symptoms and more specifically with a higher incidence of tardive dyskinesia. The C/C-genotype for CYP1A2 results in smokers in a reduction of enzyme activity, but an effect on the incidence of tardive dyskinesia is controversial. For dopamine D2 receptors the effect of the -141C Ins/Del polymorphism on efficacy is not clear yet, although the Taq I polymorphism is associated with greater improvement of positive, but not negative symptoms in acute psychosis. The Gly9-allele of the dopamine D3 receptor is associated with the response to clozapine, but in studies in which the choice of antipsychotics is not restricted, the role of this polymorphism is unclear. The reverse is applicable to the dopamine D(4.2/4.7) polymorphism. For the 5-HT2A receptor the His452Tyr polymorphism is associated with response to clozapine, the 102 T/C polymorphism leads to equivocal results. The polymorphism studied for 5-HT5A, 5-HT6, alpha1A- and alpha2A-receptors give no clear associations with the response to clozapine. The polymorphism studied of the dopamine D2 and D4 receptor are not related to extrapyramidal adverse effects and side effects, respectively. The 9Gly-variant of the dopamine D3 receptor, the 102C-variant, but not the His452Tyr polymorphism of the 5-HT2A-receptor and the 23Ser-variant (for females only) of the 5-HT2C receptor seem to increase the susceptibility to tardive dyskinesia. Weight gain induced by antipsychotics seems to be associated with the -759C-allele of the 5-HT2C receptor. CONCLUSION: The results show the first careful steps toward application of pharmacogenetics in a more individualised, tailor-made, pharmacotherapy. A pre-condition seems to be a multifactorial approach, as can be expected for multifactorial processes. Publication Types: Review

Pharmacoeconomics. 2004;22(8):481-93. Related Articles, Links The role of cost-effectiveness analysis in the era of pharmacogenomics. Flowers CR, Veenstra D. Pharmaceutical Outcomes Research and Policy Program, University of Washington Medical Center, Seattle, Washington, USA. crflowe@emory.org The broad availability of genetic information and technologies heralds an era when practitioners will utilise genomic testing to individualise patients' care. Pharmacogenomics uses a spectrum of approaches to explore the association of genetic variation with drug efficacy or toxicity. Investigators have described a broad array of genetic polymorphisms that confer inter-individual differences in drug response. Pharmacogenomics offers the potential to improve drug effectiveness, reduce adverse drug reactions and provide cost-effective care. However, it has had little impact on current clinical practice and the economic implications of pharmacogenomics remain unclear. Assessing the incremental cost effectiveness of a pharmacogenomic strategy involves examination of factors associated with the genotype of interest, the genomic test, the disease state and the treatment. A pharmacogenomic strategy is likely to be cost effective when: (i) the polymorphism under consideration is prevalent in the population and has a high degree of penetrance; (ii) genetic testing is highly sensitive and specific, and less costly alternative tests that could be used to individualise therapy are not readily available; (iii) the disease state involves outcomes with significant morbidity or mortality if left untreated; and (iv) the treatment involves significant outcomes and/or costs that can be impacted by genotype-individualised therapy. We foresee pharmacogenomic applications being particularly relevant for drugs: with a narrow therapeutic index or a high degree of variability in inter-individual response; where there are limitations in current methods for monitoring their adverse effects and treatment responses; and where there are few alternative treatment options. Because of the characteristics of chemotherapeutic agents and the severity of clinical outcomes in cancer, oncology appears to be one of the most appropriate disease areas for the application of pharmacogenomics. We have developed a framework which can assist researchers, pharmacists, physicians, and policy makers in evaluating the implications of specific strategies, and identifying when formal cost-effectiveness analyses should be conducted to quantitatively evaluate the benefits of pharmacogenomics. Publication Types: Review

Pharmacoeconomics. 2004;22(8):495-8. Related Articles, Links Comment in: Pharmacoeconomics. 2005;23(5):527. Pharmacogenomics and the evolution of healthcare : is it time for cost-effectiveness analysis at the individual level? Bala MV, Zarkin GA. Centocor Inc., Malvern, Pennsylvania 19355, USA. mbala@cntus.jnj.com The efficacy and toxicity of any given drug can vary substantially from one individual to another. The heterogeneity in individual genetics contributes, in part, to this variability. Pharmacogenomics uses each patient's individual genetic information to identify the drug with the best efficacy-safety profile for that patient. However, heterogeneity is also present in individuals' preferences for alternate efficacy-safety profiles. We argue that as healthcare evolves towards individualised drug therapy, preference elicitation and cost-effectiveness analysis should also be performed at the individual level to maximise societal welfare.

Pharmacoeconomics. 2005;23(5):445-7. Related Articles, Links Does pharmacogenomics provide an ethical challenge to the utilisation of cost-effectiveness analysis by public health systems? La Caze A. School of Pharmacy, University of Queensland, Queensland, Australia. alacaze@pharmacy.uq.edu.au Pharmacogenomics promotes an understanding of the genetic basis for differences in efficacy or toxicity of drugs in different individuals. Implementation of the outcomes of pharmacogenomic research into clinical practice presents a number of difficulties for healthcare. This paper aims to highlight one of the unique ethical challenges which pharmacogenomics presents for the utilisation of cost-effectiveness analysis by public health systems. This paper contends that pharmacogenomics provides a challenge to fundamental principles which underlie most systems for deciding which drugs should be publicly subsidised. Pharmacogenomics brings into focus the conflict between equality and utility in the context of using cost-effectiveness analysis to aid distribution of a limited national drug budget.

Pharmacoeconomics. 2005;23(5):527. Related Articles, Links Comment on: Pharmacoeconomics. 2004;22(8):495-8. On pharmacogenomics and cost-effectiveness analysis at the individual level. Bala MV, Zarkin GA. Publication Types: Comment Letter

Pharmacoepidemiol Drug Saf. 2006 Feb;15(2):99-105. Related Articles, Links Pharmacogenetics of drug-induced arrhythmias: a feasibility study using spontaneous adverse drug reactions reporting data. De Bruin ML, van Puijenbroek EP, Bracke M, Hoes AW, Leufkens HG. Utrecht Institute for Pharmaceutical Sciences (UIPS), Department of Pharmacoepidemiology and Pharmacotherapy, Utrecht, The Netherlands. m.l.debruin@pharm.uu.nl PURPOSE: The bottleneck in pharmacogenetic research on rare adverse drug reactions (ADR) is retrieval of patients. Spontaneous reports of ADRs may form a useful source of patients. We investigated the feasibility of a pharmacogenetic study, in which cases were selected from the database of a spontaneous reporting system for ADRs, using drug-induced arrhythmias as an example. METHODS: Reports of drug-induced arrhythmias to proarrhythmic drugs were selected from the database of the Netherlands Pharmacovigilance Centre (1996-2003). Information on the patient's general practitioner (GP) was obtained from the original report, or from another health care provider who reported the event. GPs were contacted and asked to recruit the patient as well as two age, gender and drug matched controls. Patients were asked to fill a questionnaire and provide a buccal swab DNA sample through the mail. DNA samples were screened for 10 missense mutations in 5 genes associated with the congenital long-QT (LQT) syndrome (KCNQ1, KCNH2, SCN5A, KCNE1, KCNE2). RESULTS: We identified 45 eligible cases, 29 GPs could be contacted of which seven were willing to participate. Four cases and five matched controls could be included in the study, giving an overall participation rate of 9% (4/45). The main reason for GPs not being willing to participate was lack of time. Variants were identified in KCNH2, SCN5A and KCNE1. CONCLUSIONS: Spontaneous reporting systems for ADRs may be used for pharmacogenetic research. The methods described, however, need to be improved to increase participation and international collaboration may be required. Copyright 2005 John Wiley and Sons, Ltd.

Pharmacogenet Genomics. 2005 Apr;15(4):193-4. Related Articles, Links Comment on: Pharmacogenet Genomics. 2005 Apr;15(4):195-200. Weight gain with antipsychotic drugs: the role of the 5-HT2C receptor (HTR2C) and other genes. Harrison PJ. University Department of Psychiatry, Warneford Hospital, Oxford, UK. paul.harrison@pysch.ox.ac.uk Publication Types: Comment

Pharmacogenet Genomics. 2005 Apr;15(4):195-200. Related Articles, Links Comment in: Pharmacogenet Genomics.

2005 Apr;15(4):193-4. Polymorphisms of the 5-HT2C receptor and leptin genes are associated with antipsychotic drug-induced weight gain in Caucasian subjects with a first-episode psychosis. Templeman LA, Reynolds GP, Arranz B, San L. Division of Psychiatry and Neuroscience, Queen's University Belfast, Whitla Medical Building, 97 Lisburn Road, Belfast BT9 7BL, UK. OBJECTIVES: Weight gain, leading to further morbidity and poor treatment adherence, is a common consequence of treatment with antipsychotic drugs. Two recent studies in the same cohort of Chinese Han subjects have shown that polymorphisms of the promoter regions of both the serotonin 5-hydroxytryptamine 2C (5-HT2C) receptor and the leptin genes, are associated with antipsychotic-induced weight gain over 10 weeks. We have investigated whether these effects remain true in a Caucasian population and following longer term treatment. METHODS: Seventy-three Spanish caucasian patients with a first-episode psychosis and initially drug-naive were genotyped for the 5-HT2C receptor -759C/T and leptin -2548A/G polymorphisms. Body mass index and plasma leptin levels were monitored after 6 weeks, 3 months and 9 months of antipsychotic treatment. RESULTS: Patients with the -759T variant allele showed significantly less weight gain than those without this allele. This effect held true in the smaller group of patients receiving olanzapine. The -2548 leptin polymorphism was not associated with short-term (6 week and 3 month) weight increases but did show significant association with 9-month antipsychotic-induced weight gain. The 5-HT2C -759 genotype was significantly associated with pre-treatment plasma leptin levels. CONCLUSIONS: These findings confirm the importance of two genetic factors associated with long-term antipsychotic-induced weight increases in schizophrenia, and implicate a role for leptin in the 5-HT receptor-mediated weight regulation.

Pharmacogenet Genomics. 2005 Apr;15(4):201-9. Related Articles, Links Functional analysis of polymorphisms in the organic anion transporter, SLC22A6 (OAT1). Fujita T, Brown C, Carlson EJ, Taylor T, de la Cruz M, Johns SJ, Stryke D, Kawamoto M, Fujita K, Castro R, Chen CW, Lin ET, Brett CM, Burchard EG, Ferrin TE, Huang CC, Leabman MK, Giacomini KM. Department of Pharmacology, Kitasato University School of Medicine, Sagamihara, Kanagawa, 228-8555, Japan. OBJECTIVES: The organic anion transporter, OAT1 (SLC22A6), plays a role in the renal elimination of many drugs and environmental toxins. The goal of this study was to identify and functionally characterize OAT1 variants as a first step towards understanding whether genetic variation in OAT1 may contribute to interindividual differences in renal elimination of xenobiotics. METHODS: As part of a larger study, 276 DNA samples from an ethnically diverse population were screened and 12 coding region variants of OAT1 were identified. The non-synonymous variants were then constructed and characterized in Xenopus laevis oocytes. A small family-based clinical study was conducted to determine the renal elimination of a model OAT1 substrate, adefovir (an antiviral agent) in human subjects who possessed a non-functional variant, OAT1-R454Q. RESULTS: Six non-synonymous variants were identified; two (OAT1-R50 H and OAT1-R293W) were present at > or = 1% in at least one ethnic population. These two variants exhibited normal uptake of p-aminohippurate, ochratoxin A and methotrexate assayed in X. laevis oocytes.

One variant, OAT1-R454Q, was non-functional with respect to the above substrates. In the clinical study, there was no significant decrease in the renal secretory clearance of adefovir in family members heterozygous for OAT1-454Q in comparison to those with the reference transporter, OAT1-454R. CONCLUSIONS: These data indicate that the coding region of OAT1 has low genetic and functional diversity and suggest that coding region variants of OAT1 may not contribute substantially to interindividual differences in renal elimination of xenobiotics.

Pharmacogenet Genomics. 2005 Apr;15(4):211-8. Related Articles, Links Influence of microsomal triglyceride transfer protein promoter polymorphism -493 GT on fasting plasma triglyceride values and interaction with treatment response to atorvastatin in subjects with heterozygous familial hypercholesterolaemia. Garcia-Garcia AB, Gonzalez C, Real JT, Martin de Llano JJ, Gonzalez-Albert V, Civera M, Chaves FJ, Ascaso JF, Carmena R. Unidad Mixta de Investigacion, Hospital Clinico Universitario de Valencia, Spain. Familial hypercholesterolaemia (FH) is an autosomal dominant disease characterized by elevated levels of low-density lipoprotein-cholesterol (LDL-C). Phenotypic expression is highly variable, being influenced by diet, age, gender, body mass index, apolipoprotein E genotype and type of LDL-receptor gene mutation. Microsomal triglyceride (TG) transfer protein (MTP) is a protein involved in lipid metabolism. Polymorphism MTP -493 GT has been shown to modulate lipid levels in several populations. To analyse the effect of this polymorphism in the lipid phenotype expression of FH and treatment response, we studied a sample of 222 Spanish FH patients, of whom 147 were studied before and after treatment with 20 mg of atorvastatin daily during 6 weeks. The variant was analysed by polymerase chain reaction amplification and single-strand confirmation polymorphism. Treatment reduced LDL-C, total cholesterol and TGs. Baseline fasting TGs and very-low-density lipoprotein cholesterol levels were lower in female T allele carriers (TG: 111+/-51 mg/dl GG, 89+/-35 mg/dl GT, 83+/-26 mg/dl TT, P=0.022; very-low-density lipoprotein cholesterol: 24+/-13 mg/dl GG, 16+/-5 mg/dl GT, 17+/-5 mg/dl TT, P=0.018). Triglyceride response to atorvastatin was modulated by this polymorphism in men (P=0.009), but not in women, although differences between genotypes were maintained after treatment. In conclusion, the MTP -493 GT polymorphism modulates pre- and post-treatment plasma TG values of FH in Spanish subjects in a gender-specific way. Other environmental and genetic factors likely also modulate this response.

Pharmacogenet Genomics. 2005 Apr;15(4):219-25. Related Articles, Links Genetic and environmental factors affecting the response to statin therapy in patients with molecularly defined familial hypercholesterolaemia. Miltiadous G, Xenophontos S, Bairaktari E, Ganotakis M, Cariolou M, Elisaf M. Department of Internal Medicine, Medical School, University of Ioannina, Ioannina, Greece. Familial hypercholesterolaemia (FH) is the most common inherited metabolic disease characterized by elevated serum levels of low-density lipoprotein cholesterol (LDL-C) and ischaemic heart disease early in life. Early diagnosis and treatment are essential to prevent premature atherosclerosis in FH patients. The aim of our study was the evaluation of the effects of genetic [class of the LDL receptor (LDLR) gene mutation, apolipoprotein (apo)E, apoA-IV and cholesterol ester transfer protein gene polymorphisms] and environmental factors (age, sex, smoking habit and body mass index) on the lipid-lowering response to statin therapy in patients with molecularly defined FH. Atorvastatin 20 mg/day was prescribed in 49 patients with heterozygous FH. The lipid profile was examined before and after 12 weeks of therapy. Statin therapy resulted in a decrease of 37% and 36% in LDL-C and apoB levels, respectively. The study population was then divided into 2 groups according to the class of the LDLR mutation [patients sharing a class V mutation (the G1775A mutation, n=21) and patients sharing class II mutations (the G1646A and the C858A mutations, n=28)]. In both groups, the percentage decrement in LDL-C and apoB levels were correlated with the initial LDL-C and apoB levels, respectively. The class of the LDLR mutation affected the LDL-C and apoB-lowering response of heterozygous FH patients to statin therapy. In detail, heterozygotes sharing a class V mutation of the LDLR showed a higher percentage decrement in LDL-C and apoB levels after atorvastatin administration compared to patients sharing class II mutations (49+/-9% versus 34+/-9%, P=0.001 for LDL-C and 42+/-16% versus 35+/-20%, P=0.001 for apoB). The influence of the classes of the LDLR gene mutations on the change of LDL-C and apoB levels to atorvastatin was still significant in a multivariate analysis. None of the other genetic and environmental factors studied affected the lipid-lowering response to atorvastatin therapy in patients with heterozygous FH in a multivariate analysis. Our data indicate that the class of the LDLR gene mutation affects the LDL-C and apoB-lowering response of heterozygous FH patients to statin therapy. Specifically, patients with a class V mutation exhibit higher percentage decrease in LDL-C and apoB levels after statin therapy compared to patients sharing class II mutations.

Pharmacogenet Genomics. 2005 Apr;15(4):227-34. Related Articles, Links
Beta1-adrenergic receptor polymorphisms and left ventricular remodeling changes in response to beta-blocker therapy. Terra SG, Hamilton KK, Pauly DF, Lee CR, Patterson JH, Adams KF, Schofield RS, Belgado BS, Hill JA, Aranda JM, Yarandi HN, Johnson JA. Department of Pharmacy Practice, University of Florida College of Pharmacy, Gainesville, FL 32610, USA. OBJECTIVE: Large variability exists in the improvement in left ventricular (LV) function from beta-blocker treatment. We hypothesized that polymorphisms at codon 389 (Arg389Gly) and 49 (Ser49Gly) in the beta1-adrenergic receptor (AR) gene were associated with LV reverse remodeling changes in response to beta-blocker therapy among heart failure patients. METHODS: We prospectively enrolled 61 beta-blocker naive patients with systolic heart failure. Patients underwent baseline echocardiography followed by metoprolol CR/XL. The dose was doubled on a biweekly basis up to 200 mg/day or attainment of maximum tolerated dose. Echocardiography was repeated after the patient received the target or highest tolerated dose for 3 months. RESULTS: Among patients with the Arg389Arg genotype, ejection fraction (EF) increased from 23+/-5 to 29+/-10 (P=0.008). Gly389 carriers did not demonstrate any significant change in EF (22+/-9 to 23+/-11; P=0.45). There was a significant between-group difference in EF by genotype (P=0.04). The Arg389Arg genotype was also associated with significantly greater reductions in LV end-diastolic and end-

systolic diameters compared to Gly389 carriers. Patients with the Gly49 variant also had a significantly greater reduction in LV end-diastolic diameter compared to Ser49 homozygotes. Multiple regression analysis modeling revealed that the codon 389 polymorphism was a significant predictor of an improvement in EF and both codon 49 and 389 polymorphisms were significant predictors of final LV end-diastolic diameter. CONCLUSIONS: Heart failure patients with the Arg389Arg genotype and Gly49 carriers had greater improvements in LV remodeling from beta-blocker treatment.

Pharmacogenet Genomics. 2005 Apr;15(4):235-44. Related Articles, Links Preferred mexiletine block of human sodium channels with IVS4 mutations and its pH-dependence. Mohammadi B, Jurkat-Rott K, Alekov A, Dengler R, Bufler J, Lehmann-Horn F. Department of Neurology, Medical School Hannover, Hannover, Germany. The effects of extracellular pH (6.2, 7.4 and 8.2) and 0.1 mM mexiletine, a channel blocker of the lidocaine type, are studied on two mutations of the fourth voltage sensor of the Nav1.4 sodium channel, R1448H/C. The fast inactivated channel state to which mexiletine preferentially binds is destabilized by the mutations. By contrast to the expected low response of R1448H/C carriers, mexiletine is particularly effective in preventing exercise-induced stiffness and paralysis from which these patients suffer. Our measurements performed in the whole-cell mode on stably transfected HEK cells show for the first time that the mutations strikingly accelerate closed-state inactivation and, as steady-state fast inactivation is shifted to more negative potentials, stabilize the fast inactivated channel state in the potential range around the resting potential. At pH 7.4 and 8.2, the phasic mexiletine block is larger for R1448C (55%) and R1448H (47%) than for wild-type channels (31%) due to slowed recovery from block (tau is approximately 520 ms for R1448C versus 270 ms for wild-type at pH 7.4) although the recovery from inactivation is slightly faster for the mutants (tau is approximately 1.9 ms for R1448C versus 3.8 ms for wild-type at pH 7.4). At pH 6.2, recovery from block is relatively fast (tau is approximately 35 ms for R1448H/C and 14 ms for wild-type) and thus shows no use-dependence. We conclude that enhanced closed-state inactivation expands the concept of a mutation-induced uncoupling of channel inactivation from activation to a new potential range and that the higher mexiletine efficacy in R1448H/C carriers compared to other myotonic patients offers a pharmacogenetic strategy for mutation-specific treatment.

Pharmacogenet Genomics. 2005 Apr;15(4):245-56. Related Articles, Links Haplotype and functional analysis of four flavin-containing monooxygenase isoform 2 (FMO2) polymorphisms in Hispanics. Krueger SK, Siddens LK, Henderson MC, Andreasen EA, Tanguay RL, Pereira CB, Cabacungan ET, Hines RN, Ardlie KG, Williams DE. Department of Environmental and Molecular Toxicology, Oregon State University, Corvallis, OR 97331, USA. OBJECTIVES: Previous work defined two flavin-containing monooxygenase 2 (FMO2) alleles. The major allele, FMO2*2 (g.23,238C>T), encodes truncated inactive protein (p.X472) whereas the minor allele, FMO2*1, present in African- and Hispanic-American populations, encodes active protein (p.Q472). Recently, four common (27 to 51% incidence) FMO2 single nucleotide polymorphisms (SNPs) were detected in African-Americans

(N=50); they encode the following protein variants: p.71Ddup, p.V113fs, p.S195L and p.N413 K. Our objectives were to: (1) determine the incidence of these SNPs in 29 Hispanic individuals previously genotyped as g.23,238C (p.Q472) and 124 previously genotyped as homozygous g.23,238 T (p.X472); (2) determine FMO2 haplotypes in this population; and (3) assess the functional impact of SNPs in expressed proteins. METHODS: SNPs were detected via allele-specific oligonucleotide amplification coupled with real-time or electrophoretic product detection, or single strand conformation polymorphism. RESULTS: The g.7,700_7,702dupGAC SNP (p.71Ddup) was absent. The remaining SNPs were present but, except for g.13,732C>T (p.S195L), were less common in the current Hispanic study population versus the previously described African-Americans. Only expressed p.N413 K was as active as p.Q472, as determined by methimazole- and ethylenethiourea-dependent oxidation. Haplotype determination demonstrated that the g.10,951delG (p.V113fs), g.13,732C>T (p.S195L) and g.22,060T>G (p.N413 K) variants segregated with g.23,238C>T (p.X472). CONCLUSIONS: SNPs would not alter FMO2 activity in individuals possessing at least one FMO2*1 allele. It is likely that these SNPs will segregate similarly in African-American populations. Therefore, estimates that 26% of African-Americans and 2-7% of Hispanic-Americans have at least one FMO2*1 allele should closely reflect the percentages producing active FMO2 protein.

Pharmacogenet Genomics. 2005 Apr;15(4):257-64. Related Articles, Links
The naturally occurring Arg219Leu variant of the human 5-HT1A receptor: impairment of signal transduction. Bruss M, Kostanian A, Bonisch H, Gothert M. Institute of Pharmacology and Toxicology, University of Bonn, Bonn, Germany. m.bruess@uni-bonn.de The present study in transfected HEK293 cells aimed to investigate whether the pharmacological and/or transductional properties of the naturally occurring Arg219Leu variant (VAR) in the third intracellular loop of the h5-HT1A receptor differ from those of the wild-type receptor. Binding of [3H]8-hydroxy-2-(di-n-propylamino)tetraline ([H]8-OH-DPAT) and of [35S]GTPgammaS to membranes, as well as inhibition of forskolin-stimulated [3H]cAMP formation by 5-HT receptor agonists in whole cells, were estimated. The VAR and wild-type h5-HT1A receptors were found to be expressed at virtually identical densities. The VAR and wild-type receptors did also not differ with respect to the potencies of 5-HT receptor agonists and antagonists in inhibiting [3H]8-OH-DPAT binding. The ability of 5-HT to stimulate [35S]GTPgammaS binding (a measure of G protein coupling) to the VAR receptor and of the agonists 5-HT, buspirone and urapidil to inhibit forskolin-stimulated cAMP accumulation in HEK293 cells expressing the VAR receptor was decreased by 60-90%. In conclusion, the Arg219Leu variation of the human 5-HT1A receptor does not change the binding properties, but is associated with a drastic impairment of signal transduction. In patients carrying this variation, disturbances of 5-HT1A receptor-mediated functions and diminished responses to drugs acting via this receptor may occur.

Pharmacogenet Genomics. 2005 Dec;15(12):883-9. Related Articles, Links
Pharmacogenetics and obesity: common gene variants influence weight loss response of the norepinephrine/dopamine

transporter inhibitor GW320659 in obese subjects. Spraggs CF, Pillai SG, Dow D, Douglas C, McCarthy L, Manasco PK, Stubbins M, Roses AD. Genetics Research, GlaxoSmithKline Research and Development, Medicines Research Centre, Stevenage, UK. colin.f.spragg@gsk.com BACKGROUND: GW320659, a highly selective neuronal norepinephrine and dopamine re-uptake inhibitor, has been evaluated for the treatment of obesity. Scrutiny of the weight loss data from a phase II study (GlaxoSmithKline study OBS20001) showed a wide variation in weight loss response following GW320659 treatment and the possibility that the study population might include subgroups with enhanced weight loss response. METHODS: Pharmacogenetic analysis was performed in 191 subjects prospectively ascertained from a Phase II dose ranging study to evaluate the influence of genotype on weight loss efficacy and safety of GW320659 in obese subjects. RESULTS: Common genetic polymorphisms in the drug target (norepinephrine transporter protein 1, SLC6A2) and mechanism pathway (NMDA receptor channel NR1 subunit, GRIN1) were associated with increased weight loss following GW320659 treatment in a proportion (36%) of the study population. In the patient subgroup selected for these genotypes, GW320659 (15 mg/day) produced a significant difference in mean weight loss of 7.84 kg (SD 5.23, n = 14), compared to 2.53 kg (SD 5.17, n = 24) in the subgroup that did not possess the genotypes (P = 0.006). This subgroup also showed a highly significant weight loss response for GW320659 compared to placebo (+0.31 kg, SD 3.32, n = 16) with the same genotypes (P < 0.0001). In addition, there was no difference in placebo response between either subgroup. CONCLUSIONS: Polymorphisms in SLC6A2 and GRIN1 could be used to maximize effective obesity pharmacotherapy by norepinephrine/dopamine transporter inhibitors by identifying patients that may be predisposed to particularly good treatment weight loss response. Publication Types: Clinical Trial, Phase II Multicenter Study Randomized Controlled Trial

Pharmacogenet Genomics. 2005 Feb;15(2):61-7. Related Articles, Links Pharmacogenetics in the treatment of depression: pharmacodynamic studies. Serretti A, Artioli P, Quartesan R. Department of Psychiatry, Vita-Salute University, San Raffaele Hospital, Milan Italy. serretti.alessandro@hsr.it The pharmacological treatment of mood disorders has reduced their morbidity and improved mental health for millions of individuals worldwide, favouring a considerable reduction of the direct and indirect costs caused by these common pathologies. Unfortunately, not all individuals benefit, and 30-40% of patients do not show a complete response to treatment. Efficient clinical predictors are not available, although genetic factors are thought to play a substantial (but complex) role in the antidepressant response. Pharmacogenetics, which investigates the influence of genetic features on the pharmacological response, has gained increasing attention and holds great promise for clinical psychiatry. Here, a brief overview is provided on the various pharmacogenetic studies published to date that analyse the commonest treatments for depression: antidepressants, sleep deprivation and lithium salts. Publication Types: Review

Pharmacogenet Genomics. 2005 Jan;15(1):1-5. Related Articles, Links Influence of CYP2B6 polymorphism on plasma and intracellular concentrations and toxicity of efavirenz and nevirapine in HIV-infected patients. Rotger M, Colombo S, Furrer H, Bleiber G, Buclin T, Lee BL, Keiser O, Biollaz J, Decosterd L, Telenti A; Swiss HIV Cohort Study. Institute of Microbiology and Section of Infectious Diseases, University Hospital, Lausanne, Switzerland. BACKGROUND: Efavirenz (EFV) and nevirapine (NVP) are metabolized by cytochrome P450 2B6 (CYP2B6). Allele 516 G>T (Gln172His) is associated with diminished activity of this isoenzyme, and may lead to differences in drug exposure. METHODS: We evaluated this allele as a pharmacogenetic marker of EFV and NVP pharmacokinetics and EFV toxicity in 167 participants receiving EFV and 59 receiving NVP recruited within the genetics project of the Swiss HIV Cohort Study. Drug concentrations were measured in plasma and in peripheral blood mononuclear cells (PBMCs) from the same sample. Neuropsychological toxicity of EFV (sleep disorders, mood disorders, fatigue) was assessed using a standardized questionnaire. RESULTS AND CONCLUSIONS: CYP2B6 516TT was associated with greater plasma and intracellular exposure to EFV, and greater plasma exposure to NVP. Intracellular drug concentration, and CYP2B6 genotype were predictors of EFV neuropsychological toxicity. CYP2B6 genotyping may be useful to complement an individualization strategy based on plasma drug determinations to increase the safety and tolerability of EFV.

Pharmacogenet Genomics. 2005 Jan;15(1):15-21. Related Articles, Links Variation in the toll-like receptor 4 gene and susceptibility to myocardial infarction. Holloway JW, Yang IA, Ye S. Human Genetics Division, School of Medicine, University of Southampton, Southampton, UK. Variation in the gene encoding toll-like receptor 4 (TLR4), a transmembrane receptor that mediates inflammatory responses to bacterial endotoxin, has been associated with susceptibility to atherosclerosis and its complications, such as myocardial infarction (MI), the pathogenesis of which involves inflammation. A recent study has also indicated that TLR4 gene variation influences the effect of statin treatment on reducing atherosclerosis complications. We studied the TLR4 gene Asp299Gly polymorphism in relation to susceptibility to myocardial infarction in a cohort of patients with angiographically documented coronary artery disease, and performed a meta-analysis using data sets from three independent studies. The meta-analysis showed that overall, odds ratio (OR) for MI was 0.73 [95% confidence interval (CI) 0.55-0.96, P=0.024] in 299Gly carriers compared to non-carriers, and there was no evidence of heterogeneity among the sample sets (P=0.679). In our patient cohort, a significant association of 299Gly bearing genotypes with lower susceptibility to myocardial infarction was observed only in patients receiving statin treatment, with 299Gly carriers having an OR of 0.49 (95% CI 0.27-0.78, P=0.015) for MI compared to non-carriers. These results are consistent with the notion that variation in the TLR4 gene contributes to inter-individual variability in susceptibility to coronary ischaemic events, and that TLR4 genotype and statin treatment may have a synergistic effect.

Pharmacogenet Genomics. 2005 Jan;15(1):23-8. Related Articles, Links Alpha2B adrenergic receptor 301-303 deletion polymorphism and vascular alpha2 adrenergic receptor response. Muszkat M, Sofowora GG, Xie HG, Wood AJ, Stein CM. Division of Clinical Pharmacology, Vanderbilt University School of Medicine,

Nashville, Tennessee 37232-6602, USA. Postsynaptic alpha2B adrenergic receptors (ARs) mediate vasoconstriction. There is more than 1000-fold variability in vascular sensitivity to an alpha2-AR agonist. Genetic variability may contribute to such interindividual differences in sensitivity. A 301-303 deletion (del) polymorphism has been identified in the coding region of the alpha2B-AR gene and has functional effects in vitro. Thus, we examined the hypothesis that the del301-303 polymorphism contributes to variability in vascular alpha2-AR responses in vivo. Healthy subjects were recruited based on their alpha2B-AR genotype. Their vascular sensitivity was determined using a linear variable differential transformer following the infusion of increasing doses (range 0.01-1000 ng/min) of the alpha2-AR agonist, dexmedetomidine, into a dorsal hand vein. The dose that produced 50% (ED50) of maximum venoconstriction (Emax) was determined for each subject. Vascular response was compared among the three genotypes. Forty-nine subjects were studied [28 wild-type wt/wt, 13 wt/del, 8 del/del]. There was no difference in dexmedetomidine ED50 and Emax among the alpha2B-AR del301-303 genotypes. The ED50 was 1.39 ng/min [95% confidence interval (CI) 0.03-63.0 ng/min] in wt/wt subjects, 1.63 ng/min (95% CI 0.01-177.8 ng/min) in wt/del and 2.37 ng/min (95% CI 0.17-33.7 ng/min) in del/del (P=0.80). The average Emax was 75.4+/-14.9% in wt/wt, 75.7+/-21.3% in wt/del and 82.2+/-12.9% in del/del subjects (P=0.26). These findings suggest that the del301-303 polymorphism does not contribute significantly to interindividual in vivo variability in response to alpha2-AR activation in the hand vein.

Pharmacogenet Genomics. 2005 Jan;15(1):29-34. Related Articles, Links Calcium-sensing receptor gene polymorphism Arg990Gly and its possible effect on response to cinacalcet HCl. Rothe HM, Shapiro WB, Sun WY, Chou SY. Division of Nephrology and Hypertension, The Brookdale University Hospital and Medical Center, Brooklyn, New York 11212, USA. rothe@doctors.org.uk Cinacalcet, a novel calcimimetic compound, is effective in reducing parathyroid hormone (PTH) levels in approximately 70% of patients with secondary hyperparathyroidism. However, interindividual variations in the dose required to achieve the treatment goal have been noted in clinical studies. Our investigation examined the genetic polymorphisms of the calcium-sensing receptor (CaSR) gene as one possible cause of the different responses to cinacalcet. We report data on seven end-stage renal failure patients who were treated with regular haemodialysis and who participated in clinical trials of cinacalcet. All patients had secondary hyperparathyroidism with baseline intact PTH (iPTH) levels greater than 600 pg/ml. Three patients were male and four female with a mean+/-SD age of 60+/-12 years. DNA was extracted from peripheral lymphocytes. An area in exon 7 of the CaSR gene was amplified by the polymerase chain reaction and sequenced. Mean+/-SD baseline iPTH was 1086+/-189 pg/ml. The five patients without Arg990Gly demonstrated a 29.7+/-4.0% (+/-SEM) reduction in iPTH from individual baseline. One patient was found to be homozygous for the Arg990Gly polymorphism and another was heterozygous for both arginine and glycine alleles. The homozygous patient showed a significantly higher sensitivity to cinacalcet compared to the other patients

(P=0.003) with a 76.3+/-7.7% reduction in iPTH from baseline. No polymorphisms were noted in codons 986 or 1011. This preliminary study points to the possibility that patients homozygous for glycine at the 990 position in exon 7 of the CaSR may be more sensitive to the calcimimetic drug cinacalcet compared to those who are homozygous for arginine at that location.

Pharmacogenet Genomics. 2005 Jan;15(1):35-41. Related Articles, Links Genetic polymorphism in the phenobarbital-responsive enhancer module of the UDP-glucuronosyltransferase 1A1 gene and irinotecan toxicity. Kitagawa C, Ando M, Ando Y, Sekido Y, Wakai K, Imaizumi K, Shimokata K, Hasegawa Y. Department of Medicine, Division of Respiratory Diseases, Nagoya University Graduate School of Medicine, Showa-ku, Nagoya, Japan. Genetic polymorphism of the UDP-glucuronosyltransferase (UGT) 1A1 gene is associated with the decreased glucuronidation activity of an active metabolite of irinotecan, SN-38, and UGT1A1*28 has been shown as a predictive factor for irinotecan toxicity. The phenobarbital-responsive enhancer module (PBREM) of the UGT1A1 promoter region has been reportedly associated with the transcriptional activity of the gene. We investigated whether the polymorphism of PBREM (T-3279G) would affect inter-patient variations in sensitivity to irinotecan toxicity. The study population comprised 119 cancer patients who had received irinotecan. We reviewed their clinical records, including patient characteristics, and observed their toxicity levels following irinotecan infusion. Genotyping was performed by sequencing analyses. Logistic regression analyses were performed to assess the relationship between genotypes and irinotecan toxicity. We identified the homozygotes of the reference allele for T-3279G in 68 patients, the heterozygotes in 37, and the homozygotes for the variant in 14. Logistic regression analysis indicated a significant association between the homozygotes for T-3279G and the severe toxicity (odds ratio 5.80; 95% confidence interval 1.67-20.1). However, multivariate analysis, including the data of UGT1A1*28 polymorphism, revealed a diminution of the association due to a highly significant linkage disequilibrium between these polymorphisms. Our results suggest that a highly significant linkage disequilibrium exists between T-3279G and UGT1A1*28 polymorphisms, and that the variants of T-3279G and UGT1A1*28 cooperatively decrease transcriptional activity of the UGT1A1 promoter. The determination of T-3279G and UGT1A1*28 genotypes might be clinically useful in predicting severe irinotecan toxicity in cancer patients.

Pharmacogenet Genomics. 2005 Jan;15(1):51-60. Related Articles, Links Genetic and other sources of variation in the activity of serum paraoxonase/diazoxonase in humans: consequences for risk from exposure to diazinon. O'Leary KA, Edwards RJ, Town MM, Boobis AR. Department of Health Toxicology Unit, Experimental Medicine and Toxicology, Imperial College London, Hammersmith Campus, London, UK. Diazinon is the only organophosphorus insecticide that is currently approved for use in sheep dip in the UK. Reports that some individuals may be genetically more susceptible to possible chronic adverse health effects, due to variations in PON1 activity, are complicated by the reliability of activity measurements. In the present study, the influence of three polymorphisms of PON1 on serum diazoxonase activity was investigated in 85 healthy volunteers.

Serum activity was assessed in as close to physiological conditions as possible (at pH 7.4, 150 mM NaCl and 37 degrees C with 50 microM diazoxon as substrate) and by quantifying pyrimidinol formation using high-performance liquid chromatography. PON1 genotypes were determined by the polymerase chain reaction and restriction enzyme digestion. For PON1 Q192R, individuals with the RR genotype had the highest serum diazoxonase activity, in contrast to some previous reports where activity was determined under less physiological conditions. Activity was slightly reduced in individuals with the QR genotype and activity was reduced even further in those with the QQ genotype. For PON1 L55 M, there was a significant decrease in mean enzyme activity from LL>LM>MM genotypes. The promoter polymorphism PON1 -108 C/T had only a slight effect on activity. Overall, intragenotype variation in PON1 activity was appreciably greater than the mean intergenotype differences. In conclusion, although there is a wide variation in activity in individuals both within and between genotypes, those individuals with a combination of Q and M alleles generally have a lower ability to detoxify diazoxon, which implies a potentially greater susceptibility to toxicity from diazinon.

Pharmacogenet Genomics. 2005 Jan;15(1):7-13. Related Articles, Links Single nucleotide polymorphisms in the CYP2J2 and CYP2C8 genes and the risk of hypertension. King LM, Gainer JV, David GL, Dai D, Goldstein JA, Brown NJ, Zeldin DC. Division of Intramural Research, National Institute of Environmental Health Sciences, National Institutes of Health, Research Triangle Park, North Carolina 27709, USA. CYP2J2 and CYP2C8 metabolize arachidonic acid (AA) to cis-epoxyeicosatrienoic acids (EETs), which play a central role in regulating renal tubular fluid-electrolyte transport and vascular tone. We hypothesized that functionally relevant polymorphisms in the CYP2J2 or CYP2C8 genes influence hypertension risk. We examined associations between CYP2J2*7 (G-50 T promoter) and CYP2C8*3 (Arg139Lys and Lys399Arg, which are in 100% linkage disequilibrium) polymorphisms and hypertension in a biethnic population from Tennessee. CYP2J2*7 variant allele frequency was significantly higher in African-Americans versus Caucasians (14.1% versus 7.7%, P=0.01), irrespective of hypertension status. When analysed separately by race, the genotype distribution of the CYP2J2*7 variant allele was not significantly different among African-Americans with/without hypertension, but was significantly different among Caucasians with/without hypertension (P=0.03). Indeed, the odds ratio of having hypertension attributable to carrying the CYP2J2*7 variant allele adjusted for age, gender, body mass index and family history was 0.39 (95% confidence interval 0.17-0.89) among Caucasians, suggesting a protective effect. Additional subgroup analyses revealed a significantly lower CYP2J2*7 variant allele frequency in hypertensive versus normotensive Caucasian males (5.6% versus 12.5%, P=0.02) and in hypertensive versus normotensive Caucasians without a family history of hypertension (1.5% versus 11.0%, P=0.03). With respect to the CYP2C8*3 variant, genotype distribution and allele frequencies were similar between normotensive and hypertensive subjects. This study provides evidence for an association between CYP2J2*7 genotype and hypertension in Caucasian males and Caucasians without a family history of hypertension, but suggests no association between CYP2C8*3 genotype and hypertension. Confirmation of these findings in additional populations is warranted.

Pharmacogenet Genomics. 2005 Jul;15(7):451-6. Related Articles, Links Significance of a common single nucleotide polymorphism in exon 10 of the follicle-stimulating hormone (FSH) receptor gene for the ovarian response to FSH: a pharmacogenetic approach to controlled ovarian hyperstimulation. Behre HM, Greb RR, Mempel A, Sonntag B, Kiesel L, Kaltwasser P, Seliger E, Ropke F, Gromoll J, Nieschlag E, Simoni M. Andrology Unit, Department of Urology, University Hospital, Halle, University Hospital, Munster, Germany. The p.N680S sequence variation of the follicle-stimulating hormone (FSH) receptor gene was previously shown to influence the ovarian response to FSH in normo-ovulatory women undergoing controlled ovarian hyperstimulation. In this prospective, randomized, controlled study, we tested whether the same daily dose of FSH results in lower levels of oestradiol in women homozygous for the p.N680S sequence variation, and whether the difference can be overcome by higher FSH doses. Women undergoing controlled ovarian hyperstimulation for in vitro fertilization or intracytoplasmic sperm injection and homozygous for the wild-type or for the p.N680S FSH receptor were randomly assigned to group I (Ser/Ser, n=24), receiving an FSH dose of 150 U/day, or group II (Ser/Ser, n=25), receiving an FSH dose of 225 U/day. In group III (Asn/Asn, n=44), the FSH dose was 150 U/day. Age and basal FSH levels were not different between groups. At ovulation induction, total FSH doses were comparable in group I (1631+/-96 U) and group III (1640+/-57 U) but significantly higher in group II (2421+/-112 U) (P<0.001). Peak oestradiol levels on the day of human chorionic gonadotrophin (hCG) administration were significantly lower in group I (5680+/-675 pmol/l) compared to group III (8679+/-804 pmol/l) (P=0.028). Increasing the FSH dose from 150 to 225 U/day overcame the lower oestradiol response in women with Ser/Ser (group II, 7804+/-983 pmol/l). In women undergoing controlled ovarian hyperstimulation, the p.N680S sequence variation results in lower oestradiol levels following FSH stimulation. This lower FSH receptor sensitivity can be overcome by higher FSH doses. Publication Types: Clinical Trial Multicenter Study Randomized Controlled Trial

Pharmacogenet Genomics. 2005 May;15(5):287-93. Related Articles, Links A multilocus approach to the antihypertensive pharmacogenetics of hydrochlorothiazide. Maitland-van der Zee AH, Turner ST, Schwartz GL, Chapman AB, Klungel OH, Boerwinkle E. Human Genetics Center, University of Texas Health Science Center, Houston, TX 77030, USA. a.h.maitland-vanderzee@pharm.uu.nl OBJECTIVES: To assess the influence of variations in multiple candidate genes on inter-individual variation in diastolic blood pressure (DBP) response to hydrochlorothiazide. METHODS: A community-based sample of 585 adults with essential hypertension underwent monotherapy with hydrochlorothiazide for 4 weeks. In a nested case-control design, 195 individuals in the highest tertile of DBP response (responders) and 195 individuals in the lowest tertile of DBP response (non-responders) were genotyped for 45 polymorphisms in 19 candidate genes. For those polymorphisms where the set association approach found to be significantly associated with DBP response, logistic regression was performed to estimate the odds ratio (OR) for response associated variation in the identified genotype/haplotype. RESULTS: Two polymorphisms in the sodium channel gamma-subunit promotor gene, and a polymorphism in the endothelial nitric oxide synthase gene, were significantly associated with blood pressure response to hydrochlorothiazide. In the final experiment for the set association model P=0.038. In the logistic regression analyses, compared to subjects with the CT/CT haplotype of the SCNN1G gene, those with the GA/GA haplotype had OR 5.21 of being a DBP responder [95% CI 1.65-16.47]. Compared to subjects with the GT genotype of the ENOSA_rs1799983 polymorphism, those with the GG genotype had an OR 2.19 of being a DBP responder [95% CI 1.27-3.77]. CONCLUSIONS: Two polymorphisms in the sodium channel gamma-subunit promotor gene, and a polymorphism in the endothelial nitric oxide synthase gene, were associated with significant differences in odds of DBP response to hydrochlorothiazide. Follow-up studies are needed to define the functional genetic variations and their mechanisms of pharmacogenetic effects.

Pharmacogenet Genomics. 2005 May;15(5):365-9. Related Articles, Links Pharmacogenetic testing for drug metabolizing enzymes: is it happening in practice? Gardiner SJ, Begg EJ. Department of Medicine, Christchurch School of Medicine and Health Sciences, Christchurch, New Zealand. sharon.gardiner@cdhb.govt.nz It is widely claimed that pharmacogenetics may form the basis of 'personalized medicine'. We sought to determine the current utilization of pharmacogenetic testing for drug metabolizing enzymes (DMEs). The hypothesis was that these tests were rarely performed clinically. Questionnaires were sent to 629 individuals representing laboratories, hospitals and universities throughout Australia and New Zealand. The questionnaires asked which facilities performed pharmacogenetic tests for selected DMEs, and details about the tests, if performed. The overall response rate was 81.1% (510/629); three respondents declined to participate. Clinical genotyping and phenotyping tests for DMEs could be performed by 10 (2.0% of 507) and 18 (3.6%) facilities, respectively. The most frequently performed genetic tests were for thiopurine methyltransferase (approximately 400 times in 2003) and pseudocholinesterase (approximately 250 times). The frequency of phenotyping exceeded genotyping by five- and eight-fold, respectively. One centre performed CYP2D6 phenotyping frequently (approximately 4200 times in 2003) for perhexiline. Genotyping and phenotyping tests for other cytochrome P450 enzymes, N-acetyltransferase-2 and dihydropyrimidine dehydrogenase were effectively never undertaken for clinical purposes. Pharmacogenetic tests for DMEs are currently performed rarely in clinical practice, despite repeated claims that they may benefit patient care. The only tests performed with any regularity in Australasia are for thiopurine methyltransferase and pseudocholinesterase, and CYP2D6 phenotyping in one centre for patients on perhexiline. The low clinical utilization reflects a poor evidence base, unestablished clinical relevance and, in the few cases with the strongest rationale, a slow translation to the clinical setting.

Pharmacogenet Genomics. 2005 Nov;15(11):769-78. Related Articles, Links Genotype-phenotype correlation between the polymorphic UGT2B17 gene deletion and NNAL glucuronidation activities in human liver microsomes. Lazarus P, Zheng Y, Aaron Runkle E, Muscat JE, Wiener D. Department of Pharmacology, Penn State University College of Medicine, Hershey, Pennsylvania 17033, USA. plazarus@psu.edu The nicotine-derived tobacco-specific nitrosamine, 4-(methylnitrosamino)-1-(3-pyridyl)-1-butanone (NNK), is one of the most potent and abundant procarcinogens found in tobacco and tobacco smoke, and glucuronidation of its major metabolite, 4-(methylnitrosamino)-1-(3-pyridyl)-1-butanol (NNAL), is an important mechanism for NNK detoxification. In cigarette smokers and tobacco chewers, there is a wide variation in the urinary levels of the ratio of NNAL to NNAL glucuronide (NNAL-Gluc). To determine whether genetic variation plays a potential role in this inter-individual variability, NNAL-glucuronidating activities were analysed in a series of human liver microsomal specimens and compared with UGT2B17 deletion genotypes in the same subjects. Assays performed in vitro demonstrated that over-expressed UGT2B17 exhibits high O-glucuronidating activity against NNAL. When stratifying subjects by UGT2B17 genotype, a significant or near-significant decrease in NNAL-O-Gluc formation was observed in liver microsomes from individuals who were either heterozygous [(+/0), P=0.07] or homozygous [(0/0), P=0.016] for the UGT2B17 deletion compared to liver microsomes from individuals with intact UGT2B17 alleles [(+/+)]. There was a significant (P<0.01) association between the level of liver microsomal NNAL-O-glucuronide formation and increasing numbers of the UGT2B17 null alleles in the liver microsomal specimens examined in this study, and a significant decrease in NNAL-O-Gluc formation was observed when comparing liver microsomes from individuals who had at least one UGT2B17 allele deleted [(+/0)+(0/0)] versus microsomes from UGT2B17 (+/+) subjects (P=0.004). When stratifying by the median value of NNAL-O-Gluc formation activity, a significantly (P=0.015) higher number of subjects with liver microsomes having low NNAL-O-Gluc formation activity contained the UGT2B17 null genotype compared to subjects with liver microsomes exhibiting high NNAL-O-Gluc formation activity. When stratifying by UGT2B7/UGT2B17 haplotypes, the association between the level of liver microsomal NNAL-O-glucuronide formation and increasing numbers of the UGT2B17 null allele was at the level of statistical significance for subjects with the UGT2B7 (*1/*2) (P=0.05) or UGT2B7 (*2/*2) (P<0.02) genotypes. These data suggest that the UGT2B17 deletion polymorphism is associated with a reduced rate of NNAL detoxification in vivo and may increase individual susceptibility to tobacco-related cancers.

Pharmacogenet Genomics. 2005 Nov;15(11):779-86. Related Articles, Links CYP2C9, CYP2C19, ABCB1 (MDR1) genetic polymorphisms and phenytoin metabolism in a Black Beninese population. Allabi AC, Gala JL, Horsmans Y. Centre d' Investigations Cliniques et de Recherches Therapeutiques, Cove, Republic of Benin. The genetically polymorphic cytochrome P450 2C9 (CYP2C9) metabolizes many important drugs. Among them, phenytoin has been used as a probe to determine CYP2C9 phenotype by measuring the urinary excretion of its major metabolite, S-enantiomer of 5-(4-hydroxyphenyl)-5-phenylhydantoin (p-HPPH). Phenytoin pharmacokinetic is also dependent on the activity of CYP2C19 and p-glycoprotein (ABCB1). To determine the influence of CYP2C9, CYP2C19 and ABCB1 genetic polymorphisms on phenytoin metabolism in a Black population, 109 healthy Beninese subjects received a single 300 mg oral dose of phenytoin. Blood was drawn 4 h after drug intake and urine was collected during the first 8 h. Plasma phenytoin and urine S- and R-enantiomers of p-HPPH were determined by high-performance liquid chromatography. Urinary excretion of (S)-p-HPPH [defined as urinary volumex(S)-p-HPPH urinary concentration] and PMR (defined as the ratio of p-HPPH in urine to 4 h phenytoin plasma concentration), both markers of CYP2C9 activity, were used to determine the functional relevance of new variants of CYP2C9 (*5, *6, *8, *9 and *11) in this population. Plasma phenytoin concentration was significantly associated with ABCB1 haplotype/genotype (P=0.05, Kruskal-Wallis test) and levels increased significantly in the genotype order: wild-type, T3421A and Block-2 genotypes (P=0.015, Jonckheere-Terpstra test). Urinary excretion of (S)-p-HPPH and PMR were significantly associated with the CYP2C9 genotype (P=0.001, analysis of variance (ANOVA) and P<0.0001, Kruskal-Wallis test, respectively) and decreased in the order: CYP2C9*1/*1, CYP2C9*1/*9, CYP2C9*9/*9, CYP2C9*1/*8, CYP2C9*8/*9, CYP2C9*9/*11, CYP2C9*1/*5, CYP2C9*6/*9, CYP2C9*1/*6, CYP2C9*8/*11, CYP2C9*5/*8 and CYP2C9*5/*6 (P<0.001, Jonckheere-Terpstra test). A combined analysis of CYP2C9, 2C19 and ABCB1 revealed that only ABCB1 predicted phenytoin concentration at 4 h and explained 8% of the variability (r=0.08, P=0.04). On the other hand, only CYP2C9 was predictive for the urinary excretion of (S)-p-HPPH and PMR (r=0.21, P=0.001 and r=0.25, P<0.001, respectively). Furthermore, significant relation was found between urinary excretion of (R)-p-HPPH and CYP2C9 genotype (P=0.035) and levels significantly increased in the genotype order: CYP2C9*1/*9, CYP2C9*1/*1, CYP2C9*9/*11, CYP2C9*1/*8 and CYP2C9*1/*5 (P<0.001, Jonckheere-Terpstra test). In summary, the present study demonstrates that, in a Black population, CYP2C9*5, *6, *8 and *11 variants, but not CYP2C9*9, are associated with a decreased phenytoin metabolism. The data also confirm the limited contribution of MDR1 gene to inter-individual phenytoin pharmacokinetic variation.

Pharmacogenet Genomics. 2005 Nov;15(11):787-800. Related Articles, Links Valproic acid-induced skeletal malformations: associated gene expression cascades. Massa V, Cabrera RM, Menegola E, Giavini E, Finnell RH. Department of Biology, University of Milan, Milan, Italy. OBJECTIVES: Valproic acid (VPA) is a widely used anticonvulsant medication with well-known teratogenic effects in both humans and in experimental animal model systems. The most commonly observed malformations induced by VPA in experimental animals include neural and skeletal defects. In this study the potential alterations in somitic tissue gene expression relative to the development of observed axial skeletal defects were examined. METHODS: SWV mice were treated at 8.5 days post coitum (d.p.c.) with 1.36 mmol/kg or 2.72 mmol/kg VPA by i.p. injection. At 18.5 d.p.c., animals were killed and stained for morphological and skeletal examination. Cervical malformations consisting of vertebral fusions and cervical ribs were consistently observed. Phenotypic analysis confirmed the presence of dose-dependent axial skeletal malformations induced by in-utero VPA-exposure. Using antisense RNA amplification and cDNA microarrays, we examined the expression of approximately 5700 genes in the first six postotic somites of control and treated embryos at 6, 12, 18 and 24 h after the 8.5 d.p.c. VPA treatment. RESULTS: Analysis indicated that several ontological groups (e.g. histone deacetylase complex, guanosine triphosphatases, cell proliferation and cytoskeletal) have significantly enriched gene expression changes in response to the teratogenic insult. The RNA from 6 h post-treatment was also subjected to a microarray cross-platform validation, and genes identified on both platforms are presented. CONCLUSION: These data were then used to deduce candidate cellular pathways that may be responsible for the VPA-induced teratogenic skeletal phenotypes.

Pharmacogenet Genomics. 2005 Nov;15(11):801-15. Related Articles, Links Thiopurine S-methyltransferase pharmacogenetics: variant allele functional and comparative genomics. Salavaggione OE, Wang L, Wiepert M, Yee VC, Weinshilboum RM. Department of Molecular Pharmacology and Experimental Therapeutics, Mayo Clinic College of Medicine-Mayo Clinic, Rochester, Minnesota 55905, USA. Thiopurine S-methyltransferase (TPMT) catalyses the S-methylation of thiopurine drugs. Genetic polymorphisms for TPMT are a major factor responsible for large individual variations in thiopurine toxicity and therapeutic effect. The present study investigated the functional effects of human TPMT variant alleles that alter the encoded amino acid sequence of the enzyme, TPMT*2, *3A, *3B, *3C and *5 to *13. After expression in COS-1 cells and correction for transfection efficiency, allozymes encoded by these alleles displayed levels of activity that varied from virtually undetectable (*3A,*3B and *5) to 98% (*7) of that observed for the wild-type allele. Although some allozymes had significant elevations in apparent Km values for 6-mercaptopurine and S-adenosyl-L-methionine (i.e. the two cosubstrates for the reaction), the level of enzyme protein was the major factor responsible for variation in activity. Quantitative Western blot analysis demonstrated that the level of enzyme protein correlated closely with level of activity for all allozymes except TPMT*5. Furthermore, protein levels correlated with rates of TPMT degradation. TPMT amino acid sequences were then determined for 16 non-human mammalian species and those sequences (plus seven reported previously, including two nonmammalian vertebrate species) were used to determine amino acid sequence conservation. Most human TPMT variant allozymes had alterations of residues that were highly conserved during vertebrate evolution. Finally, a human TPMT homology structural model was created on the basis of a Pseudomonas structure (the only TPMT structure solved to this time), and the model was used to infer the functional consequences of variant allozyme amino acid sequence alterations. These studies indicate that a common mechanism responsible for alterations in the activity of variant TPMT allozymes involves alteration in the level of enzyme protein due, at least in part, to accelerated degradation.

Pharmacogenet Genomics. 2005 Nov;15(11):817-29. Related Articles, Links St. John's wort and its constituent hyperforin concordantly regulate expression of genes encoding enzymes involved in basic cellular pathways. Krusekopf S, Roots I. Institute of Clinical Pharmacology, Charite Campus Mitte, Charite University Medical Center, Humboldt University of Berlin, Berlin, Germany. Solveigh.Krusekopf@charite.de OBJECTIVES AND METHODS: The effects of St. John's wort and hyperforin on gene expression were analysed in HepG2 cells by Affymetrix microarray hybridization and real time reverse transcription-PCR. RESULTS: Both compounds increased mRNAs of the drug metabolizing enzymes CYP3A4, CYP1A1, CYP1A2 and the flavin containing monooxygenase FMO5, and of the multidrug resistance protein MRP2. CYP4F2 and the reduced nicotinamide adenine dinucleotide dehydrogenase NQO1 were downregulated. Expression of genes mediating cholesterol biosynthesis was decreased, while facilitated glucose transporters and glycolysis genes were induced, indicating increased glucose metabolism. Changes of a considerable number of additional transcripts corresponded to reports on gene regulation by hypoxia. Endoplasmic reticulum stress-regulated genes involved in unfolded protein response and in protection of cells from apoptosis were downregulated. Other calcium binding proteins were affected by both treatments, suggesting an increase in intracellular calcium. CONCLUSIONS: St. John's wort and hyperforin concordantly affected expression of genes not only mediating metabolism and transport of exogenous and endogenous compounds, but also involved in energy metabolism, intracellular calcium regulation, cell proliferation and apoptosis.

Pharmacogenet Genomics. 2005 Oct;15(10):705-11. Related Articles, Links

The pharmacogenetics of methotrexate in inflammatory bowel disease. Herrlinger KR, Cummings JR, Barnardo MC, Schwab M, Ahmad T, Jewell DP. Gastroenterology Unit, University of Oxford, Gibson Laboratories, Radcliffe Infirmary, Oxford, UK. klaus.herrlinger@rbk.de OBJECTIVES: Methotrexate (MTX) is an effective immunosuppressive treatment in inflammatory bowel disease (IBD) but its use is limited by unpredictable toxicity and efficacy. MTX metabolism is complex involving a number of enzymes. An individual's response to MTX may in part be genetically determined by functional genetic variation in genes encoding these enzymes. We report a pharmacogenetic evaluation of MTX therapy in IBD. METHODS: We studied 102 IBD patients treated with MTX, and 202 patients with Crohn's disease (CD), 205 patients with ulcerative colitis (UC) and 189 healthy volunteers served as controls to assess allele frequencies in the disease and healthy populations. All subjects were genotyped for four polymorphisms: G80A in the reduced folate carrier (RFC1) gene, G452T in the gamma-glutamyl hydrolase (GGH) gene and C677T and A1298C in the methylenetetrahydrofolate reductase (MTHFR) gene. Three non-conservative SNPs in the RFC1 and the MTHFR gene could not be detected in our patient cohort. Genotype-phenotype associations were evaluated with respect to efficacy and toxicity of MTX therapy. RESULTS: No significant differences in the allele frequencies between CD, UC and healthy controls were detected. Overall 21% of patients experienced MTX side effects. Patients homozygous for the MTHFR 1298C allele were more likely to experience one or more side effects compared to patients with the wild-type 1298AA genotype (21.0 vs. 6.3%, $P < 0.05$). None of the genotyped SNPs or haplotypes, either alone or in combination, was associated with short-term efficacy or sustained response. CONCLUSIONS: Side effects of MTX in IBD are associated with a SNP in the MTHFR gene but response cannot be predicted by any of the investigated SNPs.

Pharmacogenet Genomics. 2005 Sep;15(9):599-608. Related Articles, Links Influence of ABCB1, ABCC1, ABCC2, and ABCG2 haplotypes on the cellular exposure of nelfinavir in vivo. Colombo S, Soranzo N, Rotger M, Sprenger R, Bleiber G, Furrer H, Buclin T, Goldstein D, Decosterd L, Telenti A; Swiss HIV Cohort Study. Division of Clinical Pharmacology, University Hospital, Lausanne, Switzerland. OBJECTIVES: The human immunodeficiency virus protease inhibitor nelfinavir is substrate of polyspecific drug transporters encoded by ABCB1 (P-glycoprotein), ABCC1 (MRP1) and ABCC2 (MRP2), and an inhibitor of BCRP, encoded by ABCG2. Genetic polymorphism in these genes may be associated with changes in transport function. METHODS: A comprehensive evaluation of single nucleotide polymorphisms (39 SNPs in ABCB1, 7 in ABCC1, 27 in ABCC2, and 16 in ABCG2), and inferred haplotypes was done to assess possible associations of genetic variants with cellular exposure of nelfinavir in vivo. Analysis used peripheral mononuclear cells from individuals receiving nelfinavir (n=28). Key results were re-examined in a larger sample size (n=129) contributing data on plasma drug levels. RESULTS AND CONCLUSIONS: There was no significant association between cellular nelfinavir area under the curve (AUC) and SNPs or haplotypes at ABCC1, ABCC2, ABCG2. There was an association with cellular exposure for two loci in strong linkage disequilibrium: ABCB1 3435C>T; AUCTT>AUCCT>AUCCC (ratio 2.1, 1.4, 1, Ptrend=0.01), and intron 26 +80T>C; AUCCC> AUCCT > AUCTT (ratio 2.4, 1.3, 1, Ptrend=0.006). Haplotypic analysis using tagging SNPs did not improve the single SNP association values.

Pharmacogenet Genomics. 2006 Jan;16(1):1-7. Related Articles, Links Pharmacogenetics of opioid receptors and addiction. Mayer P, Hollt V. Bundesinstitut fur Arzneimittel und Medizinprodukte, Bonn, Germany. It is generally assumed that combinations of polymorphic alleles of different genes contribute to polygenetic disorders. Variants of the opioid receptors are the obvious candidates underlying addiction. Most research has focused on the coding variation A118G of the mu opioid receptor (MOPr), which replaces asparagine at position 40 by aspartate (Asn40Asp). However, to date, no conclusive evidence exists regarding which physiological effects this mutation may cause. Other rare polymorphisms in the MOPr cause marked effects (e.g. impairment of G-protein coupling) but, due to their low frequency, their role in addiction is questionable. A large number of polymorphic sites have been found in the putative promoter region of the mu opioid receptor. These variations may alter the expression level of the receptors in neurones, but the functional relevance of promoter polymorphisms is hard to predict. In the delta opioid receptor, surprisingly few polymorphisms have been detected within the coding region, and a clear association with addiction has not been shown to date. The kappa opioid receptor contains mainly silent polymorphisms. Nevertheless, there are studies reporting positive associations of silent mutations in the three opioid receptors with drug addiction. The underlying mechanism remains unclear, but examples exist indicating that silent mutations affect mRNA stability. Taken together, the coding polymorphisms, which are rather frequent, reveal no convincing association. The vast number of non-coding, intronic or promoter polymorphisms in the opioid receptors may influence addictive behaviour, but these polymorphisms are far less studied, and their physiological significance remains to be demonstrated. Publication Types: Review

Pharmacogenetics. 2004 Apr;14(4):225-38. Related Articles, Links Erratum in: Pharmacogenetics. 2005 Apr;15(4):265. Pharmacogenetic determinants of interindividual variability in bupropion hydroxylation by cytochrome P450 2B6 in human liver microsomes. Hesse LM, He P, Krishnaswamy S, Hao Q, Hogan K, von Moltke LL, Greenblatt DJ, Court MH. Clinical Pharmacology Laboratory, Department of Pharmacology and Experimental Therapeutics, Tufts University School of Medicine, 136 Harrison Avenue, Boston, MA 02111, USA. Bupropion is primarily metabolized in human liver by cytochrome P450 (CYP) 2B6, an isoform that shows high interindividual variability in expression and catalysis. The aim of this study was to identify mechanisms underlying this variability through comprehensive phenotype-genotype analysis of a well-characterized human liver bank (n = 54). There was substantial variability in microsomal bupropion hydroxylation activities (over 45-fold) and CYP2B6 protein content (over 288-fold), with excellent correlation between protein and activity values (rs = 0.88). CYP2B6 mRNA levels showed less variability (13-fold) and poorer correlation (rs = 0.44) to CYP2B6 protein resulting from 20-30% of livers that contained substantial CYP2B6 mRNA, but low CYP2B6 protein. Livers were genotyped for the common coding polymorphisms (Q172H, K262R and R487C) and 14 additional variations identified by sequencing of the gene promoter to -3000 bp. Of 14 haplotypes that were inferred, *1A (reference), *1H (-2320t>c; -750t>c) and *6B (-1456t>c; -750t>c; Q172H; K262R) were most common with frequencies of 0.28, 0.20 and 0.26, respectively. Alcohol use history (P = 0.011) and *6B haplotype (P = 0.011) were identified as significant predictors of bupropion hydroxylation. A consideration of the effects of these variables on CYP2B6 mRNA and protein levels suggests that alcohol use is associated with enhanced CYP2B6 gene transcription, but the presence of at least one *6B allele reduces this effect on bupropion hydroxylation at the post-transcriptional level. In conclusion, the results of this study indicate that interindividual variability in bupropion hydroxylation is a consequence of interactions between environmental and genetic influences on CYP2B6 gene function.

Pharmacogenetics. 2004 Apr;14(4):267-9. Related Articles, Links Single nucleotide polymorphism characterization by mRNA expression imbalance assessment. Wojnowski L, Brockmoller J. Department of Clinical Pharmacology, Georg-August-Universitat, Gottingen, Germany. wojnowski@med.uni-mainz.de The functional characterization of single nucleotide polymorphism (SNPs) represents a major challenge for pharmacogenetics and related research areas. Here, we propose a procedure, termed mRNA expression imbalance assessment, that can be applied to detect cis-acting SNPs with an effect on mRNA expression. The procedure is based on the observation that the relative transcript levels derived from the two alleles of an autosomal gene are reflected in the sequence of the amplified cDNA. The key element of the procedure is the detection of a discrepancy between the specific nucleotide signal intensity of a marker SNP in the genomic DNA and in the cDNA. We used the CYP3A5*1/*3 polymorphism as a proof principle for this approach. In this case, we could even demonstrate that the procedure works equally well with the appropriate tissue samples and in silico, using the existing databanks of sequences. In conclusion, the procedure provides a fast and easy tool, which may facilitate identification of functional SNPs.

Pharmacogenetics. 2004 Aug;14(8):487-99. Related Articles, Links Human UGT1A6 pharmacogenetics: identification of a novel SNP, characterization of allele frequencies and functional analysis of recombinant allozymes in human liver tissue and in cultured cells. Nagar S, Zalatoris JJ, Blanchard RL. Department of Pharmacology, Fox Chase Cancer Center, Philadelphia, PA, USA. BACKGROUND: UDP-glucuronosyltransferase (UGT) enzymes catalyze the glucuronidation and typically inactivation of endogenous and exogenous molecules including steroid hormones, bilirubin and many drugs. The UGT1A6 protein is expressed predominantly in liver and metabolizes small phenolic drugs including acetaminophen, salicylates and many beta-blockers. Interindividual variation in the capacity of humans to glucuronidate drugs has been observed. RESULTS: We have identified a novel common single nucleotide polymorphism (SNP) in the human UGT1A6 gene resulting in a Ser7Ala change in encoded amino acid. We have further functionally characterized that polymorphism in the context of two previously reported polymorphisms, Thr181Ala and Arg184Ser. These non-synonymous cSNPs define four common haplotypes. Alleles appear with similar frequencies in Caucasian and African-American populations with distributions adhering to Hardy-Weinberg equilibrium. UGT1A6 genotype, rate of substrate glucuronidation and level of immunoreactive UGT1A6 protein was determined. A 25-fold variation in the rate of substrate glucuronidation and an 85-fold variation in level of immunoreactive protein were measured. Liver tissue samples that were homozygous for UGT1A6*2 exhibited a high rate of glucuronidation relative to tissues with other genotypes. Biochemical kinetic studies of recombinant UGT1A6 expressed in HEK293 cells indicated that the UGT1A6*2 allozyme, expressed homozygously, had almost two-fold greater activity toward p-nitrophenol than UGT1A6*1 and when expressed heterozygously (UGT1A6*1/*2) it was associated with low enzyme activity. CONCLUSIONS: These data suggest that common genetic variation in human UGT1A6 confers functionally significant differences in biochemical phenotype as assessed in human tissue and cultured cells expressing recombinant allozymes. This genetic variation might impact clinical efficacy or toxicity of drugs metabolized by UGT1A6.

Pharmacogenetics. 2004 Aug;14(8):539-47. Related Articles, Links Relative impact of covariates in prescribing warfarin according to CYP2C9 genotype. Hillman MA, Wilke RA, Caldwell MD, Berg RL, Glurich I, Burmester JK. Department of Care Management, Marshfield Clinic, Marshfield, Wisconsin, USA. Patients on warfarin anticoagulant therapy demonstrate wide variation in maintenance dose.

Patients possessing variants (*2 and *3) of the cytochrome P450 2C9 gene require reduced maintenance doses compared to those having wild-type alleles (*1). Many other clinical factors have been shown to affect warfarin dose as well. To determine the relative impact of CYP2C9 genotype, age, gender, body surface area, concomitant medication, treatment indication and comorbidity, we conducted a retrospective cohort study in 453 patients managed by the anticoagulation service of a large, horizontally integrated, multispecialty group practice. In this largely Caucasian patient population, the CYP2C9 gene frequencies for *1/*1, *1/*2, *1/*3, *2/*2, *2/*3 and *3/*3 were 65.1%, 19.0%, 12.1%, 1.6%, 1.8% and 0.4%, respectively, approximating Hardy-Weinberg equilibrium. Mean maintenance doses for these genotypes were 36.5, 29.1, 23.5, 28.0, 18.1 and 5.5 mg/week, respectively. In univariate analyses, genotype alone accounted for 19.8% of the variability in maintenance dose. Age, body surface area and male gender accounted for 14.6%, 7.5% and 4.7%, respectively, while cardiac valve replacement as the indication for warfarin accounted for 5.4% of the variability. Collectively, these factors accounted for 33.7% of all dosing variability according to multiple regression. These results will help strengthen the mathematical models that are currently being developed for prospective gene-based warfarin dosing.

Pharmacogenetics. 2004 Aug;14(8):549-56. Related Articles, Links Pharmacogenetic roles of CYP2C19 and CYP2B6 in the metabolism of R- and S-mephobarbital in humans. Kobayashi K, Morita J, Chiba K, Wanibuchi A, Kimura M, Irie S, Urae A, Ishizaki T. Laboratory of Pharmacology and Toxicology, Graduate School of Pharmaceutical Sciences, Chiba University, Chiba, Japan. OBJECTIVES AND METHODS: We assessed the relationship between the metabolism of R- and S-mephobarbital (MPB) and genetic polymorphisms of cytochrome P450 (CYP) 2C19 and CYP2B6. Nine homozygous extensive metabolizers (homo-EMs, 2C19*1/2C19*1) of CYP2C19, ten heterozygous EMs (hetero-EMs, 2C19*1/2C19*2, 2C19*1/2C19*3) and eleven poor metabolizers (PMs, 2C19*2/2C19*2, 2C19*3/2C19*3, 2C19*2/2C19*3) recruited from a Japanese population, received an oral 200 mg-dose of racemic MPB. Blood and urine samples were collected, and R-MPB, S-MPB and the metabolites, phenobarbital (PB) and 4'-hydroxy-MPB, were measured. Each subject was also genotyped for CYP2B6 gene. RESULTS: The mean area under the plasma concentration-time curve (AUC) of R-MPB was 92-fold greater in PMs than in homo-EMs. R/S ratios for AUC of MPB were much higher in PMs than in EMs (homo- and hetero-). The cumulative urinary excretion of 4'-hydroxy-MPB up to 24 h postdose was 21-fold less in PMs than in homo-EMs. The metabolic ratio of AUCPB/(AUCS-MPB + AUCR-MPB) was higher in PMs than in EMs (homo- and hetero-). In addition, this metabolic ratio was lower in the carriers of CYP2B6*6 compared with that in its non-carriers. CONCLUSIONS: Our results indicate that the 4'-hydroxylation of R-MPB is mediated via CYP2C19 and that the rapid 4'-hydroxylation of R-MPB results in a marked difference in the pharmacokinetic profiles between R-MPB and S-MPB in the different CYP2C19 genotypic individuals. In addition, a minor fraction of the interindividual variability in PB formation from MPB may be explainable by the CYP2B6*6 allele.

Pharmacogenetics. 2004 Dec;14(12):785-92. Related Articles, Links Methylenetetrahydrofolate reductase gene polymorphisms and response to fluorouracil-based treatment in advanced colorectal cancer patients. Etienne MC, Formento JL, Chazal M, Francoual M, Magne N, Formento P, Bourgeon A, Seitz JF, Delpero JR, Letoublon C, Pezet D, Milano G. Centre Antoine Lacassagne, Nice, France. Methylenetetrahydrofolate reductase (MTHFR) controls intracellular CH2FH4 concentrations (required for optimal fluoropyrimidine efficacy) by irreversibly converting CH2FH4 into 5-methyltetrahydrofolate. MTHFR 677C>T and 1298A>C polymorphisms are linked to altered enzyme activity. Thus, mutated MTHFR tumours should, in theory, be more sensitive to 5-fluorouracil (5FU) than wild-type tumours. MTHFR polymorphisms in position 677 and 1298 were analysed in 98 colorectal cancer patients with unresectable liver metastases (57 men, 41 women, mean age 64 years) receiving 5FU-folinic acid. 677C>T and 1298A>C genotypes were determined simultaneously by melting curve analyses on liver metastases. 677C>T genotype distribution was 46.9% wt/wt, 34.7% wt/mut and 18.4% mut/mut; that of 1298A>C was 52.0% wt/wt, 35.7% wt/mut and 12.3% mut/mut. The response rate was not related to 1298A>C genotype but was significantly linked to 677C>T genotype (response rate: 40%, 21% and 56% in wt/wt, wt/mut and mut/mut, respectively; P = 0.040), with an increased response rate in mut/mut tumours relative to wt/wt (odds ratio = 1.88). Thymidylate synthase activity measured in metastases was a significant predictor of 5FU responsiveness and the addition of the 677C>T genotype improved model prediction. MTHFR 1298A>C polymorphism was significantly linked to specific survival, with homozygous mutated patients having the worst prognosis (P = 0.009, relative risk = 2.48 in mut/mut versus wt/wt). MTHFR 1298A>C genotype remained a significant predictor in a multivariate analysis including metastasis characteristics. The results suggest that MTHFR genotypes are relevant and independent factors of patient outcome in 5FU-based treatment of advanced colorectal cancer.

Pharmacogenetics. 2004 Dec;14(12):841-50. Related Articles, Links Pharmacogenetics and herb-drug interactions: experience with Ginkgo biloba and omeprazole. Yin OQ, Tomlinson B, Waye MM, Chow AH, Chow MS. School of Pharmacy, the Chinese University of Hong Kong, Shatin, New Territories, Hong Kong. OBJECTIVE: Ginkgo biloba was found to exert a significant inductive effect on CYP2C19 activity. This study was designed to investigate the potential herb-drug interaction between G. biloba and omeprazole, a widely used CYP2C19 substrate, in subjects with different CYP2C19 genotypes. METHODS: Eighteen healthy Chinese subjects previously genotyped for CYP2C19 were selected. All subjects received a single omeprazole 40 mg at baseline and then at the end of a 12-day treatment period with G. biloba (140 mg, bid). Multiple blood samples were collected over 12 h, and 24 h urine was collected post omeprazole dosing. Plasma and urine concentrations of omeprazole and its metabolites, 5-hydroxyomeprazole and omeprazole sulfone, were determined, and their pharmacokinetics calculated non-compartmentally. RESULTS: Plasma concentrations of omeprazole and omeprazole sulfone were significantly decreased, and 5-hydroxyomeprazole significantly increased following G. biloba administration in comparison to baseline. A significant decrease in the ratio of area under the plasma concentration-time curve (AUC) of omeprazole to 5-hydroxyomeprazole was observed in the homozygous extensive metabolizers, heterozygous extensive metabolizers, and poor metabolizers, respectively. The decrease was greater in PMs than EMs. No significant changes in the AUC ratios of omeprazole to omeprazole sulfone were observed. Renal clearance of 5-hydroxyomeprazole was significantly decreased after G. biloba, but the change was not significantly different among the three genotype groups. CONCLUSION: Our results show that G biloba can induce omeprazole hydroxylation in a CYP2C19 genotype-dependent manner and concurrently reduce the renal clearance of 5-hydroxyomeprazole. Co-administration of G. biloba with omeprazole or other CYP2C19 substrates may significantly reduce their effect, but further studies are warranted.

Pharmacogenetics. 2004 Jul;14(7):391-3. Related Articles, Links Comment on: Pharmacogenetics. 2004 Jul;14(7):397-406. Pharmacogenetics and the regulation of gene transcription. Grant DM. Department of Pharmacology, Faculty of Medicine, Leslie Dan Faculty of Pharmacy, Institute for Drug Research, University of Toronto, Toronto, Canada. denis.grant@utoronto.ca Publication Types: Comment Review

Pharmacogenetics. 2004 Jul;14(7):395-6. Related Articles, Links Comment on: Pharmacogenetics. 2004 Jul;14(7):407-17. Closing the gap between science and clinical practice: the thiopurine S-methyltransferase polymorphism moves forward. Krynetskiy EY, Evans WE. Department of Pharmaceutical Sciences, St Jude Children's Research Hospital, Memphis, Tennessee, USA. Publication Types: Comment Review

Pharmacogenetics. 2004 Jun;14(6):333-4. Related Articles, Links Comment on: Pharmacogenetics. 2004 Jun;14(6):335-42. Bringing genomics to the bedside: a cost-effective pharmacogenomic test? Veenstra DL. School of Pharmacy, University of California, San Francisco, California 94143, USA. davidv@itsa.ucsf.edu Publication Types: Comment Editorial

Pharmacogenetics. 2004 Jun;14(6):335-42. Related Articles, Links Comment in: Pharmacogenetics. 2004 Jun;14(6):333-4. Pharmacogenetics. 2004 Nov;14(11):783-4; author reply 784. Cost-effectiveness analysis of HLA B*5701 genotyping in preventing abacavir hypersensitivity. Hughes DA, Vilar FJ, Ward CC, Alfirevic A, Park BK, Pirmohamed M. Department of Pharmacology and Therapeutics, University of Liverpool, Liverpool, L69 3GE, UK. OBJECTIVE: Abacavir, a human immunodeficiency virus-1 (HIV-1) nucleoside-analogue reverse transcriptase inhibitor, causes severe hypersensitivity in 4-8% of patients. HLA B*5701 is a known genetic risk factor for abacavir hypersensitivity in Caucasians. Our aim was to confirm the presence of this genetic factor in our patients, and to determine whether genotyping for HLA B*5701 would be a cost-effective use of healthcare resources. METHODS: Patients with and without abacavir hypersensitivity were identified from a UK HIV clinic. Patients were genotyped for HLA B*5701, and pooled data used for calculation of test characteristics. The cost-effectiveness analysis incorporated the cost of testing, cost of treating abacavir hypersensitivity, and the cost and selection of alternative antiretroviral regimens. A probabilistic decision analytic model (comparing testing versus no testing) was formulated and Monte Carlo simulations performed. RESULTS: Of the abacavir hypersensitive patients, six (46%) were HLA B*5701 positive, compared to five (10%) of the non-hypersensitive patients (odds ratio 7.9 [95% confidence intervals 1.5-41.4], P = 0.006). Pooling of our data on HLA B*5701 with published data resulted in a pooled odds ratio of 29 (95% CI 6.4-132.3; P < 0.0001). The cost-effectiveness model demonstrated that depending on the choice of comparator, routine testing for HLA B*5701 ranged from being a dominant strategy (less expensive and more beneficial than not testing) to an incremental cost-effectiveness ratio (versus no testing) of Euro 22,811 per hypersensitivity reaction avoided. CONCLUSIONS: Abacavir hypersensitivity is associated with HLA B*5701, and pre-prescription pharmacogenetic testing for this appears to be a cost-effective use of healthcare resources.

Pharmacogenetics. 2004 Sep;14(9):577-86. Related Articles, Links Extracting and characterizing gene-drug relationships from the literature. Chang JT, Altman RB. Department of Genetics, Stanford Biomedical Informatics, Stanford, CA 94305-5120, USA. A fundamental task of pharmacogenetics is to collect and classify relationships between genes and drugs. Currently, this useful information has not been comprehensively aggregated in any database and remains scattered throughout the published literature. Although there are efforts to collect this information manually, they are limited by the size of the published literature on gene-drug relationships. Therefore, we investigated computational methods to extract and characterize pharmacogenetic relationships between genes and drugs from the literature. We first evaluated the effectiveness of the co-occurrence method in identifying related genes and drugs. We then used supervised machine learning algorithms to classify the relationships between genes and drugs from the Pharmacogenetics and Pharmacogenomics Knowledge Base (PharmGKB) into five categories that have been defined by active pharmacogenetic researchers as relevant to their work. The final co-occurrence algorithm was able to extract 78% of the related genes and drugs that were published in a review article from the literature. Our algorithm subsequently classified the relationships between genes and drugs from the PharmGKB into five categories with 74% accuracy. We have made the data available on a supplementary website at http://bionlp.stanford.edu/genedrug/ Gene-drug relationships can be accurately extracted from text and classified into categories. Although the relationships that we have identified do not capture the details and fine distinctions often made in the literature, these methods will help scientists to track the ever-growing literature and create information resources to support future discoveries.

Pharmacogenetics. 2004 Sep;14(9):607-13. Related Articles, Links Pharmacogenetics of selective serotonin reuptake inhibitor response: a 6-month follow-up. Serretti A, Zanardi R, Franchini L, Artioli P, Dotoli D, Pirovano A, Smeraldi E. Department of Psychiatry, Vita-Salute University, San Raffaele Hospital, Milan, Italy. serretti.alessandro@hsr.it BACKGROUND: We previously reported the association between some genetic factors and short-term antidepressant outcome. In the present paper we investigated the same gene variants in a prospective 6-months naturalistic follow-up. METHODS: The sample included 185 inpatients affected by recurrent major depression consecutively admitted to the Psychiatric Inpatient Unit of San Raffaele Hospital from 1998 to 2003 and prospectively followed for 6 months after their recovery. All the patients were undertaking continuation therapy. The functional polymorphism in the upstream regulatory region of the serotonin transporter gene (SERTPR), the tryptophan hydroxylase A218C substitution, a VNTR polymorphism located 1.2 kb upstream of the monoamine oxidase-A coding sequences, the CLOCK gene T3111C and the PER3exon15 gene T1940G substitutions were analysed, using PCR-based techniques. RESULTS: No association was found between clinical variables and relapses; subjects showing TT genotype at CLOCK gene tended to relapse within 6 months after recovery more than TC and CC subjects taken together. A non-significant tendency of SERTPR*s/s subjects to a minor frequency of relapse was also observed. CONCLUSION: Some subjects showing remission after acute treatment relapsed within 6 months, despite undertaking a maintenance treatment; the causes could be heterogeneous, but CLOCK gene variants may influence the outcome.

Pharmacogenomics J. 2004;4(2):74-6. Related Articles, Links Representational oligonucleotide microarray analysis (ROMA) in pharmacogenomics. Liu ET. Publication Types: News

Pharmacogenomics J. 2004;4(2):77-87. Related Articles, Links Clinical implications of pharmacogenomics for tardive dyskinesia. Muller DJ, Shinkai T, De Luca V, Kennedy JL. Department of Psychiatry, University of Toronto, Centre for Addiction and Mental Health, Toronto, ON, Canada. Publication Types: Review

Pharmacogenomics J. 2004;4(3):161-70. Related Articles, Links Pharmacogenetics and bipolar disorder. Mamdani F, Groisman IJ, Alda M, Turecki G. Douglas Hospital Research Centre, McGill University, Montreal, Quebec, Canada. Bipolar disorder (BD) is a major psychiatric condition that commonly requires prophylactic and episodic treatment. There is important variability in the therapeutic response and side-effect profiles to currently available pharmacological agents. Pharmacogenetics have provided new hopes to develop more efficient treatment strategies tailored to the individual patient's needs. This review assesses nonsystematically studies using pharmacogenetic strategies in BD. Most of these studies have focused on patients selected according to lithium response, and more recently, a growing number of studies have been investigating genetic factors in mixed samples of patients classified according to response to antidepressant treatment. Although previous clinical and family studies support the use of pharmacogenetic strategies both to increase phenotype homogeneity as well as to identify genetic factors that may mediate response to treatment, most molecular studies carried out to date are still preliminary and in need of external validation. A major problem has been comparability between studies, in part, because of differences in the criteria used to define response. More attention should be paid to standardize the criteria for drug response definition. Publication Types: Review

Pharmacogenomics J. 2004;4(3):171-4. Related Articles, Links Pharmacogenomic perspectives of chronic hepatitis C virus

(HCV) infection. Tang J, Kaslow RA. Department of Medicine, University of Alabama at Birmingham, Birmingham, AL 35294, USA. jtang@uab.edu Publication Types: Review

Pharmacogenomics J. 2004;4(4):219. Related Articles, Links Old principles in new clothes. Redei EE. Publication Types: Editorial

Pharmacogenomics J. 2004;4(4):226-32. Related Articles, Links Pharmacogenomics in drug development: societal and technical aspects. Bartfai T. Department of Neuropharmacology, Harold L Dorris Neurological Research Center, The Scripps Research Institute, La Jolla, CA 92037, USA. tbartfai@scripps.edu

Pharmacogenomics J. 2004;4(4):233-44. Related Articles, Links The pharmacogenomics of selective serotonin reuptake inhibitors. Serretti A, Artioli P. Department of Psychiatry, Vita-Salute University, San Raffaele Institute, Milan Italy. serretti@alessandro@hsr.it The introduction of selective serotonin (5-HT) reuptake inhibitors (SSRIs) has significantly improved the pharmacological treatment of a range of psychiatric disorders. Nevertheless, despite the undoubted advantages of antidepressant treatment in terms of improved tolerability to therapy while maintaining a high level of efficacy, not all patients benefit from it; an appreciable proportion do not respond adequately, while others may show adverse reactions. The necessary change of the initial treatment choice often requires extended periods for the remission of symptomatology. Such difficulties could be avoided if it should be possible to determine more quickly the most suitable drug. Several factors have been thought to influence the outcome of antidepressant therapy. Among the factors influencing the interindividual variability in response to treatment with SSRI, differences in genetic features may play a significant role. Several genetic polymorphisms have been associated with therapeutic SSRI response, including genetic variants of the 5-HT transporter, 5-HT-2A-receptor, tryptophan hydroxylase, brain-derived neurotrophic factor, G-protein beta3 subunit, interleukin-1beta and angiotensin-converting enzyme, although with conflicting results; also cytochrome P450 drug-metabolising enzymes may bear a particular importance, although further corroboration of the findings is necessary, and further key participating genes remain to be identified. The hope is that the identification of these genetic components will eventually facilitate the development of a customised SSRI treatment. Publication Types: Review

Pharmacogenomics J. 2004;4(4):260-6. Related Articles, Links Variable drug metabolism genes in Arab population. Bu R, Gutierrez MI, Al-Rasheed M, Belgaumi A, Bhatia K. King Fahad National Center for Children's Cancer and Research, King Faisal Specialist Hospital and Research Center, Riyadh, Saudi Arabia. Cataloging interethnic differences in the distribution of genotypes of drug metabolic genes provides valuable information for profiling the pharmacogenetics of a population. We used PCR analysis to catalog the frequencies of alleles and genotypes for CYP1A1, NAT2, GSTs, MTHFR, MTR (MS) and NQO*1 in Arabs. The frequencies of alleles and/or genotypes for CYP1A1*2A, GSTT1 null, GSTT1 and GSTM1 double null, and GSTP1 A1578G in Arabs were significantly higher than those reported in Caucasians. However, the distribution of NAT2 acetylator phenotypes in both populations was similar. In contrast, the frequencies of MTHFR 677T allele and the combined (677+1298) genotypes for low activity were lower than those reported in Caucasians. Other alleles in Arabs, including CYP1A1 T3801C and GSTP1 A1578G were present in frequencies similar to Africans. The overall profile of variations in metabolism genes in Arabs is thus unique.

Pharmacogenomics J. 2004;4(5):288-90. Related Articles, Links Pharmacogenomics in Japan. Tamaoki M, Gushima H, Tsutani K. RandD Planning and Administration Department, Yamanouchi Pharmaceutical Co. Ltd, Tokyo, Japan. tamaoki@yamanouchi.co.jp Publication Types: Review

Pharmacogenomics J. 2004;4(6):347-8. Related Articles, Links Pharmacogenomics in admixed populations: the Brazilian pharmacogenetics/pharmacogenomics network--REFARGEN. Suarez-Kurtz G. Publication Types: Editorial

Pharmacogenomics J. 2004;4(6):350-3. Related Articles, Links Pharmacogenetic approaches to rheumatoid arthritis. Taniguchi A, Kamatani N. Institute of Rheumatology, Tokyo Women's Medical University, Tokyo, Japan. amtanigu@ior.twmu.ac.jp Publication Types: Review

Pharmacogenomics J. 2004;4(6):354-8. Related Articles, Links Availability of pharmacogenomics-based prescribing information in drug package inserts for currently approved drugs. Zineh I, Gerhard T, Aquilante CL, Beitelshees AL, Beasley BN, Hartzema AG. Department of Pharmacy Practice, University of Florida College of Pharmacy, Gainesville, FL 32610, USA. zineh@cop.ufl.edu

Pharmacogenomics J. 2004;4(6):359-61. Related Articles, Links Pharmacogenetics research network and knowledge base fourth scientific meeting. Davis AF, Long RM. Office of Communications and Public Liaison, National Institute of General Medical Sciences, National Institutes of Health, Bethesda, MD, USA. Publication Types: Congresses

Pharmacogenomics J. 2004;4(6):374-8. Related Articles, Links Identification of a pharmacogenetic effect by linkage disequilibrium mapping. Xu CF, Lewis KF, Yeo AJ, McCarthy LC, Maguire MF, Anwar Z, Danoff TM, Roses AD, Purvis IJ. Discovery and Pipeline Genetics, GlaxoSmithKline Medicines Research Centre, Stevenage, Hertfordshire, UK. cfx74267@gsk.com A practical limitation to the identification of genetic profiles predictive of drug-induced adverse events is the number of patients with the adverse event that can be tolerated before the drug is withdrawn. Whole genome screening for regions of linkage disequilibrium (LD) associated with a particular phenotype may provide the mechanism to rapidly discover specific and sensitive profiles. We have used data from a large phase III clinical trial of tranilast and typed 76 SNPs over a 2.7 megabase region flanking the uridine diphosphate glucuronosyltranserferase 1A1 gene. Three SNPs within one LD block showed strong association with tranilast-induced hyperbilirubinemia (P<10(-13)). Our data illustrated that a genome-wide LD scan of 100,000-200,000 SNPs is sufficient to identify a pharmacogenetic association with a drug-induced adverse event.

Pharmacogenomics J. 2005;5(1):2-5. Related Articles, Links Stored tissue samples: through the confidentiality maze. Joly Y, Knoppers BM, Nguyen MT. Centre de recherche en droit public, Universite de Montreal, Montreal (Quebec), Canada. yann.joly@umontreal.ca

Pharmacogenomics J. 2005;5(3):149-56. Related Articles, Links Sequencing drug response with HapMap. Lin M, Aquilante C, Johnson JA, Wu R. Department of Statistics, University of Florida, Gainesville, FL 32611, USA. The information about how DNA sequence varies across the human genome is crucial for unravelling the genetic basis of drug response. A haplotype map, or HapMap, intended to reveal such a variation pattern, has been recently developed by the International HapMap Consortium. Here, we present a conceptual model for directly characterizing specific DNA sequence variants that are responsible for drug response based on the haplotype structure provided by HapMap. Our model is developed in the maximum likelihood context, incorporated by clinically meaningful mathematical functions that model drug response and implemented with the EM algorithm. Our model is employed to a pharmacogenetic study of cardiovascular disease with 107 patients. We found that the haplotype constituted by allele Gly16 (G) at codon 16 and allele Glu27 (G) at codon 27 genotyped within the beta2AR candidate gene exhibits a different effect on heart rate curve from the rest haplotypes. Parents with the diplotype consisting of two copies of haplotype GG are more sensitive in heart rate to increasing dosages of dobutamine than those with other haplotypes. This model provides a powerful tool for elucidating the genetic variants of drug response and ultimately designing personalized medications based on each patient's genetic constitution.

Pharmacogenomics J. 2005;5(3):183-92. Related Articles, Links Systematic investigation of genetic variability in 111 human genes-implications for studying variable drug response. Freudenberg-Hua Y, Freudenberg J, Winantea J, Kluck N, Cichon S, Bruss M, Propping P, Nothen MM. Institute of Human Genetics, University of Bonn, Bonn, Germany. In order to identify single-nucleotide polymorphisms (SNPs) and analyze their characteristics in a set of 111 genes, we resequenced exons and flanking regions in an average of 170 chromosomes from individuals of European origin. Genetic variability was decreased in noncoding regions highly conserved between human and rodents, indicating functional relevance of these regions. Furthermore, diversity of coding nonsynonymous SNPs was found lower in regions encoding a known protein sequence motif. SNPs predicted to be of functional significance were more common amongst rare variants. Despite the significant recent growth of SNP numbers in public SNP databases, only a small fraction of these rare variants is represented. This may be relevant in the investigation of the genetic causes of severe side effects, for which rare variants are plausible candidates. Estimation of htSNPs reduces the genotyping effort required in capturing common haplotypes, for certain genes, however, this accounts for only a small fraction of haplotype diversity.

Pharmacogenomics J. 2005;5(4):218-20. Related Articles, Links The need for education in pharmacogenomics: a regulatory perspective. Frueh FW, Goodsaid F, Rudman A, Huang SM, Lesko LJ. Publication Types: News

Pharmacogenomics J. 2005;5(4):221-5. Related Articles, Links Pharmacogenomics education: International Society of Pharmacogenomics recommendations for medical, pharmaceutical, and health schools deans of education. Gurwitz D, Lunshof JE, Dedoussis G, Flordellis CS, Fuhr U, Kirchheiner J, Licinio J, Llerena A, Manolopoulos VG, Sheffield LJ, Siest G, Torricelli F, Vasiliou V, Wong S. Department of Human Genetics and Molecular Medicine, Sackler Faculty of Medicine, Tel-Aviv University, Tel-Aviv, Israel. gurwitz@post.tau.ac.il Pharmacogenomics would be instrumental for the realization of personalized medicine in coming decades. Efforts are evident to clarify the potential bioethical, societal, and legal implications of key pharmacogenomics-based technologies projected to be soon introduced into the core practice of medicine. In sharp contrast, a lack of sufficient attention to educational aspects of pharmacogenomics, both for professionals and for society at large, is evident. In order to contribute to this discussion, a 'Pharmacogenomics Education Forum' was held on October 2, 2004 during the 3rd Annual Meeting of the International Society of Pharmacogenomics (ISP) at Santorini, Greece. The participants, members of the ISP Pharmacogenomics Education Forum, after deliberate discussions, proposed a document of 'Background Statement' and 'Recommendations and Call for Action' addressed to Deans of Education at Medical, Pharmaceutical, and Health Schools globally. This document has been considered by the education committee of the International Society of Pharmacogenomics and the result is presented here. We hope that this call would be listened to, and soon followed by beneficial action, ultimately leading to enhanced implementation of personalized medicine into core medical education and practice.

Pharmacogenomics J. 2005;5(4):226-43.

Related Articles, Links Genetic factors influencing pyrimidine-antagonist chemotherapy. Maring JG, Groen HJ, Wachters FM, Uges DR, de Vries EG. Department of Pharmacy, Diaconessen Hospital Meppel and Bethesda Hospital Hoogeveen, Meppel, The Netherlands. maring@diacmeppel.nl Pyrimidine antagonists, for example, 5-fluorouracil (5-FU), cytarabine (ara-C) and gemcitabine (dFdC), are widely used in chemotherapy regimes for colorectal, breast, head and neck, non-small-cell lung cancer, pancreatic cancer and leukaemias. Extensive metabolism is a prerequisite for conversion of these pyrimidine prodrugs into active compounds. Interindividual variation in the activity of metabolising enzymes can affect the extent of prodrug activation and, as a result, act on the efficacy of chemotherapy treatment. Genetic factors at least partly explain interindividual variation in antitumour efficacy and toxicity of pyrimidine antagonists. In this review, proteins relevant for the efficacy and toxicity of pyrimidine antagonists will be summarised. In addition, the role of germline polymorphisms, tumour-specific somatic mutations and protein expression levels in the metabolic pathways and clinical pharmacology of these drugs are described. Germline polymorphisms of uridine monophosphate kinase (UMPK), orotate phosphoribosyl transferase (OPRT), thymidylate synthase (TS), dihydropyrimidine dehydrogenase (DPD) and methylene tetrahydrofolate reductase (MTHFR) and gene expression levels of OPRT, UMPK, TS, DPD, uridine phosphorylase, uridine kinase, thymidine phosphorylase, thymidine kinase, deoxyuridine triphosphate nucleotide hydrolase are discussed in relation to 5-FU efficacy. Cytidine deaminase (CDD) and

5'-nucleotidase (5NT) gene polymorphisms and CDD, 5NT, deoxycytidine kinase and MRP5 gene expression levels and their potential relation to dFdC and ara-C cytotoxicity are reviewed. Publication Types: Review

Pharmacogenomics J. 2005;5(6):338-45. Related Articles, Links Pharmacogenomic assessment of treatment options in gestational diabetes. Ort T, Voss M, Lichtmacher A, Saidel M, DeFrancesco M, Greenberg P, Hunt B, Eisen A. CuraGen Corporation, Branford, CT, USA. Gene expression profiles offer a multidimensional view of metabolic diseases, typically characterized by a single parameter, and can provide a basis for choosing between therapies yielding a common clinical end point. We applied such an approach in gestational diabetes mellitus (GDM). Gene expression was examined in four maternal tissues and placentas from normal patients and euglycemic GDM patients, undergoing elective Cesarean sections at term, treated either by diet or diet plus insulin. Deviations from normal were 11-fold greater for the patients treated by diet, alone, than for patients treated by diet plus insulin. Assuming the achievement of a "normal" gene expression profile, in addition to euglycemia, is a desirable outcome of treatment, insulin treatment appears to have a beneficial effect in the treatment of GDM. Subsequently, we utilized the expression data to identify serum biomarkers that provide ways to monitor the benefits of insulin treatment in GDM.

Pharmacogenomics J. 2005;5(6):374-80. Related Articles, Links Combining several polymorphisms of thymidylate synthase gene for pharmacogenetic analysis. Krajinovic M, Costea I, Primeau M, Dulucq S, Moghrabi A. Centre de Recherche, Hopital Sainte-Justine, Centre Hospitalier Universitaire Mere-Enfant, 3175 Cote-Sainte-Catherine, Montreal, Quebec, Canada H3T 1C5. maja.krajinovic@umontreal.ca Thymidylate synthase (TS) is an essential enzyme in proliferating cells and an important target for several chemotherapeutics. Several TS gene polymorphisms correlate with variable TS expression: a double (2R) and triple (3R) 28-bp repeat element, a G to C substitution of the 3R allele and a 6 bp variation in 3'UTR. We have previously shown that childhood acute lymphoblastic leukemia (ALL) patients who are homozygous for the 3R allele had reduced event-free survival (EFS) probabilities. Here, we analyzed all three polymorphisms in an extended group of ALL patients (n=259). The effect of the 3R homozygosity on ALL outcome was confirmed (P=0.006), whereas 6 bp polymorphism did not influence EFS when analyzed separately. No significant difference among 3R3R genotype subgroups, as defined by a G to C substitution, was observed. The haplotype analysis revealed the higher frequency of the 3RC/6 bp+ haplotype (P=0.04) and the protective role of the 2R/6b p- (P=0.04). Consequently, homozygosity for the 6 bp- allele appeared to reduce an event-predisposing effect of 3R variant. Although of importance for translation into the clinical practice, these findings need confirmation in larger studies.

Pharmacogenomics J. 2006 Feb 28; [Epub ahead of print] Related Articles, Links Defining the clinical role of pharmacogenetics in antiepileptic drug therapy. Dlugos DJ, Buono RJ, Ferraro TN. 1Divison of Neurology, The

Children's Hospital of Philadelphia, Philadelphia, PA, USA. y publisher]

Pharmacogenomics J. 2006 Feb 7; [Epub ahead of print] Related Articles, Links Overview of the pharmacogenetics of HIV therapy. Rodriguez-Novoa S, Barreiro P, Jimenez-Nacher I, Soriano V. 1Pharmacokinetic Unit, Hospital Carlos III, Madrid, Spain. The administration of standard doses of most antiretroviral drugs results in significant variations in plasma drug concentrations among different individuals, influencing antiviral activity as well as incidence of drug-related toxicities. The reasons for this large inter-individual variability in drug levels are multifactorial, and involve differences in metabolism related to gender, concomitant medications, drug compliance, underlying diseases and genetic factors. Pharmacogenetics is the discipline that analyses the genetic basis for the inter-individual variation in the body disposition of drugs. One of its main goals is to give grounds to individualized treatment. The majority of pharmacogenetic traits so far have involved drug metabolism. This is the case for the inherited variation in the pharmacokinetics and pharmacodynamics of drugs such as hydralazine or isoniazid, which is due to polymorphisms in the N-acetyltransferase-2 (NAT2) gene, which allows splitting the population into three categories: slow, intermediate, and fast metabolizers. Pharmacogenetic studies conducted so far with antiretroviral drugs have focussed on metabolizer enzymes at the liver and on transporter proteins on cell membranes. Herein, we review the most relevant metabolizer enzymes and protein transporters, along with the genetic polymorphisms, which seem to influence the pharmacokinetics of antiretroviral drugs, ultimately determining its efficacy and toxicity.The Pharmacogenomics Journal advance online publication, 7 February 2006; doi:10.1038/sj.tpj.6500374. y publisher]

Pharmacogenomics J. 2006 Jan 10; [Epub ahead of print] Related Articles, Links Influence of phenotype and pharmacokinetics on beta-blocker drug target pharmacogenetics. Beitelshees AL, Zineh I, Yarandi HN, Pauly DF, Johnson JA. 1Department of Pharmacy Practice and Center for Pharmacogenomics, University of Florida College of Pharmacy, Gainesville, FL, USA. Two common polymorphisms in the beta(1)-adrenergic receptor gene, Ser49Gly and Arg389Gly, are associated with variable antihypertensive response to metoprolol. We sought to determine whether similar pharmacogenetic associations were present with the negative chronotropic response phenotype to metoprolol. Metoprolol was titrated in 54 untreated hypertensive patients to achieve blood pressure control. We found no association between either resting or exercise heart rate at baseline (untreated) or in response to metoprolol by codon 389 genotype. In contrast, when compared by codon 49 genotype, Ser49 homozygotes had significantly higher resting heart rates at baseline (untreated) than Gly49 carriers (82+/-10 versus 74+/-11 bpm, respectively, P=0.016). When corrected for plasma concentration, we found no difference in reduction in exercise heart rate in response to metoprolol between Ser49 homozygotes and Gly49 carriers (0.75+/-0.11 versus 0.57+/-0.17%/ng/ml, respectively, P=0.37). However, if one fails to account for plasma concentration, trends toward a significant difference in heart rate reduction are seen between Ser49 homozygotes and Gly49 carriers (31% reduction versus 25% reduction, P=0.05). Our data suggest that neither the beta(1)-adrenergic receptor

Arg389Gly, nor the Ser49Gly polymorphisms are associated with variable negative chronotropic response to metoprolol. In addition, our data highlight the importance of measuring metoprolol concentration in order to account for variable pharmacokinetics and avoid misinterpretation of the data.The Pharmacogenomics Journal advance online publication, 10 January 2006; doi:10.1038/sj.tpj.6500354. y publisher]

Pharmacogenomics J. 2006 Jan 17; [Epub ahead of print] Related Articles, Links Pharmacogenetics and pharmacogenomics: origin, status, and the hope for personalized medicine. Kalow W. 1Department of Pharmacology, University of Toronto, Toronto, Canada. Pharmacogenetics arose with studies of single genes, which had major effects on the action of particular drugs. It turned into pharmacogenomics through realization that the controls of most drug responses are multifactorial. Then, variable gene expression posed new problems, for example what do drugs do to genes, or how useful is any genetic pretesting of a person? A common disease may be caused by different groups of genes in different people, who therefore require different drugs for treatment. Personlized medicine is currently represented by a physician's attention to a patients age, sex, or ethnic backround, that is groups showing smaller genetic variation than is typical for general humanity. Occasionally, there is also the use of single-gene pretesting of a patient before drug administration. Over time, improvements in multigenic testing promise to increase the role of personalized medicine. However, the many pharmacogenomic complexities, and particularly time-dependent changes of gene expression, will never allow personalized medicine to become an error-free entity.The Pharmacogenomics Journal advance online publication, 17 January 2006; doi:10.1038/sj.tpj.6500361. y publisher]

Pharmacogenomics J. 2006 Jan-Feb;6(1):16-21. Related Articles, Links Pharmacogenetics and the concept of individualized medicine. Shastry BS. Department of Biological Sciences, Oakland University, Rochester, MI 48309, USA. shastry@oakland.edu Adverse drug reaction in patients causes more than 2 million hospitalizations including 100,000 deaths per year in the United States. This adverse drug reaction could be due to multiple factors such as disease determinants, environmental and genetic factors. In order to improve the efficacy and safety and to understand the disposition and clinical consequences of drugs, two rapidly developing fields--pharmacogenetics (focus is on single genes) and pharmacogenomics (focus is on many genes)--have undertaken studies on the genetic personalization of drug response. This is because many drug responses appear to be genetically determined and the relationship between genotype and drug response may have a very valuable diagnostic value. Identification and characterization of a large number of genetic polymorphisms (biomarkers) in drug metabolizing enzymes and drug transporters in an ethnically diverse group of individuals may provide substantial knowledge about the mechanisms of inter-individual differences in drug response. However, progress in understanding complex diseases, its negative psychosocial consequences, violation of privacy or discrimination, associated cost and availability and its complexity (extensive geographic variations in genes) may become potential barriers in incorporating this pharmacogenetic data in risk assessment and treatment decisions. In addition, it requires increased enthusiasm and education in the clinical community and an understanding of pharmacogenetics itself by the lay public. Although individualized medications remain as a challenge for the future, the pharmacogenetic approach in drug development should be still continued. If it becomes a reality, it delivers benefits to improve public health and allow genetically subgroup diseases thereby avoiding adverse drug reactions (by knowing in advance who should be treated with what drug and how). Publication Types: Review

Pharmacogenomics J. 2006 Jan-Feb;6(1):3-7. Related Articles, Links The current clinical practice of pharmacogenetic testing in Europe: TPMT and HER2 as case studies. Woelderink A, Ibarreta D, Hopkins MM, Rodriguez-Cerezo E. 1Institute for Prospective Technological Studies, European Commission Joint Research Centre, Edificio EXPO, Seville, Spain.

Pharmacogenomics. 2004 Apr;5(3):273-82. Related Articles, Links Pharmacogenomics of the OATP and OAT families. Marzolini C, Tirona RG, Kim RB. Division of Clinical Pharmacology,Vanderbilt University School of Medicine, Nashville, TN 37232, USA. richard.kim@vanderbilt.edu Drug disposition is highly dependent on the interplay between drug metabolism and transport in organs such as the intestine, kidney, and liver. Genetically determined variation in drug transporter function or expression is now increasingly recognized to have a significant role as a determinant of intersubject variability in drug response. Similar to the discoveries of functional genetic variations in drug efflux transporters, such as multi-drug resistance proteins 1 and 2, there have been considerable advances in the identification of single nucleotide polymorphisms in transporters that facilitate cellular drug uptake. Among the uptake transporters, members of the organic anion-transporting polypeptides and organic anion transporters can mediate the cellular uptake of a large number of structurally divergent compounds. Accordingly, functionally relevant polymorphisms in these transporters may contribute to interindividual and interethnic variability in drug disposition and response. In this review, recent progress relating to pharmacogenomics of organic anion transporters will be outlined along with a compilation of currently known genetic polymorphisms. Publication Types: Review

Pharmacogenomics. 2004 Apr;5(3):283-94. Related Articles, Links Pharmacogenetics of human androgens and prostate cancer--an update. Novelli G, Margiotti K, Chiocca AM, Spera E, Micali F, Reichardt JK. Universita di Roma Tor Vergata, Roma, Italy. novelli@med.uniroma2.it Prostate cancer is the most common non-skin cancer in the US; it is the second leading cause of death from cancer among US men, and the seventh leading cause of death in the US. This review examines the recent biochemical and pharmacogenetic literature related to prostate cancer, specifically that which focused on constitutional ('germline') single nucleotide polymorphisms at 'functional candidate' genes for prostate cancer. The investigations summarized in this review demonstrate the need to study the molecular genetics at these loci to rationally develop personalized medicine. In addition, the identification of somatic pharmacogenetic alterations in one of these loci suggests that this may also be a fruitful field of investigations with important clinical applications. Pharmacogenomic investigations of constitutional and tumor DNA may lead to significant advances in chemoprevention, presymptomatic diagnosis and improved treatment of prostate cancer. Publication Types: Review

Pharmacogenomics. 2004 Apr;5(3):331-6. Related Articles, Links Role of pharmacoproteomics in the development of personalized medicine. Jain KK. Jain PharmaBiotech, Basel, Switzerland. jain@pharmabiotech.ch Pharmacoproteomics is the use of proteomic technologies in drug discovery and development. Along with pharmacogenomics and pharmacogenetics, pharmacoproteomics will play an important role in the development of personalized medicines in several ways. Proteomic technologies are contributing to molecular diagnostics, which is a basis of personalized medicine. Pharmacoproteomics is a more functional representation of patient-to-patient variation than that provided by genotyping. Proteomics-based characterization of multifactorial diseases may help to match a particular target-based therapy to a particular marker in a subgroup of patients. Individualized therapy may be based on differential protein expression rather than a genetic polymorphism. Finally, proteomic technologies would enable discovery and development of drugs suitable for personalized therapy. Protein chips will be used increasingly in clinical diagnostics in the next 5 years, particularly in the point-of-care diagnostics. This will facilitate the practice of personalized medicine in the clinic by the end of this decade. Publication Types: Review

Pharmacogenomics. 2004 Apr;5(3):337-40. Related Articles, Links Gentronix. McCulloch P. Gentronix Ltd, Manchester, UK. Gentronix is an innovative biotechnology company with the aim of providing cell-based assays and systems to ease or remove some of the current bottlenecks in preclinical drug discovery and development. Gentronix's first product, GreenScreen trade mark GC, is a combined genotoxicity and cytotoxicity test designed for high-throughput screening of new pharmaceutical lead compounds, giving drug development scientists a cost-effective preview of the battery of mandatory regulatory genotoxicity tests. Future products based on the company's extensive intellectual property rights portfolio will combine the company's expertise in cellular biosensor systems with novel optical detection technology to deliver a range of products for other applications within drug discovery, as well as industrial and environmental monitoring of toxic chemicals.

Pharmacogenomics. 2004 Dec;5(8):1019-22. Related Articles, Links Candidate gene selection in pharmacogenomics: biology leads the way. Watters JW, McLeod HL. Publication Types: Editorial

Pharmacogenomics. 2004 Dec;5(8):1023-7. Related Articles, Links Pharmacogenomics in Asia. Tamaoki M, Gushima H, Tsutani K. Product Evaluation Department, Yamanouchi Pharmaceutical Co. Ltd., Tokyo, Japan. tamaoki@yamanouchi.co.jp It is well known that genetic polymorphisms, such as SNPs, vary between races so that not only Western populations' pharmacogenetic/pharmacogenomic data but also data from Asians are viewed as vital to drug development and clinical practice. For this report, the current state of pharmacogenetic/pharmacogenomic-related activities in five Asian countries

(China, Japan, the Republic of Korea, Singapore, and Taiwan) were researched and analyzed. The results show that there are multiple efforts underway in all of these countries, including the examination of guidelines, the implementation of projects to establish foundations for pharmacogenetics/pharmacogenomics, and several clinical trials, that have hardly been recognized up to now. Publication Types: Review

Pharmacogenomics. 2004 Dec;5(8):1033-6. Related Articles, Links Genotyping for drug-metabolizing enzymes--does the promise meet the reality? Gardiner SJ, Begg EJ. Department of Medicine, Christchurch School of Medicine, Private Bag 4345, Christchurch, New Zealand. sharon.gardiner@cdhb.govt.nz Publication Types: Clinical Conference

Pharmacogenomics. 2004 Dec;5(8):1037-48. Related Articles, Links Alcoholism: genes and mechanisms. Oroszi G, Goldman D. Laboratory of Neurogenetics, NIAAA, NIH, 5625 Fishers Lane, Room 3S32, MSC9412, Rockville, MD 20852, USA. Alcoholism is a chronic relapsing/remitting disease that is frequently unrecognized and untreated, in part because of the partial efficacy of treatment. Only approximately one-third of patients remain abstinent and one-third have fully relapsed 1 year after withdrawal from alcohol, with treated patients doing substantially better than untreated [1]. The partial effectiveness of strategies for prevention and treatment, and variation in clinical course and side effects, represent a challenge and an opportunity to better understand the neurobiology of addiction. The strong heritability of alcoholism suggests the existence of inherited functional variants of genes that alter the metabolism of alcohol and variants of other genes that alter the neurobiologies of reward, executive cognitive function, anxiety/dysphoria, and neuronal plasticity. Each of these neurobiologies has been identified as a critical domain in the addictions. Functional alleles that alter alcoholism-related intermediate phenotypes include common alcohol dehydrogenase 1B and aldehyde dehydrogenase 2 variants that cause the aversive flushing reaction; catechol-O-methyltransferase (COMT) Val158Met leading to differences in three aspects of neurobiology: executive cognitive function, stress/anxiety response, and opioid function; opioid receptor micro1 (OPRM1) Asn40Asp, which may serve as a gatekeeper molecule in the action of naltrexone, a drug used in alcoholism treatment; and HTTLPR, which alters serotonin transporter function and appears to affect stress response and anxiety/dysphoria, which are factors relevant to initial vulnerability, the process of addiction, and relapse. Publication Types: Review

Pharmacogenomics. 2004 Dec;5(8):1107-16. Related Articles, Links Pharmacogenetics/pharmacogenomics and antirheumatic drugs in rheumatology. Ferraccioli G, De Santis M, Tolusso B. Division of Rheumatology, Postgraduate School in Rheumatology, Institute of Internal Medicine and Geriatrics, Catholic University of the Sacred Heart-CIC, Via Moscati 31, 00168 Rome, Italy. gf.ferraccioli@rm.unicatt.it Genomic medicine has raised many expectations with regard to individualized therapies. Drug response is a complex function of many genes interacting with environmental and behavioral factors. In addition, poor prescribing, interactions between drugs and an incomplete understanding of the metabolism of many drugs, which are administered simultaneously to treat concomitant morbidities, are leading causes of the occurrence of adverse drug reactions in chronic non-inflammatory and autoimmune rheumatic diseases. Symptomatic non-steroidal anti-inflammatory drugs, as well as disease-modifying drugs, are complicated by drop-outs (poor patient compliance) in a large percentage of patients. Even though intensive and careful monitoring is always clearly advisable, preliminary data suggest that typing of genes controlling the effects, metabolism and response of drugs might be of clinical utility to define the 'at-risk' genotype. Publication Types: Review

Pharmacogenomics. 2004 Dec;5(8):1139-49. Related Articles, Links A systematic review of cost-effectiveness analyses of pharmacogenomic interventions. Phillips KA, Van Bebber SL. School of Pharmacy, Institute of Health Policy Studies and UCSF Comprehensive Cancer Center, University of California, San Francisco, 3333 California St., UCSF Box 0613, San Francisco, CA 94143, USA. kathryn@itsa.ucsf.edu Cost-effectiveness analysis is a widely used tool to assess the value of healthcare interventions. Our objective was to conduct a systematic review of the literature on the cost effectiveness of pharmacogenomic interventions. We found 11 studies that met our inclusion criteria. The most commonly examined disease was deep vein thrombosis (n=4), followed by cancer (n=3) and viral infections (n=3); the most frequently examined mutation was factor V Leiden (n=5); and the majority of the mutations examined were inherited mutations (n=7), although several studies looked at acquired (tumor or viral) mutations (n=4). The majority of the studies reported a favorable cost-effectiveness ratio for the pharmacogenomic-based strategy (n=7), while two studies reported that the pharmacogenomic-based strategy was not cost effective and two were equivocal. We conclude that there have been few evaluations of the economic costs and benefits of pharmacogenomic interventions and they have covered a limited number of conditions. Further analyses that can be used to guide the use of pharmacogenomics in clinical practice and in developing health policies are urgently needed. Publication Types: Review

Pharmacogenomics. 2004 Dec;5(8):1151-62. Related Articles, Links Homocysteine: exploring its potential as a pharmacodynamic biomarker of antifolate chemotherapy. Valik D, Radina M, Sterba J, Vojtesek B. Department of Laboratory Medicine, Masaryk Memorial Cancer Institute, Zluty kopec 7, 656 53 Brno, Czech Republic. valik@mou.cz For decades it has been well known that elevated levels of homocysteine are harmful to humans on the basis of clinical observations derived from classical model diseases, such as inherited metabolic disorders. This group of diseases includes classical homocystinuria and several other inherited diseases affecting the so-called 'transsulfuration pathways'. Homocysteine lies in a metabolic checkpoint that interconnects one-carbon-transferring reactions with metabolism of sulfur-containing amino acids, since every molecule of 5-methyltetrahydrofolate derived either from plasma or generated from other folate species must be demethylated to liberate the reduced tetrahydrofolate. This unidirectional mechanism operates in every cell and has no alternative in eukaryotic cells. Antifolates are a group of anticancer agents targeting various metabolic steps within folate metabolism. They exert an indirect influence on the rate of appearance/disappearance of homocysteine from cellular and plasma compartments. Recently, it has been postulated that homocysteine may be a marker of the 'pharmacodynamic effect' of methotrexate, but studies attesting to this role are only now emerging. Here, we explore the genetic disease of folate and homocysteine metabolism and discuss the links between these model disorders with pharmacology and pharmacogenetics of folate antagonists used in the clinic. We outline possible ways of how homocysteine may be used as a biomarker of antifolate therapy. Publication Types: Review

Pharmacogenomics. 2004 Dec;5(8):1163-6. Related Articles, Links Toward an integrative systems toxicology. Hurban P. Icoria, Inc., 108 TW Alexander Drive, Research Triangle Park, NC 27709-4528, USA. phurban@icoria.com

Pharmacogenomics. 2004 Dec;5(8):1167-73. Related Articles, Links Molecular pathology in oncology--the AstraZeneca perspective. Campbell DA, Carmichael J, Chopra R. Experimental Medicine, AstraZeneca, Alderley Park, Macclesfield, Cheshire, SK10 4TG, UK. david.campbell@astrazeneca.com Growth of the oncology portfolio remains of strategic importance to AstraZeneca, and the adoption of new technologies to allow us to enhance this portfolio is central to this strategy. With the move away from classical hormonal and cytotoxic therapies to the development of more targeted approaches for the treatment of cancer, an understanding of the molecular pathology of the disease state is becoming vital. Our understanding of the pathogenesis of cancer has increased dramatically over the last few decades and with the publication of the human genome and the resultant explosion in the field of genetics and genomics, AstraZeneca is turning its attention to using these new technologies to enhance the oncology RandD platform. In particular, the fields of pharmacogenetics and pharmacogenomics in relation to oncology have received much attention and this has been mirrored externally both within the pharmaceutical/biotechnology and academic sectors. Future products from the AstraZeneca oncology portfolio will increasingly rely on the use of genetics and genomics for patient identification and stratification, whilst these technologies will also provide a source of novel biomarkers and diagnostics that may allow us to streamline the RandD process and help us to better understand the biological basis of the diseases we are aiming to treat. The AstraZeneca perspective is, however, pragmatic enough to appreciate the practical challenges involved in applying pharmacogenetics and genomics not only for early drug development, but also in the organization of the healthcare infrastructure to undertake timely and complex laboratory investigations. Finally, validation of this approach will require carefully controlled clinical studies.

Pharmacogenomics. 2004 Jul;5(5):451-4. Related Articles, Links Perspectives and challenges of clinical pharmacogenomics in cancer. Pusztai L. Publication Types: Editorial

Pharmacogenomics. 2004 Jul;5(5):463-77. Related Articles, Links Neuropsychiatric pharmacogenetics: moving toward a comprehensive understanding of predicting risks and response. Bishop JR, Ellingrod VL. University of Iowa College of Pharmacy, Clinical and Administrative Division, S413 Pharmacy Building, Iowa City, IA 52242-1112, USA. Pharmacogenetic research in the area of neuropsychiatric illnesses is rapidly evolving. Due to the complexity of the human brain, it is not surprising that our knowledge about the interaction between genetics and the treatment of these illnesses is very small. The Human Genome Project (HGP) has identified > 30,000 genes; several thousand of which have been found to occur in the brain or serve a role that enhances the brain's function. Much of the research in the post-HGP era is being driven by a desire to use genetics to predict which patients deviate from the norm in terms of drug response or side effects. By identifying these people, we will be able to direct clinical practice such that therapies for these disorders can be individualized. With this in mind, the following review is intended to cover a broad understanding of CNS pharmacogenetics with the goal of summarizing available literature on promising candidate gene targets, which may eventually help us predict clinical outcomes in patients taking medications commonly used to treat neuropsychiatric disorders. Publication Types: Review

Pharmacogenomics. 2004 Jul;5(5):479-86. Related Articles, Links The role of pharmacogenomics in the prediction of efficacy of anti-TNF therapy in patients with Crohn's disease. Mascheretti S, Schreiber S. 1st Department of Medicine, Christian-Albrechts-Universtitat Kiel, Schittenhelmstrasse 12, D-24105 Kiel, Germany. s.mascheretti@mucosa.de TNF-alpha plays a central role in the pathophysiology of Crohn's disease. Infliximab, a chimeric monoclonal antibody against TNF-alpha, has been shown to be effective and well-tolerated in several large placebo-controlled trials and has become a common treatment for Crohn's disease. The blockade of TNF through the infusion of infliximab is characterized by high clinical efficacy and rapid onset of action. A single infusion of infliximab results in a remission rate of 30-40%. Lack of response appears to be a stable trait even after repeated infusions, suggesting that it might be genetically determined. Mutations in the TNF-alpha gene have been extensively studied as predictors of response with various results. Polymorphisms in the TNF-alpha receptors TNF-R1 and TNF-R2 have been found not to be associated with treatment response. Similarly, the three mutations in the CARD15 gene, which are independently associated with susceptibility to Crohn's disease, have also been found not to be associated with treatment response. Publication Types: Review

Pharmacogenomics. 2004 Jul;5(5):503-5. Related Articles, Links Pharmacogenomic data: FDA voluntary and required submission guidance. Salerno RA, Lesko LJ. Worldwide Regulatory Affairs, Wyeth Research, Collegeville, PA 19426, USA. salernr@wyeth.com Publication Types: Congresses

Pharmacogenomics. 2004 Jul;5(5):507-11. Related Articles, Links Pharmacogenomic data submissions to the FDA: non-clinical case studies. Leighton JK, DeGeorge J, Jacobson-Kram D, MacGregor J, Mendrick D, Worobec A. Division of Oncology Drug Products, CDER, FDA, 5600 Fishers Lane, Rockville, MD 20850, USA. leightonj@cder.fda.gov Publication Types: Congresses

Pharmacogenomics. 2004 Jul;5(5):513-7. Related Articles, Links Pharmacogenomic data submissions to the FDA: clinical pharmacology case studies. Ruano G, Collins JM, Dorner AJ, Wang SJ, Guerciolini R, Huang SM. Genomas LLC, New Haven, CT, USA. Publication Types: Congresses

Pharmacogenomics. 2004 Jul;5(5):519-24. Related Articles, Links Pharmacogenomic data submissions to the FDA: clinical case studies. Trepicchio WL, Williams GA, Essayan D, Hall ST, Harty LC, Shaw PM, Spear BB, Wang SJ, Watson ML. Clinical Research and Pharmacogenomics, Millennium Pharmaceuticals, 40 Landsdowne Street Cambridge, MA 02139, USA. wtrepicchio @mpi.com Publication Types: Congresses

Pharmacogenomics. 2004 Jul;5(5):525-52. Related Articles, Links The genomic response of skeletal muscle to methylprednisolone using microarrays: tailoring data mining to the structure of the pharmacogenomic time series. Almon RR, DuBois DC, Piel WH, Jusko WJ. Department of Biological Sciences, SUNY at Buffalo, Buffalo, NY 14260, USA. almon@eng.buffalo.edu High-throughput data collection using gene microarrays has great potential as a method for addressing the pharmacogenomics of complex biological systems. Similarly, mechanism-based pharmacokinetic/pharmacodynamic modeling provides a tool for formulating quantitative testable hypotheses concerning the responses of complex biological systems. As the response of such systems to drugs generally entails cascades of molecular events in time, a time series design provides the best approach to capturing the full scope of drug effects. A major problem in using microarrays for high-throughput data collection is sorting through the massive amount of data in order to identify probe sets and genes of interest. Due to its inherent redundancy, a rich time series containing many time points and multiple samples per time point allows for the use of less stringent criteria of expression, expression change and data quality for initial filtering of unwanted probe sets. The remaining probe sets can then become the focus of more intense scrutiny by other methods, including temporal clustering, functional clustering and pharmacokinetic/pharmacodynamic modeling, which provide additional ways of identifying the probes and genes of pharmacological interest.

Pharmacogenomics. 2004 Jul;5(5):553-8. Related Articles, Links Frequency of compound genotypes associated with beta-blocker efficacy in congestive heart failure. Lanfear DE, Marsh S, Cresci S, Spertus JA, McLeod HL. Washington University School of Medicine, Department of Medicine, 660 S Euclid Ave, Campus Box 8069, St Louis, MO 63110-1093, USA. An important practical problem in pharmacogenetics is the integration of compound genotypes into individualized therapy. Polymorphisms in the genes encoding the angiotensin-converting enzyme, and beta(1)- and beta(2)-adrenoceptors have been identified as predictors of 'good response' to beta-adrenergic antagonists among heart failure patients. These variants were used as the basis for exploring the concept of compound genotype assessment. The frequency of compound variants in these genes was determined using PCR and pyrosequencing to genotype population samples of 95 African-Americans and 95 European-Americans. Both groups could be divided into four subgroups according to the number of favorable genotypes present. Each subgroup accounted for a significant proportion of subjects (the smallest was 7% of total). This study provides the first look into the population frequency of these compound genotypes, and it provides the necessary first step for future evaluation of polygenic strategies to individualize therapy for heart failure.

Pharmacogenomics. 2004 Jul;5(5):571-9. Related Articles, Links From pharmacogenetics to personalized medicine: a vital need for educating health professionals and the community. Frueh FW, Gurwitz D. Stepoutside Consulting, LLC, Gaithersburg, MD 20878, USA. felix@stepoutside.com The field of pharmacogenetics will soon celebrate its 50th anniversary. Although science has delivered an impressive amount of information in these 50 years, pharmacogenetics has suffered from lack of integration into clinical practice. There are several reasons for this, including the unmet need for education at medical schools and the lack of awareness about the impact of genetic medicine on healthcare in the community. Recently, the FDA announced that it considers pharmacogenomics one of three major opportunities on the critical path to new medical products. This notion by the FDA is filling the regulatory void that existed between drug developers and drug users. However, in order to bring pharmacogenetic testing to the prescription pad successfully, healthcare professionals and policy makers, as well as patients, need to have the necessary background knowledge for making educated treatment decisions. To effectively move pharmacogenetics into everyday medicine, it is therefore imperative for scientists and teachers in the field to take on the challenge of disseminating pharmacogenetic insights to a broader audience. Publication Types: Review

Pharmacogenomics. 2004 Jun;5(4):355-6. Related Articles, Links Advances in genome biology and technology. Mardis ER. Washington University School of Medicine, Department of Genetics, 4444 Forest Park Blvd, Box 8501, St Louis, MO 63108, USA. emardis@watson.wustl.edu Publication Types: Congresses

Pharmacogenomics. 2004 Jun;5(4):361-79. Related Articles, Links Pharmacogenomic strategies against resistance development in microbial infections. Ziebuhr W, Xiao K, Coulibaly B, Schwarz R, Dandekar T. Institut fur Molekulare Infektionsbiologie, Wurzburg, Germany. There are several promising new strategies against resistance development in microbial infections. This paper discusses typical experimental and bioinformatical strategies to study the impact of infectious challenges on host-pathogen interaction, followed by several novel approaches and sources for new pharmaceutical strategies against resistance development. Genomics reveals promising new targets by providing a better understanding of cellular pathways, through the identification of new pathways, and by identifying new intervention areas, such as phospholipids, glycolipids, innate immunity, and antibiotic peptides. Additional antibiotic resources come from new genomes, including marine organisms, lytic phages and probiotic strategies. A system perspective regards all interactions between the host, pathogen and environment to develop new pharmacogenomic strategies against resistance development. Publication Types: Review

Pharmacogenomics. 2004 Jun;5(4):429-32. Related Articles, Links How personalized medicine is changing the rules of drug life exclusivity. Sullivan CG. King and Spalding LLP, 191 Peachtree St, Atlanta, GA 30303, USA. csullivan@kslaw.com Personalized medicine is premised on the notion that diagnostic techniques can improve safety or effectiveness of pharmaceutical therapies based upon individual genetic or proteomic make-ups. This article explains how diagnostic techniques and pharmaceutical therapies interact during the US Food and Drug Administration's approval of branded and generic drugs in the US, and how the same labeling requirement for generic drugs of the Hatch-Waxman Act can prevent generic drugs from entering the market when proprietary pharmacogenomic techniques are incorporated into the labeling of a branded drug. Publication Types: Review

Pharmacogenomics. 2004 Jun;5(4):433-8. Related Articles, Links Solexa Ltd. Bennett S. Solexa Ltd, Chesterford Research Park, Saffron Walden, CB10 1XL, UK. simon.bennett @solexa.com Solexa Ltd is developing an integrated system, based on a breakthrough single molecule sequencing technology, to address a US$2 billion market that is expected to grow exponentially alongside and as a consequence of further technological enhancements. The system, software and consumables will initially be sold to research organizations, pharmaceutical companies and diagnostic companies that will sequence large regions of genomic DNA, including whole genomes, at costs several orders of magnitude below current levels. Solexa expects to launch its first product in 2006, and as it continues to make time and cost efficiencies, additional products will be launched into the expanding markets that will have broad applications in basic research through to healthcare management.

Pharmacogenomics. 2004 Oct;5(7):757-61. Related Articles, Links Chemical genetics: toward the next generation of molecular medicines. Halazy S. Publication Types: Editorial Review

Pharmacogenomics. 2004 Oct;5(7):775-8. Related Articles, Links Bioscience 2004. Strathdee G, Brown R. Centre for Oncology and Applied Pharmacology, Glasgow University, Cancer Research UK, Beatson Laboratories, UK. Publication Types: Congresses

Pharmacogenomics. 2004 Oct;5(7):779-802. Related Articles, Links Pharmacogenomics and drug response in cardiovascular disorders. Siest G, Jeannesson E, Berrahmoune H, Maumus S, Marteau JB, Mohr S, Visvikis S. Universite Henri Poincare, INSERM U525, Nancy I, Faculte de Pharmacie, 30 rue Lionnois, 54000 Nancy, France. gerard.siest@pharma.uhp-nancy.fr. There are a total of 17 families of drugs that are used for treating the heterogeneous group of cardiovascular diseases. We propose a comprehensive pharmacogenomic approach in the field of cardiovascular therapy that considers the five following sources of variability: the genetics of pharmacokinetics, the genetics of pharmacodynamics (drug targets), genetics linked to a defined pathology and its corresponding drug therapies, the genetics of physiologic regulation, and environmental-genetic interactions. Examples of the genetics of pharmacokinetics are presented for phase I (cytochromes P450) and phase II (conjugating enzymes) drug-metabolizing enzymes and for phase III drug transporters. The example used to explain the genetics of pharmacodynamics is glycoprotein IIIa and the response to antiplatelet effects of aspirin. Genetics linked to a defined pathology and its corresponding drug therapies is exemplified by ADRB1, ACE, CETP and APOE and drug response in metabolic syndrome. The examples of cytochrome P450s, APOE and ADRB2 in relation to ethnicity, age and gender are presented to describe genetics of physiologic regulation. Finally, environmental-genetic interactions are exemplified by CYP7A1 and the effects of diet on plasma lipid levels, and by APOE and the effects of smoking in cardiovascular disease. We illustrate this five-tiered approach using examples of cardiovascular drugs in relation to genetic polymorphism. Publication Types: Review

Pharmacogenomics. 2004 Oct;5(7):803-17. Related Articles, Links Pharmacogenomics of adrenoceptors. Flordellis C, Paris H, Karabinis A, Lymperopoulos A. University of Patras, Department of Pharmacology, School of Medicine, 26504 Rio Patras, Greece. flordell@med.upatras.gr. Adrenoceptors (ARs) consist of nine subtypes (alpha(1A)-, alpha(1B)-, alpha(1D)-, beta(1)-, beta(2)-, beta(3)-, alpha(2A)-, alpha(2B)- and alpha(2C)-AR), which are involved in a wide spectrum of physiological functions and are the site of action for a considerable percentage of currently prescribed therapeutics. With the exception of alpha(1D), all AR subtypes are polymorphic with genetic variations in the coding and non-coding regions. This review discusses the biochemical consequences of these genetic variations and their impact in receptor function, disease pathophysiology, and drug response. Pharmacogenomic principles that have been discovered are also discussed. Publication Types: Review

Pharmacogenomics. 2004 Oct;5(7):819-34. Related Articles, Links Pharmacogenetics of methotrexate. Krajinovic M, Moghrabi A. Universite de Montreal, Service d'Hematologie-Oncologie, Centre de Recherche, Hopital Sainte-Justine Departement de Pediatrie, 3175 Cote St Catherine, Montreal, Quebec, H3T 1C5, Canada. maja.krajinovic@umontreal.ca. Methotrexate (MTX) has proven efficient in the treatment of a number of malignancies, as well as non-malignant disorders characterized by a rapid cellular growth. Yet some patients might develop resistance, while others could have toxic side effects. MTX achieves its cytotoxicity through the inhibition of folate-dependent enzymes, suggesting that the genes controlling their activity or the levels of folate cofactors can modulate drug efficacy and, thus, the sensitivity of a patient to MTX. Indeed, several studies, conducted mostly in leukemia and rheumatoid arthritis patients, have addressed the potential for tailoring MTX therapy based on a patient's genetics. Several genetic variants have been shown to have a predictive role, among which the most frequently studied are those of methylenetetrahydrofolate reductase and thymidylate synthase genes. The other candidates, as well as gene-gene interactions, which may be even more important for the prediction of disease outcomes than the individual gene effects, are also briefly discussed. Publication Types: Review

Pharmacogenomics. 2004 Oct;5(7):835-43. Related Articles, Links Pharmacogenetics of irinotecan toxicity. Marsh S, McLeod HL. Washington University, School of Medicine, Division of Oncology, 660 South Euclid Avenue, Campus Box 8069, St Louis, MO 63110, USA. smarsh@im.wustl.edu. Irinotecan is an anticancer drug approved in combination therapy for advanced colorectal cancer. Severe, life-threatening toxicities can occur from irinotecan treatment. Although multiple genes may play a role in irinotecan activity, the UDP glycuronosyltransferase 1 family, polypeptide A1 (UGT1A1) enzyme has been strongly associated with toxicity. A common dinucleotide repeat polymorphism in the UGT1A1 promoter region (UGT1A1*28) has been correlated with severe toxicity in cancer patients receiving irinotecan-containing therapy. Prospective screening of patients prior to chemotherapy selection may reduce the frequency of severe toxicities by allowing alternate therapy selections for patients carrying the UGT1A1*28 polymorphism. Publication Types: Review]

Pharmacogenomics. 2004 Oct;5(7):861-78. Related Articles, Links Toward the pharmacogenomics of cystic fibrosis--an update. Sangiuolo F, D'Apice MR, Gambardella S, Di Daniele N, Novelli G. Department of Biopathology and Diagnostic Imaging, Tor Vergata University, Roma, Italy. Cystic fibrosis (CF) is the most common autosomal recessive disorder in Caucasians, with a frequency of approximately 1 in 3000 live births. The mutated gene is a defective chloride channel in epithelial cells, named cystic fibrosis transmembrane conductance regulator (CFTR). Several different protocols for the scanning of the entire gene have aided molecular diagnosis and improved our understanding of the disorder's pathophysiology, but also showed the disease's complexity. Therefore, CF phenotype remains difficult to predict from CFTR mutation data alone: several studies have suggested that additional genes could modulate its clinical outcome. Gene replacement therapy is still far from being used in patients with CF, mostly due to the difficulties with targeting the appropriate cells. In this review, we summarize recent advances, both in the pharmacological and gene therapy field, aimed for the treatment of the disease. Publication Types: Review

Pharmacogenomics. 2004 Oct;5(7):879-93. Related Articles, Links Genomics, proteomics and metabonomics in toxicology: hopefully not 'fashionomics'. Pognan F. AstraZeneca Pharmaceuticals, Safety Assessment, Wilmington, DE 19850, USA. francois.pognan@astrazeneca.com. Genomics, proteomics and metabonomics are applied to toxicology either as stand-alone technologies or in combination, with the intention of providing a more efficient assessment of the potential side effects of new chemical entities. Two different approaches are taken: a predictive/proactive strategy based on a statistical analogy of 'signatures' of drugs to many known toxicant gene or metabolite fingerprints; and a mechanistic/reactive strategy based on the in-depth biological analysis of the gene, protein or metabolite profiles induced by one or a few compounds of interest. This article focuses on the advantages and disadvantages of these technologies, as well as the many hurdles associated with both these approaches in toxicology that have to be considered before applying them to the assessment of future drugs. Publication Types: Review

Pharmacogenomics. 2004 Oct;5(7):943-7. Related Articles, Links Systems literature analysis. Persidis A, Deftereos S, Persidis A. andreasp@biovista.com. Systems literature analysis (SLA) is the literature-driven version of systems biology. It treats collections of scientific literature as a system of millions of interconnections between research parameters, such as genes, diseases, tissues, cell events, model organisms, experiment types, and reagents. SLA aims to replace the traditional keyword-based querying of literature databases, which return sorted lists of papers, with a systems-based approach that returns integrated networks of relationships. Major applications include literature-based discovery of novel targets that link, for example, previously unlinked diseases and phenotypes to common genes and cellular events, and experiment design.

Pharmacogenomics. 2004 Sep;5(6):627-41. Related Articles, Links Pharmacogenomics and stomach cancer. Toffoli G, Cecchin E. Experimental and Clinical Pharmacology, CRO--National Cancer Institute, via Pedemontana Occidentale, 12, 33081 Aviano, Italy. gtoffoli@cro.it In subgroups of gastric cancer patients, chemotherapy treatments carry a high risk of toxicity without any clear evidence of antitumor activity. Individualization of therapy is required to treat each patient with the optimal drug and dose. Genetic polymorphisms are the hereditary determinants for interindividual variations of drug effect and the genetic approach represents a new tool to design a tailored therapy. This review focuses on the relevance of the host polymorphisms involved in metabolism, cellular transport and interaction with molecular targets of the drugs used in gastric cancer in conventional or innovative chemotherapy regimens. Pharmacogenetic studies based on a single gene or multi-gene approach (pharmacogenomics) are promising to identify gastric cancer patients at risk for adverse toxicity, but larger and controlled studies are needed to justify changes in the chemotherapeutic strategies. Publication Types: Review

Pharmacogenomics. 2004 Sep;5(6):643-55. Related Articles, Links Pharmacogenetics of antiretroviral therapy: genetic variation of response and toxicity. Martin AM, Nolan D, Gaudieri S, Phillips E, Mallal S. Centre for Clinical Immunology and Biomedical Statistics, Royal Perth Hospital and Murdoch University, Perth, Western Australia. The application of a pharmacogenetic approach to antiretroviral drug therapy represents a significant challenge, as treatment involves multiple drugs and drug classes with the potential for significant variability in drug-host, as well as drug-drug, interactions. However, despite this inherent complexity, considerable gains have been made in understanding how genetic factors influence the efficacy and toxicity of HIV therapy. In this review the available evidence regarding genetic variation in drug disposition will be examined, including the potential for relatively polymorphic drug-metabolizing enzymes (e.g., cytochrome P450 isoforms) and drug transporters (e.g., P-glycoprotein) to influence the disposition of HIV protease inhibitor and non-nucleoside reverse transcriptase inhibitor drugs. In addition, the role of genetic variation in determining the immune response to drug-specific antigens will be considered as a potentially significant determinant of susceptibility to idiosyncratic drug reactions (e.g., major histocompatibility complex alleles associated with abacavir hypersensitivity). The current and potential clinical utility of pharmacogenetic testing in HIV management will also be emphasized. Publication Types: Review

Pharmacogenomics. 2004 Sep;5(6):673-89. Related Articles, Links Toward individualized pharmaceutical care of East Asians: the value of genetic testing for polymorphisms in drug-metabolizing genes. Morrison A, Levy R. SCRIBCO, P.O. Box 1525, Blue Bell, PA 19422, USA. scribbler@verizon.net Research into the relationship between genetics and drug response has focused on polymorphisms in genes that encode drug-metabolizing enzymes, particularly the genes of cytochrome P450 superfamily 2, which affect the clearance of the anticoagulant warfarin, proton pump inhibitors, tricyclic antidepressants, and many other clinically relevant drugs. Much of this work has targeted East Asians, a genetically distinguishable and populous group. Researchers have identified polymorphisms that inactivate gene function, compared polymorphism frequencies in East-Asian and Caucasian populations, and determined the effects on the pharmacokinetic parameters of drugs. Detection in an individual of polymorphisms known to inactivate a drug-metabolizing enzyme is predictive of poor metabolism of drugs processed by that pathway, which itself may be predictive of an atypical drug response. Genetic tests can be used to screen for individuals with poor metabolizer phenotypes, with the ultimate goal of predicting the clinical effects of drugs. Publication Types: Review

Pharmacogenomics. 2004 Sep;5(6):691-8. Related Articles, Links Pharmacogenetics of dopamine receptors and response to antipsychotic drugs in schizophrenia--an update. Scharfetter J. Universitatsklinik fur Psychiatrie, Abteilung fur Allgemeine Psychiatrie, Wahringer Gurtel 18-20, A-1090 Wien, Austria. joachim.scharfetter@akh-wien.ac.at A considerable number of pharmacogenetic studies have been performed in recent years to define the association of antipsychotic medication response with dopamine receptor polymorphisms and, despite contradictory results, decisive trends have emerged. For the dopamine D2 receptor (DRD2), a trend toward an association with favorable response seems to emerge for the -141C Ins allele of the DRD2 -141C Ins/Del polymorphism and the A1 allele of the Taq1A polymorphism. In the case of the D3 receptor, the Ser9Gly polymorphism has been extensively investigated and a pattern of association is seen between the Ser9 allele and a response to typical antipsychotics, and between the Gly9 allele and a response to atypical antipsychotics. For the D4 receptor, no convincing association results have been reported to date. These trends are discussed with regard to methodological directives and functional implications. Publication Types: Review

Pharmacogenomics. 2004 Sep;5(6):731-9. Related Articles, Links Report on the joint EFPIA, DIA and EMEA pharmacogenetics workshop: moving toward clinical application. McCarthy A, Kerr M, Abadie E, Chibout SD, Imbert G, Cohen N, Drakoulis N, Knudsen LE, Flamion B, Hashimoto L, Kreutz WV, McHale D, Mitchell T, Papaluca Amati M, Roberts R, Shaw P, Stuerzebecher CS, Townend D. Genetics Research, GlaxoSmithKline Research and Development, Greenford Road, Greenford, Middlesex, UB6 0HE, UK. alun.d.mccarthy@gsk.com Publication Types: Congresses

Pharmacogenomics. 2005 Apr;6(3):205-207. Related Articles, Links Pharmacogenomics and pharmacogenetics. Iqbal O. Loyola University Medical Center, MD, FACC, Department of Pathology, 2160 S, First Avenue, Maywood, IL 60153, USA. oiqbal@lumc.edu. y publisher]

Pharmacogenomics. 2005 Apr;6(3):211-223. Related Articles, Links Pharmacogenetics and nicotine addiction treatment. Munafo MR, Shields AE, Berrettini WH, Patterson F, Lerman C. 1University of Bristol, Department of Experimental Psychology, 8 Woodland Road, Bristol, BS8 ITN, UK. E-mail: marcus.munafo @bris.ac.uk , 2Georgetown University, Health Policy Institute, Georgetown Public Policy

Institute, 2233 Wisconsin Ave, NW, Suite 525, Washington DC 20007, USA, 3University of Pennsylvania, Department of Psychiatry, Center for Neurobiology and Behavior, Room 111 Clinical Research Building, 415 Curie Bvd, PA 19104, USA, 4University of Pennsylvania, Transdisciplinary Tobacco Use Research Center, Abramson Cancer Center, 3535 Market St, Suite 4100, PA 19104, USA. This review focuses on the current status of, and future directions for, pharmacogenetic research on nicotine dependence and smoking cessation treatment. Pharmacological treatment involving nicotine replacement therapy and bupropion for nicotine addiction and smoking cessation has been shown to be efficacious when provided in combination with behavioral support. Cessation rates remain somewhat modest, however, and one possibility is that success rates may be enhanced by offering treatments tailored to an individual's genotype. Nonetheless, research on this issue remains in its infancy, and although the scope for individualized treatment tailored to genotype is promising, there are substantial practical, ethical and social considerations that must be addressed before such research is translated into clinical practice. y publisher]

Pharmacogenomics. 2005 Dec;6(8):793-5. Related Articles, Links Pharmacogenetics - where are we and where are we heading? Kola I. Merck and Co., Inc., Basic Research, 126 East Lincoln Avenue, Rahway, New Jersey, USA. ismail_kola@merck.com.

Pharmacogenomics. 2005 Dec;6(8):835-847. Related Articles, Links Advances and challenges in fluoropyrimidine pharmacogenomics and pharmacogenetics. Soong R, Diasio RB. 1National University of Singapore, Oncology Research Institute and Department of Pathology, 10 Medical Drive, MD11 Level 5, Singapore 117597, Republic of Singapore. nmirs@nus.edu.sg , 2University of Alabama at Birmingham, Department of Pharmacology and Toxicology, 1670 University Boulevard VH101, Birmingham AL35294, USA. Robert.Diasio@ccc.uab.edu. In cancer pharmacogenetics (the study of how variability in a single or set of known genes influences drug response) and pharmacogenomics (the study of variability on a genome-wide scale), one of the most important fields of research focuses on the fluoropyrimdines (FPs) and, in particular, 5-fluorouracil (5-FU). After over 40 years of use, FPs remain one of the most commonly used cancer chemotherapy agents and their application includes a wide spectrum of cancer types. FPs also continue to be the baseline component for many new regimens with novel molecular-targeted agents that are being rapidly introduced. Hence, it would seem appropriate that pharmacogenetic/genomic models for optimizing cancer patient management would involve indicators of FP response. In this article, the current trends in FP pharmacogenetics and pharmacogenomics are reviewed based on the advances made to date and the challenges faced in realizing their full potential. y publisher]

Pharmacogenomics. 2005 Dec;6(8):849-56. Related Articles, Links Pharmacogenetics and anesthesiologists. Galley HF, Mahdy A, Lowes DA. University of Aberdeen, Academic Unit of Anaesthesia and Intensive Care, School of Medicine,Institute of Medical Sciences, Aberdeen, AB25 2ZD, UK. h.f.galley@abdn.ac.uk. Genetic variation contributes to an individual's sensitivity and response to a variety of drugs important to anesthetic practice. Early insights into the clinical impact of pharmacogenetics were provided by anesthesiology - investigations into prolonged apnea after succinylcholine administration, thiopental-induced porphyria and malignant hyperthermia contributed to the novel science of pharmacogenetics in the early 1960s. Genetic polymorphisms involved in pharmacokinetics (absorption, distribution, metabolism, and excretion of drugs) and pharmacodynamics (receptors, ion channels and enzymes) can affect an individual's response to the drugs used in anesthetic practice. In addition, genetic variation in proteins directly unrelated to drug action or metabolism can influence responses to environmental changes that occur during anesthesia. This review will summarize the current knowledge of genetic variation in response to drugs relevant to anesthesia, and how this impacts upon clinical practice.

Pharmacogenomics. 2005 Dec;6(8):873-7. Related Articles, Links Concordance of pharmacogenetic markers in germline and colorectal tumor DNA. Marsh S, Mallon MA, Goodfellow P, McLeod HL. Washington University School of Medicine, Campus Box 8069-660 South Euclid AvenueSt Louis, MO 63110, USA. smarsh@im.wustl.edu. Introduction: Most cancer pharmacogenetic studies use germline DNA, as tumor tissue is often inaccessible in the advanced disease setting. However, this relies on the assumption that germline DNA is representative of the tumor genotype. To date, there has been little attention paid to defining the relationship between tumor and germline genomes. Materials and methods: This study compared 28 polymorphisms in 13 genes of high importance to cancer pharmacogenetics from ten different chromosome regions, in DNA from normal mucosa and colon tumors in 44 paired samples. Results: 93% of samples had one or fewer genotype discrepancies. 77% of patients had intraindividual genotypes in complete concordance. In addition, although microsatellite instability (MSI) was identified in 20% of tumors, no significant association between MSI and genotype discrepancies was observed ($p = 0.672$). Conclusions: While this data validates the use of germline DNA pharmacogenetics in colorectal cancer, statistical analysis and modeling of pharmacogenetic data should be employed to incorporate this small, but important, source of error.

Pharmacogenomics. 2005 Jan;6(1):59-63. Related Articles, Links CEPH individuals are representative of the European American population: implications for pharmacogenetics. Meucci MA, Marsh S, Watters JW, McLeod HL. Washington University School of Medicine, Departments of Medicine, Molecular Biology and Pharmacology, and Genetics, and the Siteman Cancer Center, St. Louis, MO, USA. Previous studies have highlighted the use of phenotype generation in immortalized lymphoblastoid cells from the Centre d'Etude du Polymorphisme Humain (CEPH) pedigrees as a powerful means of discovering genes involved in complex biological and pharmacological phenotypes. However, there is no data on how representative CEPH pedigrees are of the general population of European origin for genetic variants of pharmacogenetic significance. A vast amount of data in a population of restricted applicability would be of little value. Genotype and allele frequencies of 28 variants in 15pharmacogenetically relevant genes were analyzed in germ-line DNA from European- and African-origin blood donors, and CEPH cell lines of European origin. The results demonstrate that allele frequencies for the 28 polymorphisms are highly similar between the CEPH and the European-origin populations. However, genotype frequencies in the CEPH population did not provide a high level of prediction for the African-origin population. These data support the usefulness of the CEPH panel in pharmacogenetic discovery efforts for European-derived populations.

Pharmacogenomics. 2005 Jul;6(5):503-513. Related Articles, Links The pharmacogenetics of coumarin therapy. Voora D, McLeod HL, Eby C, Gage BF. 1Washington University School of Medicine, Departments of Medicine and of Pathology, St. Louis, MO, USA, 2Washington University School of Medicine, Division of General Medical Sciences, Campus Box 8005, 660 S. Euclid Ave., St. Louis, MO, 63110, USA. bgage@im.wustl.edu. Vitamin K antagonists (coumarins) are widely-used oral anticoagulants for the prevention of venous thromboembolism and strokes. Wide inter-individual variation in dose response and frequent bleeds characterize the initiation of coumarin therapy. Over the past 10 years both genetic and nongenetic determinants of coumarin dose response have been identified. A comprehensive pharmacogenetics approach to warfarin therapy has the potential to improve the safety and efficiency of warfarin initiation. y publisher]

Pharmacogenomics. 2005 Jul;6(5):535-8. Related Articles, Links EPIDAUROS Biotechnologie AG. Arnold HP, Kluge P, Mauch S. EPIDAUROS Biotechnologie AG, Am Neuland 1,82347 Bernried, Germany. contact@epidauros.com http://www.epidauros.com. EPIDAUROS Biotechnologie AG is a leading provider of pharmacogenetic consulting, genotyping and research services to the international pharmaceutical and biotechnology industries, contract research organizations and healthcare providers. The company's mission is to improve safety, efficacy and predictability in drug development and drug therapy. EPIDAUROS determines its customers' needs in the field of pharmacogenetics using an in-depth consultancy process. The development and conduct of genotyping assays for drug-metabolizing enzymes, drug transporters and drug targets (for example, receptors) - all performed under stringent quality standards - are a major activity at EPIDAUROS. The company offers its research services to academic and industrial partners for the development of innovative diagnostic solutions by using its intellectual property.

Pharmacogenomics. 2005 Jun;6(4):317-9. Related Articles, Links Pharmacogenetics and pharmacogenomics instruction in schools of pharmacy in the USA: is it adequate? Latif DA.

Pharmacogenomics. 2005 Jun;6(4):323-337. Related Articles, Links The pharmacogenetics of calcineurin inhibitors: one step closer toward individualized immunosuppression? Hesselink DA, van Gelder T, van Schaik RH. 1Erasmus MC, Department of Internal Medicine, Room Ee 563a, Renal Transplant Unit, Dr Molewaterplein 50, 3015 GE Rotterdam, The Netherlands. d.a.hesselink@erasmusmc.nl , 2Erasmus MC, Hospital Pharmacy, Clinical Pharmacology Unit, Rotterdam, The Netherlands, 3Erasmus MC, Clinical Chemistry, Rotterdam, The Netherlands. The immunosuppressive drugs cyclosporin (CsA) and tacrolimus (Tac) are widely used to prevent acute rejection following solid-organ transplantation. However, the clinical use of these agents is complicated by their many side effects, a narrow therapeutic index and highly variable pharmacokinetics. The variability in CsA and Tac disposition has been attributed to interindividual differences in the expression of the metabolizing enzymes cytochrome P450 (CYP) 3A4 and 3A5, and in the expression of the drug transporter P-glycoprotein (encoded by the ABCB1 gene, formerly known as the multidrug resistance 1 gene). Variation in the expression of these genes could in turn be explained by several recently-identified single nucleotide polymorphisms (SNPs). Determination of these SNPs in (future) transplant recipients has the potential to identify individuals who are at risk of under-immunosuppression or the development of adverse drug reactions. Ultimately, genotyping for CYP3A and ABCB1 may lead to further individualization of immunosuppressive drug therapy for the transplanted patient. y publisher]

Pharmacogenomics. 2005 Jun;6(4):339-56. Related Articles, Links Novel technology and the development of pharmacogenetics within the pharmaceutical industry. Gibson N, Jawaid A, March R. 1AstraZeneca Pharmaceuticals, Research and Development Genetics Department, Mereside, Alderley Park, Macclesfield, Cheshire SK10 4TG, UK. neil.gibson @astrazeneca.com , 2. ansar.jawaid @astrazeneca.com , 3. ruth.march @astrazeneca.com. This article focuses on the role of pharmacogenetics (PGx) technology across the drug development pipeline. Recent technology developments in three main areas are discussed: the discovery of polymorphisms or other variants in genes of interest; genotyping technologies used in PGx research (both for candidate gene analyses and for a whole-genome association approach); and the use of genotyping in patients prior to prescription (diagnostics). Finally, the associated issues of genetic data management and analysis are addressed, and the challenges facing the pharmaceutical industry in storing, manipulating and exploiting the large and complex data sets that will be generated from emerging PGx platforms are discussed. In conclusion, it is demonstrated that, despite the failures of some technology development programs and the slow rate of progress of others, there has, in fact, been steady progress toward the implementation of PGx within the pharmaceutical industry.

Pharmacogenomics. 2005 Jun;6(4):399-410. Related Articles, Links beta(2)-adrenergic receptor polymorphisms and response to salbutamol among Indian asthmatics(). Kukreti R, Bhatnagar P, B-Rao C, Gupta S, Madan B, Das C, Guleria R, Athavale AU, Brahmachari SK, Ghosh B. 1GenoMed Lab, (Gene Quest Laboratory, Nicholas Piramal India Ltd) at Institute of Genomics and Integrative Biology (CSIR), Delhi 110007, India. ritushree @hotmail.com , 2Institute of Genomics and Integrative Biology, CSIR, Delhi University Campus, Delhi 110007, India, 3All India Institute of Medical Sciences (AIIMS), Department of Medicine, Delhi 110029, India, 4KEM hospital, Chest and EPRC Department, Parel, Mumbai 400012, India, 5Current address: ChemInformatics, Quest Institute of life Sciences, Nicholas Piramal India Ltd, Goregaon East, Bombay 400063, India. Introduction: The beta(2)-adrenergic receptor (beta(2)AR or ADRbeta(2)) is the target for beta(2)-agonist drugs used for bronchodilation in asthma and other respiratory diseases. The aim of this study was to identify common single nucleotide polymorphisms (SNPs) and haplotypes in asthmatics and healthy individuals from an Indian population, and determine the influence of beta(2)AR SNPs in responsiveness to beta(2)-agonist therapy in asthma patients. Methods: Ten variable SNP sites within a span of 2.193 kb were identified in the beta(2)AR gene by sequencing and genotyping 374 bronchial asthma patients and healthy individuals from an Indian population. Spirometry tests were performed on 80 unrelated patients before and after administration of 200 mug of salbutamol. A postbronchodilator forced expiratory volume in one second (FEV(1)) change of >/= 15.3% was considered a good response, and a change of < 15.3% was defined as a poor response, to salbutamol. Results: The pattern of linkage disequilibrium between the ten SNPs showed a single, linked SNP block consisting of sites -468, -367, -47, -20, and 79 having strong linkage disequilibrium, while the SNPs at sites -1023, -654, 46, 252, and 523 showed very low linkage with one another and with the linked region. The SNPs were found to be organized into 16 haplotypes in the studied population. We found that patients with a homozygous Arg-16 form at nucleotide position 46 are poor responders with probability of 0.81, and patients with a homozygous Gly-16 form are good responders with a probability of 0.73. The responder status to salbutamol treatment and the genotype at nucleotide position 46 in beta(2)AR gene of an asthmatic patient are significantly associated in the studied Indian population (chi2 = 9.98, df = 2, p = 0.0068). Most importantly, this association for responsiveness to salbutamol at nucleotide position 46 is independent of other SNPs in the beta(2)AR gene. Conclusion: This study suggests that the SNP at nucleotide position 46 has particular relevance to pharmacogenetics in the Indian population studied. y publisher]

Pharmacogenomics. 2005 Mar;6(2):115-38. Related Articles, Links Mechanisms of resistance to anticancer drugs: the role of the polymorphic ABC transporters ABCB1 and ABCG2. Lepper ER, Nooter K, Verweij J, Acharya MR, Figg WD, Sparreboom A. National Cancer Institute, Clinical Pharmacology Research Core, Building 10, Room 5A01, 9000 Rockville Pike, Bethesda, MD 20892, USA. sparreba @mail.nih.gov. ATP-binding cassette (ABC) genes play a role in the resistance of malignant cells to anticancer agents. The ABC gene products, including ABCB1 (P-glycoprotein) and ABCG2 (breast cancer-resistance protein [BCRP], mitoxantrone-resistance protein [MXR], or ABC transporter in placenta [ABCP]), are also known to influence oral absorption and disposition of a wide variety of drugs. As a result, the expression levels of these proteins in humans have important consequences for an individual's susceptibility to certain drug-induced side effects, interactions, and treatment efficacy. Naturally occurring variants in ABC transporter genes have been identified that might affect the function and expression of the protein. This review focuses on recent advances in the pharmacogenetics of the ABC transporters ABCB1 and ABCG2, and discusses potential implications of genetic variants for the chemotherapeutic treatment of cancer.

Pharmacogenomics. 2005 Mar;6(2):163-8. Related Articles, Links Clinical pharmacogenetics of immunosuppressive drugs in organ transplantation. Szekeres T, Haushofer A. Medical University of

Vienna, Clinical Institute for Medical and Chemical Laboratory Diagnostics 5H, General Hospital of Vienna, Waehringer Guertel 18-20, A-1090 Vienna, Austria. thomas.szekeres@meduniwien.ac.at. Organ transplantation has become an important additional option for patients with organ failure. Immunosuppressive drugs showing a very narrow therapeutic window have to be administered. Different transporters and metabolic pathways are responsible for absorption and metabolism of these drugs; for instance, the P-glycoprotein (P-gp) pump regulates the absorption of a drug, and its metabolism is catalyzed by cytochrome P450s (CYPs). As the phenotypes of P-gp or the CYPs are predetermined by their genotypes, genetic testing prior to drug therapy may help to predict the drug doses required. This review describes polymorphisms of the genes coding for P-gp and CYPs, and focuses on the compounds cyclosporin and tacrolimus. It is hoped that this information might help to judge the value of pharmacogenetic testing prior to immunosuppressive therapy in solid organ transplantation.

Pharmacogenomics. 2005 Mar;6(2):95-100. Related Articles, Links Restoring value to stalled Phase II compounds: the case for developing a novel compound for depression using pharmacogenetics. Reed C, Kalnik M, Rakin K, Athanasiou M, Judson R. Genaissance Pharmaceuticals, 5 Science Park, New Haven, CT 06511, USA. Publication Types: Editorial

Pharmacogenomics. 2005 Oct;6(7):673-689. Related Articles, Links Pharmacogenetics of folate-related drug targets in cancer treatment. Robien K, Boynton A, Ulrich CM. 1Fred Hutchinson Cancer Research Center, Cancer Prevention Program, 1100 Fairview Ave N, M4-B402, Seattle, WA 98109 1024, USA. nulrich@fhcrc.org , 2University of Washington, Department of Epidemiology, Seattle, WA 98195, USA, 3University of Washington, Interdisciplinary Graduate Program in Nutritional Sciences, Seattle, WA 98195, USA. Folate metabolism is the target of two major drug groups: folate antagonists (for example, methotrexate) and thymidylate synthase inhibitors (for example, 5-fluorouracil). These agents are used in the treatment of cancer, as well as for other conditions, such as rheumatoid arthritis. High-dose cancer treatment protocols can induce a state of acute folate depletion which may lead to significant treatment-related toxicity. Polymorphisms in folate-metabolizing enzymes may modify the therapeutic effectiveness and toxicity of these drugs. This review briefly summarizes the drugs targeting the folate pathway and describes common polymorphisms in folate-metabolizing enzymes and transport proteins. Pharmacogenetic studies investigating folate-related drug targets in the treatment of colorectal cancers and hematologic malignancies will subsequently be discussed. Findings to date illustrate a potential for targeting therapy based on patients' genotypes, in order to improve outcomes and reduce toxicity. However, larger, well-designed studies are needed to confirm these early findings. y publisher]

Pharmacogenomics. 2005 Sep;6(6):585-601. Related Articles, Links Sarcomas and pharmacogenetics. Biason P, Toffoli G. CRO - National Cancer Institute, Experimental and Clinical Pharmacology, Via Pedemontana Occidentale, 12 33081 Aviano (PN), Italy. gtoffoli@cro.it. Sarcomas are a heterogeneous group of tumors, requiring different chemotherapeutic approaches. Recently, several regimens for metastatic tumors were evaluated with respect to the different responses to conventional chemotherapy of the various histologic subtypes of sarcomas. The impact of pharmacogenetics in the progress of chemotherapy appears to be crucial in defining the clinical response to many drugs, such as anthracycline or alkylating agents, that are widely used in treatment regimens for soft tissue sarcomas (STS) or sarcomas of the bone. Polymorphisms of metabolizing enzymes (e.g., cytochrome P450 and glutathione-S-transferase), transporter proteins (reduced folate carrier and P-glycoprotein) or target proteins (thymidylate synthase, methylenetetrahydrofolate reductase, dihydrofolate reductase, and c-KIT) may be responsible for an altered clinical outcome, in terms of both response and toxicity. The administration of new chemotherapeutic agents, such as imatinib for gastrointestinal tumors (GIST), requires the study of genetic polymorphisms possibly affecting the integrity of the target (c-KIT), which may provide valid information regarding possible developments of therapy. For STS and sarcoma of the bone, the genetic markers, which could be unambiguously predictive of the phenotypic profile of patients, are as yet undetermined.

Pharmacogenomics. 2005 Sep;6(6):629-637. Related Articles, Links Pharmacogenetics of controlled ovarian hyperstimulation. de Castro F, Moron FJ, Montoro L, Real LM, Ruiz A. 1Hospital Universitario Principe de Asturias, Unidad de Reproduccion Humana Asistida, Alcala de Henares, Madrid, Spain, 2Neocodex, Departamento de Genomica Estructural, C/Charles Darwin sn, Parque Cientifico y Tecnologico Isla de la Cartuja, 41092-Sevilla, Spain. aruiz@neocodex.es. Controlled ovarian hyperstimulation (COH) is a routine treatment employed in most assisted reproductive techniques (ARTs). The existence of genetic factors involved in COH has been suspected. The main challenge for clinicians involved in ART is COH cycle cancellation, which usually occurs due to two opposing situations. On the one hand, there is the presence of a poor response during COH treatment, and on the other there is the presentation of a side effect related to gonadotropin hypersensitivity (ovarian hyperstimulation syndrome [OHSS]). Evidence for an association between single nucleotide polymorphisms and COH outcome has been obtained during the last decade. The genetic dissection of both extreme phenotypes of COH will be the main objective of this review. The development of predictive panels useful for the clinical management of COH is currently underway, and will improve the clinical management of patients undergoing ART. y publisher]

Pharmacogenomics. 2006 Jan;7(1):1-3. Related Articles, Links Comment on: Pharmacogenomics. 2006 Jan;7(1):49-59. Is primary care ready for pharmacogenetics? Voora D, Gage BF. Publication Types: Comment Editorial

Pharmacogenomics. 2006 Jan;7(1):25-9. Related Articles, Links Copy number variants and pharmacogenomics. Ouahchi K, Lindeman N, Lee C. Brigham and Women's Hospital, Department of Pathology, and Harvard Medical School, Boston, MA 02115, USA. The earliest pharmacogenomic studies focused on highly penetrant sequence polymorphisms in drug-metabolizing enzymes. The recent discovery of the widespread occurrence of copy number variants/polymorphisms in the human genome holds promise for new pharmacogenomic discoveries, aside from the commonly used single nucleotide polymorphism approach. Here we review the discovery of copy number variants and speculate on their implications for pathophysiology and pharmacogenomics. Publication Types: Review

Pharmacogenomics. 2006 Jan;7(1):31-47. Related Articles, Links Pharmacogenomics: a path to predictive medicine for schizophrenia. Gupta S, Jain S, Brahmachari SK, Kukreti R. Institute of Genomics and Integrative Biology (CSIR), Delhi University Campus, Delhi 110007, India. A significant variability is observed among patients in response to antipsychotics, and is caused by a variety of factors. This review summarizes the available knowledge of associations between pharmacogenetics and drug response in schizophrenia. The multifactorial etiology of schizophrenia makes it a complex interaction of symptoms. Adopting a pharmacogenomics approach represents a unique opportunity for the prediction of response to antipsychotic drugs by investigating genes implicated with specific symptoms and side effects. A network model of the interaction/crosstalk between the neurotransmitter signaling systems is presented to emphasize the importance of the genes associated with the molecular mechanisms of the disease and drug response. These genes may serve as potential susceptibility genes and drug targets for schizophrenia. The crucial point for the identification of a significant biologic marker(s) will include not only the experimental validation of the genes involved in the neurotransmitter signaling systems, but also the availability of large exactly comparable phenotyped patients samples. Coupling our knowledge of genetic polymorphisms with clinical response data promises a bright future for rapid advances in personalized medicine. Publication Types: Review

Pharmacogenomics. 2006 Jan;7(1):49-59. Related Articles, Links Comment in: Pharmacogenomics. 2006 Jan;7(1):1-3. Patients' and physicians' perspectives on pharmacogenetic testing. Rogausch A, Prause D, Schallenberg A, Brockmoller J, Himmel W. Georg-August-University Gottingen, Department of General Practice/Family Medicine, Humboldtallee 3837073 Gottingen, Germany. arogaus@gwdg.de INTRODUCTION: The integration of pharmacogenetic testing into routine care will, in part, depend upon the patients' and physicians' acceptance of these tests. Empirical data regarding patients' and physicians' views on pharmacogenetic testing are lacking. OBJECTIVES: To explore patients' and physicians' perspectives on the potential implications of pharmacogenetic testing, particularly focusing on asthma, and to analyze the possible determinants of their expectations, hopes and fears. METHODS: We conducted telephone interviews with patients with asthma or chronic obstructive pulmonary disease taking part in a larger pharmacogenetic study, in addition to general practitioners (GPs) from a different region in Germany. A total of 328 patients and 378 GPs were invited to participate. Determinants of their attitudes toward pharmacogenetic testing were assessed using logistic regression analysis. RESULTS: Informed consent to participate in this study was given by 196 patients (60%) and 106 GPs (28%). Most patients (96%) and physicians (52%) appreciated the availability of pharmacogenetic tests for a disease such as asthma. Approximately a third of the patients worried about potential unfavorable test results (35%) and violation of privacy (36%). Female patients were more likely to have a fearful attitude (odds ratio [OR]=2.85; 95% confidence interval [CI]=1.58-5.12). Younger patients were generally more likely to be hopeful about the usefulness of pharmacogenetic testing (OR=2.12; CI=1.01-4.46). The GPs' concerns were mainly related to the possibility that patients might either be put under pressure to be tested (72%) or be disadvantaged at private health insurance agencies (61%). The nature of the responsible institution, the clarity of the research aim and explicit informed consent from patients influenced a physicians' decision regarding whether to support a pharmacogenetic study. CONCLUSION: The concerns of patients and GPs differ somewhat with respect to negative psychosocial consequences, discrimination or violation of privacy. Development of information for physicians and patients would be helpful in preventing unrealistic fears or hopes.

Pharmacogenomics. 2006 Jan;7(1):61-5. Related Articles, Links Defining the opportunity for pharmacogenetic intervention in primary care. Grice GR, Seaton TL, Woodland AM, McLeod HL. St Louis College of Pharmacy, Division of Pharmacy Practice, St Louis, MO 63110, USA. Pharmacogenetics (PG), the study of human genome function and its effects on drug response, represents an exciting approach for reducing adverse drug events and increasing therapeutic efficacy. However, there is no clear information of the potential impact of PG in the primary care setting. Therefore, a study was conducted to determine the frequency of use of medications under PG influence, including 16 PG adverse drug reaction (ADR)-associated medications, in the primary care setting. PATIENTS AND METHODS: A cohort of 607 consecutive patients was accrued over a 3-month period from three primary care practices. Patients were asked to answer a verbal survey of demographics and medication use during the past 12 months. The survey specifically evaluated 16 drugs known to commonly cause ADRs and undergo metabolism by polymorphic enzymes. Patients also disclosed information on all other medication use in the last year. Medication use was verified by chart review. The primary outcome was the frequency of medication use. RESULTS: Among the 16 ADR-associated medications, patients used analgesics (88.5%), antihypertensives (14.3%) and antidepressants (9.6%) most commonly. Overall, 28.6% of patients took more than one of the PG ADR-associated medications. Neither gender nor race appeared to influence the frequency of use of these medications ($p=0.5$ and $p=0.08$, respectively). Patients taking one or more of the drugs were older ($p<0.001$). More patients seen for a chronic visit took one or more of the ADR-associated drugs than patients seen for an acute visit (35.8 versus 18.5%, $p<0.001$). DISCUSSION: This is the first attempt to describe the potential role of pharmacogenetics in the primary care setting. The findings indicate that at least one in four primary care patients take at least one medication that commonly causes adverse drug reactions due to genetic variability in drug metabolism, indicating that there is a potential role of pharmacogenomics in primary care. Nearly every patient was on a medication with putative PG association. CONCLUSIONS: Studies of the ability of PG should not be limited to medical subspecialties, as there is a great potential impact of PG on the primary care setting.

Pharmacogenomics. 2006 Jan;7(1):89-103. Related Articles, Links Challenges and opportunities in the application of pharmacogenetics to antiepileptic drug therapy. Ferraro TN, Dlugos DJ, Buono RJ. University of Pennsylvania, Center for Neurobiology and Behavior, Room 2209, Translational Research Laboratories, and The Children's Hospital of Philadelphia, Department of Pediatrics, Philadelphia, PA 19104, USA. TNF-@mail.med.upenn.edu The recent surge of interest in pharmacogenetics has provoked considerable thought regarding its relevance to antiepileptic drug (AED) therapy. Initial studies have focused on genes whose products play a putatively important role in AED pharmacology, particularly drug transporter proteins, drug metabolizing enzymes and ion channel subunits. However, there is a lack of good correspondence between results from different laboratories, and more recent findings are awaiting attempts at confirmation. Thus, there are currently no AED treatment guidelines that are informed by pharmacogenetic data. In order to begin to have clinical impact, standards specific to the conduct of future AED studies must be established. Of particular importance are the need for accurate epilepsy classification, appropriate AED selection and clear and objective assessment outcome measures. In addition, general standards for analysis and interpretation of genetic association data must be better codified and applied consistently across studies. Finally, extensive clinical research networks must be formulated and large numbers of well characterized patients must be recruited. Further development of these critical factors will optimize chances for overcoming current challenges posed by AED pharmacogenetic research and ultimately allow the realization of improved, more rational therapeutic strategies. Publication Types: Review

Pharmacogenomics. 2006 Mar;7(2):149-55. Related Articles, Links Pharmacogenetics: development issues and solutions for safe and effective medicines. Arnold HP, McHale D. EPIDAUROS Biotechnologie AG, Am Neuland 1, 82347 Bernried, Germany. harnold@epidauros.com

Pharmacogenomics. 2006 Mar;7(2):247-53. Related Articles, Links Clinical genomics data standards for pharmacogenetics and pharmacogenomics. Shabo A. IBM Research Lab in Haifa, Haifa University Campus, Mount Carmel, Haifa, 31905, Israel. This special report concerns a talk on data standards given at a workshop entitled 'An International Perspective on Pharmacogenetics: The Intersections between Innovation, Regulation and Health Delivery', which was held by the Organization for Economic Co-operation and Development (OECD) on October 17-19, 2005, in Rome, Italy. The worlds of healthcare and life sciences (HCLS) are extremely fragmented in terms of their underlying information technology, making it difficult to semantically exchange information between disparate entities. While we have reached the point where functional interoperability is ubiquitous, we are still far from achieving true semantic interoperability where a receiving system can use incoming data as though it was created internally. The critical enablers of semantic interoperability are information standards dedicated to HCLS data, spanning all the way from biological research data to clinical research and clinical trials, and finally to healthcare clinical data. The challenge lies in integrating various data standards based on predetermined goals, thereby improving the quality of care provided to patients.

Pharmacol Rep. 2005 Jan-Feb;57(1):1-13. Related Articles, Links Genetic factors underlying differential blood platelet sensitivity to inhibitors. Rozalski M, Boncler M, Luzak B, Watala C. Department of Hemostasis and Hemostatic Disorders, Medical University of Lodz, Zeromskiego 113, PL 90-549 Lodz, Poland. Blood platelets are not only the primary defence mechanism involved in physiological hemostasis, but also their disorders constitute a crucial risk factor in arterial thrombosis. As arterial thrombi are composed of predominantly platelets formed under conditions of elevated shear stress at sites of atherosclerotic vascular injury and disturbed blood flow, the prevention of arterial thrombosis has been for years the main target for antiplatelet therapy. Individual differences in the rate of platelet activation and reactivity markedly influence normal hemostasis and the pathological outcome of thrombosis. Such an individual variability is largely determined by environmental and genetic factors. These are known to either hamper platelets' response to agonists, and thereby mimic the pharmacological modulation of platelet function or mask therapy effect and sensitize platelets. Some clinical studies have indicated that platelet glycoprotein polymorphisms are genetic factors contributing to arterial thrombosis. In spite of some discrepancies between different studies, there is substantial evidence that the integrin beta3 P1(A2) allele, the variants GPIbalpha Met145 and GPIbalpha (-5C) haplotype or the integrin alpha2 haplotype 1 (807T) each contribute to the risk for and morbidity of thrombotic disease. In this article, we reviewed a role of the aforementioned polymorphisms in modulating platelet function and platelet response to inhibitors. The paper focuses on the association between Pl(A1/A2) polymorphism and sensitivity (or resistance) to aspirin and the inhibitory efficacy of GPIIb-IIIa antagonists. Additionally, a potential role of 807C/T polymorphism (GPIa), polymorphisms of GPIb and platelet purinoreceptor P2Y12 in affecting platelet sensitivity to blocking agents is discussed. Publication Types: Review

Pharmacol Rep. 2005 Jan-Feb;57(1):124-7. Related Articles, Links Prophylactic effect of lithium in bipolar affective illness may be related to serotonin transporter genotype. Rybakowski JK, Suwalska A, Czerski PM, Dmitrzak-Weglarz M, Leszczynska-Rodziewicz A, Hauser J. Department of Adult Psychiatry, Poznan University of Medical Sciences, Szpitalna 27/33, 60-572 Poznan, Poland. rybakows@wlkp.top.pl Serotonin transporter promoter length polymorphism (5-HTTLPR) has been implicated in the pathogenesis of mood disorders and in the therapeutic response to serotonergic drugs. In this study, the 5-HTTLPR was estimated in 67 patients with bipolar mood disorder, receiving lithium carbonate for prophylactic purposes for the period of more than 5 years (mean 15 years). The patients were divided into excellent responders (n = 18), partial responders (n = 35) and poor responders (n = 14). In lithium non-responders, the genotype s/s and the allele s was significantly more frequent than in excellent and partial responders. The obtained results are discussed in view of other studies showing an association of S genotype with worse response to serotonergic drugs. A supposition is made that prophylactic management of bipolar illness can be optimized by defining 5-HTTLPR genotype. Publication Types: Clinical Trial

Pharmacol Res. 2004 Apr;49(4):303-8. Related Articles, Links DNA microarrays and pharmacogenomics. Meloni R, Khalfallah O, Biguet NF. Laboratoire de Genetique de la Neurotransmission et des Processus Neurodegeneratifs, CNRS UMR 7091, Bat CERVI, Hopital de la Pitie-Salpetriere, 83 Boulevard de l'Hopital, 75013 Paris, France. meloni@infobiogen.fr The DNA microarrays have proven to be a state of the art technique for high throughput comprehensive analysis of thousand of genes in parallel. The application of a DNA microarray to compare normal and pathological cells, tissues or organs may allow, along with classical positional cloning techniques, to speed up the discovery of genes and gene pathways implicated in several diseases. This in turn will result in further application of the DNA microarray technique in the field of pharmacogenomics in order to characterize and validate new therapeutic targets, their mechanism of action, metabolic pathways and unwanted secondary effects. However, the lack of standardized criteria for the analysis and interpretation of the huge amount of data generated by DNA microarrays may hamper its utilization on a routine basis in the human health domain. Publication Types: Review

Pharmacol Res. 2004 Apr;49(4):309-29. Related Articles, Links Pharmacogenetics of antipsychotic-induced weight gain. Muller DJ, Muglia P, Fortune T, Kennedy JL. Neurogenetics Section, Centre for Addiction and Mental Health, Department of Psychiatry, University of Toronto, 250 College Street, Toronto, Ont., Canada M5T 1R8. daniel_mueller@camh.net Weight gain appears to be a serious side effect encountered during treatment with many antipsychotic drugs. Although the propensities of inducing weight gain vary considerably between antipsychotics, weight gain is mostly observed in atypical antipsychotics, increasingly prescribed for a variety of psychiatric disorders. Beside the psychological consequences weight gain may influence patients' compliance and secondary medical comorbidities related to being overweight may arise, including diabetes, hypertonia, respiratory problems, and some types of cancer. Obesity research generally suggests that a complex system of neurotransmitters, neuropeptides, hormones and immune related factors interact in neural circuits involving at least the hypothalamus, the solitary tract and cortical structures to regulate energy homeostasis and body weight. Antipsychotics that have weight gain inducing properties may disrupt associated pathways at any of these levels, although it remains unclear what the mechanisms of action might be. Given the potential deleterious effects of weight gain, individual predictors of weight gain would be extremely helpful at the beginning of pharmacological treatment with atypical antipsychotics, allowing obesity to be avoided or for counteractive steps such as dietary restrictions to be taken in predisposed individuals. So far, only a few predictors to detect individuals at high risk have been reported and these have limited power. It is likely that genetic factors play a major role in determining individual response to antipsychotics as well as their side effect profile. In this article, we have reviewed literature related to antipsychotic-induced weight gain and have discussed the major issues, before updating the reader on current obesity research findings. Finally, we emphasize previous studies relating to the pharmacogenetics of antipsychotic-induced weight gain. Publication Types: Review

Pharmacol Res. 2004 Apr;49(4):331-42. Related Articles, Links Pharmacogenetics of neoplastic diseases: new trends. Di Paolo A, Danesi R, Del Tacca M.

Department of Oncology, Transplants and Advanced Technologies in Medicine, Division of Pharmacology and Chemotherapy, University of Pisa, 55 Via Roma, 56126 Pisa, Italy. r.danesi@med.unipi.it The study of the influence of genotype on drug activity and efficacy (pharmacogenetics) and the genome-wide approach to drug discovery and interpretation of complex pharmacological responses (pharmacogenomics) are gaining momentum in current molecular medicine. The reasons of the variable activity and tolerability of cancer chemotherapy are being unraveled by the discovery of genotypic alterations affecting pharmacokinetics and pharmacodynamics of drugs. Indeed, genetic variability may alter drug catabolism (i.e. dihydropyrimidine dehydrogenase for 5-fluorouracil, thiopurine-S-methyl transferase for thiopurines, aldehyde dehydrogenase for cyclophosphamide) and anabolism (i.e. thymidine phosphorylase for capecitabine, deoxycitidine kinase for gemcitabine). Moreover, increased expression of transporter systems (i.e. the ATP binding cassette (ABC) superfamily) is associated with reduction of the cytoplasmic levels of drugs which may be unable to exert a cytotoxic effect. Additional systems could protect tumor cells from drug cytotoxicity, including the DNA repair machinery (nucleotide excision repair (NER) and DNA alkyltransferases) and antiapoptotic systems (i.c. bcl-2). Finally, alterations of drug targets may be associated with a decrease in the effectiveness of chemotherapy (i.e. mutations affecting tubulin and topoisomerase I for taxanes and irinotecan, respectively, and increased expression of thymidilate synthase for 5-fluorouracil). Therefore, genetic analysis has the potential to predict treatment efficacy and tolerability. However, major problems encountered in pharmacogenetic and pharmacogenomic studies are the need of extensive validation of available technology, the difficulties in obtaining a suitable amount of tissue from patients during the course of their disease and the extremely complex regulation of gene function. From this perspective, the evaluation of the cellular effect of drugs in relation to protein expression and function (pharmacoproteomics) may be able to overcome these obstacles, and allow the optimisation of cancer chemotherapy in association with a pharmacogenetic approach. Publication Types: Review

Pharmacol Res. 2004 Apr;49(4):343-9. Related Articles, Links Trends in pharmacogenomics of drugs used in the treatment of asthma. Pignatti PF. Section of Biology and Genetics, Department of Mother and Child, Biology and Genetics, University of Verona, Strada Le Grazie 8, 37134 Verona, Italy. pierfranco.pignatti@univr.it Pharmacogenetic studies of drugs used in the treatment of asthma have produced a few examples of reduced response in patients carrying specific genotypes in genes involved in the action of beta-2 agonists or leukotriene modifiers. Other candidate genes related to these drugs, as well as glucocorticoids, theophilline, anticholinergics, antihistaminics, and drug-metabolizing enzymes, may be proposed. Statistical power and population stratification may be issues of importance in case-control association studies. Future developments include expanded gene knowledge from asthma genetic and genomic studies, the development of new preventive and curative treatments, multiple contemporary genotyping methods for pharmacogenetically important genes in a given individual, and the construction of asthma functional pharmacogenomic profiles. In conclusion, it seems that asthma pharmacogenetic studies need to be replicated in prospective clinical trials in different populations with a large number of subjects being genotyped. It is suggested that large clinical trials which are proposed for asthma drugs experimentation should include a pharmacogenetic study as well. Publication Types: Review

Pharmacol Res. 2004 Apr;49(4):351-6. Related Articles, Links Trends in pharmacogenomics of drugs acting on hypertension. Trotta R, Donati MB, Iacoviello L. Angela Valenti Laboratory of Genetic and Environmental Risk Factors for Thrombotic Disease, Consorzio Mario Negri Sud, 66030 Santa Maria Imbaro, Italy. With the recent rapid increase in scientific understanding of the human genome it is becoming possible to identify the extent to which genetic variations influence drug response. The emergence of pharmacogenetics heralds a new era in which drug therapies will be selected on the basis of differences in individuals' genotypes, enhancing drug safety and efficacy. The major focus of this review is pharmacogenetics of antihypertensive drugs. Genetics can influence the pharmacokinetics and pharmacodynamics of such drugs at different levels. The presently available applications of genetic concepts to some drugs commonly used in the treatment of hypertension (ACE-inhibitors, diuretics, beta-blockers...) will be summarized. Also sensitivity to salt intake will be considered as an example of pharmacogenetics. The identification of genetic markers of drug response will help to achieve a better control of blood pressure in the population, by allowing a better tailor of antihypertensive therapy to individual patients. Publication Types: Review

Pharmacol Res. 2004 Apr;49(4):357-61. Related Articles, Links Pharmacogenetics and pharmacogenomics: are they still promising? Pirazzoli A, Recchia G. GlaxoSmithKline Spa, Via Alessandro Fleming 2, 37135 Verona, Italy. ap3563@gsk.com In the last several years pharmacogenetics and pharmacogenomics have attracted the interest of the scientific community and of important pharmaceutical groups. What is the consequence for medicine and for the pharmaceutical industry? What has emerged from this investment, and what can we expect for the future? As with many new technologies, pharmacogenetics and pharmacogenomics were first adapted with much enthusiasm, and then found to require time and experience, together with sustained investment, before they could take their full place in drug discovery and development. The benefits of these technologies are now emerging, however, and they have become essential tools for the pharmaceutical industry. Publication Types: Review

Pharmacol Res. 2004 Apr;49(4):363-73. Related Articles, Links Adverse drug reactions: role of pharmacogenomics. Severino G, Del Zompo M. Section of Clinical Psychopharmacology, Department of Neurosciences B.B. Brodie, University of Cagliari, Cagliari, Italy. Adverse drug reactions (ADRs) are a significant cause of morbidity and mortality. The majority of ADRs can be considered common disorders with considerable clinical variability (clinical phenotype) in which many different genes are involved together with environmental variables. Pharmacogenomics is the study of how genes affect the individual response to drugs. There is some evidence that in the future the use of pharmacogenomics could help to reduce ADRs, as it aims to predict which patients are likely to respond to a particular drug and which patients are likely to have significant ADRs. In this article some examples of genetic polymorphisms affecting drug kinetics, drug toxicity and hypersensitivity related to ADRs are illustrated. Publication Types: Review

Pharmacol Res. 2004 Apr;49(4):375-9. Related Articles, Links Ethical considerations on pharmacogenomics. Mordini E. Secretary of the Bioethical Commission of the National Research Council Centre for Science, Society and Citizenship, Rome, Italy. e.mordini@bioethics.it Pharmacogenetics offers the prospect of an era of safer and more effective drugs, as well as more individualized use of drug therapies. The effect of human genetic variance on responses to therapy will influence drug-development clinical trials and the use of products in clinical practice. It also promises to raise new ethical challenges, in particular in the fields of research and therapy. Last but not least, pharmacogenetics is likely to fulfil the old dream of an individualised medicine, but in a totally unexpected way. Publication Types: Review

Pharmacol Res. 2004 Aug;50(2):195-200. Related Articles, Links Allele and genotype frequencies of CYP2C9, CYP2C19 and CYP2D6 in an Italian population. Scordo MG, Caputi AP, D'Arrigo C, Fava G, Spina E. Department of Experimental and Clinical Medicine and Pharmacology, Section of Pharmacology, University of Messina, Torre Biologica, Policlinico Universitario, Via Consolare Valeria-Gazzi, 98125 Messina, Italy. The polymorphic cytochrome P450 isoenzymes (CYPs) 2C9, 2C19 and 2D6 metabolise many important drugs, as well as other xenobiotics. Their polymorphism gives rise to important interindividual and interethnic variability in the metabolism and disposition of several therapeutic agents and may cause differences in the clinical response to these drugs. In this study, we determined the genotype profile of a random Italian population in order to compare the CYP2C9, CYP2C19 and CYP2D6 allele frequencies among Italians with previous findings in other Caucasian populations. Frequencies for the major CYP2C9, CYP2C19 and CYP2D6 mutated alleles and genotypes have been evaluated in 360 unrelated healthy Italian volunteers (210 males and 150 females, aged 19-52 years). Genotyping has been carried out on peripheral leukocytes DNA by molecular biology techniques (PCR, RFLP, long-PCR). CYP2C9, CYP2C19 and CYP2D6 allele and genotype frequencies resulted in equilibrium with the Hardy-Weinberg equation. One hundred and fourteen subjects (31.7%) carried one and 23 subjects (6.4%) carried two CYP2C9 mutated alleles. Sixty-eight (18.9%) volunteers were found to be heterozygous and six (1.7%) homozygous for the CYP2C19*2, while no CYP2C19*3 was detected in the evaluated population. Volunteers could be divided into four CYP2D6 genotypes groups: 192 subjects (53.3%) with no mutated alleles (homozygous extensive metabolisers, EM), 126 (35.0%) with one mutated allele (heterozygous EM), 12 (3.4%) with two mutated alleles (poor metabolisers, PM) and 30 (8.3%) with extracopies of a functional gene (ultrarapid metabolisers, UM). Frequencies of both CYP2C9 and CYP2C19 allelic variants, as well as CYP2D6 detrimental alleles, in Italian subjects were similar to those of other Caucasian populations. Conversely, the prevalence of CYP2D6 gene duplication among Italians resulted very high, confirming the higher frequency of CYP2D6 UM in the Mediterranean area compared to Northern Europe. Copyright 2004 Elsevier Ltd.

Pharmacol Res. 2006 Feb;53(2):162-5. Epub 2005 Dec 6. Related Articles, Links No association between CYP2D6 polymorphism and Alzheimer's disease in an Italian population. Scordo MG, Dahl ML, Spina E, Cordici F, Arena MG. Department of Medical Sciences, Clinical Pharmacology, University of Uppsala, Akademiska sjukhuset, Ing. 61, 75185 Uppsala, Sweden. gabriella.scordo@medsci.uu.se Allelic variation at the CYP2D6 gene has been suggested to be associated with CNS disorders, including Parkinson's disease and Lewy body dementia. In order to elucidate whether a relationship exists between CYP2D6 polymorphism and the risk of developing Alzheimer's disease (AD), CYP2D6 allele and genotype frequencies have been evaluated in 94 patients from Southern Italy (29 men and 65 women, aged 74+/-8 years) with AD, and in 350 healthy controls (204 men, 146 women, aged 33+/-9 years) from the same geographical region. Allele frequencies among AD patients were not significantly different from those in healthy controls. Subjects could be divided in four CYP2D6 genotype groups: 52 (56%) patients and 205 (59%) controls carried no mutated alleles (homozygous extensive metabolizers (EM)), 33 (35%) patients and 109 (31%) controls carried one mutated allele (heterozygous EM), while 4 (4%) patients and 11 (3%) controls were found to have two mutated alleles (poor metabolizers (PM)). Five (5%) patients and 25 (7%) controls carried extra copies of a functional gene (ultrarapid metabolizers (UM)). Our results indicate that CYP2D6 polymorphism is unlikely to represent a major risk factor in susceptibility to Alzheimer's disease.

Pharmacol Rev. 2005 Mar;57(1):1-26. Related Articles, Links Pharmacogenetics and human molecular genetics of opiate and cocaine addictions and their treatments. Kreek MJ, Bart G, Lilly C, LaForge KS, Nielsen DA. The Laboratory of the Biology of Addictive Diseases, The Rockefeller University, Box 171, 1230 York Avenue, New York, New York 10021, USA. kreek@rockefeller.edu Opiate and cocaine addictions are major social and medical problems that impose a significant burden on society. Despite the size and scope of these problems, there are few effective treatments for these addictions. Methadone maintenance is an effective and most widely used treatment for opiate addiction, allowing normalization of many physiological abnormalities caused by chronic use of short-acting opiates. There are no pharmacological treatments for cocaine addiction. Epidemiological, linkage, and association studies have demonstrated a significant contribution of genetic factors to the addictive diseases. This article reviews the molecular genetics and pharmacogenetics of opiate and cocaine addictions, focusing primarily on genes of the opioid and monoaminergic systems that have been associated with or have evidence for linkage to opiate or cocaine addiction. This evidence has been marshalled either through identification of variant alleles that lead to functional alterations of gene products, altered gene expression, or findings of linkage or association studies. Studies of polymorphisms in the mu opioid receptor gene, which encodes the receptor target of some endogenous opioids, heroin, morphine, and synthetic opioids, have contributed substantially to knowledge of genetic influences on opiate and cocaine addiction. Other genes of the endogenous opioid and monoaminergic systems, particularly genes encoding dopamine beta-hydroxylase, and the dopamine, serotonin, and norepinephrine transporters have also been implicated. Variants in genes encoding proteins involved in metabolism or biotransformation of drugs of abuse and also of treatment agents are reviewed. Publication Types: Review

Pharmacol Ther. 2005 Apr;106(1):19-38. Epub 2004 Dec 15. Related Articles, Links Polymorphisms affecting gene regulation and mRNA processing: broad implications for pharmacogenetics. Johnson AD, Wang D, Sadee W. Integrated Biomedical Sciences Graduate Program, Department of Pharmacology, College of Medicine and Public Health, The Ohio State University, 5072 Graves Hall, 333 W. 10th Avenue, Columbus, OH 43210-1239, USA. johnson.2060@osu.edu Functional polymorphisms that alter gene expression and mRNA processing appear to play a critical role in shaping human phenotypic variability. Intensive studies on polymorphisms affecting drug response have revealed multiple modes of altered gene function, frequently involving cis-acting regulatory sequence variants. Experimental and in silico methods have advanced the search for such polymorphisms, but considerable challenges remain. Here, a survey of polymorphisms in drug-related genes indicates that: (a) a substantial proportion of genetic variability still remains unaccounted for; (b) a majority of these genes harbors known regulatory polymorphisms; and (c) a portion of polymorphisms affect splicing and mRNA turnover. Pharmacogenetic optimiziation of individual drug therapy may require a complete understanding of all functional sequence variants in key genes. This review surveys known noncoding polymorphisms in genes encoding cytochrome P450s and other drug-metabolizing enzymes, drug transporters, and drug targets and receptors. Current methods and challenges associated with the identification and characterization of functional polymorphisms are also discussed. Publication Types: Review

Pharmacol Ther. 2005 Apr;106(1):97-132. Epub 2005 Jan 12. Related Articles, Links UDP-glucuronosyltransferases and clinical drug-drug interactions. Kiang TK, Ensom MH, Chang TK. Faculty of Pharmaceutical Sciences, The University of British Columbia, 2146 East Mall, Vancouver, British Columbia, V6T 1Z3, Canada. UDP-glucuronosyltransferase (UGT) enzymes catalyze the conjugation of various endogenous substances (e.g., bilirubin) and exogenous compounds (e.g., drugs). The human UGT superfamily is comprised of 2 families (UGT1 and UGT2) and 3 subfamilies (UGT1A, UGT2A, and UGT2B). Many of the individual UGT enzymes are expressed not only in liver but also in extrahepatic tissues, where the extent of glucuronidation can be substantial. Several others (e.g., UGT1A7, UGT1A8, and UGT1A10) are expressed only in extrahepatic tissues. The molecular regulation of UGT enzyme is still not fully understood, but various transcription factors appear to play a regulatory role. The expression of individual UGT enzymes is subject to genetic polymorphism and these enzymes can be inhibited or induced by xenobiotics. Experimental evidence in humans indicates that the glucuronidation of acetaminophen, codeine, zidovudine, carbamazepine, lorazepam, and propafenone can influenced by specific interacting drugs. In contrast, the glucuronidation of diflunisal, morphine, naproxen, and temazepam is not affected appreciably by the drugs investigated to date. In general, UGT-mediated human drug interaction studies are difficult to interpret. The factors that complicate the interpretation of this type of drug interaction data are discussed. Publication Types: Review

Pharmacol Ther. 2005 Aug;107(2):155-76. Related Articles, Links Pharmacogenetics for individualized cancer chemotherapy. Efferth T, Volm M. German Cancer Research Center, M070, Im Neuenheimer Feld 282, 69120 Heidelberg, Germany. thomas.efferth@web.de The same doses of medication cause considerable heterogeneity in efficacy and toxicity across human populations. Genetic factors are thought to represent important determinants of drug efficacy and toxicity. Pharmacogenetics focuses on the prediction of the response of tumor and normal tissue to standard therapy by genetic profiling and, thereby, to select the most appropriate medication at optimal doses for each individual patient. In the present review, we discuss the relevance of single nucleotide polymorphisms (SNP) in genes, whose gene products act upstream of the actual drug target sites, that is, drug transporters and drug metabolizing phase I and II enzymes, or downstream of them, that is, apoptosis-regulating genes and chemokines. SNPs in relevant genes, which encode for proteins that interact with anticancer drugs, were also considered, that is, enzymes of DNA biosynthesis and metabolism, DNA repair enzymes, and proteins of the mitotic spindle. A significant body of evidence supports the concept of predicting drug efficacy and toxicity by SNP genotyping. As the efficacy of cancer chemotherapy, as well as the drug-related toxicity in normal tissues is multifactorial in nature, sophisticated approaches such as genome-wide linkage analyses and integrate drug pathway profiling may improve the predictive power compared with genotyping of single genes. The implementation of pharmacogenetics into clinical routine diagnostics including genotype-based recommendations for treatment decisions and risk assessment for practitioners represents a challenge for the future. Publication Types: Review

Pharmacotherapy. 2004 Jun;24(6):720-6. Related Articles, Links Comparison of cytochrome P450 2C9 genotyping methods and implications for the clinical laboratory. Aquilante CL, Lobmeyer MT, Langaee TY, Johnson JA. Department of Pharmacy Practice, College of Pharmacy, University of Florida, Gainesville 32610, USA. STUDY OBJECTIVE: To compare the accuracy, speed, and cost of two methodologies used for genotyping known variants in the cytochrome P450 (CYP) 2C9 metabolizing enzyme gene. DESIGN: Comparative study. SETTING: University research center. SAMPLES: Fifteen-milliliter mouthwash samples collected from 253 subjects participating in a warfarin pharmacogenomic study. INTERVENTION: Genotyping for the isoleucine-to-leucine change at codon 359 (Ile359Leu [*3] polymorphism) was performed by using the Pyrosequencing and polymerase chain reaction (PCR)-restriction fragment length polymorphism (RFLP) methods in all 253 samples. Genotyping for the arginine-to-cysteine change at codon 144 (Arg144Cys [*2] polymorphism) was performed by using Pyrosequencing in all samples and by PCR-RFLP in a random subset of 136 samples. MEASUREMENTS AND MAIN

RESULTS: Comparisons of genotyping success rates, time efficiency, and cost analyses were conducted for Pyrosequencing and PCR-RFLP at each variant site. Pyrosequencing and PCR-RFLP produced similar success rates on the first genotyping attempt for the Arg144Cys variant (93.3% vs 90.4%, respectively) and the Ile359Leu variant (83.8% vs 79.1%, respectively). With Pyrosequencing, genotyping 96 samples for either polymorphism could be performed in 1 hour. In contrast, genotyping 96 samples by RFLP took 10 hours for the Arg144Cys variant and 20 hours for the Ile359Leu variant. Total cost/sample for Arg144Cys genotyping was dollars 1.90 with PCR-Pyrosequencing and dollars 3.14 with PCR-RFLP. Total cost/sample for Ile359Leu genotyping was dollars 1.88 with PCR-Pyrosequencing and dollars 10.18 with PCR-RFLP CONCLUSION: Compared with RFLP, genotype determination by Pyrosequencing is a more time-efficient, cost-effective, and robust method for CYP2C9 genotyping. Because of its wide applicability and ease of use, Pyrosequencing is a promising technology for future pharmacogenomic investigations.

Pharmacotherapy. 2004 May;24(5):688-9; discussion 691-3. Related Articles, Links Comment on: Pharmacotherapy. 2003 Nov;23(11):1381-90. The future of pharmacy education: back to which basics? Sansgiry SS. Department of Clinical Sciences and Administration, College of Pharmacy, University of Houston, Houston, Texas 77030-3407, USA. ssansgiry@uh.edu Publication Types: Comment

Philos Trans R Soc Lond B Biol Sci. 2005 Aug 29;360(1460):1563-70. Related Articles, Links Pharmacogenetics of drug-metabolizing enzymes: implications for a safer and more effective drug therapy. Ingelman-Sundberg M, Rodriguez-Antona C. Division of Molecular Toxicology, IMM, Karolinska Institutet, Nobels vag 13, 171 77 Stockholm, Sweden. maging@ki.se The majority of phase I- and phase II-dependent drug metabolism is carried out by polymorphic enzymes which can cause abolished, quantitatively or qualitatively decreased or enhanced drug metabolism. Several examples exist where subjects carrying certain alleles do not benefit from drug therapy due to ultrarapid metabolism caused by multiple genes or by induction of gene expression or, alternatively, suffer from adverse effects of the drug treatment due to the presence of defective alleles. It is likely that future predictive genotyping for such enzymes might benefit 15-25% of drug treatments, and thereby allow prevention of adverse drug reactions and causalities, and thus improve the health of a significant fraction of the patients. However, it will take time before this will be a reality within the clinic. We describe some important aspects in the field with emphasis on cytochrome P450 and discuss also polymorphic aspects of foetal expression of CYP3A5 and CYP3A7. Publication Types: Review

Philos Trans R Soc Lond B Biol Sci. 2005 Aug 29;360(1460):1571-2. Related Articles, Links The genetics of human drug response. Goldstein DB. Department of Biology, Darwin Building, University College London, Gower Street, London WC1E 6BT, UK. d.goldstein@duke.edu The genetics of variable drug response appears to be a more tractable complex trait than common disease predisposition. This has implications for prioritizing research and for experimental design, and in particular argues for extensive use of candidate gene based approaches in pharmacogenetic association studies. Eventually, when whole genome scanning becomes feasible, it may be appropriate to consider weighting schemes that assign higher prior probabilities of variants in genes related to the mode of action of metabolism of medicines. Publication Types: Review

Philos Trans R Soc Lond B Biol Sci. 2005 Aug 29;360(1460):1579-88. Related Articles, Links Pharmacogenetics in drug development. McCarthy AD, Kennedy JL, Middleton LT. Translational Medicine and Genetics, GlaxoSmithKline, Greenford Road, Greenford, Middlesex UB6 0HE, UK. Over the last two decades, identification of polymorphisms that influence human diseases has begun to have an impact on the provision of medical care. The promise of genetics lies in its ability to provide insights into an individual's susceptibility to disease, the likely nature of the disease and the most appropriate therapy. For much of its history, pharmacogenetics (PGx-the use of genetic information to impact drug choice) has been limited to comparatively simple phenotypes such as plasma drug levels. Progress in genetics technologies has broadened the scope of PGx efficacy and safety studies that can be implemented, impacting on a broad spectrum of drug discovery and development activities. Recent PGx data show the ability of this approach to generate information that can be applied to dose selection, efficacy determination and safety issues. This in turn will lead to significant opportunities to affect both the approach to clinical development and the probability of success--the latter being an important aspect for pharmaceutical companies and for the patients who will benefit from these new medicines. Publication Types: Review

Philos Trans R Soc Lond B Biol Sci. 2005 Aug 29;360(1460):1617-38. Related Articles, Links Pharmacogenetics in drug regulation: promise, potential and pitfalls. Shah RR. clin.safety@lineone.net Pharmacogenetic factors operate at pharmacokinetic as well as pharmacodynamic levels-the two components of the dose-response curve of a drug. Polymorphisms in drug metabolizing enzymes, transporters and/or pharmacological targets of drugs may profoundly influence the dose-response relationship between individuals. For some drugs, although retrospective data from case studies suggests that these polymorphisms are frequently associated with adverse drug reactions or failure of efficacy, the clinical utility of such data remains unproven. There is, therefore, an urgent need for prospective data to determine whether pre-treatment genotyping can improve therapy. Various regulatory guidelines already recommend exploration of the role of genetic factors when investigating a drug for its pharmacokinetics, pharmacodynamics, dose-response relationship and drug interaction potential. Arising from the global heterogeneity in the frequency of variant alleles, regulatory guidelines also require the sponsors to provide additional information, usually pharmacogenetic bridging data, to determine whether data from one ethnic population can be extrapolated to another. At present, sponsors explore pharmacogenetic influences in early clinical pharmacokinetic studies but rarely do they carry the findings forward when designing dose-response studies or pivotal studies. When appropriate, regulatory authorities include genotype-specific recommendations in the prescribing information. Sometimes, this may include the need to adjust a dose in some genotypes under specific circumstances. Detailed references to pharmacogenetics in prescribing information and pharmacogenetically based prescribing in routine therapeutics will require robust prospective data from well-designed studies. With greater integration of pharmacogenetics in drug development, regulatory authorities expect to receive more detailed genetic data. This is likely to complicate the drug evaluation process as well as result in complex prescribing information. Genotype-specific dosing regimens will have to be more precise and marketing strategies more prudent. However, not all variations in drug responses are related to pharmacogenetic polymorphisms. Drug response can be modulated by a number of non-genetic factors, especially co-medications and presence of concurrent diseases. Inappropriate prescribing frequently compounds the complexity introduced by these two important non-genetic factors. Unless prescribers adhere to the prescribing information, much of the benefits of pharmacogenetics will be squandered. Discovering highly predictive genotype-phenotype associations during drug development and demonstrating their clinical validity and utility in well-designed prospective clinical trials will no doubt better define the role of pharmacogenetics in future clinical practice. In the meantime, prescribing should comply with the information provided while pharmacogenetic research is deservedly supported by all concerned but without unrealistic expectations. Publication Types: Review

PLoS Med. 2005 Oct;2(10):e342. Epub 2005 Oct 25. Related Articles, Links Pharmacogenetics in the management of coumarin anticoagulant therapy: the way forward or an expensive diversion? Greaves M. School of Medicine, University of Aberdeen, Aberdeen, United Kingdom. m.greaves@abdn.ac.uk Publication Types: Comment

Pol Arch Med Wewn. 2004 Jan;111(1):119-31. Related Articles, Links [Fundamentals of pharmacogenetics in clinical practice] [Article in Polish] Prandota J. Wydzial Lekarsko-Stomatologiczny AM we Wroclawiu. Publication Types: Review

Pol Arch Med Wewn. 2005 Jul;114(1):644-51. Related Articles, Links [Pharmacogenetics of the local thrombolysis in patients with deep vein thrombosis] [Article in Polish] Falkowski A, Kaczmarczyk M, Goracy I, Gorecka-Szyld B, Poncyljusz W, Parczewski M, Ciechanowicz A. Katedra i Zaklad Radiologii Ogolnej i Stomatologicznej Pomorskiej AM w Szczecinie. Thrombophilia, the state of increased tendency for blood clotting, is considered the disorder of a complex etiology, caused by both environmental and genetic factors. As gene variants predisposing to thrombophilia and influencing the increased risk of vein thrombosis might influence response to local thrombolysis, the aim of the work was to characterize the pharmacogenetic conditions for local streptokinase treatment in patients with a deep vein thrombosis (DVT) of lower extremities based on the following polymorphism analyses: G1691A polymorphism of factor V (FV), G20210A polymorphism of prothrombin (PT), A4250G (Thr312Ala) polymorphism of fibrinogen-alpha (FGA), G(-455)A polymorphism of fibrinogen-beta (FGB), 4G/5G polymorphism of plasminogen activator inhibitor type 1(PAI-1) and insertion/deletion (I/D) polymorphism of tissue plasminogen activator (t-PA). The study included 40 DVT patients who underwent a local thrombolytic treatment within 14-day period from diagnosis. Full recanalization was achieved in 20 subjects (50%) [group R(+)], whereas incomplete or total lack of recanalization was identified in the remaining 20 patients [group R(-)]. No major complications of thrombolytic treatment occurred in the studied group. In the case of prothrombin gene all individuals carried homozygous wild type genotype (GG). Prevalence of the genotypes and alleles of the remaining five polymorphisms did not differ significantly between the groups R(+) and R(-). Neither sex nor age, smoking or time period from diagnosis to introduction of the thrombolytic treatment significantly influenced treatment efficacy. The results of the study suggest that a local thrombolysis with streptokinase introduced within two week period from the diagnosis is a safe and efficient method of treatment for deep vein thrombosis of lower extremities. However, size of the group is insufficient to clearly determine the association between investigated polymorphisms and efficacy of local treatment with streptokinase.

Prim Care. 2004 Sep;31(3):543-59, ix. Related Articles, Links Pharmacogenetics. David SP. Department of Family Medicine, Brown Medical School, Brown University Center for Primary Care and Prevention, Primary Care Genetics Laboratory, Translational Research Center, Memorial Hospital of Rhode Island USA. Sean_David@brown.edu This article provides an introduction to the discipline of pharmacogenetics and discusses the implications of pharmacogenetics research for primary care practice. Examples are given of how genetic information can predict and inform; drug interactions influencing drug efficacy, metabolism, dosing, and toxicity. Caveats on the need for vigilance in the interpretation of pharmacogenetics studies are discussed briefly, together with the need for a convergence of biomolecular research, translational research, education,and policy to promote evidence-based genetic medicine. Publication Types: Review

Proc Am Thorac Soc. 2004;1(4):364-7. Related Articles, Links Asthma steroid pharmacogenetics: a study strategy to identify replicated treatment responses. Weiss ST, Lake SL, Silverman ES, Silverman EK, Richter B, Drazen JM, Tantisira KG. Respiratory, Genetic, and Environmental Epidemiology, Channing Laboratory, Brigham and Women's Hospital, 75 Francis Street, Boston, MA 02115. restw@channing.harvard.edu Asthma treatment with inhaled steroids demonstrates significant between-person variability. Genetic variation could contribute to this response to inhaled glucocorticosteroids. Difficulties in performing genetic association studies are well known. We designed a test and validation strategy to assess steroid pathway candidate genes. One hundred thirty-one single nucleotide polymorphisms in 14 candidate genes in the steroid pathway were genotyped in an 8-week clinical trial of 470 adults with moderate to severe asthma. We then validated our findings in a second population of individuals with childhood asthma in a 4-year clinical trial of inhaled corticosteroids and a third population of adults with asthma. One gene, corticotrophin-releasing hormone receptor 1 (CRHR1, NM_004382), demonstrated multiple single nucleotide polymorphism associations within each of the three populations. The approach of a test and multiple replication populations is a valuable strategy in asthma pharmacogenetics, which can insure valid association findings. Publication Types:

Clinical Trial Multicenter Study Randomized Controlled Trial

Proc Natl Acad Sci U S A. 2004 Aug 10;101(32):11725-30. Epub 2004 Aug 2. Related Articles, Links Breed distribution and history of canine mdr1-1Delta, a pharmacogenetic mutation that marks the emergence of breeds from the collie lineage. Neff MW, Robertson KR, Wong AK, Safra N, Broman KW, Slatkin M, Mealey KL, Pedersen NC. Veterinary Genetics Laboratory, School of Veterinary Medicine, University of California, Davis, CA 95616, USA. mwneff@ucdavis.edu A mutation in the canine multidrug resistance gene, MDR1, has previously been associated with drug sensitivities in two breeds from the collie lineage. We exploited breed phylogeny and reports of drug sensitivity to survey other purebred populations that might be genetically at risk. We found that the same allele, mdr1-1Delta, segregated in seven additional breeds, including two sighthounds that were not expected to share collie ancestry. A mutant haplotype that was conserved among affected breeds indicated that the allele was identical by descent. Based on breed histories and the extent of linkage disequilibrium, we conclude that all dogs carrying mdr1-1Delta are descendants of a dog that lived in Great Britain before the genetic isolation of breeds by registry (ca. 1873). The breed distribution and frequency of mdr1-1Delta have applications in veterinary medicine and selective breeding, whereas the allele's history recounts the emergence of formally recognized breeds from an admixed population of working sheepdogs. Publication Types: Historical Article

Proc Natl Acad Sci U S A. 2004 Aug 10;101(32):11809-14. Epub 2004 Jul 28. Related Articles, Links Genome-wide discovery of loci influencing chemotherapy cytotoxicity. Watters JW, Kraja A, Meucci MA, Province MA, McLeod HL. Department of Medicine, Siteman Cancer Center, Washington University School of Medicine, 660 South Euclid Avenue, Campus Box 8069, St. Louis, MO 63110, USA. Little is known about the heritability of chemotherapy activity or the identity of genes that may enable the individualization of cancer chemotherapy. Although numerous genes are likely to influence chemotherapy response, current candidate gene-based pharmacogenetics approaches require a priori knowledge and the selection of a small number of candidate genes for hypothesis testing. In this study, an ex vivo familial genetics strategy using lymphoblastoid cells derived from Centre d'Etude du Polymorphisme Humain reference pedigrees was used to discover genetic determinants of chemotherapy cytotoxicity. Cytotoxicity to the mechanistically distinct chemotherapy agents 5-fluorouracil and docetaxel were shown to be heritable traits, with heritability values ranging from 0.26 to 0.65 for 5-fluorouracil and 0.21 to 0.70 for docetaxel, varying with dose. Genome-wide linkage analysis was also used to map a quantitative trait locus influencing the cellular effects of 5-fluorouracil to chromosome 9q13-q22 [logarithm of odds (LOD) = 3.44], and two quantitative trait loci influencing the cellular effects of docetaxel to chromosomes 5q11-21 (LOD = 2.21) and 9q13-q22 (LOD = 2.73). Finally, 5-fluorouracil and docetaxel were shown to cause apoptotic cell death involving caspase-3 cleavage in Centre d'Etude du Polymorphisme Humain lymphoblastoid cells. This study identifies genomic regions likely to harbor genes important for chemotherapy cytotoxicity using genome-wide linkage analysis in human pedigrees and provides a widely applicable strategy for pharmacogenomic discovery without the requirement for a priori candidate gene selection.

Proc Natl Acad Sci U S A. 2005 Jun 28;102(26):9394-9. Epub 2005 Jun 20. Related Articles, Links Human thiopurine S-methyltransferase pharmacogenetics: variant allozyme misfolding and aggresome formation. Wang L, Nguyen TV, McLaughlin RW, Sikkink LA, Ramirez-Alvarado M, Weinshilboum RM. Department of Molecular Pharmacology and Experimental Therapeutics, Mayo Clinic College of Medicine, Rochester, MN 55905, USA. Thiopurine S-methyltransferase (TPMT) catalyzes the S-methylation of thiopurine drugs. TPMT genetic polymorphisms represent a striking example of the potential clinical value of pharmacogenetics. Subjects homozygous for TPMT*3A, the most common variant allele for low activity, an allele that encodes a protein with two changes in amino acid sequence, are at greatly increased risk for life-threatening toxicity when treated with standard doses of thiopurines. These subjects have virtually undetectable levels of TPMT protein. In this study, we tested the hypothesis that TPMT*3A might result in protein misfolding and aggregation. We observed that TPMT*3A forms aggresomes in cultured cells and that it aggregates in vitro, functional mechanisms not previously described in pharmacogenetics. Furthermore, there was a correlation among TPMT half-life values in rabbit reticulocyte lysate, aggresome formation in COS-1 cells, and protein aggregation in vitro for the three variant allozymes encoded by alleles that include the two TPMT*3A single-nucleotide polymorphisms. These observations were compatible with a common structural explanation for all of these effects, a conclusion supported by size-exclusion chromatography and CD spectroscopy. The results of these experiments provide insight into a unique pharmacogenetic mechanism by which common polymorphisms affect TPMT protein function and, as a result, therapeutic response to thiopurine drugs.

Proc Natl Acad Sci U S A. 2005 May 17;102(20):7215-20. Epub 2005 May 9. Related Articles, Links Insights into TOR function and rapamycin response: chemical genomic profiling by using a high-density cell array method. Xie MW, Jin F, Hwang H, Hwang S, Anand V, Duncan MC, Huang J. Department of Molecular, David Geffen School of Medicine, University of California, Los Angeles, CA 90095, USA. With the advent of complete genome sequences, large-scale functional analyses are generating new excitement in biology and medicine. To facilitate genomewide functional analyses, we developed a high-density cell array with quantitative and automated readout of cell fitness. Able to print at > x 10 higher density on a standard microtiter plate area than currently possible, our cell array allows single-plate screening of the complete set of Saccharomyces cerevisiae gene-deletion library and significantly reduces the amount of small molecules and other materials needed for the study. We used this method to map the relation between genes and cell fitness in response to rapamycin, a medically important natural product that targets the eukaryotic kinase Tor. We discuss the implications for pharmacogenomics and the uncharted complexity in genotype-dependent drug response in molecularly targeted therapies. Our analysis leads to several basic findings, including a class of gene deletions that confer better fitness in the presence of rapamycin. This result provides insights into possible therapeutic uses of rapamycin/CCI-779 in the treatment of neurodegenerative diseases (including Alzheimer's, Parkinson's, and Huntington's diseases), and cautions the possible existence of similar rapamycin-enhanceable mutations in cancer. It is well established in yeast that although TOR2 has a unique rapamycin-insensitive function, TOR1 and TOR2 are interchangeable in the rapamycin-sensitive functions. We show that even the rapamycin-sensitive functions are distinct between TOR1 and TOR2 and map the functional difference to a approximately 120-aa region at the N termini of the proteins. Finally, we discuss using cell-based genomic pattern recognition in designing electronic or optical biosensors.

Prog Neuropsychopharmacol Biol Psychiatry. 2005 Jul;29(6):1010-6. Related Articles, Links New drug targets in the signaling pathways activated by antidepressants. Paez-Pereda M. Max Planck Institute of Psychiatry, Kraepelinstr. 10, 80804, Munich, Germany. paez-pereda@affectis.de Studies of twins, genetic linkage and association support the existence of a genetic component to the susceptibility to depression. Biochemical parameters that change in depressive patients are also observed in their relatives. This indicates that genetic factors control these physiological changes and the susceptibility to depression. The study of the mechanisms by which different genetic factors affect the organism's response to drugs can identify better diagnostic tools as well as drug targets. Pharmacogenomics can, therefore, help to find the most efficacious treatment for patients with specific genetic profiles. However, the genetic factors that determine the susceptibility to depression and the different responses to antidepressant treatment are largely unknown. Pharmacogenetic studies have used three different categories of genes to search for associations with the outcome of drug treatments. These gene categories are drug-metabolizing enzymes, known drug targets and known susceptibility genes. The present review will explore the different signal transduction pathways involved in antidepressant action and their possible use in psychopharmacogenomics and drug discovery. Publication Types: Review

Prog Neuropsychopharmacol Biol Psychiatry. 2005 Jul;29(6):1021-8. Related Articles, Links The role of 5-HT2C receptor polymorphisms in the pharmacogenetics of antipsychotic drug treatment. Reynolds GP, Templeman LA, Zhang ZJ. Division of Psychiatry and Neuroscience, Queen's University Belfast, Whitla Medical Building, 97 Lisburn Road, Belfast BT9 7BL, UK. G.Reynolds@qub.ac.uk The development of novel, atypical antipsychotics has been welcomed due to their lower incidence of extrapyramidal side effects. However, as with all pharmacotherapy, patient response is often varied and these novel compounds are not without their own side effect profile, most notably weight gain. Inter-individual variations in response to drug treatment are, in part, due to polymorphisms of the genes encoding drug targets. The importance of the serotonin system in psychiatric symptomatology and several side effects of antipsychotic drugs is well established. Thus genetic polymorphisms of two central 5-HT receptors (5-HT2A and 2C), at which many of the newer antipsychotic drugs act, are prime candidates for pharmacogenetic analysis of the effects of these drugs in the treatment of schizophrenia. To date, much work has focussed on the 5-HT2A receptor subtype.

However, pharmacological evidence and recent molecular genetic studies would suggest a role for the 5-HT2C receptor in the consequences of antipsychotic treatment, particularly in relation to the development of both drug-induced dyskinesias and weight gain. This review briefly examines the pharmacology and physiology of the 5HT2C receptor in the context of its genetics, with discussion of known polymorphisms of this receptor gene and its promoter region. Associations between these polymorphisms and the development of schizophrenia, the symptom responses to antipsychotic treatment and side effects of such treatment, notably tardive dyskinesia and weight gain, are assessed and related to the presumed functionality of these polymorphisms. Such studies clearly demonstrate the potential of pharmacogenetics in optimising treatment for the individual patient. Publication Types: Review

Prog Neuropsychopharmacol Biol Psychiatry. 2005 Jul;29(6):1029-37. Related Articles, Links Pharmacogenetics in model systems: defining a common mechanism of action for mood stabilisers. Williams RS. Department of Biology and Wolfson Institute for Biomedical Research, University College London, Gower St., London WC1E 6BT, United Kingdom. robin.williams@ucl.ac.uk Defining the underlying causes of psychiatric disorders has provided an ongoing and intractable problem. The analysis of the genetic basis of manic depression, in particular, has been impeded by the absence of a suitable model system and by the lack of candidate causative genes. One recent approach to overcome these problems has involved identifying those genes which control the sensitivity to anti-manic drugs in a model organism. Characterisation of the role of these genes and their encoded proteins in this model has allowed the analysis of their mammalian homologues to elucidate the therapeutic role of these drugs and the possible aetiology of manic depression. This approach has been used successfully with the cellular slime mould, Dictyostelium discoideum. This article introduces the use of model systems for pharmacogenetics research. It describes the identification of prolyl oligopeptidase in D. discoideum as a modulator of inositol phosphate signalling, and the subsequent identification of a common mechanism of action of three anti-manic drugs in mammalian neurons. The use of pharmacogenetics in model systems will provide a powerful tool for the ongoing analysis of both the treatment and cause of psychiatric disorders. Publication Types: Review

Prog Neuropsychopharmacol Biol Psychiatry. 2005 Jul;29(6):1062-73. Related Articles, Links Pharmacogenetics of the serotonin transporter. Lesch KP, Gutknecht L. Molecular and Clinical Psychobiology, Department of Psychiatry and Psychotherapy, University of Wuerzburg, Fuechsleinstr. 15, 97080 Wuerzburg, Germany. kplesch@mail.uni-wuerzburg.de Response to psychopharmacologic drugs is genetically complex, results from an interplay of multiple genomic variations with environmental influences, and depends on the structure or functional expression of gene products, which are direct drug targets or indirectly modify the development and synaptic plasticity of neural networks critically involved in their effects. During brain development, the serotonin (5HT) system, which is commonly targeted by antidepressant, anxiolytic, and antipsychotic drugs, controls neuronal specification, differentiation, and phenotype maintenance. While formation and integration of these neural networks is dependent on the action of multiple proteins, converging lines of evidence indicate that genetically controlled variability in the expression of the 5HT transporter (5HTT) is critical to the development and plasticity of distinct neurocircuits. The most promising finding to date indicate an association between the response time as well as overall response to serotonin reuptake inhibitors (SSRIs) and a common polymorphism (5HTTLPR) within the transcriptional control region of the 5HTT gene (SLC6A4) in patients with depressive disorders. The formation and maturation of serotonergic and associated systems, in turn, are influencing the efficacy of serotonergic compounds in a variety of psychiatric conditions. Based on the notion that complex gene x gene and gene x environment interactions in the regulation of brain plasticity are presumed to contribute to individual differences in psychopharmacologic drug response, the concept of developmental psychopharmacogenetics is emerging. Publication Types: Review

Prog Neuropsychopharmacol Biol Psychiatry. 2005 Jul;29(6):1074-84. Related Articles, Links The influence of Serotonin Transporter Promoter Polymorphism (SERTPR) and other polymorphisms of the serotonin pathway on the efficacy of antidepressant treatments. Serretti A, Benedetti F, Zanardi R, Smeraldi E. Department of Psychiatry, Istituto Scientifico H San Raffaele, Vita-Salute University, Centro San Raffaele del Monte Tabor Foundation, Via Stamira D'Ancona 20, 20127 Milano, Italy. serretti.alessandro@hsr.it The definition of a genetic liability profile for specific antidepressant treatment will soon be available offering considerable help in early detection of effective therapy in affective disorders. The search for genetic factors predisposing to drug response or side-effects in affective disorders started only in the last few years. The efficacy of antidepressant action was associated with several polymorphisms, located on coding genes of proteins thought to be involved in the different mechanisms of action of antidepressant treatments. Among these, gene variants in sequences of serotonin pathway proteins were candidate, both for the well known evidence of its involvement in the development of depressive symptomathology and for the wide-world use of selective serotonin reuptake inhibitors as first choice treatment of depression. A polymorphism in the promoter region of the serotonin transporter (SERTPR) was independently associated with efficacy for a range of treatments, other polymorphism located on the tryptophan hydroxylase gene, 5-HT2a receptor and G-protein beta 3 showed some association, while other candidate genes were not associated with treatment efficacy. Possible liability genes controlling at least to some extent both acute and long-term treatment were identified, and the further objective is to identify other candidate genes in order to define individualized treatments according to genetic profile in a future. The present paper reviews the pharmacogenetic studies published to date, focusing the attention on the serotonergic pathway. Publication Types: Review

Prog Neuropsychopharmacol Biol Psychiatry. 2005 Jul;29(6):996-8. Related Articles, Links The future of antidepressant pharmacogenetics is arriving. Introduction. Holsboer F. Max Planck Institute Psychiatry, Kraepelinstrasse 2-10, Munich 8-80806, Germany. holsboer@mpipsykl.mpg.de

Prog Neuropsychopharmacol Biol Psychiatry. 2005 Jul;29(6):999-1009. Related Articles, Links Antidepressant-elicited changes in gene expression: remodeling of neuronal circuits as a new hypothesis for drug efficacy. Yamada M, Yamada M, Higuchi T. Department of Psychogeriatrics, National Institute of Mental Health, National Center of Neurology and Psychiatry, Tokyo 187-8553, Japan. mitsu@ncnp-k.go.jp Although antidepressants have been used clinically for more than 50 years, no consensus has been reached concerning their precise molecular mechanism of action. Pharmacogenomics is a powerful tool that can be used to identify genes affected by antidepressants or by other effective therapeutic manipulations. Using this tool, others and we have identified as candidate molecular targets several genes or expressed sequence tags (ESTs) that are induced by chronic antidepressant treatment. In this article, we review antidepressant-elicited changes in gene expression, focusing especially on the remodeling of neuronal circuits that results. This refocusing motivates our hypothesis that this plasticity represents the mechanism for drug efficacy, and thus a causal event for clinical improvement. Defining the roles of these molecules in drug-induced neural plasticity is likely to transform the course of research on the biological basis of antidepressants. Such detailed knowledge will have profound effects on the diagnosis, prevention, and treatment of depression. Consideration of novel biological approaches beyond the "monoamine hypothesis" of depression is expected to evoke paradigm shifts in the future of antidepressant research. Publication Types: Review

Psychiatr Genet. 2005 Sep;15(3):155-6. Related Articles, Links The Third Annual Pharmacogenetics in Psychiatry Meeting, 2004. Hassoun Y, Razi K, Malhotra AK. Department of Psychiatry Research, The Zucker Hillside Hospital, North Shore-Long Island Jewish Health System, Glen Oaks, NY 11004, USA. Publication Types: Congresses

Psychopharmacology (Berl). 2004 Aug;174(4):477-89. Epub 2004 Jul 8. Related Articles, Links Pharmacogenetics of antipsychotic-induced weight gain. Correll CU, Malhotra AK. Department of Psychiatry Research, The Zucker Hillside Hospital, North Shore-Long Island Jewish Health System, Glen Oaks, NY 11004, USA. RATIONALE: Antipsychotic medications have been associated with considerable weight gain. The degree of inter-individual variability and known genetic contributions to obesity suggest a combination of genetic and environmental factors. In the absence of established mechanisms and valid predictors for this relevant adverse effect, pharmacogenetic studies may provide the basis for the development of individualized treatment and preventive interventions. OBJECTIVE: The aim of the present review is to analyze the theoretical and empirical knowledge base for the selection of the most promising target genes that may contribute to antipsychotic-induced weight gain. METHODS: Examination of the preclinical and clinical literature that can inform the rational choice of target genes that may play a role in the development of adverse changes in body composition associated with antipsychotic treatment. RESULTS: Theoretically, candidate gene selection can be guided by knowledge about molecular pathways associated with obesity, receptors modulated by antipsychotic drugs, and enzymes implicated in their metabolism and bioavailability. While most available data relate to the general mechanisms of obesity and few studies have directly examined the genetic contributions to antipsychotic-induced weight gain, several genes warrant further investigation. These include the 5-HT(2C), pro-opiomelanocortin, leptin, ghrelin, tumor necrosis factor alpha, adiponectin, dopamine D(2) receptor, histamine-H(1) receptor, and alpha(1), beta(2) and beta(3) adrenergic receptor genes. CONCLUSIONS: Pharmacogenetic studies can provide powerful tools for the pre-treatment identification of individuals at high risk for antipsychotic-induced weight gain, to uncover biological mechanisms that may even generalize to non-drug-induced weight gain, and to isolate novel targets for treatments of weight gain and obesity. To enhance power, future studies should pay close attention to population selection and avoidance/control of confounds, particularly past treatment exposure. Publication Types: Review

Psychopharmacology (Berl). 2004 Aug;174(4):512-24. Epub 2004 Jul 13. Related Articles, Links Implications of genetic research on the role of the serotonin in depression: emphasis on the serotonin type 1A receptor and the serotonin transporter. Neumeister A, Young T, Stastny J. Clinical Neuroscience Division, Department of Psychiatry, VA National Center for PTSD (116-A), Yale University School of Medicine, 950 Campbell Avenue, West Haven, CT 06516, USA. Alexander.Neumeister@yale.edu Serotonin systems appear to play a key role in the pathophysiology of major depressive disorder. Consequently, ongoing research determines whether serotonin related genes account for the very robust differential behavioral and neural mechanisms that discriminate patients with depression from healthy controls. Serotonin type 1(A) receptors and the serotonin transporters are reduced in depression, and recent genetic research in animals and humans has implicated both in depression. Preclinical studies have utilized a variety of animal models that have been used to explain pathophysiological mechanisms in humans, although it is not clear at all whether these models constitute relevant models for depression in humans. However, data from preclinical studies can generate hypotheses that are tested in humans by combining genetic data with behavioral and physiological challenge paradigms and neuroimaging. These studies will enhance our understanding about combined influences from multiple interacting genes, as well as from environmental factors on brain circuits and their function, and about how these mechanisms may contribute to the pathophysiology of neuropsychiatric disorders. Publication Types: Review

Psychopharmacology (Berl). 2004 Aug;174(4):561-70. Epub 2004 May 18. Related Articles, Links Pharmacogenetic insights to monoaminergic dysfunction in alcohol dependence. Heinz A, Goldman D, Gallinat J, Schumann G, Puls I. Department of Psychiatry, Campus Charite Mitte, Charite-University Medicine Berlin, Schumannstrasse 20/21, 10117 Berlin, Germany. andreas.heinz@charite.de RATIONALE: Alcohol dependence is characterized by the development of tolerance, withdrawal symptoms, and craving for alcohol. Chronic alcohol consumption causes neuroadaptive changes in the central dopaminergic and serotonergic system, which are partially reversible after detoxification. The severity and time-course of recovery of these neuroadaptive changes may depend on the genetic constitution of monoamine transporters and receptors and contribute to the relapse risk of alcoholics. OBJECTIVES: To assess the interaction between the genetic constitution and the in vivo availability of dopamine and serotonin transporters and receptors, chronic alcohol intake, alcohol craving and withdrawal. METHODS: Review of brain imaging studies that assess the genotype and availability of dopamine and serotonin transporters in detoxified alcoholics and healthy control subjects. RESULTS: Chronic alcohol intake induced neuroadaptive reductions in striatal dopamine transporter (DAT) availability, which were reversible during early abstinence. A polymorphism of the DAT gene (SLC6A3) was associated with the in vivo transporter availability and with the severity of alcohol withdrawal. Neurotoxic reductions in 5-HTT protein expression were limited to homozygous carriers of the long allele in the 5-HTT gene (SCL6A4) regulatory region and correlated with negative mood states. CONCLUSION: Genetic constitution interacts with the in vivo availability of central dopamine and serotonin transporters during alcohol detoxification and may affect the severity of alcohol withdrawal and clinical depression. Publication Types: Review

Psychopharmacology (Berl). 2004 Aug;174(4):571-7. Epub 2004 Apr 27. Related Articles, Links Changes in food reward following smoking cessation: a pharmacogenetic investigation. Lerman C, Berrettini W, Pinto A, Patterson F, Crystal-Mansour S, Wileyto EP, Restine SL, Leonard DG, Shields PG, Epstein LH. Department of Psychiatry, Abramson Cancer Center, University of Pennsylvania, 3535 Market Street, Suite 4100, Philadelphia, PA 19104, USA. clerman@mail.med.upenn.edu RATIONALE: Despite the high prevalence and public health significance of weight gain following smoking cessation, little is known about the underlying bio-behavioral mechanisms or effective therapies. OBJECTIVES: We evaluated the effects of bupropion on food reward following smoking abstinence and the moderating influence of genotype. METHODS: Seventy-one smokers of European ancestry were genotyped for the dopamine D2 receptor (DRD2) Taq1 polymorphism and randomized to treatment with bupropion (300 mg) or placebo for smoking cessation. Subjects participated in two behavioral laboratory sessions during which the rewarding value of food was assessed using a behavioral economics measure: session 1 occurred prior to medication and before cessation of smoking; session 2 occurred following 3 weeks of medication and 1 week of sustained abstinence. RESULTS: Carriers of the DRD2 A1 minor allele exhibited significant increases in the rewarding value of food following abstinence from smoking, and these effects were attenuated by bupropion treatment ($P=0.03$ for medication by genotype interaction). Further, higher levels of food reward at session 2 (post-quit) predicted a significant increase in weight by 6-month follow-up in the placebo group, but not in the bupropion-treated group ($P=0.006$ for medication by food reward interaction). CONCLUSIONS: These results provide new evidence that the increase in body weight that occurs following smoking cessation is related to increases in food reward, and that food reward is partly determined by genetic factors. Bupropion's efficacy in attenuating abstinence-induced weight gain may be attributable, in part, to decreasing food reward. Publication Types: Clinical Trial Randomized Controlled Trial

Psychosomatics. 2006 Jan-Feb;47(1):75-85. Related Articles, Links Clinical guidelines for psychiatrists for the use of pharmacogenetic testing for CYP450 2D6 and CYP450 2C19. de Leon J, Armstrong SC, Cozza KL. University of Kentucky Mental Health Research Center at Eastern State Hospital, Lexington, KY 40508, USA. jdeleon@uky.edu Pharmacogenetics has arrived in clinical psychiatric practice with the FDA approval of the AmpliChip CYP450 Test that genotypes for two cytochrome P450 2D6 (CYP2D6) and 2C19 (CYP2C19) genes. Other pharmacogenetic tests, including those focused on pharmacodynamic genes, are far from ready for clinical application. CYP2D6 is important for the metabolism of many antidepressants and antipsychotics, and CY2C19 is important for some antidepressant metabolism. Poor metabolizers (PMs), lacking the enzyme, account for up to 7% of Caucasians for CYP2D6 and up to 25% of East Asians for CYP2C19. Patients having three or more active CYP2D6 alleles (up to 29% in North Africa and the Middle East), are called CYP2D6 ultra-rapid metabolizers (UMs). CYP2D6 phenotypes (particularly PMs) are probably important in patients taking tricyclic antidepressants (TCAs), venlafaxine, typical antipsychotics, and risperidone. The CYP2C19 PM phenotype is probably important in patients taking TCAs and perhaps citalopram, escitalopram, and sertraline. On the basis of the literature and the authors' clinical experience, the authors provide provisional recommendations for identifying and treating CYP2D6 PMs, CYP2C19 PMs, and CYP2D6 UMs. The next few years will determine whether CYP2D6 genotyping is beneficial for patients taking the new drugs aripiprazole, duloxetine, and atomoxetine. Practical recommendations for dealing with laboratories offering CYP2D6 and CYP2C29 genotyping are provided. Publication Types: Review

Radiology. 2004 Jun;231(3):613-6. Related Articles, Links Personalized medicine. Thrall JH. Department of Radiology, Massachusetts General Hospital, Harvard Medical School, 14 Fruit Street, FND-216, Boston, MA 02114, USA. thrall.james@mgh.harvard.edu

Reprod Biomed Online. 2005 Nov;11(5):589-600. Related Articles, Links Pharmacogenetics in ovarian stimulation - current concepts and future options. Greb RR, Behre HM, Simoni M. Muenster University Hospital, Germany. robert.greb@uni-muenster.de Tailoring ovarian stimulation to the individual patient can be challenging because the ovarian response varies substantially between patients. Pharmacogenetics has emerged as a new area of research to improve the balance between desired and undesired actions of drugs, based upon the genetic predisposition of the individual patient. Clinical studies have demonstrated that the p.N680S polymorphism of the FSH-receptor gene determines the ovarian response to FSH stimulation in patients undergoing IVF. In homozygous Ser(680)/Ser(680) type women, the FSH receptor appears to be more resistant to FSH action even in normal menstrual cycles. Therefore, genotyping of patients scheduled for ovarian stimulation could be an attractive tool to individualize FSH dosing according to genetic differences in ovarian sensitivity. More clinical studies are warranted to investigate the usefulness of genotyping for the p.N680S polymorphism as a routine diagnostic test before ovarian stimulation. Publication Types: Review

Reprod Toxicol. 2005 Sep-Oct;20(3):433-40. Related Articles, Links Mapping molecular responses to xenoestrogens through Gene Ontology and pathway analysis of toxicogenomic data. Currie RA, Orphanides G, Moggs JG. Syngenta Central Toxicology Laboratory, Alderley Park, Macclesfield SK10 4TJ, UK. richard.currie@syngenta.com The recent sequencing of mammalian genomes has driven the development of genomic technologies, including microarray-based gene expression profiling, that allow simultaneous measurement of the expression levels of thousands of genes. Gene expression profiling applied to toxicology (toxicogenomics) has the potential to reveal, holistically, the molecular pathways and cellular processes that mediate the adverse responses to a toxicant. However, the initial output of a toxicogenomics experiment consists of a list of genes whose expression is altered upon toxicant exposure. In order to interpret these data in a biological context, new bioinformatic methods must be developed to place gene expression changes in the context of the underlying pathways and processes affected. One emerging approach is the application of Gene Ontology (GO) mapping and pathway analysis to gene expression profiling data. The utility of this in mechanistic toxicology will be illustrated using examples in which GO mapping of toxicogenomic data has provided novel insights into the molecular mechanisms induced by exposure to xenoestrogens.

Respirology. 2004 Nov;9(4):426-7. Related Articles, Links A molecular chink in the lung cancer armour. Fong KM, Bowman R. Publication Types: Editorial Review

Rev Epidemiol Sante Publique. 2005 Jun;53(3):267-82. Related Articles, Links [Molecular biology in clinical cancer research: the example of digestive cancers] [Article in French] Lievre A, Laurent-Puig P. INSERM U 490, Universite Paris-V, Paris. Pole Biologie, Hopital Europeen Georges-Pompidou, AP-HP, 20, rue Leblanc, 75015 Paris. Cancer is a DNA disease characterized by uncontrolled cell proliferation due to the accumulation of genetic alterations. Recent progress in molecular biology allowed the identification of markers potentially usefull for patients management through the identification of these genetic alterations and a best understanding of chemotherapy molecular targets. Several examples in digestive oncology underline the relevance of molecular biology in clinical research. If almost all colorectal cancers (CRC) correspond to the same histopathological type (adenocarcinoma), molecular biology allowed the identification of two different molecular mechanisms of colorectal carcinogenesis: chromosomal instability characterized by recurrent allelic losses on chromosomes 17, 5, 18, 8 and 22 that contribute to the inactivation of tumor suppressor genes, and genetic instability characterized by the instability of microsatellite loci due to an alteration of DNA mismatch repair leading to the accumulation of mutations in genes involved in the control of cell cycle and apoptosis. These data are potentially interesting for the management of CRC patients. Indeed, microsatellite instability seems not only to be a good prognostic factor but also a molecular factor that can predict response to adjuvant 5-fluorouracil based chemotherapy. Therapeutic clinical trials taking into account these molecular parameters are still going on. DNA microarray-based gene expression profiling technology that allows the simultaneous analysis of thousand of tumor genes represents also an interesting approach in oncology with the recent identification of a "genetic signature" as a risk factor of tumor recurrence in stage II CRC, a setting in which the benefit of adjuvant chemotherapy remains on debate. At last, a best understanding of chemotherapy molecular targets allowed the identification of genetic markers that can predict the response and/or the toxicity of anti-cancer drugs used in gastrointestinal cancers, which could be helpful in the future to propose for each patient a personalized treatment. Mutations that can predict the response of new target therapies such as the inhibitors of the c-KIT tyrosine kinase activity in gastrointestinal stromal tumors have also been found and will allow the selection of patients who can have benefit from these new therapeutic drugs. Publication Types: Review

Rev Esp Cardiol. 2004 Apr;57(4):331-46. Related Articles, Links [Pediatric cardiology in the genomic era] [Article in Spanish] Marin-Garcia J. The Molecular Cardiology and Neuromuscular Institute. Highland Park. New Jersey 08904, USA. tmci@att.net While congenital heart disease, cardiomyopathy, arrhythmias and acquired cardiac diseases are common causes of mortality and morbidity in infants and children, the basic underlying mechanisms of many specific pediatric cardiovascular diseases still remains undetermined. Breakthroughs in molecular genetic technology have just begun to be applied in pediatric cardiology stemming from the use of chromosomal mapping and the identification of genes involved in both the primary etiology and as significant risk factors in the development of cardiac and vascular abnormalities. This review will focus on information obtained thus far by molecular genetic analysis in the diagnosis, treatment and overall understanding of pediatric cardiovascular disease pathogenesis examining both the more prevalent congenital/inherited heart defects, arrhythmias and cardiomyopathies, as well as sporadic and acquired disorders. In addition, a survey of the pediatric cardiologist's armamentarium with regards to molecular and genetic analysis is presented highlighting the current use of molecular diagnostic methods including microarray, gene-mapping, proteomic, transgenic and stem cell technologies as well as future directions in both clinical application and research. Publication Types: Review

Rev Esp Cardiol. 2005 Jun;58(6):745-8. Related Articles, Links [Pharmacogenetic study of the response to flecainide and propafenone in patients with atrial fibrillation] [Article in Spanish] Martinez-Selles M, Castillo I, Montenegro P, Martin ML, Almendral J, Sanjurjo M. Servicio de Cardiologia, Hospital Universitario Gregorio Maranon, Madrid, Spain. We analyzed cytochrome P450 2D6 polymorphism by determining phenotype as the metabolic ratio between dextromethorphan and its main metabolite, dextrorphan. We studied 18 men and 22 women in whom mean age was 54.6+/-11.9 years. In 9 patients metabolic ratio was determined before antiarrhythmic treatment and again during treatment, with a mean increase of 0.13+/-0.15 (P=.03). We found 19 poor metabolizers and 21 extensive metabolizers. Adverse effects were more frequent in poor metabolizers (21.1%) than in extensive metabolizers (4.8%; P=.12). Antiarrhythmic treatment was effective in 27 patients (67.5%), with no difference between poor and extensive metabolizers.

Rev Gastroenterol Disord. 2004;4 Suppl 1:S8-S13. Related Articles, Links Viral factors affecting the outcome of therapy for chronic hepatitis C. Fried MW.

Department of Medicine, Division of Digestive Diseases, University of North Carolina, Chapel Hill, NC, USA. The advent of sensitive virologic assays to quantify hepatitis C virus (HCV) RNA and to differentiate specific genotypes of HCV has greatly expanded our understanding of the pathogenesis of chronic hepatitis C. These molecular virologic techniques are regularly employed to assist with management decisions regarding antiviral therapy. Genotype is the strongest predictor of a sustained virologic response (SVR). The dynamic change of HCV RNA during treatment, defined at week 12 as early virologic response (EVR), is useful for identifying individuals who are unlikely to have an SVR. Discontinuation of therapy can be considered for those patients with genotype 1 when an EVR is not achieved. However, limitations exist regarding interpretation of EVR and treatment decisions must be individualized, particularly when other endpoints of therapy, such as histological response or treatment of extrahepatic manifestations are being considered. Publication Types: Review

Rev Invest Clin. 2004 Jul-Aug;56(4):554-60.· Related Articles, Links [Genomic medicine. Myths and reality] [Article in Spanish] Lisker R. Direccion de Investigacion, Instituto Nacional de Ciencias Medicas y Nutricion Salvador Zubiran. rlisker@quetzal.innsz.mx Genomic medicine is simply the routine use of genomic analysis, preferably by direct DNA studies, to improve the quality of medical care. A likely consequence will be to increase the predictive and prevention capacities of medicine, including common diseases, such as cancer, diabetes and others. The most common variability of the genome are the SNPs (single nucleotide polymorphisms), every person having between 3 and 10 million of them. SNPs may or not be harmless, and studies are in progress in cases and controls studies to answer the question of whether they determine why some persons have a given disease and others do not, and if they have something to do with that the individual variation in the response to drugs. We discuss in the same context the haplotype map project (HapMap) as a tool to facilitate the study of possible associations of genome changes and common diseases. We discuss the most successful effort in gene therapy, that of severe combined immunodeficiency, in which 17 out of 18 patients responded well to the procedure, although 2 of them developed late side effects in the form of acute leukemia, very likely related to the therapy. The ethical social and legal problems of genomic medicine are discussed very lightly and several references are given to readers interested in this matter. Publication Types: Review

Rev Med Interne. 2005 Sep;26(9):725-32. Epub 2005 Mar 17. Related Articles, Links [Pharmacogenetics and antiplatelet drugs] [Article in French] Fontana P, Reny JL. Service d'angiologie et d'hemostase, departement de medecine interne, faculte de medecine, hopital cantonal universitaire, 24, rue Micheli-du-Crest, 1211 Geneve 14, Suisse. pierre.fontana@medecine.unige.ch PURPOSE: The observation of inherited drug response variability gave rise to the field of pharmacogenetics. Pharmacogenetic research on drug targets, particularly platelet enzymes and receptors, is more recent and is becoming an emerging field. CURRENT KNOWLEDGE AND KEY POINTS: In the Framingham study, the heritability of platelet aggregation response ranges from

44 to 62%, depending on the agonists used. The gene coding for GPIIIa, a sub-unit of the fibrinogen receptor GPIIbIIIa, is one of the most extensively studied gene in relation with aggregation tests and antiplatelet drugs. The GPIIIa PLA1/PLA2 polymorphism has been associated with clopidogrel and orbofiban platelet response. However, data are more controversial concerning the association with aspirin response. Recently, Cox-1 and GPIa (part of the GPIaIIa collagen receptor) genetic variations have also been pointed out as possible candidates to explain part of the variability of the response to antiplatelet agents. Finally, the H1/H2 polymorphism of the platelet ADP receptor P2Y12 gene has been associated with ADP-induced platelet aggregation response and peripheral arterial disease. This polymorphism may modulate the effect of P2Y12 antagonists like clopidogrel and its clinical implication is currently under study. FUTURE PROSPECTS AND PROJECTS: Gene-expression profiling and proteomics may allow the identification of new candidate genes whose variations may be associated with the heritability of platelet aggregation response. In the next future, phenotypic or genotypic studies could be available to tailor the prescription of antiplatelet drugs. Publication Types: Review

Rev Med Liege. 2005 Dec;60(12):918-22. Related Articles, Links [Integration of pharmacogenetics in the medical practice] [Article in French] Dideberg V, Bours V. Service de Genetique, Humaine, CHU Sart-Tilman, 4000 Liege. vinciane.dideberg@chu.ulg.ac.be Today, the initiation of any medical treatment still raises questions about its efficacy and safety. Indeed, therapeutic responses vary over time and between individuals and are influenced by age, sex, other treatments and the pathology itself. Genetic factors are thought to be responsible for 20 to 95% of these individual variations. Recent advances in biotechnology, molecular genetics and genomics allow a better understanding of drug metabolism and action. Pharmacogenetics, compiling phenotypic and genotypic data, may lead to a more personalized treatment. To allow a better approach of pharmacogenetics and pharmacogenomics, we will define these two terms and describe their actual and future clinical application. Publication Types: Review

Rev Neurol. 2004 Dec 1-15;39(11):1063-71. Related Articles, Links [Pharmacogenomics: the quest for individualized therapy] [Article in Spanish] Lopez-Lopez M, Guerrero-Camacho JL, Familiar-Lopez IM, Jung-Cook H, Corona-Vazquez T, Alonso-Vilatela ME. Departamento de Sistemas Biologicos, Universidad Autonoma Metropolitana, Unidad Xochimilco, Mexico. AIM: Different patients exhibit wide variability in the way they respond to medications. Individual differences in drug response can result from environmental factors, as well as genetic determinants. In particular, inherited differences in the metabolism and disposition of drugs can have a great influence on the efficacy and toxicity of medications, so herein we focus on the pharmacogenetics of drug metabolism. DEVELOPMENT: Clinical observations of inherited differences in drug effects were first documented in the 1950s, giving rise to the field of pharmacogenetics. These observations were then followed by population studies of drug disposition phenotype, then biochemical, and eventually molecular elucidation of the genetic defect associated with the inherited trait. Genetic polymorphisms have been described for many phase I and phase II drug-metabolizing enzymes including several cytochromes P450, N-acetyltransferases, and thiopurine S-methyltransferase. Rapid advances in human genomics gave birth to pharmacogenomics, an emerging discipline that uses genome-wide approaches to study the entire spectrum of genes involved in drug response. High-through-put genomic technologies will serve as the foundation of personalized therapies. CONCLUSIONS: Knowledge of an individual's genetic variability in drug response may be clinically and economically important and could provide the basis for a rational approach to drug prescription in neuropsychiatric disorders. Publication Types: Review

Rev Port Cardiol. 2004 Dec;23(12):1621-30. Related Articles, Links Antihypertensive pharmacogenetics. [Article in English, Portuguese] Nogueira JB. Medicina 1, Hospital de Santa Maria, Faculdade de Medicina de Lisboa Lisboa, Portugal. braznogueira@fm.ul.pt Essential hypertension is a complex disease in which multiple genetic and environmental factors interact to produce the phenotype. The genetic contribution to blood pressure variations is estimated to range from 30% to 50%. In this review we describe some of the genes and genetic polymorphisms that have been most consistently related to blood pressure elevation and also the importance of pharmacogenetics and the emerging evidence of genetic influences on antihypertensive drug responses, with the potential for getting the right drug into the right patient based on the individual genetic profile. Publication Types: Review

Rheumatology (Oxford). 2005 Aug;44(8):1051-5. Epub 2005 May 18. Related Articles, Links Methotrexate-induced pancytopenia: serious and under-reported? Our experience of 25 cases in 5 years. Lim AY, Gaffney K, Scott DG. Rheumatology Department, Norfolk and Norwich University Hospital, Norwich NR4 7UY, UK. anitalim@doctors.org.uk OBJECTIVE: To ascertain the extent of methotrexate (MTX)-related pancytopenia at the Norfolk and Norwich University Hospital (NNUH) between 1999 and 2004. METHODS: Patients were identified by a department database search, review of pharmacy records and personal communication. Pancytopenia was defined as white blood cell count (WBC) <3.5 x 10(9)/l, haemoglobin (Hb) <11 g/dl and platelet count <130 x 10(9)/l. Severe pancytopenia was defined as WBC <2.0 x 10(9)/l, Hb <10 g/dl and platelet count <50 x 10(9)/l. RESULTS: Twenty-five patients had MTX-induced pancytopenia. Eleven patients were taking folic acid and one folinic acid. The median dose of MTX was 12.5 mg weekly (interquartile range 5.625 mg) and median duration of treatment 36 months (interquartile range 40.5 months). The severity of pancytopenia correlated with the dose (P = 0.04). The numbers of patients with potential risk factors were: renal insufficiency, 8; pre-existing folate deficiency, 7; age >75 yr, 15; hypoalbuminaemia, 18; pre-existing infection with hip prosthesis, 1; possible drug interactions, 18; dosing errors, 1; and polypharmacy, 15. Pancytopenia was detected by routine blood monitoring in nine patients. There were seven deaths (28% mortality), five from sepsis and two from acute myeloid leukaemia. CONCLUSION: This is the largest reported individual case series of MTX-induced pancytopenia. With the increasing long-term use of MTX, it is important that patients be monitored for haematological side-effects as pancytopenia can be a late manifestation. Pharmacogenetics may hold the answer to predicting who is at risk of this potentially fatal complication of MTX.

Rinsho Ketsueki. 2005 Jun;46(6):433-8. Related Articles, Links [Development of personalized peptide vaccines for advanced cancer patients] [Article in Japanese] Yamada A. Publication Types: Review

S Afr Med J. 2005 Jan;95(1):19-20. Related Articles, Links Pharmacogenetics offers hope. Bateman C. Publication Types: News

Schizophr Bull. 2004;30(3):577-86. Related Articles, Links The international suicide prevention trial (interSePT): rationale and design of a trial comparing the relative ability of clozapine and olanzapine to reduce suicidal behavior in schizophrenia and schizoaffective patients. Alphs L, Anand R, Islam MZ, Meltzer HY, Kane JM, Krishnan R, Green AI, Potkin S, Chouinard G, Lindenmayer JP, Kerwin R. larry.alphs@pfizer.com Suicidal behavior in patients with psychotic disorders represents a seriously undertreated life-threatening condition. The International Suicide Prevention Trial (InterSePT) is the first large-scale, prospective study designed to evaluate the potential of antipsychotic medications to reduce suicidal behaviors in patients with schizophrenia or schizoaffective disorder who are known to be at high risk for suicide. The unique challenges to study design and the solutions identified for the InterSePT study are described. These challenges included defining suicidal behavior in patients with psychosis, endpoint selection, determination of analytic strategy, and development of scales to assess suicidal behavior. Given the life-threatening nature of suicidal behavior, ethical considerations required that the design minimize suicide attempts and deaths. While the study focused primarily on treatment of suicide, opportunities were used to collect data in related areas of interest, including suicide risk factors, other efficacy measures (e.g., Positive and Negative Syndrome Scale, Covi Anxiety Scale, Calgary Depression Scale), adverse events, pharmacoeconomics, and pharmacogenetics. Because of the complexity of the design issues, a steering committee, suicide monitoring board, and publication committee were established to assist with their management. Publication Types: Clinical Trial Multicenter Study Randomized Controlled Trial

Schizophr Res. 2005 Jun 1;75(1):21-6. Related Articles, Links Genetic susceptibility to tardive dyskinesia in chronic schizophrenia subjects: III. Lack of association of CYP3A4 and CYP2D6 gene polymorphisms. Tiwari AK, Deshpande SN, Rao AR, Bhatia T, Lerer B, Nimgaonkar VL, Thelma BK. Department of Genetics, University of Delhi South Campus, New Delhi 110021, India. Tardive dyskinesia is a severe debilitating movement disorder characterized by choreoathetotic movements developing in one-fifth of the patients with schizophrenia. In this study we have investigated the significance of CYP3A4*1B and CYP2D6*4 polymorphisms in TD susceptibility among chronic schizophrenia patients (n = 335) from north India. Tardive dyskinesia was diagnosed in approximately 29% (96/335) of these patients. No significant association of either of the two SNPs with TD (CYP3A4*1B chi2 = 0. 308, df = 1, p = 0.579; CYP2D6*4 chi2 = 0.006, df = 1, p = 0.935) was observed. However a trend towards increased severity of TD in patients heterozygous for the CYP2D6*4 mutation was observed.

Schmerz. 2005 Oct;19(5):372-7. Related Articles, Links [Does genomics determine efficacy of analgesics?] [Article in German] Stamer U, Stuber F. Klinik und Poliklinik fur Anasthesiologie und operative Intensivmedizin, Rheinische Friedrich-Wilhelms-Universitat Bonn. ulrike.stamer@ukb.uni-bonn.de Recent advances in knowledge about gene structure derived from the human genome project has also revealed data on genomic variation and their possible impact on complex and acute diseases as well as pharmacotherapy. The hypothesis of a genetic predisposition for complex diseases such as pain syndromes, side effects, and adverse outcomes challenging the clinician is ready to be tested by advanced genetic-epidemiologic study designs employing the latest genotyping technology. In pain therapy, the genetic background of the efficacy of analgesics, especially of opioids, is of particular interest. Genetic differences in drug kinetics and dynamics, e.g., differences in metabolism or genetic variations of the drug target (e.g., receptors) will be of importance in the future. Pharmacogenetics can individualize pharmacotherapy and improve care by predicting the optimal dose and avoiding side effects and toxicity in individual patients.

Schweiz Rundsch Med Prax. 2004 Mar 3;93(10):359-65. Related Articles, Links [Pharmacogenetics. Tailored therapy in medicine -- opportunities and challenges] [Article in German] Scharplatz M, Puhan M, Steurer J, Bachmann LM. Horten-Zentrum fur praxisorientierte Forschung und Wissenstransfer, Zurich. madlaina.scharplatz@usz.ch This article provides a general introduction into the field of pharmacogenetics and discusses its opportunities and limits. Pharmacogenetic research explores genetic variability between patients to explain observed differences in effectiveness of a drug therapy or adverse event profiles. Sometimes drug therapy is unfavourable: Patients may respond only partially to a drug therapy, do not respond at all, or suffer from serious adverse events. The reasons for the varying effectiveness of a drug therapy are due to factors like absorption; metabolism, elimination and target interaction. Recent research has led to a better understanding of the molecular genetic mechanisms behind those factors. Numerous new polymorphisms have been described, for example for the beta 2-adrenergic receptor or the cytochrome which can either improve or reduce the response to drug therapy. Two polymorphisms for the tumour necrosis factor alpha have shown to be associated with an increased risk of serious adverse events (hypersensibility: fever, rash, gastrointestinal symptoms) if treated with abacavir (HIV-treatment). Pharmacogenetic tests provide information about certain polymorphisms and raise the hope for an individualized pharmacotherapy. Yet, not only genetic but also environmental factors influence the effectiveness of a therapy. Even though results from research implies that pharmacogenetics has a great potential to maximize the effectiveness of pharmacotherapy and to reduce the incidence of drug-related adverse events, extensive clinical research both on effectiveness and costs is required to assess the true benefits of these exciting new technologies. Publication Types: Review

Science. 2004 Aug 27;305(5688):1222-3. Related Articles, Links Pharmacogenomics. Cancer sharpshooters rely on DNA tests for a better aim. Couzin J. Publication Types: News

Science. 2004 Jul 9;305(5681):183. Related Articles, Links Comment in: Science. 2005 Feb 25;307(5713):1200-1; author reply 1200-1. Science. 2005 Feb 25;307(5713):1200-1; author reply 1200-1. Genetics. Genomic research and human subject privacy. Lin Z, Owen AB, Altman RB. Department of Genetics, Stanford University School of Medicine, CA 94305-5120, USA.

Science. 2004 Oct 22;306(5696):575. Related Articles, Links Genomics and drug toxicity. Lord PG, Papoian T. Publication Types: Editorial

Science. 2005 Dec 9;310(5754):1605. Related Articles, Links Indian Ocean tsunami. In the wake: looking for keys to posttraumatic stress. Stone R. Publication Types: News

Science. 2005 Feb 18;307(5712):1050-1. Related Articles, Links Medicine. Race and reification in science. Duster T. Institute for the History of the Production of Knowledge, New York University, 269 Mercer Street, New York, NY 10003-6687, USA. troy.duster@nyu.edu

Science. 2005 Feb 25;307(5713):1191. Related Articles, Links American Association for the Advancement of Science meeting. DNA tells story of heart drug failure. Couzin J. Publication Types: News

Science. 2005 Jul 1;309(5731):81. Related Articles, Links To what extent are genetic variation and personal health linked? Couzin J. Publication Types: News

Science. 2005 Jun 10;308(5728):1572. Related Articles, Links Gender in the pharmacy: does it matter? Kaiser J. Publication Types: News

Science. 2005 Jun 24;308(5730):1858-60. Related Articles, Links Pharmacogenomics. Going from genome to pill. Service RF. Publication Types: News

Seishin Shinkeigaku Zasshi. 2004;106(1):38-41. Related Articles, Links [Future antidepressant research and pharmacogenomics] [Article in Japanese] Yamada M. Department of Psychiatry, Showa University Karasuyama Hospital. Although antidepressants have been used clinically for more than 50 years, no consensus has been reached concerning their precise molecular mechanism of action. Using pharmacogenomics tools, we and other investigators have identified as candidate molecular targets several genes or expressed sequence tags (ESTs) that are induced by chronic antidepressant treatment. In this article, we review antidepressant-elicited changes in gene expression, focusing especially on the remodeling of neuronal circuits that results. This refocusing motivates our hypothesis that this plasticity represents the mechanism for drug efficacy, and thus a causal event for clinical improvement. Consideration of novel biological approaches beyond the "monoamine hypothesis" of depression is expected to evoke paradigm shifts in the future of antidepressant research. Publication Types: Review

Seishin Shinkeigaku Zasshi. 2004;106(8):1050-5. Related Articles, Links [Front line of therapies for depression] Nomura S. Publication Types: Review

Semin Oncol. 2004 Feb;31(1 Suppl 3):39-53. Related Articles, Links Molecular therapeutics: promise and challenges. Kohn EC, Lu Y, Wang H, Yu Q, Yu S, Hall H, Smith DL, Meric-Bernstam F, Hortobagyi GN, Mills GB. Laboratory of Pathology, Center for Cancer Research, National Cancer Institute, Bethesda, MD, USA. The ability to analyze the genetic and epigenetic aberrations present in a particular patient's tumor on a global basis is rapidly maturing. The emerging fields of functional genomics and functional proteomics offer the opportunity to translate these advances into a full comprehension of the pathophysiology of cancer. Linking these approaches to chemical genomics and molecular therapeutics should provide an expanding repertoire of targeted therapeutics for clinical evaluation. Novel clinical trial designs that can determine the efficacy of targeted therapeutics in patients selected for aberrations in the target are needed to evaluate the wealth of new drugs becoming available. The promise of these technologies and advances in our understanding of cancer is immense, making it our responsibility to see them to fruition. These technologies should lead to a new era of individualized molecular medicine, wherein we will treat each patient with a "prescription" based on the genetic changes in each patient's tumor and their own genetic make-up, resulting in more effective and less toxic therapy. Publication Types: Review

Semin Oncol. 2005 Dec;32(6 Suppl 8):15-20. Related Articles, Links Metastatic colorectal cancer: first- and second-line treatment in 2005. Rougier P, Lepere C. Hopital Ambroise Pare, Boulogne Billancourt, France. phillipe.rougier@apr.ap-hop-paris.fr First-, second-, and third-line therapies for the treatment of metastatic colorectal cancer may influence choices for subsequent therapy. First-line treatment for metastatic colorectal cancer depends largely on combination chemotherapy regimens that have been proven to prolong survival, control disease progression, and improve quality of life, without excessive toxicity. Standard therapies include 5-fluorouracil, irinotecan, and oxaliplatin, but other combination therapies are currently under investigation. An upcoming area of study includes agents that target vascular endothelial growth factor and epidermal growth factor receptor. While doublet therapy is more active than 5-fluorouracil alone, triplet therapy is also emerging. Second-line therapy is dependent upon prior treatment, and second-line FOLFIRI or FOLFOX regimens that incorporate 5-fluorouracil, leucovorin, and either irinotecan or oxaliplatin, respectively, are still in question because of residual toxicities. After combination chemotherapy, a non-cross-resistant chemotherapy is the best choice. Second-line targeted therapy has been well-tolerated and active in several trials. Future developments will most likely occur in the areas of pharmacogenetics (eg, toxicity, age, comorbidities, patient choice, strategy of cure, palliation) and pharmacogenomics (eg, resistance/activity, gene expression) to produce individualized therapies for patients. The type of adjuvant treatment, genomic consideration, and genetic predisposition will be determining factors in the ideal protocol for first-line therapy. Publication Types: Review

Semin Oncol. 2005 Dec;32(6 Suppl 9):S87-9. Related Articles, Links Pharmacogenetics in esophageal cancer. Wu X, Lu C, Chiang SS, Ajani JA. Department of Epidemiology, The University of Texas M.D. Anderson Cancer Center, Houston, 77030, USA. xwu@mdanderson.org The current oncology practice of treating cancer with aggressive doses of radiation and chemotherapy is potentially disastrous, as response and side effects vary depending on several factors including pharmacogenetics. This study is the first to evaluate esophageal cancer treatment with a pharmacogenetic paradigm and its application of pharmacogenetic analysis to multiple genes in each drug action pathway as a means of developing a more accurate and consistent risk prediction model. This study has enrolled 235 patients with resectable adenocarcinoma or squamous cell carcinoma of the esophagus who had been treated with chemoradiation followed by esophagectomy. The preliminary finding that methylenetetrahydrofolate reductase polymorphisms modify 5-fluorouracil response supports the hypothesis that response or resistance to therapy in esophageal cancer patients may be modulated by genetic variants involved in the metabolism or mechanism of chemotherapy drug action. Our ongoing esophageal cancer research aims to determine individual pharmacogenetic profiles to identify patients most likely to have chemotherapeutic benefit and patients with the highest risk of suffering genotoxic side effects. These profiles will ideally lead to individualized therapies, improved treatment outcomes, and a movement toward clinically applied pharmacogenetics. This emergent area of biomedicine could lead to substantially improved clinical outcomes for patients with adenocarcinoma or squamous cell carcinoma of the esophagus.

Semin Oncol. 2005 Feb;32(1):113-9. Related Articles, Links Pharmacogenetic influences on treatment response and toxicity in colorectal cancer. Tan BR, McLeod HL. Department of Medicine and The Siteman Cancer Center, Washington University School of Medicine, St Louis, MO, USA. Current use of chemotherapeutic and targeted agents for advanced colorectal cancer (CRC) results in high tumor response rates and relatively long overall patient survival. Fluoropyrimidines, irinotecan, and oxaliplatin are highly active in first-line and salvage therapy of colorectal cancer. Targeted therapies, including anti-angiogenesis agents and anti-epidermal growth factor receptor antibodies, have been incorporated with traditional chemotherapy and offer additional options for patients with CRC. However, there is marked variability in response to therapy, as well as frequency and severity of toxicities. Molecular markers and pharmacogenomic profiling may improve prediction of patients who will experience significant benefit or toxicity from currently available agents. Validation of these predictive factors in prospective clinical trials is now necessary to allow for a rational and systematic individualization of cancer therapy. Publication Types: Review

Semin Oncol. 2005 Oct;32(5):437-42. Related Articles, Links Epigenetic drugs: a longstanding story. de Vos D. Pharmachemie BV, PO Box 552, 2003 RN Haarlem, The Netherlands. dick.d.vos@pharmachemie.com In this chapter, the development of decitabine from its synthesis in 1964 to the submission of a registration file in 2004 is reviewed. The proper application of the unique properties of decitabine took quite some time to elucidate. In addition, the practical handling in the clinic was not easy as the prolonged myelosuppression of decitabine made it difficult to determine the preferred dose and schedule. Laboratory studies on DNA methylation and cell differentiation showed possible applications in solid and hematologic malignancies. However, despite many attempts, results in solid tumors have been disappointing thus far. After thorough investigation, decitabine achieved therapeutic application in myelodysplastic syndrome (MDS), in particular in patients with a poor prognosis. Further indications may include acute myeloid leukemia (AML), chronic myelogenous leukemia (CML), hematopoietic stem cell transplantation, sickle cell anemia, and thalassemia. Whereas most drugs are already at the end of their life cycle after 40 years, decitabine is only at the beginning. Its application will broaden with the increase in knowledge of epigenetic mechanisms and their relationship to drug therapy. Publication Types: Historical Article Review

Semin Perinatol. 2004 Apr;28(2):132-40. Related Articles, Links Pharmacogenomics and renal drug disposition in the newborn. Kapur G, Mattoo T, Aranda JV. Department of Pediatric Nephrology, Pediatric Pharmacology Research Unit Network, Wayne State University School of Medicine, Children's Hospital of Michigan, Detroit, MI 48201, USA. Genetic polymorphisms in the genes coding for drug metabolizing enzymes, drug transporters, and drug receptors are major determinants of an individual's response to drugs. The potential interactions of pharmacogenomics of renal drug transporters and drug receptors with renal drug disposition and the immature kidneys are briefly reviewed. Examples of gene polymorphisms seen in the RAAS (renin angiotensin system), beta-adrenergic receptors, dopamine receptors and cytochrome P450 and their potential clinical impact are discussed. The human newborn has deficient hepatic and renal drug metabolism and disposition. This immaturity in drug-handling capacity may potentially be superimposed to genetic polymorphisms determining drug metabolism and transport thereby substantially increasing interpatient variability in drug dose requirements and in drug responses in the newborn. Pharmacogenomics is a tool that can be used to individualize drug therapy in newborns to minimize adverse drug effects and to optimize efficacy.
Publication Types: Review

Semin Thromb Hemost. 2004 Oct;30(5):591-600. Related Articles, Links Clinical and functional consequences of platelet membrane glycoprotein polymorphisms. Yee DL, Bray PF. Department of Pediatrics, Hematology/Oncology Section, Baylor College of Medicine, Houston, Texas, USA. The last several years have seen an abundance of studies of genetic risk factors for vascular disease, and platelet glycoprotein (GP) polymorphisms have been a primary focus of this area of research. This article reviews GP receptor polymorphisms, particularly those on GPIa-IIa (integrin alpha2beta1), GPIb-IX-V, GPIIb-IIIa (integrin alpha(IIb)beta3), and GPVI, and summarizes clinical and functional studies that have attempted to clarify their roles in human disease. Our focus is on recent work relevant to thrombotic and hemostatic processes and advances in pharmacogenetics. We consider issues affecting our ability to derive firm conclusions from these studies, and discuss future directions in this rapidly evolving area. Publication Types: Review

Soc Sci Med. 2005 Sep;61(6):1201-10. Related Articles, Links 'At the point at which you can do something about it, then it becomes more relevant': informed consent in the pharmacogenetic clinic. Hedgecoe A. Department of Sociology, University of Sussex, Falmer, Brighton BN1 6JQ, UK. a.m.hedgecoe@sussex.ac.uk Sociological investigation of informed consent has generated rich and complex descriptions of the clinical encounter, often challenging the straightforward picture painted by medical ethicists. This paper builds on this work, drawing on ideas from the Sociology of Science and Technology, to explore informed consent issues surrounding the use of the drug Herceptin, widely cited as an example of a novel approach to drug development called pharmacogenetics. Drawing on qualitative semi-structured interviews with 25 UK-based breast cancer specialists, this paper explores Herceptin's disputed epistemological status, as an example of pharmacogenetics or as something out of the ordinary in terms of clinical practice. It considers how, in turn, this impacts on the way in which informed consent is sought and influenced by clinicians' desire to protect patients from possibly distressing test results. It highlights the flexible, contingent and context dependent nature of informed consent in the clinical setting.

Soc Stud Sci. 2005 Jun;35(3):367-403. Related Articles, Links The emergence of toxicogenomics: a case study of molecularization. Shostak S. This paper described the efforts of scientists at the National Institute of Environmental Health Sciences (NIEHS) and their allies in the National Toxicology Program to molecularize toxicology by fostering the emergence of a new discipline: toxicogenomics. I demonstrate that the molecularization of toxicology at the NIEHS began in a process of 'co-construction'. However, the subsequent emergence of the discipline of toxicogenomics has required the deliberate development of communication across the myriad disciplines necessary to produce toxicogenomic knowledge; articulation of emergent forms, standards, and practices with extant ones; management of the tensions generated by grounding toxicogenomics in traditional toxicological standards and work practices even it transforms those standards and practices; and identification and stabilization of roles for toxicogenomic knowledge in markets and service sites, such as environmental health risk assessment and regulation. This paper describes the technological, institutional, and inter-sectoral strategies that scientists have pursued in order to meet these challenges. In so doing, this analysis offers a vista into both the means and meanings of molecularization. Publication Types: Historical Article

Southeast Asian J Trop Med Public Health. 2003;34 Suppl 3:234-8. Related Articles, Links The human genome project: opportunities, challenges and consequences for population screening. Christodoulou J. Western Sydney Genetics Program, The Children's Hospital at Westmead, Sydney, NSW, Australia. It is widely agreed that the Human Genome Project represents one of the most successful international collaborative research efforts of the last millennium. The fruits of the Human Genome Project have paved the way for a revolution in future health care, built on the foundations of an improved understanding of the molecular pathogenesis of human disease, and new and emerging technologies that will allow the rapid throughput of sophisticated gene-based testing. In this review some practical examples of these advances will be outlined, touching on such areas as pharmacogenetics, pharmacogenomics, and microarray technologies. In addition, some of the legal, ethical and social issues that have arisen from the Human Genome Project will be discussed. It is argued that in embracing the new knowledge afforded by the Human Genome Project, we must maintain a cautious approach to help minimise the potential risks in order to reap the potentially enormous benefits to society. Publication Types: Review

Stat Med. 2004 Aug 15;23(15):2413-27. Related Articles, Links Imputing gene-treatment interactions when the genotype distribution is unknown using case-only and putative placebo analyses--a new method for the Genetics of Hypertension Associated Treatment (GenHAT) study. Davis BR, Ford CE, Boerwinkle E, Arnett D, Eckfeldt J, Black H. University of Texas School of Public Health, Houston, TX 77030, USA. bdavis@sph.uth.tmc.edu There is a sizeable literature on methods for detecting gene-environment interaction in the framework of case-control studies, particularly with reference to the assumption of independence of genotype and exposure. In the context of a clinical trial, wherein gene-drug interactions with regard to outcomes are examined, these methods may be readily applied, as gene and drug are independent by randomization. In an active-controlled trial (experimental treatment vs standard) that has collected genotype information, gene-drug interactions can be estimated. In addition, the effect of the experimental treatment vs placebo can be imputed by using data from a historical placebo-controlled trial (standard vs placebo) if either (a) genotype information is available from the historical trial or (b) assumptions are made about the prevalence of genotype and the odds ratios of genotype and disease in the historical trial using information from other studies. Motivation for these procedures is provided by the Genetics of Hypertension Associated Treatment, a large pharmacogenetics, ancillary study of a hypertension clinical trial, and examples from published hypertension trials will be used to illustrate the methods.

Stat Med. 2005 May 30;24(10):1495-508. Related Articles, Links Statistical design and analysis of pharmacogenetic trials. Kelly PJ, Stallard N, Whittaker JC. Medical and Pharmaceutical Statistics Research Unit, The University of Reading, Reading RG6 6FN, UK. patrick.kelly@reading.ac.uk Pharmacogenetic trials investigate the effect of genotype on treatment response. When there are two or more treatment groups and two or more genetic groups, investigation of gene-treatment interactions is of key interest. However, calculation of the power to detect such interactions is complicated because this depends not only on the treatment effect size within each genetic group, but also on the number of genetic groups, the size of each genetic group, and the type of genetic effect that is both present and tested for. The scale chosen to measure the magnitude of an interaction can also be problematic, especially for the binary case. Elston et al. proposed a test for detecting the presence of gene-treatment interactions for binary responses, and gave appropriate power calculations. This paper shows how the same approach can also be used for normally distributed responses. We also propose a method for analysing and performing sample size calculations based on a generalized linear model (GLM) approach. The power of the Elston et al. and GLM approaches are compared for the binary and normal case using several illustrative examples. While more sensitive to errors in model specification than the Elston et al. approach, the GLM approach is much more flexible and in many cases more powerful.

Stroke. 2004 Nov;35(11 Suppl 1):2735-9. Epub 2004 Sep 9. Related Articles, Links Clinically translated ischemic stroke genomics. Meschia JF. Department of Neurology, Mayo Clinic, 4500 San Pablo Road, Jacksonville, FL 32224, USA. meschia.james@mayo.edu Cohort studies show that having a positive family history of stroke increases the odds of having a stroke by approximately 30%. The heritability of stroke appears to be heterogeneous across ischemic stroke subtypes, with cardioembolic stroke being least heritable. The relative influence of stroke risk attenuates with age, but genetics does not cease to be relevant in later adulthood. Recent family history and twin studies suggest that genetic factors remain relevant even beyond the seventh decade of life. One of the challenges of gene discovery in stroke relates to the complexities of phenotype. The complexities of phenotype can be addressed by focusing on individual ischemic stroke subtypes or by studying intermediate phenotypes like leukaraiosis, which has a heritability of approximately 70%. Although most stroke genetics research has focused on the identification of risk factor genes, an independent set of genes likely influences poststroke outcomes (for example, apolipoprotein E) and response to drug therapies (example, alpha-adducin and diuretic therapy). Publication Types: Review

Suppl Tumori. 2004 Mar-Apr;3(2):S31-2. Related Articles, Links [Pharmacogenetics in tumors of the lung] [Article in Italian] Altavilla G, Marabello G. Universita degli Studi di Messina. Publication Types: Review

Support Care Cancer. 2005 Mar;13(3):153-9. Epub 2004 Dec 21. Related Articles, Links Advances in opioid pharmacology. Gourlay GK. Pain Management Unit, Department of Anaesthesia and Pain Management, Flinders Medical Centre, The Flinders University of South Australia, 5042, Bedford Park, South Australia, Australia. Geoff.Gourlay@Flinders.edu.au Natural and synthetic opioid compounds, either alone or in combination with other drugs, are widely used analgesics for patients with both acute and chronic pain. Decades of extensive pharmacologic investigations have characterized three high-affinity cell-surface neuronal receptors, the activation of which is responsible for both the desirable properties (antinociception) and undesirable properties (respiratory depression, nausea and vomiting, dependence, etc.) of opioid drugs. Recent research in molecular biology and pharmacogenetics in relation to opioids and their receptors has helped clarify previous pharmacologic observations and has laid the groundwork for new analgesic therapies with improved therapeutic outcomes. Publication Types: Review

Swiss Med Wkly. 2004 Nov 27;134(47-48):685-94. Related Articles, Links Molecular and clinical determinants of drug-induced long QT syndrome: an iatrogenic channelopathy. Abriel H, Schlapfer J, Keller DI, Gavillet B, Buclin T, Biollaz J, Stoller R, Kappenberger L. Service of Cardiology, CHUV, Lausanne, Switzerland. Hugues.Abriel@unil.ch More than 70 drugs present on the Swiss market can cause drug-induced long QT syndrome (LQTS), which is associated with torsades de pointes (TdP) arrhythmias, potentially leading to sudden cardiac death. Basic and clinical investigations performed during the last decade have helped a better understanding of the mechanisms and risk factors of this serious public health problem. In their vast majority, QT interval prolonging drugs block the human ERG (hERG) channel involved in the repolarisation phase of the cardiac action potential, and thus lengthen the QT interval. Beside the well-known QT interval prolonging action of class IA, IC and III anti-arrhythmic drugs, many antibiotics, neurotropic, antifungal, and antimalarial drugs are also able to cause drug-induced LQTS. Reviewing the literature indicates that the risk of QT interval prolongation and TdP is increased in females, in patients with organic heart diseases and hypokalaemia. Furthermore in a few cases, genetic factors have also been reported. However thus far, no genetic test is available to detect at-risk patients, and in consequence, drug prescribers are still relying only on the clinical history and findings to perform an evaluation of the risk. Treatment of drug-induced LQTS and TdP includes identifying and withdrawing the culprit drug(s), infusing magnesium and, in resistant cases acceleration of the heart rate. In this review article we provide a list of QT interval prolonging drugs adapted to the pharmaceuticals found on the Swiss market that can be used as a check-list for drug prescribers and at-risk patients. Publication Types: Review

Tanpakushitsu Kakusan Koso. 2004 May;49(6):781-6. Related Articles, Links [Bioinformatics in medicine] [Article in Japanese] Mizushima H. hmizushi@ncc.go.jp Publication Types: Review

Tanpakushitsu Kakusan Koso. 2004 Sep;49(12):2024-34. Related Articles, Links [The pharmacogenomics of drug transporters: functional analysis approaches] [Article in Japanese] Ishikawa T, Endou H, Inui K, Tsuji A, Wada M, Sumino Y. tishikaw@bio.titech.ac.jp Publication Types: Review

Tanpakushitsu Kakusan Koso. 2005 Aug;50(9):1070-7. Related Articles, Links [Chemical genomics by post-genomic approaches using Schizosaccharomyces pombe] [Article in Japanese] Nishimura S, Matsuyama A, Yoshida M. nshin@riken.jp Publication Types: Review

Tanpakushitsu Kakusan Koso. 2005 Dec;50(16 Suppl):2084-9. Related Articles, Links [Search for type 2 diabetes susceptibility genes] [Article in Japanese] Hirota Y, Kasuga M. hirota@med.kobe-u.ac.jp Publication Types: Review

Tanpakushitsu Kakusan Koso. 2005 Dec;50(16 Suppl):2090-6. Related Articles, Links [Advanced genomic analyses for hypertension] [Article in Japanese] Tetsuro M. tmiki@m.ehime-u.ac.jp Publication Types: Review

Technol Eval Cent Asses Program Exec Summ. 2004 Dec;19(9):1-2. Related Articles, Links Special report: genotyping for cytochrome P450 polymorphisms to determine drug-metabolizer status. [No authors listed]

Ther Drug Monit. 2004 Apr;26(2):137-44. Related Articles, Links Human pharmacology of MDMA: pharmacokinetics, metabolism, and disposition. de la Torre R, Farre M, Roset PN, Pizarro N, Abanades S, Segura M, Segura J, Cami J. Unitat de Recerca en Farmacologia, Institut Municipal d'Investigacio Medica, Barcelona, Spain. rtorre@imim.es MDMA (3,4-methylenedioxymethamphetamine, ecstasy) is a widely misused psychostimulant drug abused among large segments of the young population. Pharmacologically it displays effects related to amphetamine-type drugs and a set of distinctive effects (closeness to others, facilitation to interpersonal relationship, and empathy) that have been named by some authors "entactogen" properties. MDMA is a potent releaser and/or reuptake inhibitor of presynaptic serotonin (5-HT), dopamine (DA), and norepinephrine (NE). These actions result from the interaction of MDMA with the membrane transporters involved in neurotransmitter reuptake and vesicular storage systems. The most frequent effects after MDMA/ecstasy administration are euphoria, well-being, happiness, stimulation, increased energy, extroversion, feeling close to others, increased empathy, increased sociability, enhanced mood, mild perceptual disturbances, changed perception of colors and sounds, somatic symptoms related to its cardiovascular and autonomic effects (blood pressure and heart rate increase, mydriasis), and moderate derealization but not hallucinations. Acute toxic effects are related to its pharmacologic actions. The serotonin syndrome (increased muscle rigidity, hyperreflexia, and hyperthermia), among others, is characteristic of acute toxicity episodes. MDMA metabolism is rather complex and includes 2 main metabolic pathways: (1) O-demethylenation followed by catechol-O-methyltransferase (COMT)-catalyzed methylation and/or glucuronide/sulfate conjugation; and (2) N-dealkylation, deamination, and oxidation to the corresponding benzoic acid derivatives conjugated with glycine. The fact that the polymorphic enzyme CYP2D6 partially regulates the O-demethylenation pathway prompted some expectations that subjects displaying the poor metabolizer phenotype may be at higher risk of acute toxicity episodes. In this metabolic pathway a mechanism-based inhibition of the enzyme operates because the formation of an enzyme-metabolite complex that renders all subjects, independently of genotype, phenotypically poor metabolizers after the administration of 2 consecutive doses. Therefore, the impact of CYP2D6 pharmacogenetics on acute toxicity is limited. One of the interesting features of MDMA metabolism is its potential involvement in the development of mid- to long-term neurotoxic effects as a result of progressive neurodegeneration of the serotonergic neurotransmission system. Publication Types: Review

Ther Drug Monit. 2004 Apr;26(2):152-5. Related Articles, Links Therapeutic monitoring of antidepressants in the era of pharmacogenetics studies. Eap CB, Jaquenoud SE, Baumann P. Unite de Biochimie et Psychopharmacologie Clinique, Centre de Neurosciences Psychiatriques, Departement Universitaire de Psychiatrie Adulte, Hopital de Cery, CH-1008 Prilly-Lausanne, Switzerland. Chin.Eap@inst.hospvd.ch As for other drugs, there is a large interindividual variability of the plasma concentrations of antidepressants for a given dose. Within the last 2 decades, a very large number of pharmacogenetic studies have made it possible to understand the importance of genetic factors on the disposition of drugs in the organism, many of them at the levels of drug metabolism. Polymorphism of CYP2D6 and of other drug-metabolizing enzymes may thus lead to very large differences in drug exposure between patients and possibly also to toxicity or ineffective drug concentrations in some subjects. In consequence, dose recommendations of antidepressants based on genotypes, justified by the principle of administering bioequivalent individualized drug doses, are now proposed. However, blood (and thus possibly brain) concentrations also depend on other factors than the genetic makeup of the patients. Therapeutic drug monitoring of antidepressants allows us to take into account the influence of factors such as comedications, diet, smoking habit, impaired organ function, and compliance. Therapeutic drug monitoring and genotyping are thus complementary, and their combined use contributes to improve pharmacotherapy with antidepressants and other drugs. Publication Types: Review

Ther Drug Monit. 2004 Apr;26(2):186-91. Related Articles, Links Pharmacogenetics of thiopurine S-methyltransferase and thiopurine therapy. Evans WE. St. Jude Children's Research Hospital and University of Tennessee Health Sciences Center, Memphis, TN 38101-0318, USA. william.evans@stjude.org Most medications exhibit wide interpatient variability in their efficacy and toxicity. For many medications, these interindividual differences result in part from polymorphisms in genes encoding drug-metabolizing enzymes, drug transporters, and/or drug targets (eg, receptors, enzymes). Pharmacogenomics is a burgeoning field aimed at elucidating the genetic basis of differences in drug efficacy and toxicity, using genome-wide approaches to identify the network of genes that govern an individual's response to drug therapy. For some genetic polymorphisms, such as thiopurine S-methyltransferase (TPMT), monogenic traits have a marked effect on the pharmacokinetics of medications, such that individuals who inherit an enzyme deficiency must be treated with markedly different doses of the affected medications (eg, 5-10% of the standard thiopurine dose). This review uses the TPMT polymorphism and thiopurine therapy (eg, azathioprine, mercaptopurine) to illustrate the potential of pharmacogenomics to elucidate genetic determinants of drug response, and optimize the selection of drug therapy for individual patients. Publication Types: Review

Ther Drug Monit. 2004 Apr;26(2):231-5. Related Articles, Links Pharmacogenetics in cancer chemotherapy: balancing toxicity and response. Donnelly JG. Department of Pathology, New York University School of Medicine, and South Manhattan and North Manhattan Generations Plus Health Care Networks, New York, NY 10016, USA. James.Donnelly@med.nyu.edu The goal of chemotherapy is the elimination of tumor cells from the host. This is achieved by the use of therapeutic agents that are often more harmful to normal tissues than to the targeted tumor. Many chemotherapeutic agents are designed to damage cell replication machinery either directly at the level of DNA or indirectly, by inhibiting enzymes involved with DNA repair and synthesis. Novel therapeutic agents that exert their effects at signal transduction pathways have advanced chemotherapy; however, a role for the classic chemotherapeutic agents remains. These classic agents are associated with tumor cell resistance, toxicity, and occasionally secondary neoplasia. Current practices for the dosing of therapeutic agents rely on height and body surface measurements or drug monitoring and Bayesian adaptive control. Pharmacogenetics is emerging as an alternate approach to managing chemotherapy that may prevent undertreatment while avoiding overtreatment and associated toxicities. By determining the polymorphic genetic makeup of the host and, in some instances, the altered genetic expression of the tumor, chemotherapy can be tailored for interindividual response and toxicity avoidance. Chemotherapy is particularly applicable to the pharmacogenetic approach to tailored therapy for a number of reasons. The margin of safety is low with chemotherapeutic agents. Some drugs require biotransformation for activation. Drug activation correlates with toxicity. The pathways of drug clearance or inactivation exhibit polymorphic differences. Interindividual, race-specific, and age-related responses to chemotherapeutic agents are common. Last, drug resistance can be inherent to the tumor as a result of the suppression of apoptosis. Variations in response and toxicity to a specific drug can be caused by alterations in drug-metabolizing enzymes or receptor expression. These effects can be classed as pharmacokinetic and pharmacogenetic differences. Some of the genes known to display polymorphic differences include FLT3 receptor tyrosine kinase, FCG3RA IgG FC receptor, thymidylate synthase, methylenetetrahydrofolate reductase, thiopurine S-methyltransferase, dihydropyrimidine dehydrogenase, aldehyde dehydrogenase, glutathione S-transferase, uridine diphosphate glyuronosyl transferases, N-acetyl transferases, cytochrome P450, and the DNA repair enzymes XPD and XRCC1. To be successful a pharmacogenetic approach to individualized chemotherapy must selectively take advantage of a determination of direct enzyme activity, gene expression, and genotype. Publication Types: Review

Ther Drug Monit. 2004 Aug;26(4):343-6. Related Articles, Links Pharmacogenetics in immunosuppressive therapy: the best thing since TDM? van Gelder T, Hesselink DA, van Hest RM, Mathot RA, van Schaik R. Department of Hospital Pharmacy, Erasmus Medical Center, 3000 CA Rotterdam, The Netherlands. t.vangelder@erasmusmc.nl Publication Types: Review

Ther Drug Monit. 2005 Apr;27(2):208-10. Related Articles, Links Genetic polymorphism of CYP2C9 in a Vietnamese Kinh population. Lee SS, Kim KM, Thi-Le H, Yea SS, Cha IJ, Shin JG. Pharmacogenomics Research Center and Department of Pharmacology, Inje University College of Medicine, 633-165 Gaegum-dong, Jin-gu, Busan 614-735 Korea. Cytochrome P450 2C9 (CYP2C9) shows genetic polymorphism with high interethnic variation, but no report has addressed the genetic polymorphism in the Vietnamese population. In the present study, the distribution of 2 common allelic variations of CYP2C9 was investigated in Vietnamese Kinh population, a major ethnic group in Vietnam. Genomic DNA from 157 Vietnamese subjects was amplified by polymerase chain reaction, and the presence of CYP2C9*2 and CYP2C9*3 allelic variants was determined by pyrosequencing. Among 157 Vietnamese subjects, no subject with the CYP2C9*2 allele was detected, but 7 subjects were heterozygous for the CYP2C9*3 allele. The allele frequency of CYP2C9*3 was 2.2% in the Vietnamese Kinh population. This genotype distribution was well correlated with previous reports suggesting no occurrence of CYP2C9*2 in Asians. These results suggest that CYP2C9*2 may be absent in Vietnamese Kinh population and that CYP2C9*3 is major allelic variant that causes interindividual variation of drug responses to CYP2C9 substrate drugs in the Vietnamese Kinh population.

Ther Drug Monit. 2006 Feb;28(1):23-30. Related Articles, Links Pharmacogenetics in transplant patients: can it predict pharmacokinetics and pharmacodynamics? Burckart GJ, Liu XI. University of Southern California School of Pharmacy, Los Angeles, USA. burckart@usc.edu Pharmacogenetics holds the potential to allow individualized dosing of immunosuppressive agents to optimize their therapeutic effect while minimizing adverse effects. As more pharmacogenetic information accumulates, the prospect of reducing or discontinuing the intensive therapeutic drug monitoring of immunosuppressants looks attractive. However, the long process of developing useful clinical information from basic information on the genes of interest is at a very early stage, and our present information does not supercede pharmacokinetic or blood concentration monitoring of immunosuppressants. The most extensive blood concentration/dose information available is on tacrolimus and its dosing related to CYP3A5 and ABCB1 gene polymorphisms. Although CYP3A5 genotype is definitely associated with tacrolimus dosing, the only recommendation presently published is for an arbitrary doubling of the starting tacrolimus dose in CYP3A5 expressors. For cyclosporine, sirolimus, and corticosteroids, the presently available pharmacogenetic information does not permit pharmacokinetic predictions. The pharmacodynamics of immunosuppressants, as evidenced by effects on acute rejection or adverse drug effects, have considerably more potential for prediction by pharmacogenetic models. Drug-resistant rejection, nephrotoxicity, steroid resistance and osteonecrosis, and even patient survival may ultimately be predicted by models incorporating multiple gene polymorphisms and other critical patient information. At this point, treatment algorithms can be developed that will allow us to individualize a transplant patient's immunosuppressive therapy.

Thromb Haemost. 2004 Jun;91(6):1123-8. Related Articles, Links Warfarin dosing and cytochrome P450 2C9 polymorphisms. Joffe HV, Xu R, Johnson FB, Longtine J, Kucher N, Goldhaber SZ. Department of Medicine, Brigham and Women's Hospital, Harvard Medical School, Boston, MA 02115, USA. Two cytochrome P450 2C9 (CYP2C9) polymorphisms, CYP2C9*2 and *3, metabolize warfarin inefficiently. We assessed the extent to which these polymorphisms explain very low warfarin dose requirements and hemorrhagic complications after excluding non-genetic determinants of warfarin dosing. In this retrospective observational study, 73 patients with stable warfarin doses for > or =1 month and International Normalized Ratios (INR) of 2.0-3.0 were enrolled from our Anticoagulation Clinic. Seventeen patients required < or =2 mg (low-dose), 41 required 4-6 mg (moderate-dose), and 15 required > or =10 mg (high-dose) of daily warfarin. CYP2C9 genotyping was assessed by PCR amplification and restriction enzyme digestion analysis of DNA isolated from circulating leukocytes. The CYP2C9 polymorphisms independently predicted low warfarin requirements after adjusting for Body Mass Index, age, acetaminophen use, and race (OR 24.80; 95% CI 3.83-160.78). At least one polymorphism was present in every patient requiring < or =1.5 mg of daily warfarin, and 88%, 37%, and 7% of the low-, moderate-, and high-dose groups, respectively. All homozygotes and compound-heterozygotes for the variant alleles were in the low-dose group. Rates of excessive (INR>6.0) anticoagulation (and bleeding) were 4.5 (6.0), 7.9 (7.9), and 14.7 (0) per 100 patient-years in the wild-types, heterozygotes, and compound heterozygotes/homozygotes, respectively. In conclusion, CYP2C9*2 or *3 compound heterozygotes and homozygotes have low warfarin requirements even after excluding liver disease, excessive alcohol or acetaminophen consumption, low body weight, advancing age, and drug interactions. These polymorphisms increase the rate of excessive anticoagulation, but this risk does not appear to be associated with higher bleeding rates when anticoagulation status is closely monitored.

Thromb Haemost. 2004 May;91(5):986-90. Related Articles, Links Pharmacogenetics of the CD14 endotoxin receptor polymorphism and progression of coronary atherosclerosis. Agema WR, Wouter Jukema J, de Maat MP, Zwinderman AH, Kastelein JJ, Rabelink TJ, van der Wall EE. Leiden University Medical Center, Department of Cardiology, C5-P, Albinusdreef 2, PO Box 9600, 2300 RC Leiden, The Netherlands. Atherosclerosis is at least in part an inflammatory disease. CD14 is an endotoxin receptor that after binding of lipopolysaccharides evokes endothelial activation and secretion of several cytokines. A polymorphism of CD14 has been associated with myocardial infarction.We evaluated the role of the -159 T/C polymorphism in the promoter region of the CD14 gene in relation to severity and progression of coronary atherosclerosis and response to the HMG CoA reductase inhibitor pravastatin. We recruited patients from the multi-center double-blind randomized placebo controlled REGRESS trial and genotyped the -159T/C CD14 polymorphism. DNA and angiographic follow-up were available from 759 patients with objectivated coronary artery disease. We measured changes in mean segment diameter (MSD) and minimum obstruction diameter (MOD) with quantitative coronary angiography and noted the occurrence of major adverse cardiac events. The genotype distribution was 28% TT, 49% CT, 23% CC. We did not find any association between genotype and MSD and MOD at baseline, frequency of previous myocardial infarction, changes in MSD and MOD or major clinical events. Treatment with the HMG CoA reductase inhibitor pravastatin reduced progression of coronary atherosclerosis and adverse events equally for all genotypes. We conclude, that the -159T/C polymorphism in the CD14 monocyte receptor gene was not associated with progression of coronary atherosclerosis in this population nor did it influence the efficacy of pravastatin in the treatment of atherosclerosis. Publication Types: Clinical Trial Multicenter Study Randomized Controlled Trial

Thromb Haemost. 2004 Sep;92(3):590-7. Related Articles, Links The potential clinical and economic outcomes of pharmacogenetics-oriented management of warfarin therapy - a decision analysis. You JH, Chan FW, Wong RS, Cheng G. Centre for Pharmacoeconomics Research, School of Pharmacy, Faculty of Medicine, The Chinese University of Hong Kong Shatin, N.T., Hong Kong, China. joyceyou@cuhk.edu.hk Variant cytochrome P450 (CYP) 2C9 genotypes are associated with low maintenance dose requirement of warfarin therapy and increased risk of major bleeding events. The objective of the present study was to evaluate the potential clinical and economic outcomes of using CYP2C9 genotype data to guide the management of anticoagulation therapy and to identify influential factors affecting the cost-effectiveness of this treatment scheme. A decision tree was designed to simulate, over 12 months, the clinical and economic outcomes of patients newly started on warfarin associated with two alternatives: (1) no genotyping (non-genotyped group) and (2) CYP2C9 genotyping prior to initiation of warfarin therapy (genotyped group). Non-genotyped group patients would receive standard care of an anticoagulation clinic (AC). In the genotyped group, patients with at least one variant CYP2C9 allele would receive intensified anticoagulation service. Most of the clinical probabilities were derived from literature. The direct medical costs were estimated from the Diagnosis-Related Group charges and from literature. The total number of events and the direct medical cost per 100 patient-years in the genotyped and non-geno-typed groups were 9.58 and USD155,700, and, 10.48 and USD 150,500, respectively. The marginal cost per additional major bleeding averted in the genotyped group was USD 5,778. The model was sensitive to the variation of the cost and reduction of bleeding rate in the intensified anticoagulation service. In conclusion, the pharmacogenetics-oriented management of warfarin therapy is potentially more effective in preventing bleeding with a marginal cost. The cost-effectiveness of this treatment scheme depends on the relative cost and effectiveness of a pharmacogenetics-oriented intensified anticoagulation service comparing to the standard AC care. Publication Types: Clinical Trial Controlled Clinical Trial

Thromb Haemost. 2005 Apr;93(4):700-5. Related Articles, Links Prospective dosing of warfarin based on cytochrome P-450 2C9 genotype. Voora D, Eby C, Linder MW, Milligan PE, Bukaveckas BL, McLeod HL, Maloney W, Clohisy J, Burnett RS, Grosso L, Gatchel SK, Gage BF. Department of Medicine, Washington University School of Medicine, St. Louis, MO 63110, USA. Cytochrome P-450 2C9 (CYP2C9) polymorphisms (CYP2C9*2 and CYP2C9*3) reduce the clearance of warfarin, increase the risk of bleeding, and prolong the time to stable dosing. Whether prospective use of a retrospectively developed algorithm that incorporates CYP2C9 genotype and nongenetic factors can ameliorate the propensity to bleeding and delay in achieving a stable warfarin dose is unknown. We initiated warfarin therapy in 48 orthopedic patients tailored to the following variables: CYP2C9 genotype, age, weight, height, gender, race, and use of simvastatin or amiodarone. By using pharmacogenetics-based dosing, patients with a CYP2C9 variant achieved a stable, therapeutic warfarin dose without excessive delay. However compared to those without a CYP2C9 variant, patients with a variant continued to be at increased risk (hazard ratio 3.6, 95% confidence interval 1.4-9.5, $p = 0.01$) for an adverse outcome (principally INR > 4), despite pharmacogenetics-based dosing. There was a linear relationship ($R(2) = 0.42$, $p < 0.001$) between the pharmacogenetics-predicted warfarin doses and the warfarin maintenance doses, prospectively validating the dosing algorithm. Prospective, perioperative pharmacogenetics-based dosing of warfarin is feasible; however, further evaluation in a randomized, controlled study is recommended. Publication Types: Validation Studies

Thromb Haemost. 2005 Feb;93(2):396-7. Related Articles, Links Comment on: Thromb Haemost. 2004 Jul;92(1):61-6. Retrospective analyses of acenocoumarol doses and bleeding complications in patients with wild type or variant cytochrome P450 CYP2C9 alleles. Mark L, Marki-Zay J, Paragh G, Katona A. Publication Types: Comment Letter

Thromb Res. 2003;112(5-6):273-4. Related Articles, Links Comment on: Thromb Res. 2003;112(5-6):275-83. The epidemiological night where all patients are black: will pharmacogenetics shed some light? de Gaetano G, Cerletti C, Iacoviello L, Donati MB. Publication Types: Comment Editorial

Thromb Res. 2003;112(5-6):275-83. Related Articles, Links Comment in: Thromb Res.

2003;112(5-6):273-4. Mutations within the cyclooxygenase-1 gene in aspirin non-responders with recurrence of stroke. Hillarp A, Palmqvist B, Lethagen S, Villoutreix BO, Mattiasson I. Department of Clinical Chemistry, Malmo University Hospital, SE-20502 Malmo, Sweden. andreas.hillarp@klkemi.mas.lu.se INTRODUCTION: Aspirin is a common antiplatelet drug used in the prevention of ischemic stroke due to its inhibitory effect on platelet cyclooxygenase-1 (Cox-1). Patients can be categorized as either aspirin 'responders' or 'non-responders' depending on whether they are protected against a secondary stroke event or not. In this study, we have searched for variants of the Cox-1 gene that could possibly result in an unblocked and thus, aspirin-resistant Cox-1 enzyme and phenotype. MATERIALS AND METHODS: The Cox-1 gene was sequenced in 68 patients with recurrent ischemic stroke despite taking aspirin. The genotype distribution of identified variants was determined and compared with healthy control subjects. Mutations that involved amino acid substitutions of the mature Cox-1 molecule were analysed by molecular modelling and functional analysis using whole blood aggregometry. RESULTS: Fourteen variants of the Cox-1 gene were identified. Seven of the variants involved amino acid substitutions of the Cox-1 molecule. None of the mutations were located near the catalytic site as judged from a three-dimensional model of the human Cox-1. Carriers and non-carriers of one of the mutations behaved similarly when aggregation and granule content release function were studied using collagen, ADP and arachidonic acid as agonists. CONCLUSION: The results do not support the hypothesis that common variants of the Cox-1 gene results in unblocked Cox-1 molecules in aspirin non-responders.

Thromb Res. 2005;117(1-2):55-9; discussion 65-7. Epub 2005 Jul 25. Related Articles, Links Pharmacology and pharmacogenetics of warfarin and other coumarins when used with supplements. Gage BF, Milligan PE. Division of General Medical Sciences, Washington University School of Medicine, Campus Box 8005, 660 S. Euclid, St. Louis, MO 63110, USA. bgage@im.wustl.edu Publication Types: Review

Tidsskr Nor Laegeforen. 2004 Nov 18;124(22):2921-3. Related Articles, Links [P-glycoprotein--a pump of significance for drug response] [Article in Norwegian] Molden E. Farmasoytisk institutt, Universitetet i Oslo, Postboks 1068 Blindern, 0316 Oslo. espen.molden@farmasi.uio.no

Tidsskr Nor Laegeforen. 2005 Nov 3;125(21):2953-5. Related Articles, Links Comment in: Tidsskr Nor Laegeforen. 2006 Feb 9;126(4):480; author reply 480. [CYP genotyping in psychopharmacological treatment] [Article in Norwegian] Rudberg I, Solberg DK, Refsum H. Psykofarmakologisk avdeling, Diakonhjemmet sykehus, 0319 Oslo. ida.rudberg@diakonsyk.no

Tidsskr Nor Laegeforen. 2005 Oct 6;125(19):2655-8. Related Articles, Links [Genetic variation-- important for the clinical effect of opioids?] [Article in Norwegian] Klepstad P, Dale O, Borchgrevink PC, Kaasa S, Skorpen F. Avdeling for anestesi og akuttmedisin, St. Olavs Hospital, 7006 Trondheim. pal.klepstad@ntnu.no The individual variability of opioid pharmacology suggests that the patients' genetic disposition influences the response to opioids. Given the complexity of morphine pharmacology, variability may be caused by several genes. Data suggest that variability in genes encoding the enzyme metabolising morphine (UGT2B7 gene), mu-opioid receptors (OPRM1 gene) and BBB transport of morphine by multidrug resistance transporters (MDR1 gene) influence the clinical efficacy of morphine. Furthermore, variability in an enzyme-degrading catecholamines (COMT gene) may also alter the efficacy of morphine, which shows that genetic variability in non-opioid systems may indirectly influence the clinical opioid efficacy. Results obtained so far strongly suggest that opioid efficacy is partly related to inborn properties caused by genetic variability.

Tidsskr Nor Laegeforen. 2006 Feb 9;126(4):480; author reply 480. Related Articles, Links Comment on: Tidsskr Nor Laegeforen. 2001 Nov 20;121(28):3296-8. Tidsskr Nor Laegeforen. 2002 Nov 30;122(29):2781-3. Tidsskr Nor Laegeforen. 2005 Nov 3;125(21):2953-5. [CYP genotyping in psychopharmacological treatment] [Article in Norwegian] Bramness JG. Publication Types: Comment Letter

Top HIV Med. 2005 Aug-Sep;13(3):90-5. Related Articles, Links Will pharmacogenomic discoveries improve HIV therapeutics? Haas DW. AIDS Clincal Trials Center, Vanderbilt University, Nashville, TN, USA. Pharmacogenomic studies are contributing to our understanding of interindividual differences in response to antiretroviral drugs. Genetic polymorphism in major histocompatibility complex genes predict likelihood of hypersensitivity reactions in persons prescribed abacavir, and perhaps nevirapine. Recent studies have shown that a polymorphisms in the CYP2B6 gene is associated with higher plasma efavirenz concentrations and increased efavirenz central nervous system side effects. Polymorphisms in the MDR1 gene encoding the drug pump, P-glycoprotein, may predict nevirapine-associated hepatoxicity and long-term virologic response to efavirenz. CYP2C19 polymorphisms predict nelfinavir plasma levels and, possibly, risk of virologic failure on this drug. A European mitochondrial haplogroup may predict increased risk of peripheral neuropathy associated with nucleoside reverse transcriptase inhibitors. Expansion and refinement of knowledge regarding associations between human genetics and response to antiretroviral drugs may ultimately permit individualization of therapy based on genotyping. This article summarizes a presentation on HIV therapeutics and pharmacogenomics by David W. Haas, MD, at the International AIDS Society-USA course in Atlanta in March 2005.

Toxicol Appl Pharmacol. 2005 Apr 15;204(2):101-8. Related Articles, Links Use of toxicogenomics for identifying genetic markers of pulmonary oedema. Balharry D, Oreffo V, Richards R. Cardiff School of Biosciences, Cardiff University, Museum Avenue, Cardiff, CF10 3US, United Kingdom. balharry@cf.ac.uk This study was undertaken primarily to identify genetic markers of oedema and inflammation. Mild pulmonary injury was induced following the instillation of the oedema-producing agent, bleomycin (0.5 units). Oedema was then confirmed by conventional toxicology (lavage protein levels, free cell counts and lung/body weight ratios) and histology 3 days post-bleomycin instillation. The expression profile of 1176 mRNA species was determined for bleomycin-exposed lung (Clontech Atlas macroarray, n=9). To obtain pertinent results from these data, it was necessary to develop a simple, effective method for bioinformatic analysis of altered gene expression. Data were log10 transformed followed by global normalisation. Differential gene expression was accepted if: (a) genes were statistically significant (P < or = 0.05) from a two-tailed t test; (b) genes were consistently outside a two standard deviation (SD) range from control levels. A combination of these techniques identified 31 mRNA transcripts (approximately 3%) which were significantly altered in bleomycin treated tissue. Of these genes, 26 were down-regulated whilst only five were up-regulated. Two distinct clusters were identified, with 17 genes classified as encoding hormone receptors, and nine as encoding ion channels. Both these clusters were consistently down-regulated. The magnitude of the changes in gene expression were quantified and confirmed by Q-PCR (n = 6), validating the macroarray data and the bioinformatic analysis employed. In conclusion, this study has developed a suitable macroarray analysis procedure and provides the basis for a better understanding of the gene expression changes occurring during the early phase of drug-induced pulmonary oedema.This work has been presented orally, in part at the British Association for Lung Research Summer Meeting, University of Brighton, 3-5 September, 2003 and in full at the British Toxicology Society Annual Congress, Heriot Watt University, Edinburgh, 21-24 April 2004.

Toxicol Appl Pharmacol. 2005 Sep 1;207(2 Suppl):679-83. Related Articles, Links Global gene mining and the pharmaceutical industry. Knudsen LE. Institute of Public Health, University of Copenhagen, Blegdamsvej 3, DK2100 Copenhagen O, Denmark. Worldwide efforts are ongoing in optimizing medical treatment by searching for the right medicine at the right dose for the individual. Metabolism is regulated by polymorphisms, which may be tested by relatively simple SNP analysis, however requiring DNA from the test individuals. Target genes for the efficiency of a given medicine or predisposition of a given disease are also subject to population studies, e.g., in Iceland, Estonia, Sweden, etc. For hypothesis testing and generation, several bio-banks with samples from patients and healthy persons within the pharmaceutical industry have been established during the past 10 years. Thus, more than 100,000 samples are stored in the freezers of either the pharmaceutical companies or their contractual partners at universities and test institutions. Ethical issues related to data protection of the individuals providing samples to bio-banks are several: nature and extent of information prior to consent, coverage of the consent given by the study person, labeling and storage of the sample and data (coded or anonymized). In general, genetic test data, once obtained, are permanent and cannot be changed. The test data may imply information that is not beneficial to the patient and his/her family (e.g., employment opportunities, insurance, etc.). Furthermore, there may be a long latency between the analysis of the genetic test and the clinical expression of the disease and wide differences in the disease patterns. Consequently, information about some genetic test data may stigmatize patients leading to poor quality of life. This has raised the issue of 'genetic exceptionalism' justifying specific regulation of use of genetic information. Discussions on how to handle sampling and data are ongoing within the industry and the regulatory sphere, the European Agency for the Evaluation of Medicinal Products (EMEA) having issued a position paper, the Council for International Organizations of Medical Sciences (CIOMS) having a working group on this issue, and the European Society of Human Genetics preparing background paper on 'Polymorphic sequence variants in medicine: Technical, social, legal and ethical issues. Pharmacogenetics as an example'. Within the European project Privacy in Research Ethics and Law (PRIVIREAL), recommendations for common European guidelines for membership in research ethical committees have been discussed, balancing the interests and assuring independence and legal competence. Good decision making, assuring legality of protocols and assessment of data protection is suggested to be part of any evaluation of protocols.

Toxicol In Vitro. 2005 Aug;19(5):603-19. Related Articles, Links Altered gene expression in human hepatoma HepG2 cells exposed to low-level 2,4-dichlorophenoxyacetic acid and potassium nitrate. Bharadwaj L, Dhami K, Schneberger D, Stevens M, Renaud C, Ali A. Department of Medicine and Toxicology Group, Institute of Agricultural Rural and Environmental Health, University of Saskatchewan, 103 Hospital Drive, P.O. Box 120, Royal University Hospital, Saskatoon, Sask., Canada S7N 0W8. bharadwaj@sask.usask.ca 2,4-dichlorophenoxyacetic acid (2,4-D) and nitrate are agricultural contaminants found in rural ground water. It is not known whether levels found in groundwater pose a human or environmental health risk, nor is the mechanism of toxicity at the molecular/cellular level understood. This study focused on determining whether 2,4-D or nitrate at environmentally realistic levels elicit gene expression changes in exposed cells. cDNA microarray technology was used to determine the impact of 2,4-D and nitrate in an in vitro model of exposure. Human hepatoma HepG2 cells were incubated with 2,4-D or nitrate alone for 24 h. Cell viability (neutral red assay) and proliferation (BrdU incorporation) were assessed following exposure. Total RNA from treated and control cells were isolated, reverse transcribed and reciprocal labelled with Cy3 or Cy5 dyes, and hybridized to a human cDNA microarray. The hybridized microarray chips were scanned, quantified and analyzed to identify genes affected by 2,4-D or nitrate exposure based on a two-fold increase or decrease in gene expression and reproducibility (affected in three or more treatments). Following filtering, normalization and hierarchical clustering initial data indicate that numerous genes were found to be commonly expressed in at least three or more treatments of 2,4-D or nitrate tested. The affected genes indicate that HepG2 cells respond to environmental, low-level exposure and produce a cellular response that is associated with alterations in the expression of many genes. The affected genes were characterized as stress response, cell cycle control, immunological and DNA repair genes. These findings serve to highlight new pathway(s) in which to further probe the effects of environmental levels of 2,4-D and nitrate.

Toxicol In Vitro. 2006 Mar;20(2):163-75. Epub 2005 Nov 3. Related Articles, Links Pharmacogenetics of irinotecan metabolism and transport: an update. Smith NF, Figg WD, Sparreboom A. Molecular Pharmacology Section, Medical Oncology Branch, National Cancer

Institute, Bethesda, MD, USA. The anticancer agent irinotecan (CPT-11) is converted to SN-38, which is approximately 100 to 1,000-fold more cytotoxic than the parent drug. The pharmacokinetics of irinotecan are extremely complex and have been the subject of intensive investigation in recent years. Irinotecan is subject to extensive metabolism by various polymorphic enzymes, including CES2 to form SN-38, members of the UGT1A subfamily, and CYP3A4 and CYP3A5, which form several pharmacologically inactive oxidation products. Elimination of irinotecan is also dependent on drug-transporting proteins, notably ABCB1 (P-glycoprotein), ABCC2 (cMOAT) and ABCG2 (BCRP), present on the bile canalicular membrane. The various processes mediating drug elimination, either through metabolic breakdown or excretion, likely impact substantially on interindividual variability in drug handling. This report provides an update on current strategies to individualize irinotecan chemotherapy based on each patient's genetic constitution, which may ultimately lead to more selective use of this agent.

Toxicol Lett. 2004 Apr 1;149(1-3):371-5. Related Articles, Links Progress in applying genomics in drug development. Lord PG. Johnson and Johnson Pharmaceutical Research and Development LLC, 1000 Route 202, P.O. Box 300, Raritan, NJ 08869, USA. plord@prdus.jnj.com Genomics has had an impact on two areas of drug development, "predictive" toxicology and mechanism-based risk assessment. Predictive toxicology studies are aimed at identifying the potential for a compound to be toxic. By developing databases of expression profiles for a wide variety of toxic compounds and toxic models it has been possible to create statistical and computational methods which provide an indication of the toxic potential of a drug from the pattern of gene expression changes it elicits in in vitro or in vivo systems. Because gene expression is central to many responses to xenobiotics, genomic approaches lend themselves very readily to mechanistic toxicology studies. By examining changes in gene expression in cells and tissues in response to drugs it is possible to generate hypotheses as to the underlying mechanism and in some cases it is possible to evaluate hypotheses of toxic mechanism. Some concerns remain about the use of the technology but toxicogenomics can no longer be regarded as "new" technology in drug development. The investments made in applying the technology are maturing and there is a determined effort to bring the full power of the technology into drug development. Publication Types: Review

Toxicol Pathol. 2004 Mar-Apr;32 Suppl 1:13-25. Related Articles, Links Complementary roles for toxicologic pathology and mathematics in toxicogenomics, with special reference to data interpretation and oscillatory dynamics. Morgan KT, Pino M, Crosby LM, Wang M, Elston TC, Jayyosi Z, Bonnefoi M, Boorman G. Aventis Pharmaceuticals, Bridgewater, New Jersey, USA. kevin.morgan@aventis.com Toxicogenomics is an emerging multidisciplinary science that will profoundly impact the practice of toxicology. New generations of biologists, using evolving toxicogenomics tools, will generate massive data sets in need of interpretation. Mathematical tools are necessary to cluster and otherwise find meaningful structure in such data. The linking of this structure to gene functions and disease processes, and finally the generation of useful data interpretation remains a significant challenge. The training and background of pathologists make them ideally suited to contribute to the field of toxicogenomics, from experimental design to data interpretation. Toxicologic pathology, a discipline based on pattern recognition, requires familiarity with the dynamics of disease processes and interactions between organs, tissues, and cell populations. Optimal involvement of toxicologic pathologists in toxicogenomics requires that they communicate effectively with the many other scientists critical for the effective application of this complex discipline to societal problems. As noted by Petricoin III et al (Nature Genetics 32, 474-479, 2002), cooperation among regulators, sponsors and experts will be essential for realizing the potential of microarrays for public health. Following a brief introduction to the role of mathematics in toxicogenomics, "data interpretation" from the perspective of a pathologist is briefly discussed. Based on oscillatory behavior in the liver, the importance of an understanding of mathematics is addressed, and an approach to learning mathematics "later in life" is provided. An understanding of pathology by mathematicians involved in toxicogenomics is equally critical, as both mathematics and pathology are essential for transforming toxicogenomics data sets into useful knowledge. Publication Types: Review

Toxicol Pathol. 2004 Mar-Apr;32 Suppl 1:72-83. Related Articles, Links Application of toxicogenomics to toxicology: basic concepts in the analysis of microarray data. Irwin RD, Boorman GA, Cunningham ML, Heinloth AN, Malarkey DE, Paules RS. Environmental Toxicology Program, National Institute of Environmental Health Sciences, Research Triangle Park, North Carolina 27709, USA. Irwin@niehs.nih.gov Toxicology and the practice of pathology are rapidly evolving in the postgenomic era. Observable treatment related changes have been the hallmark of toxicology studies. Toxicogenomics is a powerful new tool that may show gene and protein changes earlier and at treatment levels below the limits of detection of traditional measures of toxicity. It may also aid in the understanding of toxic mechanisms. It is important to remember that it is only a tool and will provide meaningful results only when properly applied. As is often the case with new experimental tools, the initial utilization is driven more by the technology than application to problem solving. Toxicogenomics is interdisciplinary in nature including at a minimum, pathology, toxicology, and genomics. Most studies will require the input from the disciplines of toxicology, pathology, molecular biology, bioinformatics, biochemistry, and others depending on the types of questions being asked. Publication Types: Review

Toxicol Pathol. 2004 Mar-Apr;32 Suppl 1:9-12. Related Articles, Links Pharmacogenetics to predict drug-related adverse events. Hosford DA, Lai EH, Riley JH, Xu CF, Danoff TM, Roses AD. Department of Genetics Research, GlaxoSmithKline RandD, Research Triangle Park, North Carolina 27709, USA. david.hosford@gsk.com Identification of reliable markers to predict drug-related adverse events (DRAEs) is an important goal of the pharmaceutical industry and others within the healthcare community. We have used genetic polymorphisms, including the most frequent source of variation (single nucleotide polymorphisms, SNPs) in the human genome, in pharmacogenetic approaches designed to predict DRAEs.

Three studies exemplify the principles of using polymorphisms to identify associations in progressively larger genomic regions: polymorphic repeats within the UDP-glucuronysltransferase I (UGT1A1) gene in patients experiencing hyperbilirubinemia after administration of tranilast, an experimental drug to prevent re-stenosis following coronary revascularization; high linkage disequilibrium within the Apolipoprotein E (ApoE) gene in patients with Alzheimer Disease (AD); and the polymorphic variant HLA-B57 in patients with hypersensitivity reaction after administration of abacavir, a nucleoside reverse transcriptase inhibitor for the treatment of HIV. Together, these studies demonstrate in a stepwise manner the feasibility of using pharmacogenetic approaches to predict DRAEs. Publication Types: Review

Toxicol Pathol. 2005;33(3):343-55. Related Articles, Links Prediction of nephrotoxicant action and identification of candidate toxicity-related biomarkers. Thukral SK, Nordone PJ, Hu R, Sullivan L, Galambos E, Fitzpatrick VD, Healy L, Bass MB, Cosenza ME, Afshari CA. Amgen Inc., Thousand Oaks, California 91320, USA. A vast majority of pharmacological compounds and their metabolites are excreted via the urine, and within the complex structure of the kidney,the proximal tubules are a main target site of nephrotoxic compounds. We used the model nephrotoxicants mercuric chloride, 2-bromoethylamine hydrobromide, hexachlorobutadiene, mitomycin, amphotericin, and puromycin to elucidate time- and dose-dependent global gene expression changes associated with proximal tubular toxicity. Male Sprague-Dawley rats were dosed via intraperitoneal injection once daily for mercuric chloride and amphotericin (up to 7 doses), while a single dose was given for all other compounds. Animals were exposed to 2 different doses of these compounds and kidney tissues were collected on day 1, 3, and 7 postdosing. Gene expression profiles were generated from kidney RNA using 17K rat cDNA dual dye microarray and analyzed in conjunction with histopathology. Analysis of gene expression profiles showed that the profiles clustered based on similarities in the severity and type of pathology of individual animals. Further, the expression changes were indicative of tubular toxicity showing hallmarks of tubular degeneration/regeneration and necrosis. Use of gene expression data in predicting the type of nephrotoxicity was then tested with a support vector machine (SVM)-based approach. A SVM prediction module was trained using 120 profiles of total profiles divided into four classes based on the severity of pathology and clustering. Although mitomycin C and amphotericin B treatments did not cause toxicity, their expression profiles were included in the SVM prediction module to increase the sample size. Using this classifier, the SVM predicted the type of pathology of 28 test profiles with 100% selectivity and 82% sensitivity. These data indicate that valid predictions could be made based on gene expression changes from a small set of expression profiles. A set of potential biomarkers showing a time- and dose-response with respect to the progression of proximal tubular toxicity were identified. These include several transporters (Slc21a2, Slc15, Slc34a2), Kim 1, IGFbp-1, osteopontin, alpha-fibrinogen, and Gstalpha.

Toxicol Rev. 2004;23(4):239-49. Related Articles, Links Herbal interactions involving cytochrome p450 enzymes: a mini review. Delgoda R, Westlake AC.

Natural Products Institute and Faculty of Pure and Applied Sciences, University of the West Indies, Mona, Kingston, Jamaica, West Indies. thejani.delgoda@uwimona.edu.jm The metabolism of a drug can be altered by another drug or foreign chemical, and such interactions can often be clinically significant. Cytochrome P450 (CYP) enzymes, a superfamily of enzymes found mainly in the liver, are involved in the metabolism of a plethora of xenobiotics and have been shown to be involved in numerous interactions between drugs and food, herbs and other drugs. The observed induction and inhibition of CYP enzymes by natural products in the presence of a prescribed drug has (among other reasons) led to the general acceptance that natural therapies can have adverse effects, contrary to the popular beliefs in countries where there is an active practice of ethnomedicine. Herbal medicines such as St. John's wort, garlic, piperine, ginseng, and gingko, which are freely available over the counter, have given rise to serious clinical interactions when co-administered with prescription medicines. Such adversities have spurred various pre-clinical and in vitro investigations on a series of other herbal remedies, with their clinical relevance remaining to be established. Although the presence of numerous active ingredients in herbal medicines, foods and dietary supplements complicate experimentation, the observable interactions with CYP enzymes warrant systematic studies, so that metabolism-based interactions can be predicted and avoided more readily. This article highlights the involvement of CYP enzymes in metabolism-related drug-herb interactions and the importance of gaining a mechanism-based understanding to avoid potential adverse drug reactions, in addition to outlining other contributory factors, such as pharmacogenetics and recreational habits that may compound this important health issue. Publication Types: Review

Toxicol Sci. 2005 Aug;86(2):453-69. Epub 2005 May 18. Related Articles, Links Gene ontology mapping as an unbiased method for identifying molecular pathways and processes affected by toxicant exposure: application to acute effects caused by the rodent non-genotoxic carcinogen diethylhexylphthalate. Currie RA, Bombail V, Oliver JD, Moore DJ, Lim FL, Gwilliam V, Kimber I, Chipman K, Moggs JG, Orphanides G. Syngenta Central Toxicology Laboratory, Alderley Park, Cheshire SK10 4TJ, United Kingdom. richard.currie@syngenta.com Toxicogenomics has the potential to reveal the molecular pathways and cellular processes that mediate the adverse responses to a toxicant. However, the initial output of a toxicogenomic experiment often consists of large lists of genes whose expression is altered after toxicant exposure. To interpret gene expression changes in the context of underlying biological pathways and processes, new bioinformatics methods must be developed. We have used global gene expression profiling combined with an evaluation of Gene Ontology (GO) and pathway mapping tools as unbiased methods for identifying the molecular pathways and processes affected upon toxicant exposure. We chose to use the acute effects caused by the non-genotoxic carcinogen and peroxisome proliferator (PP) diethylhexylphthalate (DEHP) in the mouse liver as a model system. Consistent with what is known about the mode of action of DEHP, our GO analysis of transcript profiling data revealed a striking overrepresentation of genes associated with the peroxisomal cellular component, together with genes involved in carboxylic acid and lipid metabolism. Furthermore we reveal gene expression changes associated with additional biological functions, including complement activation, hemostasis, the endoplasmic reticulum overload response, and circadian rhythm. Together, these data reveal potential new pathways of PP action and shed new light on the mechanisms by which non-genotoxic carcinogens control hepatocyte hypertrophy and proliferation. We demonstrate that GO mapping can identify, in an unbiased manner, both known and novel DEHP-induced molecular changes in the mouse liver and is therefore a powerful approach for elucidating modes of toxicity based on toxicogenomic data.

Toxicol Sci. 2005 Dec;88(2):585-601. Epub 2005 Sep 8. Related Articles, Links Chemical effects in biological systems--data dictionary (CEBS-DD): a compendium of terms for the capture and integration of biological study design description, conventional phenotypes, and 'omics data. Fostel J, Choi D, Zwickl C, Morrison N, Rashid A, Hasan A, Bao W, Richard A, Tong W, Bushel PR, Brown R, Bruno M, Cunningham ML, Dix D, Eastin W, Frade C, Garcia A, Heinloth A, Irwin R, Madenspacher J, Merrick BA, Papoian T, Paules R, Rocca-Serra P, Sansone AS, Stevens J, Tomer K, Yang C, Waters M. LIMT Lockheed Martin Information Technology (LMIT), Research Triangle Park, NC 27709, USA. fostel@niehs.nih.gov A critical component in the design of the Chemical Effects in Biological Systems (CEBS) Knowledgebase is a strategy to capture toxicogenomics study protocols and the toxicity endpoint data (clinical pathology and histopathology). A Study is generally an experiment carried out during a period of time for the purpose of obtaining data, and the Study Design Description captures the methods, timing, and organization of the Study. The CEBS Data Dictionary (CEBS-DD) has been designed to define and organize terms in an attempt to standardize nomenclature needed to describe a toxicogenomics Study in a structured yet intuitive format and provide a flexible means to describe a Study as conceptualized by the investigator. The CEBS-DD will organize and annotate information from a variety of sources, thereby facilitating the capture and display of toxicogenomics data in biological context in CEBS, i.e., associating molecular events detected in highly-parallel data with the toxicology/pathology phenotype as observed in the individual Study Subjects and linked to the experimental treatments. The CEBS-DD has been developed with a focus on acute toxicity studies, but with a design that will permit it to be extended to other areas of toxicology and biology with the addition of domain-specific terms. To illustrate the utility of the CEBS-DD, we present an example of integrating data from two proteomics and transcriptomics studies of the response to acute acetaminophen toxicity (A. N. Heinloth et al., 2004, Toxicol. Sci. 80, 193-202).

Toxicol Sci. 2005 Feb;83(2):205-6. Related Articles, Links Comment on: Toxicol Sci. 2005 Feb;83(2):282-92. Applying toxicogenomics in mechanistic and predictive toxicology. Cunningham ML, Lehman-McKeeman L. National Toxicology, National Institute of Environmental Health Sciences, Research Triangle Park, North Carolina 27709, USA. cunningl@niehs.nih.gov Publication Types: Comment Editorial

Toxicol Sci. 2005 Feb;83(2):282-92. Epub 2004 Sep 1. Related Articles, Links

Erratum in: Toxicol Sci. 2006 Feb;89(2):554. Comment in: Toxicol Sci. 2005 Feb;83(2):205-6. A toxicogenomic approach to drug-induced phospholipidosis: analysis of its induction mechanism and establishment of a novel in vitro screening system. Sawada H, Takami K, Asahi S. Biomedical Research Laboratories, Pharmaceutical Research Division, Takeda Pharmaceutical Company Limited, Osaka 532-8686, Japan. Sawada_Hiroshi@takeda.co.jp Phospholipidosis is a lipid storage disorder in which excess phospholipids accumulate within cells. Some cationic amphiphilic compounds are known to have the potential to induce phospholipidosis. This study was undertaken to examine the molecular mechanisms that contribute to the development of phospholipidosis and to identify specific markers that might form the basis of an in vitro screening test. Specifically, we performed a large-scale gene expression analysis using DNA microarrays on human hepatoma HepG2 cells after they were treated with each of 12 compounds known to induce phospholipidosis. In electron microscopy, HepG2 cells developed lamellar myelin-like bodies in their lysosomes, the characteristic change of phospholipidosis, after treatment with these compounds for 72 h. DNA microarray analysis performed 6 and 24 h after treatment showed alterations in gene expression reflecting the inhibition of lysosomal phospholipase activity and lysosomal enzyme transport, and the induction of phospholipid and cholesterol biosynthesis. Seventeen genes that showed a similar expression profile following treatment were selected as candidate markers. Real-time PCR analysis confirmed that 12 gene markers showed significant concordance with lamellar myelin-like body formation. Furthermore, the average fold change values of these markers correlated well with the magnitude of this pathological change. In conclusion, microarray analysis revealed that factors such as alterations in lysosomal function and cholesterol metabolism were involved in the induction of phospholipidosis. Furthermore, comprehensive gene expression analysis enabled us to identify biomarkers of this condition that we then used to develop a rapid and sensitive in vitro screening test for drug-induced phospholipidosis.

Toxicol Sci. 2005 Jul;86(1):185-93. Epub 2005 Apr 6. Related Articles, Links Hepatic gene expression changes throughout the day in the Fischer rat: implications for toxicogenomic experiments. Boorman GA, Blackshear PE, Parker JS, Lobenhofer EK, Malarkey DE, Vallant MK, Gerken DK, Irwin RD. Environmental Toxicology Program, National Institute of Environmental Health Sciences, Research Triangle Park, North Carolina 27709, USA. boorman@niehs.nih.gov There is increasing use of transcriptional profiling in hepatotoxicity studies in the rat. Understanding hepatic gene expression changes over time is critical, since tissue collection may occur throughout the day. Furthermore, when comparing results from different data sets, times of dosing and tissue collection may vary. Circadian effects on the mouse hepatic transcriptome have been well documented. However, limited reports exist for the rat. In one study approximately 7% of the hepatic genes showed a diurnal expression pattern in a comparison of rat liver samples collected during the day versus livers collected at night. The results of a second study comparing rat liver samples collected at multiple time points over a circadian day suggest only minimal variation of the hepatic transcriptome. We studied temporal hepatic gene expression in 48 untreated F344/N rats using both approaches employed in these previous studies. Statistical analysis of microarray (SAM) identified differential expression in day/night comparisons, but was less sensitive for liver samples collected at multiple times of day. However, a Fourier analysis identified numerous periodically expressed genes in these samples including period genes, clock genes, clock-controlled genes, and genes involved in metabolic pathways. Furthermore, rhythms in gene expression were identified for several circadian genes not previously reported in the rat liver. Transcript levels for twenty genes involved in circadian and metabolic pathways were confirmed using quantitative RT-PCR. The results of this study demonstrate a prominent circadian rhythm in gene expression in the rat that is a critical factor in planning toxicogenomic experiments.

Toxicol Sci. 2006 Feb;89(2):352-60. Epub 2005 Oct 12. Related Articles, Links Toxicogenomics in risk assessment: applications and needs. Boverhof DR, Zacharewski TR. Department of Biochemistry and Molecular Biology, National Food Safety and Center for Integrative Toxicology, Michigan State University, East Lansing Michigan 48824, USA. Since its inception, there have been high expectations for the science of toxicogenomics to decrease the uncertainties associated with the risk assessment process by providing valuable insights into toxic mechanisms of action. However, the application of these data into risk assessment practices is still in the early stages of development, and proof of principle experiments have yet to emerge. The following discusses some potential applications as well as impediments that warrant a concerted investigation from all stakeholders in order to facilitate the acceptance and subsequent incorporation of toxicogenomics into regulatory decision making. Publication Types: Review

Toxicol Sci. 2006 Jan;89(1):120-34. Epub 2005 Oct 26. Related Articles, Links A toxicogenomics approach to identify new plausible epigenetic mechanisms of ochratoxin a carcinogenicity in rat. Marin-Kuan M, Nestler S, Verguet C, Bezencon C, Piguet D, Mansourian R, Holzwarth J, Grigorov M, Delatour T, Mantle P, Cavin C, Schilter B. Nestle Research Center, PO Box 44, Vers-chez-les-Blanc, CH-1000 Lausanne 26, Switzerland. maricel.marin-kuan@rdls.nestle.com Ochratoxin A (OTA) is a mycotoxin occurring naturally in a wide range of food commodities. In animals, it has been shown to cause a variety of adverse effects, nephrocarcinogenicity being the most prominent. Because of its high toxic potency and the continuous exposure of the human population, OTA has raised public health concerns. There is significant debate on how to use the rat carcinogenicity data to assess the potential risk to humans. In this context, the question of the mechanism of action of OTA appears of key importance and was studied through the application of a toxicogenomics approach. Male Fischer rats were fed OTA for up to 2 years. Renal tumors were discovered during the last 6 months of the study. The total tumor incidence reached 25% at the end of the study. Gene expression profile was analyzed in groups of animals taken in intervals from 7 days to 12 months. Tissue-specific responses were observed in kidney versus liver. For selected genes, microarray data were confirmed at both mRNA and protein levels. In kidney, several genes known as markers of kidney injury and cell regeneration were significantly modulated by OTA. The expression of genes known to be involved in DNA synthesis and repair, or genes induced as a result of DNA damage, was only marginally modulated. Very little or no effect was found amongst genes associated with apoptosis. Alterations of gene expression indicating effects on calcium homeostasis and a disruption of pathways regulated by the transcription factors hepatocyte nuclear factor 4 alpha (HNF4alpha) and nuclear factor-erythroid 2-related factor 2 (Nrf2) were observed in the kidney but not in the liver. Previous data have suggested that a reduction in HNF4alpha may be associated with nephrocarcinogenicity. Many Nrf2-regulated genes are involved in chemical detoxication and antioxidant defense. The depletion of these genes is likely to impair the defense potential of the cells, resulting in chronic elevation of oxidative stress in the kidney. The inhibition of defense mechanism appears as a highly plausible new mechanism, which could contribute to OTA carcinogenicity.

Toxicology. 2005 Oct 1;213(3):177-93. Related Articles, Links Molecular responses to xenoestrogens: mechanistic insights from toxicogenomics. Moggs JG. Syngenta Central Toxicology Laboratory, Alderley Park, Cheshire SK10 4TJ, UK. jonathan.moggs@syngenta.com The xenoestrogen group of endocrine disruptors has the potential to cause reproductive and developmental effects through stimulation or disruption of sex steroid nuclear receptor signalling pathways. A more detailed understanding of the ways in which xenoestrogens interact with biological systems at the molecular level will provide a mechanistic basis for improved safety assessment. The recent sequencing of mammalian genomes has driven the development of toxicogenomic technologies, including microarray based gene expression profiling, which allow the expression levels of thousands of genes to be measured simultaneously. Since the cellular responses to xenoestrogens are predominantly mediated by estrogen receptors, which function as ligand-activated transcription factors to regulate gene expression, the application of toxicogenomics has great potential for providing insights into the molecular mechanisms of xenoestrogen action. A major challenge in applying toxicogenomics to the field of endocrine disruption is the need to define how xenoestrogen-induced changes in gene expression relate to conventional physiological and toxicological endpoints. Gene Ontology Mapping, Pathway Mapping and Phenotypic Anchoring of xenoestrogen-induced gene expression changes to cellular pathways and processes represent key steps in defining these relationships. Mechanistic insights into how xenoestrogens target specific genes and into the functional significance of xenoestrogen-induced alterations in gene expression can be further enhanced by combining transcript profiling with transgenic animal models or cell-based systems in which the estrogen receptor signalling pathways have been modified experimentally. This review illustrates how these toxicogenomic approaches are providing an unprecedented amount of mechanistic information on the molecular responses to xenoestrogens and how they are likely to impact on hazard and risk assessment. Publication Types: Lectures

Transpl Immunol. 2005 Mar;14(1):37-42. Epub 2004 Dec 7. Related Articles, Links The impact of pharmacogenomic factors on acute persistent rejection in adult lung transplant patients. Zheng HX, Zeevi A, McCurry K, Schuetz E, Webber S, Ristich J, Zhang J, Iacono A, Dauber J, McDade

K, Zaldonis D, Lamba J, Burckart GJ. School of Pharmacy, University of Southern California, 1985 Zonal Avenue, PSC-100, Los Angeles, CA 90033, USA. Persistent rejection in the face of treatment and multiple episodes of rejection are associated with the development of chronic rejection and graft loss in solid organ transplantation. The factors that create an environment for rejection that persists in the face of treatment are as yet not understood. The objective of this study was to evaluate the risk factors, including human multidrug resistance gene (MDR1), cytochrome P4503A5 (CYP3A5) and cytokine gene polymorphisms, associated with acute persistent rejection (APR) in lung transplant patients. One hundred and twenty-five adult lung transplant patients were studied. MDR1 G2677T, C3435T and CYP3A5 polymorphisms were assessed by direct sequencing of the polymorphic region in patient DNA. Cytokine genotyping for five cytokines was performed using the polymerase chain reaction-sequence specific primers (PCR-SSP) technique. Multivariate regression analysis was used to identify the predictors of acute persistent rejection. The dependent variable was the presence or absence of acute persistent rejection based on lung biopsies during the first postoperative year. The independent variables were MDR1 G2677T and C3435T, CYP4503A5 and cytokine polymorphisms, survival status, age, gender, survival days and HLA mismatches. The MDR1 C3435T polymorphism and age were independently associated with acute persistent rejection (p = 0.025, odds ratio = 0.29, 95% CI 0.1-0.86 and p = 0.016, odds ratio = 0.94, 95% CI 0.89-0.98, respectively). For the MDR1 C3435T polymorphism, 72% of patients with the C allele had acute persistent rejection in comparison to 52% for TT patients (p = 0.04). For age, a significant difference was found between the nonrejection group and the rejection group (mean+/-S.D. 52.1+/-11.2 vs. 44.4+/-12.3, p = 0.01). This is the first report of the association of a drug disposition genotype with drug-resistant acute rejection in organ transplant patients. The major predictor of acute persistent rejection in the first postoperative year for lung transplant patients was the MDR1 C3435T genotype. This association could be due to drug resistance, altered drug disposition or other immunologic effects associated with P-glycoprotein (P-gp) function. Future prospective treatment algorithms should be developed that will incorporate the knowledge of gene polymorphisms into treatment regimens to improve the outcome following lung transplantation.

Transplant Proc. 2004 Apr;36(3):687-9. Related Articles, Links Prospects for personalized immunosuppression: pharmacologic tools--a review. Del Tacca M. Division of Pharmacology and Chemotherapy, Department of Oncology, Transplants and Advanced Technologies in Medicine, University of Pisa, Pisa, Italy. m.deltacca@med.unipi.it In the last few years, novel immunosuppressive agents and new formulations, including sirolimus, mycophenolic acid (the active metabolite of mycophenolate mofetil), tacrolimus, and microemulsion cyclosporine, have significantly improved the clinical outcome of transplant recipients. However, the majority of immunosuppressive agents need a constant monitoring of drug levels to reduce the risk of graft rejection as well as drug-induced toxicities. Many factors may affect the pharmacokinetic characteristics of immunosuppressive agents, potentially reducing treatment effectiveness. Absorption and metabolism of immunosuppressive drugs are influenced by patient genotype and comedications, while comorbidities (ie, diabetes and cystic fibrosis) are responsible for altered pharmacokinetics. Dose individualization in transplant recipients is performed according to their health status, graft function, and drug therapeutic range. With respect to the last issue, therapeutic drug monitoring (TDM) plays a crucial role in achieving optimal immunosuppression, improving the efficacy of drugs, and lowering toxic effects. Pharmacokinetic analysis allowed the identification of specific parameters, such as plasma or blood levels, immediately before dosing (C(min) or trough levels) or 2 hours after administration (C(2)), which are significantly related to tissue exposure to the drug. More recently, studies have investigated treatment individualization by evaluating drug pharmacogenetics based on the expression level or mutations of their molecular targets, including calcineurin for cyclosporine and tacrolimus, and inosine monophosphate dehydrogenase for mycophenolic acid. Although no conclusive data may be drawn from these preliminary trials, further studies are underway to address the role of pharmacogenetics in clinical decision making. Publication Types: Review

Transplant Proc. 2004 Nov;36(9):2787-90. Related Articles, Links An exploratory study on pharmacogenetics of inosine-monophosphate dehydrogenase II in peripheral mononuclear cells from liver-transplant recipients. Vannozzi F, Filipponi F, Di Paolo A, Danesi R, Urbani L, Bocci G, Catalano G, De Simone P, Mosca F, Del Tacca M. Division of Pharmacology and Chemotherapy, Department of Oncology, Transplants and Advanced Technologies in Medicine, University of Pisa, 56126 Pisa, Italy. Mycophenolate mofetil (MMF) is an immunosuppressant used for the prophylaxis of rejection in renal, pancreas, and liver transplantation. It inhibits the inducible isoform of the enzyme inosine-monophosphate dehydrogenase (IMPDH II) via its active metabolite mycophenolic acid (MPA). IMPDH II is necessary for de novo purine synthesis in activated lymphocytes. The aims of the present study were to evaluate the feasibility of a real-time polymerase chain reaction (PCR) quantitative assessment of IMPDH II gene expression in liver transplant recipients as well as to provide a preliminary evaluation of possible correlations with drug tolerability. RNA was extracted from peripheral blood mononuclear cells of liver recipients after at least 6 months of MMF administration. IMPDH II gene expression was assessed using quantitative, real-time PCR and normalized using glyceraldheyde-3-phosphate dehydrogenase (GAPDH). Finally, adverse events associated with MMF administration were recorded. Real-time PCR quantitation of IMPDH II gene expression was reliable, sensitive, and specific. The intrapatient variability for both IMPDH II and GAPDH assays was lower than 0.6% in all patients. The results demonstrated a wide interpatient variability, with the mean value +/- standard deviation of 0.949 +/- 0.525 (95% confidence interval, 0.669-1.229) and a median value of 0.797. Patients with treatment-related toxicities displayed a trend to a higher level of IMPDH II expression than those without toxicity (mean, 1.126 vs 0.771). In conclusion, pharmacogenetic analysis of IMPDH II may represent a novel approach to MMF therapeutic monitoring.

Transplant Proc. 2005 Jul-Aug;37(6):2675-8. Related Articles, Links New strategies in immunosuppression. Regazzi MB,

Alessiani M, Rinaldi M. Department of Pharmacology, IRCCS Policlinico S. Matteo, Pavia, Italy. regazzim@smatteo.pv.it New immunosuppressive strategies that can prevent both acute and chronic rejection are being investigated to achieve graft tolerance and to minimize side effects and toxicity that may lead to graft loss. Drug pharmacokinetics and pharmacodynamics, as well as pharmacogenetics, all play a role in customizing treatment to the individual patient. To improve patient compliance, new drug formulations are on trial, such as the modified- release oral form of tacrolimus MR4 for once daily administration, which seems to be equivalent to bid administration in terms of steady-state exposure. Monoclonal/polyclonal antibodies are increasingly used in the induction phase in protocols where steroids are discontinued early. However, discontinuing steroids carries a high risk of acute rejection or organ failure in some subgroups of patients. The supposed benefit of steroid discontinuation may not be enjoyed by all patients. Minimizing anticalcineurin agents may prove to be similarly or even more advantageous. The use of new drugs and new combinations has greatly improved short-term transplant outcomes. The new goal is, therefore, to improve long-term results and particularly to prevent chronic rejection, thus increasing patient and organ survival. Publication Types: Review

Transplant Proc. 2005 Sep;37(7):2911-2.
Related Articles, Links Low tacrolimus dose requirements in renal transplant recipients in the omani population: implications for pharmacogenetics? Mohsin N, Pakkyara A, Budruddin M, Obaid F, Kumar A, Malvathu S, Kalankara S, Amitabh A, Daar A. Department of Nephrology and Biochemistry, Royal Hospital, Muscat, Oman. nabmoh@omantel.net.com Clinical observations suggested that the dose requirements for some immunosuppressive drugs might be lower in some Eastern populations. We performed a study of 50 among 162 patients who were converted from a cyclosporine-based immunosuppression regimen to one based on tacrolimus. The reasons for conversion were as follows: acute rejection (n = 23), hirsutism and gingival hypertrophy (n = 12), chronic allograft nephropathy (n = 4), hypertension (n = 3), and other reasons (n = 8). Target levels were 10-15 ng/mL for patients with acute rejection and 5-8 ng/mL for patients after the first year of transplantation. We measured 180 tacrolimus blood levels in 44 patients using the IMx Abbott system of mean weight 64.5 kg and mean daily dose of 4.89 +/- 2.56 mg with mean blood levels of 11.31 +/- 5.22 ng/mL. Thus, to achieve the above-mentioned levels the average dose was 0.076 mg/kg, which is lower than that generally recommended to achieve 5-8 ng/mL levels, namely, 0.15 mg/kg. In this study, we did not address the reasons for these findings. The possibilities include dietary factors influencing the absorption of tacrolimus, and genetic polymorphisms in the Omani population that affect drug levels through several possible pharmacogenetic/genomic mechanisms. We intend to perform such studies in the future.

Transplantation. 2004 Aug 15;78(3):311-5.
Related Articles, Links Pharmacogenetics in solid organ transplantation: present knowledge and future perspectives. Anglicheau D, Legendre C, Thervet E. Service de Nephrologie et de Transplantation Renale, Hopital Saint Louis, Paris, France. The promise of pharmacogenetics is to elucidate the

inherited basis of differences between individual responses to drugs, in order to identify the right drug and dose for each patient. Genetic polymorphisms are implicated in the interindividual variability of the pharmacokinetic or pharmacodynamic characteristics of immunosuppressive drugs. The first pharmacogenetic trait identified was monogenic, and concerned the prototypic example of thiopurine methyltransferase (TPMT) implicated in azathioprine metabolism. Individuals with low TPMT activity, inherited in an autosomal codominant fashion, are at risk of drug-induced myelosuppression. TPMT activity determination and DNA-based tests are now used in clinical practice. It has been also demonstrated that there is a link between the polymorphisms of the cytochrome P450 3A5, 3A4 and the multidrug resistance-1 (MDR1) genes, and the daily dose necessary to achieve adequate blood tacrolimus levels. Analysis of MDR1 haplotypes or using the association of the different genes might further improve predictions. Since genotyping methods improve rapidly, it will soon be easy to test for thousands of single nucleotide polymorphisms in one assay. Present challenges are to determine the genes of interest and to validate such determination prospectively in clinical practice. Publication Types: Review

Transplantation. 2005 Feb 27;79(4):499-502. Related Articles, Links Tacrolimus pharmacogenetics: the CYP3A5*1 allele predicts low dose-normalized tacrolimus blood concentrations in whites and South Asians. Macphee IA, Fredericks S, Mohamed M, Moreton M, Carter ND, Johnston A, Goldberg L, Holt DW. Cellular and Molecular Medicine, Renal Medicine, St. George's Hospital Medical School, Cranmer Terrace, London SW17 0RE, UK. imacphee@sghms.ac.uk Previously, we demonstrated that the dose-normalized tacrolimus blood concentration after renal transplantation was associated with a single nucleotide polymorphism (SNP) in the CYP3AP1 gene, probably through linkage with an SNP in the CYP3A5 gene. Individuals with at least one CYP3A5*1 allele synthesize CYP3A5 and CYP3A5*3/*3 homozygotes do not. We now present results with direct typing of the CYP3A5 genotype for this group of 180 kidney-only transplant recipients from a single center. South Asian and white patients with at least one CYP3A5*1 allele achieved twofold lower dose-normalized tacrolimus blood concentrations compared with CYP3A5*3/*3 homozygotes, confirming our previous findings for the CYP3AP1 SNP. There was a significant delay in achieving target blood concentrations in those with at least one CYP3A5*1 allele. Determination of the CYP3A5*1/*3 genotype could be used to predict the tacrolimus dose requirement and, given incomplete linkage, would be better than determination of the CYP3AP1 genotype.

Treat Respir Med. 2004;3(3):161-71. Related Articles, Links Therapeutic response to asthma medications: genotype predictors. Wallace AM, Sandford AJ. University of British Columbia, James Hogg iCapture Centre, St Paul's Hospital, Vancouver, British Columbia, Canada. Asthma is a major social and economic burden. Studies have shown that genetic polymorphisms can influence drug efficacy and/or toxicity. The understanding of the pharmacogenetics of asthma will allow therapeutic regimens to be tailored on an individual basis. It is hoped that linkage and association studies will define new therapeutic targets for asthma but until then, studies have focused on improving response to beta(2)-adrenoceptor agonist and leukotriene modifier therapy. Genetic polymorphism may account for interindividual differences in toxicity and efficacy of asthma medications. To date, single nucleotide polymorphism and limited haplotype analysis have provided inconclusive evidence as to how genotype predictors can be used to optimize current asthma therapies based on each patient's genetic profile. Publication Types: Historical Article Review

Treat Respir Med. 2005;4(1):9-20. Related Articles, Links Asthma management issues in infancy and childhood. Yang KD. Department 4 Medical Research, Chang Gung Children's Hospital at Kaohsiung, 123 Ta-Pei Road, Niao-Sung, Kaohsiung 833, Taiwan. yangkd@adm.cgmh.org.tw The prevalence of asthma has been increasing worldwide over the past 2 decades, especially the prevalence of childhood asthma. Currently, the prevalence of childhood asthma is around 3-20% in different countries based on the report from the International Study of Asthma and Allergies in Children (ISAAC). Asthma in childhood is predominantly an extrinsic asthma. In general, countries in the coastal, temperate, and subtropical zones have the highest prevalence of mite- and cockroach-sensitive asthma. Countries in the sub-arctic or semi-arid areas have a lower prevalence of childhood asthma, mostly associated with sensitization to pet dander, moulds, and pollens. Many genes have been linked to asthma in different ethnic populations. A global consensus for the management of asthma in adults and children >5 years of age has been made possible in the Global Initiative for Asthma (GINA) guidelines, where a step-wise management program using inhaled medication with and without oral anti-inflammatory drugs is recommended. The management of asthma in children <5 years of age remains inconclusive. Recent studies suggest that inherited susceptibility associated with risk factors from the prenatal and postnatal environment is likely to promote allergic sensitization and development of asthma. Consequently, early prevention of prenatal sensitization in utero and environmental control of early life exposure to various allergens may decrease the incidence of childhood asthma. In the management of moderate persistent asthma in infants and young children <5 years of age, airway resistance tests (FEV(1) or PEF) are not of significance, but assessment of respiratory rate and skin pulse oximeter measurements of arterial oxygen saturation are helpful. Moreover, recent advances in pharmacogenetics and pharmacogenomics may provide better individualized care for early pharmacological prevention of childhood asthma via selective modulation of airway remodeling. Publication Types: Review

Trends Biotechnol. 2006 Jan;24(1):15-21. Epub 2005 Nov 23. Related Articles, Links Zebrafish in functional genomics and aquatic biomedicine. Alestrom P, Holter JL, Nourizadeh-Lillabadi R. Department of Basic Sciences and Aquatic Medicine, Norwegian School of Veterinary Science, PO Box 8146 Dep, N-0033 Oslo, Norway. peter.alestrom@veths.no The zebrafish (Danio rerio) has many features that make it an ideal model for the study of developmental biology. It is small and easy to contain, it has transparent embryos, it is easy to breed and its early development is well characterized; these same characteristics have also made it an ideal vertebrate model in the areas of biomedicine and biotechnology. In aquaculture, the need for a well-characterized fish model has been satisfied by the zebrafish owing to the availability of functional genomics and molecular biology data to facilitate studies of growth, reproduction, meat quality and disease biology, with the corresponding development of vaccines and therapies. Zebrafish are also increasingly used in toxicogenomics to analyze the effects of toxins and pollutants in the environment, and for creating biomonitors that emit alarm signals when a toxic compound is detected. As detailed in this review, the zebrafish is a versatile and well-characterized model with applications in many fields of study. Publication Types: Review

Trends Mol Med. 2005 Nov;11(11):485-6. Epub 2005 Oct 12. Related Articles, Links Response to Sykiotis and Papavassiliou: Professional education in molecular medicine--pharmacogenetics first. Lunshof JE, Gurwitz D. Publication Types: Comment Letter

Trends Parasitol. 2005 Jul;21(7):302-5. Related Articles, Links Model-organism genomics in veterinary parasite drug-discovery. Gilleard JS, Woods DJ, Dow JA. Division of Infection and Immunity, Institute of Comparative Medicine, Faculty of Veterinary Medicine, University of Glasgow, Glasgow, UK, G61 1QH. A recent article about genomic filtering highlights exciting new opportunities for antiparasitic drug discovery resulting from major advances in genomic technologies. In this article, we discuss several approaches in which model-organism genomics and proteomics could be applied to the identification and validation of novel targets for antiparasitic drug discovery in veterinary medicine. Publication Types: Review

Trends Pharmacol Sci. 2004 Apr;25(4):193-200. Related Articles, Links Pharmacogenetics of cytochrome P450 and its applications in drug therapy: the past, present and future. Ingelman-Sundberg M. Division of Molecular Toxicology, IMM, Karolinska Institutet, SE-171 77 Stockholm, Sweden. maging@ki.se The field of cytochrome P450 pharmacogenetics has progressed rapidly during the past 25 years. All the major human drug-metabolizing P450 enzymes have been identified and cloned, and the major gene variants that cause inter-individual variability in drug response and are related to adverse drug reactions have been identified. This information now provides the basis for the use of predictive pharmacogenetics to yield drug therapies that are more efficient and safer. Today, we understand which drugs warrant dosing based on pharmacogenetics to improve drug treatment. It is anticipated that, in the future, genotyping could be used to personalize drug treatment for vast numbers of subjects, decreasing the cost of drug treatment and increasing the efficacy of drugs and health in general. I estimate that such personalized P450 gene-based treatment would be relevant for 10-20% of all drug therapy. Publication Types: Review

Trends Pharmacol Sci. 2004 Sep;25(9):457-64. Related Articles, Links Pharmacogenomics in cancer therapy: is host genome variability important? Petros WP, Evans WE. Mary Babb Randolph Cancer Center and West Virginia University School of Pharmacy, WV 26506, USA. wpetros@hsc.wvu.edu Pharmacogenomics aims to elucidate the genomic determinants of drug disposition and effect. Because cancer chemotherapy is relatively nonspecific and has narrow therapeutic indices, there is great potential for pharmacogenomics to improve treatment outcomes by either reducing toxicity or increasing efficacy. The diversity of therapeutic targets for anticancer drugs and the intensity of clinical pharmacology research in oncology have provided many examples of clinically relevant pharmacogenomic applications. Important elements that are discussed in this article include the association of genetic variability in the metabolism, intracellular transport and targets of anticancer drugs. In addition, we summarize where the field stands currently, and how information from the host and tumor might be integrated into decision making. Publication Types: Review

Trends Pharmacol Sci. 2005 Apr;26(4):196-201. Related Articles, Links Pharmacogenomics in admixed populations. Suarez-Kurtz G. Division of Pharmacology, Instituto Nacional de Cancer, Rio de Janeiro, RJ 22290-290, Brazil. kurtz@inca.gov.br Personalized drug therapy proffered by pharmacogenomics must be based on the recognition of inherent genetic individuality, rather than relying on inter-ethnic differences in the frequency of polymorphisms that affect the pharmacokinetics and targets of drugs. This is particularly significant in admixed populations, in which the substructure created by inter-ethnic crosses further increases the fluidity of racial and/or ethnic labels. Inter-ethnic admixture is either common or increasing quickly in many, if not most, populations, and so extrapolation on a global scale of pharmacogenomic data from well-defined ethnic groups is plagued with uncertainty. To impact positively on global health, pharmacogenomics must broaden its scope of investigation with respect to both target and population diversity, and avoid the risk of contributing to the creation of a genomics divide between regions and nations. In this review, I examine the challenges and advantages of studying pharmacogenomics in admixed populations, drawing examples mainly from the trihybrid populations of the Americas. Publication Types: Review

Trends Pharmacol Sci. 2005 Apr;26(4):202-9. Related Articles, Links Techniques: application of systems biology to absorption, distribution, metabolism, excretion and toxicity. Ekins S, Nikolsky Y, Nikolskaya T. GeneGo, 500 Renaissance Drive, Suite 106, St Joseph, MI 49085, USA. sean@genego.com It is widely recognized that either predicting or determining the absorption, distribution, metabolism, excretion and toxicity (ADME/Tox) properties of molecules helps to prevent the failure of some compounds before they reach the clinic. Consequently, there has been considerable research into developing better in silico, in vitro and in vivo methods and models. Toxicogenomics, proteomics, metabonomics and pharmacogenomics represent the latest experimental approaches that can be combined with high-throughput molecular screening of targets to provide a view of the complete biological system that is modulated by a compound. The functional interpretation and relevance of these complex multidimensional data to the phenotype observed in humans is the focus of current research in toxicology. Multiple content databases, data mining and predictive modeling algorithms, visualization tools, and high-throughput data-analysis solutions are being integrated to form systems-ADME/Tox. In this review, we focus on the most recent advances and applications in this area. Publication Types: Review

Trends Pharmacol Sci. 2005 Aug;26(8):391-7. Related Articles, Links New ideas on the origin of L-dopa-induced dyskinesias: age, genes and neural plasticity. Linazasoro G. Centro de Investigacion Parkinson, Policlinica Gipuzkoa, San Sebastian, Spain. glinazasoro@terra.es More than 50% of Parkinson's disease (PD) patients treated with L-dopa develop L-dopa-induced dyskinesias (LIDs) in the long term. Some patients exhibit severe dyskinesias soon after starting low doses of L-dopa, whereas other patients remain free of this disabling complication despite treatment with L-dopa. Avoiding or delaying the appearance of LIDs is one of the main objectives of the management of PD. Plasticity of the brain to adapt to a progressive disease, together with a non-physiological treatment strategy, might be the key physiopathological element that underlies LIDs. Neural plasticity varies among patients according to age and genetics. Thus, I propose that this variation explains the observed differences in the occurrence of LIDs in PD patients. Furthermore, I suggest that denervation and L-dopa treatment act as modulating and triggering factors of LIDs, respectively. In this article, the practical implications of these ideas and the role of pharmacogenetics in PD treatment are discussed. Treatment decisions are likely to rely on this information, challenging the relevance of current 'hot' debates about how to start treatment in PD. Publication Types: Review

Trends Pharmacol Sci. 2005 Nov;26(11):558-63. Epub 2005 Sep 26. Related Articles, Links Therapeutic wisdom in traditional Chinese medicine: a perspective from modern science. Jiang WY. Department of Integrated Traditional Chinese and Western Medicine, Peking University Health Science Center, Beijing 100083, PR China. Wyjiang@bjmu.edu.cn The reasons why the standards of evaluating Western medicine are not suitable for testing traditional Chinese medicine (TCM) are explicit in the therapeutic objective and principles of TCM. TCM aims to correct maladjustments and restore the self-regulatory ability of the body, and not to antagonize specific pathogenetic targets. Maladjustments in a disease can be classified into several 'patterns' according to TCM theory. Multiple diseases might share one 'pattern' and be treated by the same herbal formula whereas one disease might display several different 'patterns' and be treated by multiple formulae. These principles are supported by evidence that multi-system changes in one pattern can be modulated by a herbal formula. The approaches used in systems biology and pharmacogenetics are similar to the practices of TCM. I propose that a combined approach using specific parameters associated with modern medicine, the general condition of individuals, as outlined by TCM, and pattern stratification of diseases should be employed to re-evaluate herbal formulae.

Trends Pharmacol Sci. 2005 Sep;26(9):443-7. Related Articles, Links Using genotyping to predict responses to anti-hypertensive treatment. Kurland L, Lind L, Melhus H. Department of Medical Sciences, Uppsala University Hospital, 751 85 Uppsala, Sweden. lisa.kurland@medsci.uu.se Hypertension is prevalent and affects approximately 1 in every 4 adults in the Western world. Although many drugs are effective in treating hypertension, an individual's response to treatment is unpredictable. Pharmacogenetics holds the promise of becoming a tool to predict this response but obstacles and shortcomings need to be overcome. Significant developments in molecular biology, including the sequencing of the genome, the cataloguing of genetic variation and the development of microarray techniques, enable analysis of many genotypes simultaneously. However, despite these technical advances there are, as yet, no clinical applications of pharmacogenetics in anti-hypertensive treatment. It is therefore necessary to design prospective pharmacogenetic studies that aim to identify a genetic profile that will predict the response to anti-hypertensive treatment.

Trends Pharmacol Sci. 2006 Feb;27(2):92-6. Epub 2006 Jan 6. Related Articles, Links Recent developments in constitutive receptor activity and inverse agonism, and their potential for GPCR drug discovery. Bond RA, Ijzerman AP. Department of Pharmacological and Pharmaceutical Sciences, University of Houston, 4800 Calhoun, Houston, TX 77204-5037, USA. The concept of constitutively active G-protein-coupled receptors is now firmly rooted in receptor pharmacology. Many independent research groups have contributed to its acceptance since its introduction by Costa and Herz in 1989. This concept necessitated a revised ligand classification, and a new category of inverse agonists was introduced alongside existing agonist and antagonist ligands. Initially, it was hoped that new therapeutic modalities would become available. However, the drug industry has not adopted inverse agonism as a design criterion and instead accepted that some compounds emerge as (neutral) antagonists in compound screening, whereas other compounds possess inverse agonistic activity. In this article, we summarize aspects of the impact of constitutive activity on the drug-discovery process: for example, its use in orphan receptor assays, its link with pharmacogenetics and genomics, and its relevance for currently marketed drugs.

Tumori. 2004 Jul-Aug;90(4):13-27. Related Articles, Links [ASCO Annual Meeting 2004, New Orleans. Therapeutic options in colorectal cancer] [Article in Italian] Longo F, Mansueto G. Oncologia Medica, Policlinico Umberto I, Roma. Publication Types: Congresses

Tumori. 2005 Nov-Dec;91(6):suppl 11-22. Related Articles, Links [Docetaxel and novel strategies in the treatment of NSCLC] [Article in Italian] Longo F, Mansueto G. Servizio di Oncologia Medica, Policlinico Umberto I, Roma. Publication Types: Review

Turk J Gastroenterol. 2004 Mar;15(1):21-6. Related Articles, Links The mutations in ISDR of NS5A gene are not associated with response to interferon treatment in Turkish patients with chronic hepatitis C virus genotype 1b infection. Aslan N, Bozdayi AM, Cetinkaya H, Sarioglu M, Turkay C, Bozkaya H, Karayalcin S, Yurtaydin C, Uzunalimoglu O. Institute of Hepatology, School of Medicine, Ankara University, Ankara, Turkey. BACKGROUND/AIMS: A significant association between variations in amino acid sequences resides between 2209-2248 nucleotides of HCV non-structural 5A (NS5A) gene, and response to interferon treatment has been proposed. The aim of this study was to determine whether the amino acid sequence changes in ISDR could be correlated to response to alpha interferon treatment in Turkish patients infected with HCV genotypes 1b and 1a. METHODS: Thirty-nine patients with chronic C virus infection (35 and 4 patients with genotype 1b and 1a, respectively), receiving 3x3-5 MU of interferon a-2b for six months were included in the study. Following PCR amplification of the region from pre-treatment serum samples, the products were directly sequenced. The amino acid sequence of NS5A was compared with the published sequence for HCV-J (AA 2209-2248). Mutant type was defined as three or more amino acid mutations, and intermediate type as 1-3 amino acids in this region. Otherwise, they were defined as the wild type (no amino acid mutations). HCV RNA serum viremia levels were analyzed by branched DNA assay. RESULTS: Eighteen patients were responders (R; 46%), whereas 21 patients were non-responders (NR; 54%). Amino acid changes in both R and NR groups did not show significant difference. Intermediate or wild type strains were detected in both groups. CONCLUSIONS: In this study, we could not determine a significant association between number of amino acid changes in NS5A2209-2248 and response to interferon treatment. In the majority of the patients, it seems that amino acid sequences in this region are well conserved.

Twin Res. 2004 Oct;7(5):435-48. Related Articles, Links Pharmacogenetics of nicotine metabolism in twins: methods and procedures. Swan GE, Benowitz NL, Jacob P 3rd, Lessov CN, Tyndale RF, Wilhelmsen K, Krasnow RE, McElroy MR, Moore SE, Wambach M. Center for Health Sciences, SRI International, Menlo Park, California 94025, USA. gary.swan@sri.com This article describes a pharmacogenetic investigation of nicotine metabolism in twins. One hundred and thirty-nine twin pairs (110 monozygotic and 29 dizygotic) were recruited and assessed for smoking status, zygosity, and health conditions known or suspected to affect drug metabolism. Participants underwent a 30-minute infusion of stable isotope-labeled nicotine and its major metabolite, cotinine, followed by an 8-hour in-hospital stay. Blood and urine samples were taken at regular intervals for analysis of nicotine, cotinine, and metabolites by gas chromatography-mass spectrometry or liquid chromatography-mass spectrometry and subsequent characterization of pharmacokinetic phenotypes. DNA was genotyped to confirm zygosity and for variation in the primary gene involved in nicotine metabolism, CYP2A6. Univariate and multivariate biometric analyses planned for the future will determine genetic and environmental influences on each pharmacokinetic measure individually and in combination with each other, and in the presence and absence of covariates, including measured genotype. When the analyses are completed, this study will result in a more complete characterization of the impact of genetic and environmental influences on nicotine and cotinine metabolic pathways than has heretofore been reported. The approach taken, with its use of a quantitative model of nicotine metabolism, highly refined metabolic phenotypes, measured genotype, and advanced tools for biometric genetic analysis, provides a model for the use of twins in next-generation studies of complex drug-metabolism phenotypes. Publication Types: Twin Study

Ugeskr Laeger. 2005 May 16;167(20):2141. Related Articles, Links [Pharmacogenetics--new therapeutic possibilities] [Article in Danish] Ainsworth MA, Nielsen OH. Publication Types: Editorial

Ugeskr Laeger. 2005 May 16;167(20):2143-6. Related Articles, Links [Classical pharmacogenetics] [Article in Danish] Brosen K. Syddansk Universitet, Institut for Sundhedstjenesteforskning, Klinisk Farmakologi, Odense C. kbrosen@health.sdu.dk

Ugeskr Laeger. 2005 May 16;167(20):2146-50. Related Articles, Links [Pharmacogenetic-assisted drug development. Regulatory aspects from the viewpoint of the Medical Products Agency] [Article in Danish] Theilade MD. mdt@dkma.dk Publication Types: Review

Ugeskr Laeger. 2005 May 16;167(20):2150-3. Related Articles, Links [Lifestyle medicine and pharmacogenetics--individualised drug therapy] [Article in Danish] Moldrup C. Danmarks Farmaceutiske Universitet, Institut for Samfundsfarmaci, Kobenhavn O. cm@dfuni.dk Publication Types: Review

Ugeskr Laeger. 2005 May 16;167(20):2153-5. Related Articles, Links [The future of pharmacogenetics--cost-effectiveness and barriers] [Article in Danish] Gyrd-Hansen D. Syddansk Universitet, Institut for Sundhedstjenesteforskning, Enhed for Sundhedsokonomi. dgh@sam.sdu.dk

Ugeskr Laeger. 2005 May 16;167(20):2156-60. Related Articles, Links [Drug targets: identification and evaluation] [Article in Danish] Mikkelsen JD. Neurosearch A/S, Ballerup. JDM@Neurosearch.dk Publication Types: Review

Ugeskr Laeger. 2005 May 16;167(20):2160-4. Related Articles, Links [Pharmacogenetic/regulatory aspects seen from the viewpoint of the industry] [Article in Danish] Hansen L, Andersen D. Novo Nordisk A/S, Malov. larh@novonordisk.Com Publication Types: Review

Ugeskr Laeger. 2005 May 16;167(20):2164-7. Related Articles, Links [Genomic classification of diseases] [Article in Danish] Orntoft TF. Arhus Universitetshospital, Skejby Sygehus, Klinisk Biokemisk Afdeling.

Ugeskr Laeger. 2005 May 16;167(20):2168-70. Related Articles, Links [How far are we from the clinical use of array technology?] [Article in Danish] Csillag C, Nielsen OH, Borup R, Nielsen FC. Amtssygehuset i Herlev, Medicinsk Gastroenterologisk Afdeling C. claudio@dadlnet.dk

Ugeskr Laeger. 2005 May 16;167(20):2170-2. Related Articles, Links [Toxicology and pharmacogenetics] [Article in Danish] Dalhoff KP, Poulsen HE. H:S Rigshospitalet, Klinisk Farmakologisk Afdeling Q 7642, Kobenhavn. dalhoff@rh.dk

Ugeskr Laeger. 2005 May 16;167(20):2173-6. Related Articles, Links [Genetic variations in the metabolism of environmental toxins] [Article in Danish] Autrup H. Aarhus Universitet, Det Sundhedsvidenskabelige Fakultet, Institut for Folkesundhed, Afdelingen for Miljo- og Arbejdsmedicin. ha@mil.au.dk Publication Types: Review

Ugeskr Laeger. 2005 May 16;167(20):2177-9. Related Articles, Links [Individual monitoring of thiopurine and methotrexate treatment] [Article in Danish] Baslund B, Dalhoff KP, Schmiegelow K. H:S Rigshospitalet, Reumatologisk Klinik, Klinisk Farmakologisk Afdeling. baslund@rh.hosp.dk

Ugeskr Laeger. 2005 May 16;167(20):2180-3. Related Articles, Links [Designer drugs and their rational use in clinical hematology] [Article in Danish] Bukh A, D'Amore FA, Gimsing P, Hasselbalch HC, Johnsen HE, Kerndrup GB, Kristensen JS, Peterslund NA; Dansk Haematologisk Selskabs arbejdsgruppe vedr; DMCG Haematologi. Arhus Universitetshospital, Aalborg Sygehus, Haematologisk Afdeling.

Ugeskr Laeger. 2005 May 16;167(20):2183-5. Related Articles, Links [Biomarkers: medical tradition and a brave new world] [Article in Danish] Hansen L. Novo Nordisk A/S, Malov. larh@novonordisk.com

Ugeskr Laeger. 2005 May 16;167(20):2191-3. Related Articles, Links [Status of and perspectives on psychiatric genomic medicine] [Article in Danish] Mors NP, Borglum AD. Arhus Universitetshospital, Psykiatrisk Hospital i Arhus, Center for Psykiatrisk Grundforskning, Risskov. om@psykiatri.aaa.dk

Ugeskr Laeger. 2005 May 16;167(20):2194-6. Related Articles, Links [Psychopharmacology in a genomic perspective] [Article in Danish] Werge T, Kessing LV. H:S Sct. Hans Hospital, Forskningsinstitut for Biologisk Psykiatri. thomas.werge@shh.hosp.dk

Ugeskr Laeger. 2005 May 16;167(20):2199-200. Related Articles, Links [Future expectations when it comes to pharmacogenetics] [Article in Danish] Anderson T. Publication Types: Letter

Vascul Pharmacol. 2006 Feb;44(2):107-18. Epub 2005 Dec 13. Related Articles, Links Pharmacogenetics of antihypertensive treatment. Arnett DK, Claas SA, Glasser SP. Department of Epidemiology, University of Alabama, RPHB 220E, 1530 3rd Avenue South, Birmingham, 55294-0022, USA. arnett@uab.edu Hypertension is a common disorder associated with increased cardiovascular morbidity and mortality. Unfortunately, in the US only about one-third of those who are aware of their hypertensive status have their blood pressure adequately controlled. One reason for this is the variable and unpredictable response individuals have to pharmacologic treatment. Clinicians often resort to "trial-and-error" to match patients with effective drug treatment. Hypertension pharmacogenetics seeks to find genetic predictors of drug response. To date, more than forty studies have investigated associations between genetic polymorphisms and response to antihypertensive drugs. Angiotensin-converting enzyme inhibitors and beta blockers have been most frequently studied, followed by angiotensin II blockers, diuretics, adrenergic alpha-agonists, and calcium channel blockers. Renin-angiotensin-aldosterone system genes have been the most widely studied, with the angiotensin-converting enzyme I/D variant being typed in about one-half of all hypertension pharmacogenetic studies. In total, 160 possible gene polymorphism-drug interactions have been explored, with about one-quarter of these showing that genes predict drug response. However, disparate and conflicting findings have been the rule rather than the exception, and the discovery of clinically relevant antihypertensive drug-response genes remains elusive. While there is a growing enthusiasm that pharmacogenetics of hypertension is important, the translation of pharmacogenetic findings to clinical practice in the future will depend on additional studies to enhance our pharmacogenetics knowledge base, the availability of pharmacogenetic screening tests that are affordable and easy to implement in clinical practice, a cohort of clinicians who are trained to interpret genetic test results, and health care systems that pay for them. Caution regarding the future of hypertension pharmacogenetics is warranted.

Vascul Pharmacol. 2006 Feb;44(2):119-25. Epub 2005 Dec 15. Related Articles, Links Pharmacogenetics: progress, pitfalls and clinical potential for coronary heart disease. Humphries SE, Hingorani A. Centre for Cardiovascular Genetics, British Heart Foundation Laboratories Rayne Building, Royal Free and University College London Medical School, London WC1E 6JF, UK. Much has been written about the potential of pharmacogenetic testing to inform therapy based on an individual's genetic makeup, and to decide the most effective choice of available drugs, or to avoid dangerous side effects. Currently, there is little hard data for either in the field of cardiovascular disease. The usual approach has been opportunistic use of drug trials in unrelated patients, and to look for differences in response or outcome by "candidate gene" genotype, for example genes coding for drug metabolising enzymes (activators and metabolisers), and enzymes and receptors involved in lipid metabolism, adrenergic response, etc. As with all association studies, initially promising results have often failed the test of replication in larger studies, and the relationship between the CETP Taq-I variant and response to statins has now been disproved. The strongest data to date is the report [Chasman, D.I., Posada, D., Subrahmanyan, L., Cook, N.R., Stanton Jr., V.P., Ridker, P.M., 2004. Pharmacogenetic study of statin therapy and cholesterol reduction. J. Am. Med. Assoc. 291, 2821-2827] of a poorer cholesterol-lowering response to Pravastatin in the 7% of patients carrying a certain haplotype of the HMG CoA reductase gene (14% fall versus 19%), but if this is overcome simply by a higher dose, it is of little clinical relevance. Currently, the best example of avoiding side effects is determining genotype at the CYP2C9 locus with respect of warfarin treatment, since carriers for functional variants (>20% of the population) require lower doses for optimal anticoagulation, and homozygotes, although rare, may well experience serious bleeding if given a usual dose. The full potential of this field will only be realised with much further work.

Vascul Pharmacol. 2006 Feb;44(2):65. Epub 2005 Dec 15. Related Articles, Links Pharmacogenetics and Heart disease. Talmud PJ. Department of Medicine, University College London, 5 University St., London WC1E 6JF, UK. Publication Types: Editorial

Vascul Pharmacol. 2006 Feb;44(2):66-74. Epub 2005 Dec 22. Related Articles, Links Pharmacogenetics of multigenic disease: heart disease as an example. Cooke GE. Davis Heart and Lung Research Institute and Division of Cardiovascular Medicine, Department of Internal Medicine, College of Medicine, The Ohio State University, 235 DHLRI, 473 W. 12th Ave., Columbus, 43210-1252, USA. glen.cooke@osumc.edu We now have a greater understanding of the workings of the human genome as well as a wide assortment of pharmacological and mechanical therapies that clearly improve mortality and quality of life for our patients with cardiovascular disease, but these areas of therapeutics and genomics have essentially advanced independently with little interaction up until recently. Pharmacogenetics is the study of the effect of a medication as it relates to single or defined sets of genes. A major goal will be to integrate the two so that true personalized therapy can be delivered. This review explores the clinical implications of the complex interactions in multigenic disease and pharmacology with examples of atherosclerosis and heart failure. The therapies of today are the direct result of understanding the epidemiological, molecular and genetic basis of cardiovascular disease with the application to clinical practice. The complexity of multigenic disease and the promise of pharmacogenetics will require that we improve on the methods of drug evaluation and this includes the need for new statistical methods, bioinformatics, and novel clinical trial design with sufficient power to detect differences in therapy. There must be a continued effort to apply biological and mechanistic plausibility in understanding disease and pharmacology but openness to new ideas and concepts, especially in understanding the workings of the genome.

Vascul Pharmacol. 2006 Feb;44(2):90-106. Epub 2005 Dec 15. Related Articles, Links Pharmacogenetics and cardiac ion channels. Roepke TK, Abbott GW. Greenberg Division of Cardiology, Department of Medicine, Cornell University, Weill Medical College, 520 East 70th Street, New York, NY 10021, USA. Ion channels control electrical excitability in living cells. In mammalian heart, the opposing actions of Na(+) and Ca(2+) ion influx, and K(+) ion efflux, through cardiac ion channels determine the morphology and duration of action potentials in cardiac myocytes, thus controlling the heartbeat. The last decade has seen a leap in our understanding of the molecular genetic origins of inherited cardiac arrhythmia, largely through identification of mutations in cardiac ion channels and the proteins that regulate them. Further, recent advances have shown that 'acquired arrhythmias', which occur more commonly than inherited arrhythmias, arise due to a variety of environmental factors including side effects of therapeutic drugs and often have a significant genetic component. Here, we review the pharmacogenetics of cardiac ion channels-the interplay between genetic and pharmacological factors that underlie human cardiac arrhythmias.

Versicherungsmedizin. 2006 Mar 1;58(1):9-13. Related Articles, Links [Biochips--tools of 21st century medicine] [Article in German] Burger J. Kompetenzzentrum Biowissenschaften der Munchener Ruckversicherungs-Gesellschaft. In the next years biochips will enter into clinical medicine. Each larger diagnostics laboratory will offer genetic tests with this method. In this article the potential of biochips is shown by two examples: Differentiation and prognosis in breast cancer and individualized drug therapy (pharmacogenetics). In cancer the gene expression profile permits an accuracy of differentiation and prognosis that was impossible so far. Already soon oncologists will make their therapeutic decisions on the basis of biochip-based gene expression profiles. For an individualized drug therapy extensive genetic tests must be accomplished, above all of the cytochrome P450 system. An already available biochip seems to make this possible reliably and economically. Moreover, in science biochips will play a substantial role in the analysis of the genetic basis of common diseases. If these diseases are understood once, the clinical use of biochips will open an enormous potential for a predictive medicine. Biochips are a relevant topic for insurers--partially already today, much more however in the future.

Vestn Ross Akad Med Nauk. 2004;(10):40-5. Related Articles, Links [Pharmacogenetics and modern medicine] [Article in Russian] Liakhovich VV, Vavilin VA, Grishanova AIu, Makarova SI, Kovalenko SP.

Washburn Law J. 2003 Spring;42(3):575-99. Related Articles, Links Comment in: Washburn Law J. 2003 Spring;42(3):601-

14. Washburn Law J. 2003 Spring;42(3):615-21. Pushing drugs: genomics and genetics, the pharmaceutical industry, and the law of negligence. Feldman HL. Georgetown University Law Center, Washington, DC, USA.

Washburn Law J. 2003 Spring;42(3):601-14. Related Articles, Links Comment on: Washburn Law J. 2003 Spring;42(3):575-99. Causes for concern and causes of action: a comment on "Pushing drugs". Brownsword R. University of Sheffield, England. Publication Types: Comment

Washburn Law J. 2003 Spring;42(3):615-21. Related Articles, Links Comment on: Washburn Law J. 2003 Spring;42(3):575-99. Genomic torts: a response to Professor Feldman. Rich WJ. Washburn University School of Law, USA. Publication Types: Comment

Washington Post. 2004 Nov 16;:F1, F4. Related Articles, Links A cure for a race? Heart drug findings set off ethics debate. Payne JW. Publication Types: Newspaper Article

Wien Med Wochenschr. 2005 Feb;155(3-4):44. Related Articles, Links [Pharmacogenomics] [Article in German] Hitzenberger G. Publication Types: Editorial

Wien Med Wochenschr. 2005 Feb;155(3-4):45-9. Related Articles, Links [Drug therapy and pharmacogenomics--hopes and facts] [Article in German] Muller-Zellenberg U, Muller M. Universitatsklinik fur Klinische Pharmakologie, Medizinische Universitat Wien, Wien, Osterreich. Recent achievements in molecular genetics, in particular the characterization of a large number of non-synonymous single-nucleotide polymorphisms (ns-SNPs) have led to a substantial accumulation of knowledge about the mechanisms of interindividual variability in drug response. The concept of elucidating drug reactions by genetic analysis is termed "pharmacogenomics". Pharmacogenomics is set to provide a relevant contribution to our understanding of adverse drug reactions and non-responsiveness to drug therapy and may help realize the vision of providing individualized therapies. The greatest challenges for the field of pharmacogenomics relate to the issues of genotype-phenotype- and genotype-environment- interactions, optimal selection of study designs, predictivity and ethical aspects. Although its current impact on the routine of medicine is minimal, it is likely that pharmacogenomics will provide important contributions to the practice of drug therapy. Pharmacogenetic concepts may prove important for approximately 20% of therapeutic drugs.

Wien Med Wochenschr. 2005 Feb;155(3-4):54-8. Related Articles, Links [Therapeutic implications of polymorphisms in cytochromes and drug transporters] [Article in German] Munster E, Ziegler S, Brunner M. Universitatsklinik fur Klinische Pharmakologie, Medizinische Universitat Wien, Wien, Osterreich. There is great heterogeneity in the way individuals respond to drug therapy. Reasons for this variability include pathophysiological or environmental factors, drug interactions or genetic influences. Among those influences are polymorphisms in drug-metabolizing enzymes, such as Cytochrom-P-450 (CYP) 2D6, CYP2C9 or CYP2C19 or genetic variants in enzymes coding for drug transporters, such as P-Glycoprotein. Polymorphisms might cause changes in drug pharmacokinetics and consequently drug efficacy after administration of recommended standard drug doses.

Reduced enzyme activity can either result in a higher percentage of drug side-effects, or an augmented drug response due to increased target site concentrations. Conversely, intensified catalytic enzymatic activity might lead to subtherapeutic drug concentrations. In the future, genetic screening by genotyping before the initiation of pharmacotherapy might help to identify responders or non-responders and might it offer individualized therapies to select patient populations.

WMJ. 2005 Aug;104(6):61-6. Related Articles, Links Gene-based drug prescribing: clinical implications of the cytochrome P450 genes. Musana AK, Wilke RA. Department of General Internal Medicine, Marshfield Clinic, WI, USA. The Institute of Medicine recently mandated an increased effort to improve patient safety and reduce medical error. With the description of genetic polymorphisms in the drug metabolizing enzymes, the field of pharmacogenetics may improve medical care through a reduction in both therapeutic failure and adverse drug reaction. Investigators at the Marshfield Clinic in central Wisconsin are piloting the process of gene-based drug prescribing in a variety of contexts. This paper reviews the field of cytochrome P450 (CYP) genetics and explores factors that impact the utility of this information in clinical practice. Publication Types: Review

World J Biol Psychiatry. 2005;6 Suppl 2:23-30. Related Articles, Links Some biological correlates of drug resistance in schizophrenia: a multidimensional approach. Altamura AC, Bassetti R, Cattaneo E, Vismara S. Department of Psychiatry, Hospital Luigi Sacco, University of Milan, Via G.B. Grassi 74, 20157 Milan, Italy. c.altamura@hsacco.it Drug resistance in schizophrenic disorders treated with an antipsychotic medication is highly problematic, lacking sound criteria to define it, and to discriminate between drug response and clinical remission. This article reviews some neurochemical, psychoimmunological, pharmacogenetic and neuromorphological patterns which can affect drug response and determine drug-resistance phenomena in schizophrenia. Several neurochemical abnormalities have been reported to be relevant for the pathogenesis of schizophrenic disorders and have been related to clinical symptoms as well as to the quality of response to antipsychotics: most of the findings come from studies on DA and 5HT brain metabolism, but more recently other non-dopaminergic pathways have been implicated (e.g., glutamatergic ones). Literature data suggest that schizophrenia may be associated with significant alterations of T-cell functions, showing the activation of the inflammatory response system (IRS), particularly in treatment-resistant schizophrenia, and differential effects on IRS have been reported for conventional and atypical antipsychotics. Furthermore molecular genetic approaches provide a novel method of dissecting the heterogeneity of psychotropic drug response, providing the means of determining the molecular substrates of drug efficacy and drug-induced adverse events. On the other hand, functional neuroimaging techniques, including single photon emission computed tomography (SPECT), positron emission tomography (PET) and functional magnetic resonance imaging (FMRI), providing an in vivo assessment of the expression and function of neuroreceptors, transporters and enzymes, seem to be particularly promising for a better understanding of 'real' drug resistance. Finally, a multidimensional approach taking into account all these variables in the future would likely be the more valuable strategy to optimise response, reducing relapses or resistant clinical situations. Publication Types: Lectures

World J Gastroenterol. 2005 Sep 28;11(36):5721-4. Related Articles, Links Relationship of human leukocyte antigen class II genes with the susceptibility to hepatitis B virus infection and the response to interferon in HBV-infected patients. Han YN, Yang JL, Zheng SG, Tang Q, Zhu W. Research Unit of Liver Diseases, Shanghai 8th People's Hospital, Shanghai 200235, China. hanyn88@163.com AIM: To study the relationship of human leukocyte antigen (HLA)-DRB1 and -DQB1 alleles with the genetic susceptibility to HBV infection and the response to interferon (IFN) in HBV-infected patients. METHODS: Low-resolution DNA typing kit was used to determine HLA-DR-1 and -DQB1 genes in 72 patients with chronic hepatitis B (CHB) and HLA-DRB1 in 200 healthy people ready to donate their bone marrow in Shanghai. Among CHB patients, 35 were treated with IFNalpha-1b for 24 wk. RESULTS: The frequencies of HLA-DRB1*06, DRB1*08 and DRB1*16 alleles in 72 patients were higher than in 200 healthy people (2.08% vs 0%, OR = 3.837, P = 0.018; 11.11% vs 5.50%, OR = 2.148, P = 0.034; and 6.94% vs 3.00%, OR = 0.625, P = 0.049, respectively); whereas that of DRB1*07 allele was lower (2.78% vs 7.75%, OR = 0.340, P = 0.046). The frequency of HLA-DRB1* 14 allele was higher in 11 responders to IFN compared with 24 non-responders (18.18% vs 2.08%, OR = 10.444, P = 0.031), whereas that of DQB1*07 allele was inverse (9.09% vs 37.50%, OR = 0.167, P = 0.021). CONCLUSION: The polymorphism of HLA class II may influence the susceptibility to HBV infection and the response to IFN in studied CHB patients. Compared with other HLA-DRB1 alleles, HLA-DRB1*06, DRB1*08, and DRB1*16 may be associated with chronicity of HBV infection, HLA-DRB1*07 with protection against HBV infection, and HLA-DRB1*14 allele may be associated with a high rate of the response of CHB patients to IFN treatment. Compared with other HLA-DQB1 alleles, HLA-DQB1*07 may be associated with low response rate to IFN. Publication Types: Clinical Trial

Yakugaku Zasshi. 2004 Jun;124(6):293-9. Related Articles, Links [Analysis and its application for prevention of side-effects of drugs and for evaluation of drug responsiveness] [Article in Japanese] Inoue K. Department of Pharmaceutical Science, Akita University Hospital, Japan. kazinoue@hos.akita-u.ac.jp The response of patients to drugs can be affected by genetic polymorphisms/defects in drug metabolizing enzymes, transporters, and receptors. Genetic polymorphisms/defects are generated by mutation of coding regions and/or noncoding regions of target genes, such as single-point mutations, deletions/insertions, variation in the number of tandem repeats, etc. If a genetic defect in a patient which affects drug response were known, it would be possible to optimize medications individually. The author developed two improved methods for detecting CYP2C19(*)2 and CYP2C19(*)3. Using the methods, the type of CYP2C19 gene was examined in 80 inpatients, and the medication status of patients with the mutation was examined focusing on dosage and side effects. The author also examined polymorphisms of the serotonin transporter/biosynthetic or metabolizing enzymes in depressive patients treated with fluvoxamine, a selective serotonin reuptake inhibitor, and the relationship between clinical efficacy and polymorphisms was investigated. As a result, patients with the S/S genotype of 5-HTTLPR were found to experience better clinical efficacy. Publication Types: Review

Yakugaku Zasshi. 2005 Apr;125(4):337-47. Related Articles, Links From physical pharmacy to clinical pharmacology. Nakano M. Department of Clinical Pharmaceutics, Graduate School of Pharmaceutical Sciences, University of Shizuoka, Shizuoka 422-8526, Japan. nakano_mshr@yahoo.co.jp Research works on molecular interactions in solutions were carried out at School of Pharmacy, the University of Wisconsin under the direction of Prof. T. Higuchi and at Faculty of Pharmaceutical Sciences, Kyoto University under the direction of Prof. H. Sezaki. Studies on permeation of drugs through polymer membranes were carried out at Faculty of Pharmacy and Pharmaceutical Sciences, University of Alberta, Edmonton, Canada and at Pharmaceutical Chemistry Research Laboratories at Food and Drug Directorate, Department of Health and Welfare, Canada. Studies on modification of delivery patterns by means of pharmaceutical approaches were carried out at Faculty of Pharmaceutical Sciences, Hokkaido University. Topics related to modification of drug delivery patterns include employment of amorphous forms such as ground mixture with micro-crystalline cellulose and coprecipitate with polyvinylpyrrolidone, use of biodegradable polymers such as polylactic acid and polycarbonates, gel-forming materials such as konjac, agar and hydroxypropylcellulose, and physicochemical systems such as complexation. Works related to drug delivery and disposition of drugs in humans were carried out at Department of Pharmacy, Kumamoto University Hospital. Topics related to drug delivery in humans include injections containing anticancer drugs for intra-arterial administration, lidocaine gels for dermal anesthesia, glucagon solution for nasal administration. Topics related to disposition of drugs in humans include clinical pharmacokinetic studies in infants and elderly and medical uses of adsorbents. Publication Types: Review

Yi Chuan Xue Bao. 2006 Feb;33(2):93-104. Related Articles, Links MDR1 gene polymorphisms and clinical relevance. Li YH, Wang YH, Li Y, Yang L. Laboratory of Pharmaceutical Resource Discovery, Dalian Institute of Chemical Physics, Chinese Academy of Sciences, Dalian 116023, China. In vivo and in vitro studies have demonstrated that P-glycoprotein (P-gp) plays a very significant role in the ADME processes (absorption, distribution, metabolism, excretion) and drug-drug interaction (DDI) of drugs in humans. P-gp is the product of multidrug resistance gene (MDR1/ABCB1). Pharmacogenomics and pharmacogenetics studies have revealed that genetic polymorphisms of MDR1 are associated with alteration in P-gp expression and function in different ethnicities and subjects. By now, 50 single nucleotide polymorphisms (SNPs) and 3 insertion/deletion polymorphisms have been found in the MDR1 gene. Some of them, such as C3435T, have been identified to be a risk factor for numerous diseases. It is believed that further understanding of the physiology and biochemistry of P-gp with respect to its genetic variations may be important for individualized pharmacotherapy. Therefore, based on the latest public information and our studies, this review focuses on the following four aspects: 1) the impact of P-gp on pharmacokinetics; 2)

MDR1 genetic polymorphisms and their impacts on pharmacogenetics; 3) relationship between altered P-gp expression and function and the MDR1(C3435T) SNP, and 4) relevance of MDR1 polymorphisms to certain human diseases.

Zh Nevrol Psikhiatr Im S S Korsakova. 2004;104(8):83-6. Related Articles, Links [Pharmacogenetic challenges in the treatment of mental diseases] [Article in Russian] Sukhanov VA, Piruzian LA. Publication Types: Review

Index

A

acceptance, 15, 175, 217, 245, 282, 285, 320, 341, 373, 399, 509, 561, 564, 574
access, 50, 147, 183, 290, 309, 349, 400, 406, 449
accounting, 348, 384
accumulation, 14, 20, 95, 205, 211, 282, 300, 357, 462, 533, 580
accuracy, 281, 293, 302, 311, 358, 360, 361, 375, 399, 416, 426, 448, 454, 480, 519, 579
acetaminophen, 385, 476, 518, 551, 562
acetone, 281
acetonitrile, 217, 358
achievement, 165, 442, 486
acid, 31, 41, 42, 43, 74, 76, 88, 107, 110, 113, 170, 195, 196, 217, 227, 229, 232, 233, 262, 264, 279, 281, 288, 331, 334, 337, 382, 385, 392, 394, 434, 444, 467, 471, 472, 476, 478, 525, 537, 548, 554, 557, 562, 566, 567, 574, 583
acidosis, 42
action potential, 324, 546, 579
activation, 14, 45, 76, 141, 161, 165, 181, 203, 211, 224, 229, 280, 300, 326, 338, 345, 360, 361, 362, 402, 443, 461, 465, 485, 512, 546, 549, 552, 562, 581
active transport, 357
activity level, 141, 187
acute asthma, 98
acute leukemia, 160, 248, 535
acute lymphoblastic leukemia, 15, 160, 181, 250, 325, 371, 486
acute renal failure, 261
adaptability, 253
adaptation, 147
addiction, 149, 390, 435, 474, 491, 501, 502, 517
adenine, 230, 473
adenocarcinoma, 187, 196, 533, 542
adenoma, 196
adenopathy, 261
adenosine, 131, 180
adenosine triphosphate, 131
ADHD, 175, 277, 412
adhesion, 199
adiponectin, 530
adiposity, 272
adjustment, 165, 187, 219, 364
administrators, 313
adolescence, 266
adolescents, 255, 325
ADP, 70, 536, 554
adrenoceptors, 205, 206, 495, 498
adrenocorticotropic hormone, 330
adsorption, 249
adulthood, 546
adults, 116, 120, 139, 149, 189, 197, 236, 285, 346, 377, 390, 431, 468, 523, 570, 573
adverse event, 147, 148, 162, 185, 189, 216, 233, 246, 247, 251, 321, 326, 338, 347, 366, 374, 390, 395, 428, 450, 483, 538, 539, 552, 559, 567, 581
advertisements, 373
advertising, 373
advocacy, 147
aetiology, 86, 303, 527
affect, 11, 13, 19, 22, 24, 45, 65, 85, 93, 124, 128, 130, 131, 153, 160, 172, 183, 196, 197, 203, 220, 221, 225, 227, 228, 238, 240, 242, 248, 251, 253, 264, 283, 293, 311, 334, 339, 344, 347, 351, 356, 361, 362, 379, 382, 390, 391, 392, 395, 408, 417, 419, 425, 427, 431, 466, 475, 477, 485, 491, 501, 503, 506, 515, 518, 521, 525, 526, 531, 566, 568, 572, 575, 581

affective disorder, 363, 528
African Americans, 211, 419, 422, 434
agar, 583
age, 7, 125, 136, 145, 147, 150, 163, 165, 182, 189, 207, 208, 212, 224, 236, 250, 252, 262, 266, 277, 285, 298, 303, 325, 327, 339, 364, 374, 375, 434, 438, 445, 452, 457, 459, 460, 465, 467, 477, 478, 488, 497, 523, 534, 536, 537, 541, 546, 549, 551, 553, 566, 570, 573
agent, 18, 23, 87, 97, 110, 129, 132, 195, 200, 210, 212, 261, 307, 350, 364, 369, 401, 418, 458, 555, 558
aggregates, 525
aggregation, 180, 209, 392, 405, 525, 536, 554
aging, 245, 437
aging population, 245
agonist, 14, 87, 143, 206, 220, 231, 236, 237, 243, 263, 273, 331, 392, 465, 505, 570, 574
agranulocytosis, 84, 90, 96, 99
AIDS, 128, 129, 164, 223, 265, 378, 555
airway epithelial cells, 279
airway inflammation, 399
akathisia, 99
alanine, 41, 52
albumin, 42
alcohol, 130, 134, 303, 384, 475, 491, 530, 551
alcohol consumption, 130, 384, 530
alcohol dependence, 130, 134, 530
alcohol use, 384, 475
alcohol withdrawal, 531
alcoholic cardiomyopathy, 130
alcoholics, 531
alcoholism, 101, 130, 134, 149, 389, 390, 491
aldosterone, 137, 138, 202, 207, 577
algorithm, 12, 51, 56, 80, 123, 209, 314, 319, 320, 347, 353, 399, 480, 484, 553
allele, 27, 37, 91, 92, 93, 94, 101, 125, 140, 145, 149, 151, 152, 153, 154, 156, 162, 164, 168, 178, 180, 183, 191, 196, 197, 203, 208, 210, 211, 212, 213, 215, 216, 218, 219, 222, 224, 226, 228, 229, 230, 232, 236, 239, 262, 267, 270, 275, 278, 291, 293, 296, 297, 302, 311, 319, 322, 329, 331, 339, 341, 343, 344, 359, 362, 367, 368, 374, 375, 379, 383, 386, 389, 390, 391, 410, 421, 431, 432, 434, 435, 455, 458, 459, 461, 464, 466, 467, 470, 472, 473, 475, 476, 477, 483, 484, 486, 501, 503, 512, 516, 517, 524, 525, 531, 550, 552, 566, 569, 582
allergens, 205, 570
allergic reaction, 19
allergy, 323
alpha interferon, 574
ALT, 327
alternative, 23, 33, 89, 127, 131, 143, 163, 173, 216, 234, 264, 311, 357, 388, 456, 479, 492
alternatives, 242, 552
alters, 53, 200, 278, 369, 390, 392, 491
altruism, 434
Alzheimer's disease, 127, 517
American Psychiatric Association, 97
amines, 244
amino acids, 42, 124, 170, 382, 394, 492, 575
aminoglycosides, ix, 103, 104, 105, 109, 113, 355
ammonia, 41, 42, 74
ammonium, 42, 217
amphiphilic compounds, 563
anabolism, 140, 514
analgesic, 154, 155, 194, 226, 380, 546
analgesic agent, 154, 155
anaphylaxis, 248
androgen, 315, 358, 380
androgens, 315, 489
anemia, 137
anesthetics, 89
angiogenesis, 23, 199, 272, 334, 542
angiography, 552
angiotensin converting enzyme, 32, 74, 138, 185
angiotensin II, 11, 183, 255, 276, 376, 436, 577
angiotensin receptor blockers, 139, 377
animals, viii, 40, 44, 50, 63, 71, 75, 78, 341, 416, 471, 530, 560, 564
annotation, 72, 174, 333, 393, 449
anorexia, 340
anorexia nervosa, 340
ANOVA, 191, 213, 236, 353, 471
antagonism, 87
anti-asthma, 14, 37
antibiotic, ix, 104, 115, 116, 117, 118, 370, 496
antibiotic resistance, ix, 104, 115, 117, 118
antibody, 132, 139, 177, 262
anticancer activity, 352, 394
anticancer drug, 14, 35, 132, 198, 256, 257, 308, 318, 331, 338, 343, 356, 364, 393, 394, 397, 409, 412, 442, 443, 445, 451, 498, 506, 519, 572, 583
anticoagulant, 136, 164, 188, 325, 391, 476, 501, 522
anticoagulation, 163, 164, 180, 182, 188, 230, 477, 551, 552, 578
anticonvulsant, 471

antidepressant, 148, 149, 162, 184, 293, 304, 340, 366, 412, 414, 424, 434, 463, 480, 481, 482, 526, 527, 528, 529, 532, 540
antiemetics, 212, 306
antigen, 9, 24, 139, 251
antihistamines, 307
antihypertensive agents, 255
antihypertensive drugs, 138, 437, 515, 577
anti-inflammatory agents, 40
anti-inflammatory drugs, 43, 133, 197, 261, 423, 570
antimicrobial therapy, x, 104, 114
antioxidant, 137, 315, 565
antipsychotic, 84, 94, 95, 96, 99, 147, 148, 303, 309, 420, 433, 457, 458, 501, 509, 513, 526, 527, 529, 538, 581
antipsychotic drugs, 84, 147, 309, 433, 457, 458, 501, 509, 513, 526, 527, 529
antiretrovirals, 129, 244
antisense, 10, 78, 144, 336, 370, 402, 446, 472
antisense oligonucleotides, 10, 144, 370
antisense RNA, 472
antitumor, 224, 355, 500
antiviral therapy, 535
anxiety, 133, 340, 390, 491
apnea, 503
apoptosis, 16, 20, 22, 23, 35, 36, 210, 257, 272, 370, 411, 413, 473, 519, 533, 550, 565
appropriate technology, 214
arginine, 231, 447, 465, 519
argument, 57, 340
aripiprazole, 134, 532
Aristotle, 1, 241
arrest, 137
arrhythmia, 85
ARs, 421, 465, 498
arsenic, 281, 285, 350
arterial hypertension, 255
arteriosclerosis, 44, 74
artery, 163
arthritis, 38, 40, 261, 275
articulation, 544
aryl hydrocarbon receptor, 279
Asia, 91, 125, 490
Asian Americans, 419
Asian countries, 490
aspartate, 37, 76, 474
assessment, 88, 119, 142, 144, 166, 185, 187, 188, 202, 205, 210, 238, 246, 253, 255, 265, 284, 285, 294, 295, 308, 313, 316, 326, 330, 341, 346, 368, 369, 387, 401, 411, 412, 422, 426, 445, 475, 486, 495, 499, 511, 557, 564, 565, 567, 570, 581
assignment, 70
association, viii, ix, 12, 37, 62, 79, 83, 88, 91, 92, 93, 94, 95, 98, 100, 101, 102, 104, 133, 139, 141, 142, 156, 157, 159, 163, 165, 177, 180, 191, 194, 199, 207, 213, 217, 220, 227, 235, 236, 254, 258, 259, 262, 274, 277, 285, 289, 290, 291, 292, 293, 294, 297, 304, 309, 315, 320, 329, 330, 331, 332, 333, 340, 342, 344, 359, 368, 373, 375, 384, 388, 396, 397, 398, 408, 409, 414, 420, 422, 431, 433, 435, 442, 455, 458, 464, 466, 467, 468, 470, 474, 480, 483, 487, 501, 503, 505, 506, 508, 510, 511, 512, 514, 517, 521, 523, 526, 528, 536, 538, 552, 566, 569, 572, 574, 578
assumptions, 145, 433, 545
asthenia, 187
asthma, 7, 11, 12, 14, 32, 40, 75, 137, 150, 151, 152, 205, 217, 220, 237, 240, 241, 253, 254, 313, 330, 331, 336, 337, 345, 399, 505, 509, 514, 523, 569, 570
asthmatic children, 331
asymptomatic, 159
atherosclerosis, 40, 43, 206, 347, 459, 464, 552, 578
ATP, 13, 195, 199, 202, 210, 258, 262, 264, 278, 312, 343, 404, 506, 514
atrial fibrillation, 163, 534
atrophy, 77, 98
attention, 90, 124, 149, 172, 173, 175, 185, 219, 222, 250, 259, 277, 292, 317, 333, 403, 423, 451, 463, 481, 485, 488, 493, 503, 528, 530
attitudes, 320, 351, 509
auditing, 316
Australasia, 221, 469
Australia, 125, 129, 151, 161, 168, 186, 272, 289, 396, 398, 400, 415, 456, 469, 500, 544, 546
Austria, 257, 406, 501, 507
authority, 225
autism, 358, 412
autoimmune disease, 261, 350
automation, 214, 418
autonomy, 292
autopsy, 89, 349
autosomal dominant, 89, 125, 459
autosomal recessive, 91, 314, 499
availability, 10, 40, 50, 101, 142, 158, 172, 176, 192, 198, 250, 292, 336, 340, 398, 455, 488, 509, 531, 571, 577
aversion, 147
avoidance, 364, 530, 549

awareness, 28, 85, 88, 235, 400, 496
Azathioprine, 9, 372, 397

B

BAC, 68, 282
bacteremia, 105, 111, 113, 116
bacteria, 104, 115, 118, 120, 265, 276, 288
bacterial infection, ix, 103
banking, 217, 267, 434
banks, 158, 556
barriers, 128, 253, 284, 290, 442, 488, 576
basal ganglia, 96
base pair, 6, 384
basic research, 17, 338, 423, 425, 497
Bayesian methods, 184
BBB, 555
behavior, 134, 175, 220, 236, 361, 385, 390, 433, 538, 559
behavioral genetics, 435
Beijing, 157, 326, 573
Belgium, 124, 238, 300, 338, 417
beneficial effect, 18, 310, 486
benign, 125, 369, 380
benign prostatic hyperplasia, 380
benzodiazepine, 383
beta blocker, 202, 203, 577
beta-2 agonist, 514
bias, 140, 289, 360
bile, 41, 43, 144, 558
bile acids, 41
bile duct, 144
bilirubin, 301, 339, 476, 518
binding, ix, 13, 24, 28, 41, 42, 49, 65, 69, 70, 76, 79, 88, 93, 101, 103, 104, 106, 110, 113, 114, 119, 121, 131, 167, 195, 200, 201, 210, 240, 258, 280, 312, 333, 334, 340, 343, 393, 394, 404, 436, 444, 462, 473, 506, 514, 552
bioavailability, 10, 253, 332, 355, 529
biodiversity, 28
bioethics, 516
bioinformatics, 6, 11, 21, 31, 32, 148, 175, 203, 204, 257, 283, 335, 353, 389, 393, 401, 409, 444, 559, 561, 579
biological activity, 177
biological consequences, 177
biological processes, 22, 72, 75
biological systems, viii, 39, 192, 427, 495, 562, 565
biomarkers, 25, 30, 133, 142, 144, 177, 179, 193, 198, 211, 222, 233, 246, 249, 251, 267, 280, 288, 294, 316, 317, 338, 341, 346, 366, 386, 401, 416, 425, 433, 486, 488, 493, 560, 563
biopsy, 151
biosensors, 126, 133, 526
biosynthesis, 77, 167, 473, 519, 563
biotechnology, vii, 1, 3, 10, 25, 144, 147, 183, 241, 246, 259, 335, 372, 401, 433, 490, 493, 504, 536, 570
bipolar disorder, 143, 193, 278, 412, 434, 481
bipolar illness, 434, 512
birth, 179, 266, 279, 400, 537
births, 499
bleeding, 163, 164, 318, 319, 551, 552, 553, 578
blends, 10
blocks, 157, 263, 297, 333, 362
blood, 13, 40, 42, 43, 44, 68, 69, 74, 78, 85, 116, 136, 138, 145, 151, 153, 183, 200, 207, 211, 215, 233, 234, 236, 244, 254, 255, 267, 276, 290, 297, 308, 349, 372, 375, 376, 377, 396, 415, 431, 439, 446, 447, 469, 478, 487, 504, 512, 515, 522, 537, 548, 551, 554, 567, 568, 569, 577
blood clot, 42, 522
blood cultures, 116
blood flow, 44, 74, 512
blood pressure, 42, 43, 85, 136, 138, 145, 183, 207, 236, 244, 254, 255, 276, 376, 377, 431, 439, 469, 487, 515, 537, 548, 577
blood pressure reduction, 376
blood-brain barrier, 13, 200, 290
bloodstream, 68
BMI, 262
body, vii, 1, 3, 5, 6, 10, 19, 22, 25, 26, 41, 84, 90, 128, 143, 147, 148, 182, 190, 233, 243, 275, 281, 285, 303, 359, 386, 390, 392, 427, 436, 439, 441, 459, 460, 467, 477, 487, 513, 517, 519, 529, 531, 549, 551, 555, 563, 573
body composition, 529
body mass index, 303, 459, 460, 467
body size, 182
body weight, 84, 90, 281, 392, 513, 531, 551, 555
bonding, 37
bone marrow, 40, 87, 97, 141, 222, 372, 397, 402, 582
bone marrow transplant, 87, 97
bone mass, 371
bounds, 184
bowel, 266, 318, 361, 448
brain, 7, 13, 40, 87, 88, 94, 98, 130, 143, 156, 175, 258, 291, 340, 360, 361, 390, 404, 409, 414, 433,

436, 438, 444, 482, 494, 527, 530, 531, 548, 573, 581
brain damage, 88, 98
brain tumor, 438
Brazil, 191, 219, 265, 359, 452, 572
breakdown, 77, 558
breast cancer, 23, 32, 36, 132, 136, 146, 186, 191, 192, 199, 210, 227, 252, 272, 306, 322, 362, 369, 506, 544, 579
breast milk, 221, 453
breastfeeding, 366
breeding, 268, 524
bronchial asthma, 506
bronchitis, 111
bronchoconstriction, 205
bronchodilator, 14, 205, 331
brothers, 88
browser, 334
buccal swabs, 273
buffer, 215, 217
burn, 372
business model, 146

C

C++, 174
caffeine, 89, 298
calcium, 201, 240, 276, 465, 473, 565, 577
calcium channel blocker, 577
calibration, 358
California, 126, 131, 136, 144, 157, 174, 175, 206, 211, 236, 248, 283, 309, 318, 340, 380, 388, 409, 414, 423, 425, 426, 427, 449, 452, 479, 492, 524, 525, 550, 560, 566, 575
Canada, 140, 141, 147, 174, 240, 255, 256, 292, 310, 319, 328, 379, 407, 429, 435, 441, 479, 481, 484, 486, 488, 498, 513, 518, 557, 569, 583
cancer, 3, 7, 12, 14, 15, 17, 22, 23, 29, 32, 34, 35, 36, 80, 87, 126, 127, 128, 130, 132, 136, 140, 142, 144, 146, 158, 161, 172, 187, 192, 194, 197, 198, 199, 200, 201, 204, 207, 208, 210, 211, 212, 222, 224, 227, 232, 233, 246, 247, 248, 251, 252, 254, 255, 256, 268, 271, 272, 273, 282, 294, 300, 301, 305, 307, 309, 312, 315, 316, 317, 330, 332, 338, 339, 343, 344, 352, 355, 356, 362, 363, 369, 380, 382, 397, 401, 403, 404, 411, 422, 423, 438, 441, 442, 443, 444, 445, 446, 449, 450, 451, 452, 456, 466, 478, 489, 492, 493, 499, 500, 502, 503, 506, 507, 513, 514, 519, 524, 526, 533, 534, 535, 538, 541, 542, 549, 571, 579
cancer cells, 142, 194, 195, 210, 257, 312, 352, 397, 402, 404
cancer progression, 24, 32, 198, 315
candida, 265
candida albicans, 265
candidates, 7, 22, 25, 144, 166, 167, 176, 205, 226, 254, 257, 271, 342, 365, 414, 474, 484, 498, 526, 536
CAP, 131, 337
capillary, 414
carbohydrate, 41, 76
carbohydrate metabolism, 76
carbon, 41, 42, 43, 74, 382, 441, 492
carcinogen, 561
carcinogenesis, 282, 351, 382, 442, 444, 533
carcinogenicity, 341, 564
carcinoma, 187, 211, 354, 542
CARD15, 494
cardiac arrhythmia, 579
cardiac muscle, 77
cardiomyopathy, 11, 239, 240, 534
cardiovascular disease, 11, 32, 35, 126, 136, 163, 185, 192, 207, 222, 241, 245, 303, 308, 327, 336, 347, 348, 392, 396, 484, 497, 534, 578
cardiovascular morbidity, 577
cardiovascular physiology, 308
cardiovascular risk, 207, 391
cardiovascular system, 347
Caribbean, 422
carrier, 41, 42, 200, 229, 295, 357, 473, 508
case study, 164, 235, 267, 324, 435, 544
catabolism, 131, 140, 514
catalytic activity, 91, 213, 260, 331
catatonic, 97
catecholamines, 170, 555
categorization, 404
catheter, 110, 116
cation, 200
Caucasian population, 296, 334, 458, 501, 516
Caucasians, 91, 130, 211, 215, 270, 296, 297, 321, 349, 435, 467, 479, 482, 499, 532
causal relationship, 53
causation, 291, 428
cDNA, 81, 182, 192, 257, 268, 282, 287, 288, 289, 350, 352, 393, 394, 409, 472, 476, 557, 560
cell, 15, 17, 22, 23, 29, 36, 44, 45, 80, 104, 127, 129, 132, 145, 146, 167, 169, 181, 195, 198, 203, 205, 210, 211, 224, 249, 251, 253, 257, 261, 272, 274, 278, 280, 284, 300, 305, 315, 325, 334, 345, 351, 357, 369, 370, 387, 398, 402, 409, 410, 411, 413,

417, 426, 444, 445, 448, 449, 454, 461, 472, 473, 485, 487, 490, 492, 499, 504, 524, 525, 533, 534, 542, 546, 549, 555, 557, 559, 564, 565, 581
cell culture, 44, 249, 409, 426
cell cycle, 23, 145, 210, 305, 402, 533, 557
cell death, 524
cell fate, 300
cell line, 195, 210, 211, 272, 300, 351, 357, 370, 413, 417, 504
cell membranes, 487
cell surface, 448
cellulose, 583
central nervous system, 84, 88, 129, 182, 200, 360, 361, 555
cerebellum, 89
cerebrospinal fluid, 88, 119
changing environment, 5, 25
channel blocker, 461
channels, 264, 274, 461, 579
chemical reactions, 284
chemokine receptor, 142
chemokines, 392, 519
chemoprevention, 248, 362, 380, 442, 490
chemopreventive agents, 423
chemotaxis, 392
chemotherapeutic agent, 9, 15, 24, 141, 194, 397, 400, 445, 451, 456, 508, 549
chemotherapy, 14, 87, 140, 161, 171, 186, 190, 191, 192, 195, 197, 198, 201, 207, 208, 211, 220, 227, 252, 255, 256, 271, 272, 306, 309, 317, 325, 330, 338, 339, 343, 344, 354, 355, 356, 363, 364, 398, 400, 401, 410, 413, 423, 445, 446, 449, 451, 485, 492, 499, 500, 502, 508, 514, 519, 524, 533, 541, 542, 549, 558, 571
childhood, 160, 197, 198, 250, 266, 277, 314, 325, 371, 400, 486, 523, 570
children, 15, 120, 150, 160, 161, 181, 189, 197, 220, 250, 255, 266, 274, 277, 285, 298, 314, 325, 346, 354, 359, 390, 400, 421, 423, 431, 450, 452, 534, 570
China, 123, 125, 157, 267, 326, 341, 416, 491, 552, 573, 582, 583
Chinese medicine, 573
chirality, 176
cholesterol, 41, 43, 76, 79, 131, 132, 167, 168, 190, 191, 219, 241, 337, 347, 379, 459, 473, 563, 578
cholinesterase, 12
cholinesterase inhibitors, 12
chromatography, 177, 216, 217, 525, 575
chromosome, 23, 27, 91, 117, 135, 169, 171, 263, 358, 359, 412, 503, 524
chronic illness, 222
chronic myelogenous, 23, 36, 132, 543
chronic obstructive pulmonary disease, 509
chronic renal failure, 110
cigarette smoke, 470
cigarette smokers, 470
cimetidine, 364
circadian rhythm, 76, 562, 564
circulation, 40, 41, 43
cirrhosis, 125, 130
citalopram, 294, 366, 532
classes, 5, 10, 84, 128, 147, 148, 238, 241, 249, 251, 253, 254, 259, 272, 280, 337, 348, 353, 363, 377, 386, 402, 460, 500, 560
classification, 126, 205, 215, 225, 248, 251, 252, 254, 278, 280, 281, 294, 307, 316, 326, 349, 351, 360, 361, 380, 383, 412, 511, 574, 576
cleavage, 524
clients, 441
clinical depression, 531
clinical diagnosis, 6, 21, 242
clinical trials, 3, 22, 27, 80, 114, 142, 147, 149, 160, 166, 175, 181, 192, 204, 246, 247, 260, 267, 269, 274, 290, 299, 301, 308, 316, 325, 329, 337, 340, 342, 351, 355, 358, 377, 391, 398, 404, 423, 426, 432, 445, 465, 491, 511, 515, 516, 522, 533, 542
clone, 393
cloning, 339, 350, 353, 434, 513
closure, 280
clozapine, 38, 84, 90, 96, 98, 99, 341, 367, 455, 538
cluster analysis, viii, 40
clustering, 51, 52, 54, 55, 56, 57, 58, 60, 75, 174, 238, 256, 279, 352, 399, 413, 495, 557, 560
clusters, viii, ix, 40, 52, 56, 57, 72, 104, 113, 174, 209, 374, 399, 556
CNS, 84, 88, 90, 96, 105, 107, 114, 336, 433, 494, 517
cocaine, 99, 149, 517
cocaine abuse, 99
coding, ix, 13, 33, 93, 104, 107, 117, 125, 134, 157, 167, 184, 196, 201, 203, 227, 232, 259, 265, 331, 334, 343, 347, 406, 434, 458, 465, 474, 475, 481, 484, 498, 507, 528, 536, 543, 578, 580, 582
codominant, 569
codon, 231, 234, 447, 460, 484, 487, 519
coefficient of variation, 54
coenzyme, 131
cognition, 236

cognitive function, 373, 390, 491
cogwheel rigidity, 86
cohort, 129, 140, 152, 165, 182, 212, 262, 299, 315, 391, 450, 458, 464, 473, 477, 510, 577
colitis, 332
collaboration, 292, 457
collagen, 180, 255, 536, 554
colon, 197, 247, 276, 364, 423, 444, 503
colon cancer, 197, 247, 276, 364, 444
colorectal cancer, 132, 140, 157, 186, 198, 200, 201, 212, 220, 229, 247, 308, 309, 333, 339, 354, 356, 363, 364, 382, 478, 498, 503, 507, 533, 541, 542, 574
coma, 86
combination therapy, 144, 336, 498
combined effect, 139
commitment, 428
communication, 22, 147, 165, 292, 299, 361, 373, 402, 439, 537, 544
communication skills, 361
community, 105, 111, 115, 192, 283, 285, 310, 337, 395, 404, 406, 416, 450, 468, 489, 496, 515, 559
comorbidity, 477
compatibility, 21, 22, 242
competence, 180, 367, 557
competition, 307
competitiveness, 25
compilation, 489
complement, 73, 245, 302, 381, 464, 562
complex interactions, 185, 193, 284, 578
complexity, 12, 17, 18, 19, 22, 23, 28, 30, 125, 140, 175, 244, 251, 257, 308, 320, 332, 352, 387, 405, 417, 423, 427, 488, 494, 499, 500, 522, 525, 538, 555, 579
compliance, 128, 162, 217, 325, 342, 372, 487, 492, 513, 548, 568
complications, 139, 163, 164, 180, 195, 222, 244, 249, 263, 321, 337, 372, 438, 464, 523, 551, 553
components, 72, 124, 128, 138, 202, 225, 262, 268, 293, 300, 325, 393, 420, 454, 482, 521
composition, 128, 176, 255, 441
compounds, 10, 45, 104, 134, 142, 176, 177, 181, 205, 218, 243, 249, 250, 256, 260, 280, 286, 289, 324, 335, 337, 353, 356, 374, 381, 386, 387, 393, 394, 405, 408, 416, 426, 433, 454, 473, 485, 489, 490, 499, 507, 518, 522, 526, 528, 546, 558, 560, 563, 572, 574
comprehension, 541
computational modeling, 283
computed tomography, 88, 98, 581
computing, 406
COMT inhibitor, 143
concentration, 40, 46, 47, 62, 63, 65, 66, 67, 69, 107, 129, 151, 212, 215, 216, 217, 223, 228, 231, 236, 237, 258, 265, 288, 294, 295, 306, 309, 314, 345, 349, 362, 365, 372, 411, 415, 435, 453, 464, 471, 477, 479, 487, 551, 569
conception, 266
conceptual model, 484
concordance, 233, 287, 362, 427, 503, 563
conduct, 272, 277, 398, 492, 504, 511
conduct disorder, 278
confidence, 142, 165, 196, 199, 229, 234, 280, 281, 295, 298, 347, 367, 368, 428, 464, 465, 466, 467, 480, 510, 553, 567
confidence interval, 165, 196, 199, 229, 234, 295, 298, 347, 367, 368, 464, 465, 466, 467, 480, 510, 553, 567
confidentiality, 188, 217, 250, 351, 483
configuration, 170
conflict, 88, 457
confusion, 203
congenital heart disease, 534
congestive heart failure, 206, 495
conjugation, 105, 170, 186, 402, 518, 548
connectivity, 393
consciousness, viii, 83, 85, 98
consensus, vii, 85, 88, 139, 147, 159, 178, 281, 311, 448, 529, 540, 570
consent, 173, 250, 316, 434, 509, 544, 556
conservation, 472
consolidation, 325
construction, 50, 158, 393, 515
consulting, 504
consumers, 373
consumption, 370, 551
contact dermatitis, 323
contraceptives, 431
contracture, 89
control, 35, 41, 43, 47, 51, 52, 54, 63, 66, 71, 79, 88, 91, 93, 94, 97, 128, 136, 139, 140, 145, 150, 164, 179, 184, 191, 196, 197, 198, 199, 213, 231, 232, 253, 262, 271, 273, 278, 286, 289, 290, 300, 320, 327, 329, 344, 358, 363, 366, 369, 371, 375, 376, 396, 397, 399, 400, 414, 422, 439, 454, 468, 472, 487, 514, 515, 526, 527, 528, 530, 531, 533, 541, 545, 549, 554, 556, 557, 562, 579
control group, 94, 213, 232, 289, 366, 375
controlled studies, 255, 358, 446, 500
controlled trials, 95, 140, 185, 494

convergence, 29, 418, 424, 523
conversion, 41, 164, 176, 217, 380, 418, 485, 568
conversion rate, 418
cooling, 87
copolymers, 369
copper, 151
coronary angioplasty, 163
coronary artery bypass graft, 391
coronary artery disease, 124, 131, 240, 241, 464, 552
coronary heart disease, 167, 207, 245, 378, 379, 578
coronary thrombosis, 209
corporations, 373
correlation, 8, 13, 18, 51, 54, 55, 56, 57, 58, 60, 152, 154, 158, 170, 232, 233, 250, 279, 281, 295, 297, 302, 333, 356, 357, 369, 374, 409, 411, 413, 447, 452, 469, 475, 525
correlation coefficient, 56
cortex, 315, 360, 361, 381
corticosteroid therapy, 330
corticosteroids, 40, 43, 44, 45, 49, 50, 63, 70, 71, 74, 75, 76, 79, 254, 306, 330, 448, 452, 523, 551
corticotropin, 330
cortisol, 42, 71, 76, 77, 218, 330
cost effectiveness, 400, 456, 492
costs, 136, 140, 224, 245, 248, 273, 275, 300, 323, 345, 368, 374, 386, 418, 433, 441, 456, 463, 492, 497, 539, 553
cough, 337
coumarins, 504, 554
counseling, 292
coupling, 14, 167, 240, 454, 462, 474
coverage, 81, 184, 556
covering, 2, 11, 73
craving, 134, 149, 530
creatine, 94
creatinine, 165
critical analysis, 256
criticism, 19, 27
Croatia, 213
Crohn's disease, 40
cross-validation, 280, 281
CSF, 98
culture, 110, 119, 121, 294, 331
culture conditions, 331
curing, 423
curriculum, 33
Cushing's syndrome, 439
cycles, 303, 532
cyclins, 272
cyclooxygenase, 261, 272, 392, 423, 554
cyclophosphamide, 165, 301, 343, 443, 514
cyclosporine, 79, 551, 566, 568
cysteine-rich protein, 393
cystic fibrosis, 8, 178, 288, 312, 357, 370, 499, 567
cytochrome, viii, 8, 29, 30, 31, 33, 37, 83, 90, 91, 100, 129, 131, 134, 138, 141, 145, 148, 153, 154, 160, 164, 165, 166, 178, 194, 200, 202, 213, 214, 218, 223, 226, 227, 228, 229, 230, 232, 233, 234, 235, 244, 251, 259, 260, 267, 268, 269, 273, 294, 306, 307, 308, 316, 318, 323, 334, 338, 342, 343, 344, 349, 362, 366, 367, 368, 378, 403, 406, 410, 432, 435, 438, 464, 469, 470, 475, 477, 482, 497, 500, 501, 505, 507, 508, 516, 518, 519, 520, 532, 534, 539, 543, 547, 550, 551, 552, 553, 560, 566, 569, 571, 579, 581
cytochrome p450, 138, 166, 244, 366, 560
cytogenetics, 312, 441
cytokines, 130, 239, 244, 371, 392, 424, 454, 552, 566
cytometry, 210
cytotoxicity, 210, 334, 413, 486, 490, 498, 514, 524
Czech Republic, 336, 492

D

damage, 201, 245, 275, 436, 549
data analysis, 51, 94, 126, 166, 257, 283, 287, 352, 409
data collection, 51, 316, 495
data generation, 80
data mining, viii, 11, 20, 40, 51, 54, 73, 352, 388, 389, 495, 572
data processing, 407, 409
data set, 51, 52, 54, 55, 56, 62, 70, 142, 253, 279, 281, 283, 287, 295, 311, 320, 353, 393, 399, 449, 452, 453, 464, 505, 558, 563
data transfer, 189
database, 51, 71, 72, 73, 157, 183, 188, 193, 195, 201, 222, 273, 287, 325, 331, 333, 349, 393, 405, 406, 413, 424, 449, 457, 480, 537
database management, 71, 393, 406
DBP, 468
death, 140, 142, 199, 234, 241, 252, 364, 411, 421, 449, 450, 489, 546
deaths, 7, 18, 115, 349, 375, 488, 537, 538
decision making, 166, 204, 311, 329, 412, 557, 564, 567, 572
decision-making process, 249, 328, 433

decisions, 166, 173, 255, 280, 306, 324, 336, 348, 354, 360, 398, 401, 453, 489, 496, 519, 535, 573, 579
deep brain stimulation, 373
defects, 266, 278, 279, 471, 534, 582
defense, 128, 139, 201, 243, 288, 290, 312, 565
defense mechanisms, 201, 243, 288
deficiency, 5, 15, 30, 208, 278, 312, 321, 323, 328, 359, 537, 549
deficit, 175, 277, 435
definition, vii, 85, 199, 292, 360, 361, 481, 528
degradation, 42, 45, 62, 65, 67, 68, 74, 141, 170, 402, 411, 414, 472
degradation rate, 45, 68
dehydration, 87
delirium, 86, 87
delivery, 2, 3, 5, 8, 13, 14, 15, 21, 28, 40, 136, 232, 242, 306, 315, 369, 370, 429, 583
deltaF508, 357
delusions, 88, 93
demand, 226, 239, 245, 257, 373, 402
dementia, 517
demographic characteristics, 132
demographic factors, 12
demographics, 510
Denmark, 233, 295, 306, 336, 556
density, 11, 62, 79, 101, 131, 132, 168, 178, 180, 183, 206, 312, 336, 359, 394, 459, 525
deoxyribonucleic acid, 229, 236, 348
Department of Agriculture, 328, 378
Department of Health and Human Services, 283, 284, 286
dependent variable, 262, 367, 452, 566
dephosphorylation, 210
deposition, 44
deposits, 430
depressants, 194, 366
depression, 7, 91, 124, 133, 148, 149, 160, 162, 193, 216, 265, 340, 423, 424, 463, 507, 526, 527, 528, 529, 530, 540, 546
deprivation, 434, 463
deregulation, 300
derivatives, 140, 272, 548
dermatology, 189, 322, 323, 371
dermatomyositis, 40
desensitization, 231, 240, 304
desire, 494, 544
desmosome, 444
desorption, 388
destruction, 89
detection, 6, 15, 24, 80, 85, 88, 105, 106, 107, 113, 114, 116, 117, 118, 119, 121, 125, 135, 138, 143, 152, 176, 178, 193, 205, 217, 224, 233, 246, 264, 279, 288, 311, 312, 313, 328, 358, 362, 405, 410, 453, 462, 476, 490, 528, 559
determinism, 126
developed countries, 241, 371
developing countries, 104, 429
developmental disorder, 358
diabetes, 7, 43, 44, 50, 73, 74, 96, 110, 185, 225, 244, 262, 263, 264, 278, 312, 332, 403, 422, 437, 438, 513, 535, 567
diabetic nephropathy, 431, 437, 438
diabetic patients, 225, 261, 278, 431
diagnostic criteria, 85, 94, 96, 127
dialysis, 111
diaphoresis, 85, 86, 94
diarrhea, 161, 200, 212, 220, 261, 270
diastolic blood pressure, 431, 468
diet, 33, 85, 147, 262, 339, 445, 459, 486, 498, 548
differential equations, 62
differential treatment, 382, 390, 425
differentiation, 6, 16, 20, 22, 23, 35, 163, 176, 199, 242, 248, 278, 527, 542, 579
diffusion, 45
digestion, 135, 359, 467, 551
dilated cardiomyopathy, 11
dimensionality, 389, 427
dioxin, 279
diploid, 246
directives, 501
disability, 450
discipline, 2, 5, 6, 128, 179, 249, 268, 316, 350, 403, 425, 487, 523, 537, 544, 559
discourse, 373
discriminant analysis, 352
discrimination, 77, 147, 217, 245, 320, 332, 402, 488, 510
disease activity, 440
disease gene, 371, 389, 416
disease model, 166, 251
disease progression, 11, 136, 138, 411, 430, 541
disequilibrium, 130, 141, 157, 209, 227, 263, 277, 297, 304, 374, 381, 384, 414, 422, 466, 467, 474, 483, 506, 524, 560
disorder, 5, 89, 127, 143, 149, 175, 193, 216, 261, 277, 309, 371, 376, 396, 423, 433, 481, 499, 512, 522, 538, 563, 577
displacement, 363

disposition, 3, 12, 13, 30, 48, 128, 155, 167, 190, 191, 193, 196, 199, 201, 202, 208, 210, 211, 221, 231, 233, 235, 242, 243, 245, 249, 258, 270, 273, 275, 306, 418, 427, 440, 443, 445, 452, 487, 488, 489, 500, 505, 506, 516, 536, 543, 547, 548, 554, 566, 571, 583
dissociation, 444
distress, 87
distributed memory, 407
distribution, 25, 40, 41, 43, 44, 51, 81, 91, 116, 135, 151, 203, 209, 211, 213, 234, 244, 249, 270, 271, 273, 293, 295, 306, 347, 360, 387, 389, 404, 412, 420, 422, 424, 427, 443, 457, 467, 478, 482, 503, 524, 545, 550, 552, 554, 572, 583
distribution function, 81
distributive justice, 150, 310
diuretic, 254, 546
divergence, 13, 124
diversity, 104, 137, 157, 251, 278, 281, 322, 334, 374, 375, 396, 451, 459, 484, 572
division, 420
dizygotic, 575
DNA, ix, 5, 6, 9, 10, 15, 17, 18, 22, 27, 31, 34, 45, 63, 72, 81, 103, 104, 105, 106, 107, 109, 113, 114, 116, 117, 120, 125, 129, 133, 135, 141, 145, 152, 153, 155, 156, 167, 171, 173, 178, 183, 186, 192, 201, 208, 210, 211, 212, 215, 217, 224, 238, 241, 242, 246, 251, 256, 257, 258, 259, 267, 273, 279, 280, 282, 286, 288, 289, 291, 297, 300, 303, 310, 311, 312, 316, 319, 320, 322, 325, 331, 339, 346, 350, 352, 353, 354, 355, 356, 359, 369, 370, 382, 383, 395, 399, 401, 403, 411, 412, 416, 420, 425, 426, 428, 430, 446, 451, 452, 457, 458, 465, 476, 484, 490, 497, 503, 512, 513, 514, 516, 519, 533, 535, 539, 540, 542, 549, 550, 551, 552, 556, 557, 563, 565, 566, 569, 575, 582
DNA damage, 145, 370, 565
DNA microarray systems, x, 104, 105
DNA repair, 141, 201, 208, 224, 258, 339, 354, 402, 411, 446, 451, 514, 519, 549, 557
DNA sequencing, 6, 22, 297, 311, 353, 355
docetaxel, 358, 524
doctors, 465, 537
dogs, 152, 524
domain, 33, 71, 111, 181, 224, 280, 281, 357, 403, 443, 444, 491, 513, 562
dominant strategy, 480
donors, 375, 434, 504
dopamine, viii, 83, 87, 88, 90, 93, 98, 99, 100, 101, 102, 143, 148, 150, 156, 240, 277, 304, 306, 341, 342, 368, 372, 414, 420, 432, 435, 436, 450, 455, 462, 463, 501, 518, 530, 531, 543, 547
dopamine agonist, 87, 88
dopamine antagonists, 435
dosage, 15, 24, 26, 163, 209, 269, 314, 345, 363, 379, 412, 426, 440, 582
dosing, viii, 12, 39, 44, 49, 50, 51, 52, 74, 133, 147, 151, 162, 182, 188, 200, 203, 217, 221, 239, 275, 308, 321, 325, 339, 372, 394, 415, 418, 425, 432, 477, 478, 522, 523, 532, 537, 549, 550, 551, 553, 563, 567, 571
down-regulation, 48, 52, 54, 58, 78, 79, 80, 220, 231
draft, 311
dream, 257, 516
drinking water, 50, 281, 285
Drosophila, 28, 444
drought, 288
drug abuse, 85, 176, 547
drug action, vii, 1, 3, 5, 6, 10, 16, 20, 24, 48, 202, 256, 265, 293, 294, 307, 332, 349, 407, 408, 428, 448, 503, 542
drug addict, 474
drug addiction, 474
drug delivery, vii, 2, 3, 5, 7, 8, 10, 12, 15, 20, 21, 25, 26, 28, 29, 31, 36, 200, 241, 242, 306, 356, 369, 411, 583
drug design, 24, 144, 150, 335, 439
drug discovery, vii, 5, 6, 7, 11, 29, 30, 31, 32, 34, 36, 37, 132, 133, 141, 142, 144, 147, 166, 175, 188, 203, 204, 205, 240, 242, 249, 251, 260, 266, 267, 271, 280, 306, 308, 335, 386, 405, 408, 421, 423, 424, 425, 426, 427, 428, 429, 436, 437, 454, 490, 514, 515, 521, 526, 571, 574
drug efflux, ix, 103, 107, 308, 489
drug interaction, 3, 33, 34, 140, 160, 193, 195, 210, 226, 235, 243, 244, 251, 252, 253, 274, 302, 307, 344, 365, 402, 404, 431, 445, 478, 518, 519, 521, 523, 537, 545, 551, 577, 580, 583
drug metabolism, vii, 2, 12, 33, 90, 91, 96, 100, 128, 138, 152, 153, 154, 155, 161, 164, 190, 197, 208, 213, 224, 232, 236, 243, 253, 259, 260, 270, 303, 306, 329, 335, 343, 366, 372, 380, 390, 413, 422, 438, 451, 452, 482, 487, 489, 510, 520, 536, 543, 548, 575
drug reactions, viii, 2, 29, 30, 34, 35, 83, 90, 91, 96, 99, 137, 142, 155, 160, 164, 170, 181, 189, 205, 227, 238, 245, 248, 251, 258, 259, 266, 270, 273, 274, 275, 300, 322, 342, 354, 365, 366, 367, 382, 395, 396, 397, 418, 427, 450, 456, 457, 489, 492, 500, 505, 510, 515, 520, 521, 561, 571, 580

drug resistance, 22, 23, 29, 33, 128, 137, 172, 182, 194, 223, 225, 256, 257, 290, 292, 306, 307, 309, 312, 325, 344, 355, 356, 401, 402, 440, 443, 448, 489, 550, 566, 581
drug safety, 246, 271, 274
drug targets, vii, 1, 2, 10, 12, 17, 30, 35, 127, 147, 160, 220, 221, 258, 259, 305, 308, 328, 332, 355, 363, 371, 427, 433, 443, 448, 451, 452, 497, 504, 507, 509, 514, 518, 526, 527, 535, 549
drug therapy, 2, 8, 11, 12, 16, 24, 25, 29, 30, 31, 38, 99, 124, 131, 155, 159, 160, 167, 170, 178, 189, 219, 221, 227, 230, 244, 251, 254, 258, 274, 275, 291, 293, 302, 305, 323, 327, 332, 364, 389, 402, 424, 425, 426, 429, 430, 441, 442, 452, 456, 486, 500, 504, 505, 507, 511, 518, 520, 539, 543, 549, 571, 572, 576, 579, 580
drug toxicity, 2, 15, 138, 194, 197, 232, 258, 322, 343, 372, 424, 446, 516, 540
drug treatment, viii, 2, 29, 39, 54, 86, 134, 136, 140, 155, 186, 208, 209, 226, 238, 269, 272, 274, 291, 321, 342, 373, 408, 433, 520, 526, 571, 577
drug use, 314, 390, 407, 441, 491, 496, 554
drug withdrawal, 18
DSM, 341, 375
DSM-IV, 341, 375
duodenal ulcer, 7
duplication, 99, 100, 160, 170, 171, 294, 517
duration, 49, 158, 163, 180, 233, 247, 262, 341, 363, 415, 450, 537, 579
dyslipidemia, 40, 74
dysphagia, 86
dysphoria, 390, 491
dyspnea, 85
dystonia, 84
dystonic reactions, 307

E

earthworm, 288
East Asia, 500, 501, 532
Eastern Europe, 120
EBV infection, 261
economic problem, 321
economics, 179, 266, 426, 531
ecstasy, 547
efflux transporters, 206, 290, 365
EKG, 101
elaboration, 205
elderly, 145, 188, 274, 431, 437, 438, 583
electrodes, 346
electroencephalography, 87
electrolyte, 467
electron microscopy, 563
electrophoresis, 108, 135, 252, 354, 370, 414
ELISA, 195
email, 453
embryogenesis, 444
embryology, 314
emergence, ix, 2, 3, 5, 7, 8, 18, 23, 103, 111, 112, 118, 119, 121, 132, 144, 190, 223, 264, 308, 317, 326, 373, 374, 378, 382, 435, 515, 524, 544
emission, 88, 98, 581
empathy, 547
employment, 36, 123, 556, 583
empyema, 111
enantiomers, 176, 471
encephalitis, 97
encephalomyelitis, 81
encephalopathy, 315
encoding, ix, 8, 12, 13, 14, 23, 24, 103, 110, 117, 124, 125, 138, 143, 155, 164, 183, 199, 201, 213, 221, 226, 229, 242, 258, 262, 263, 265, 269, 270, 289, 291, 297, 308, 339, 342, 343, 350, 355, 374, 378, 397, 403, 419, 421, 444, 447, 451, 464, 473, 484, 495, 518, 526, 549, 555, 556
endocarditis, 113
endocrine, 243, 278, 281, 432, 565
endocrine glands, 243
endocrinology, 315
endonuclease, 135
endothelial cells, 439
endothelium, 76, 290
end-stage renal disease, 165
energy, 40, 41, 74, 76, 405, 473, 513, 548
energy transfer, 405
England, 139, 168, 278, 379, 580
enthusiasm, 222, 422, 425, 489, 515, 577
environment, 3, 20, 25, 50, 71, 117, 124, 130, 133, 139, 140, 150, 181, 222, 237, 245, 260, 283, 284, 293, 313, 316, 328, 348, 395, 406, 422, 496, 528, 545, 566, 570, 571, 580
environmental change, 503
environmental control, 570
environmental factors, 17, 168, 182, 193, 200, 241, 285, 292, 324, 346, 354, 384, 385, 401, 407, 424, 459, 460, 529, 530, 536, 537, 539, 579, 580
environmental impact, 5
environmental influences, 127, 259, 319, 527, 575
Environmental Protection Agency, 283

enzymatic activity, 15, 27, 91, 164, 186, 268, 269, 343, 344, 450, 581
enzyme induction, 48, 50, 80, 196, 268, 431
enzyme-linked immunosorbent assay, 413
enzymes, ix, 8, 12, 14, 23, 29, 33, 41, 42, 72, 74, 76, 79, 85, 103, 104, 106, 115, 117, 125, 126, 129, 130, 134, 138, 140, 152, 155, 160, 161, 164, 165, 166, 168, 169, 170, 171, 190, 196, 197, 200, 201, 202, 210, 213, 214, 216, 219, 220, 224, 226, 227, 235, 242, 243, 249, 251, 252, 258, 259, 263, 265, 269, 270, 271, 273, 275, 276, 298, 301, 305, 306, 308, 311, 316, 322, 327, 332, 338, 339, 342, 343, 354, 355, 356, 363, 365, 371, 372, 374, 375, 383, 385, 387, 402, 403, 406, 411, 427, 435, 440, 442, 443, 445, 446, 448, 451, 469, 473, 476, 482, 485, 487, 488, 491, 497, 498, 500, 503, 504, 505, 507, 508, 510, 511, 514, 518, 519, 520, 521, 526, 529, 535, 537, 543, 548, 549, 558, 560, 561, 571, 578, 580, 581, 582
epidemiology, 115, 116, 118, 121, 124, 191, 315, 361, 362, 382
epigenetics, 17, 143, 305
epilepsy, 33, 125, 126, 289, 290, 291, 292, 293, 300, 309, 333, 396, 511
epinephrine, 450
epithelial cells, 200, 370, 499
Epstein-Barr virus, 261
equality, 457
equilibrium, 157, 184, 213, 360, 476, 477, 516
equipment, 193, 406
erythrocytes, 30, 217
escitalopram, 532
esophageal cancer, 541
esophagus, 542
EST, 444
ester, 219, 460
estimating, 14, 182, 221, 320
Estonia, 174, 556
estrogen, 168, 280, 281, 321, 410, 565
ethical issues, 26, 124, 173, 174, 217, 250, 292, 323, 379, 427, 429, 434, 557
ethics, 172, 250, 283, 415, 435, 580
ethnic diversity, 130
ethnic groups, 156, 169, 237, 270, 321, 331, 572
ethnicity, 125, 130, 151, 235, 327, 415, 497
ethylene, 369
ethylene oxide, 369
etiology, 99, 126, 133, 143, 278, 315, 373, 410, 509, 522, 534
EU, 307, 315
eugenics, 400
eukaryotic cell, 492
euphoria, 373, 548
Euro, 480
Europe, 114, 118, 124, 132, 142, 190, 326, 374, 489, 517
European Commission, 241, 286, 489
European Union, 315
evidence, 13, 17, 18, 87, 96, 127, 136, 137, 139, 140, 143, 158, 180, 185, 192, 193, 197, 201, 208, 222, 247, 251, 255, 261, 271, 275, 290, 291, 305, 307, 308, 309, 310, 313, 315, 317, 318, 329, 332, 334, 336, 340, 344, 348, 350, 352, 366, 374, 376, 382, 392, 394, 397, 402, 404, 414, 418, 433, 441, 451, 464, 467, 469, 474, 500, 512, 516, 517, 518, 519, 523, 527, 528, 531, 537, 570, 573
evolution, 2, 5, 28, 115, 133, 134, 176, 237, 244, 407, 408, 414, 425, 429, 456, 472
exaggeration, 40
excision, 9, 15, 201, 514
excitability, 579
exclusion, 352, 525
excretion, 13, 25, 195, 200, 243, 249, 271, 275, 338, 387, 404, 412, 420, 422, 470, 477, 503, 558, 572, 583
execution, 329
exercise, 84, 147, 461, 487
exons, 93, 229, 295, 297, 347, 350, 444, 484
exonuclease, 125
expectations, 20, 29, 137, 157, 185, 302, 317, 408, 427, 439, 491, 509, 522, 548, 564, 577
expenditures, 158
experimental design, vii, 2, 23, 329, 388, 409, 417, 520, 559
expertise, 173, 490
experts, 150, 165, 185, 284, 286, 318, 334, 559
exploitation, vii, 1, 17, 22, 23, 28
exposure, 88, 129, 139, 156, 180, 188, 196, 198, 212, 223, 231, 233, 237, 251, 256, 279, 281, 284, 286, 287, 288, 302, 314, 316, 338, 343, 362, 365, 366, 378, 384, 392, 402, 409, 417, 441, 453, 464, 466, 472, 474, 530, 533, 545, 548, 557, 561, 564, 567, 568, 570
expressed sequence tag, 288, 529, 540
extensor, 86
external environment, 286
external influences, 324
external validation, 481
extracellular matrix, 199
extraction, 3, 217, 273, 311

extrapolation, 205, 280, 281, 572
extroversion, 548

F

fabrication, 193
FAD, 127
failure, 85, 104, 128, 139, 143, 153, 155, 165, 173, 202, 203, 207, 234, 240, 249, 253, 256, 261, 271, 305, 313, 322, 325, 337, 340, 354, 372, 378, 387, 402, 418, 426, 429, 437, 451, 460, 495, 507, 521, 540, 555, 568, 572, 581
falciparum malaria, 396
false positive, 348
family, 24, 88, 131, 137, 138, 152, 159, 173, 179, 200, 225, 235, 243, 260, 262, 292, 306, 320, 342, 343, 357, 359, 442, 444, 454, 458, 467, 481, 498, 545, 556
family history, 159, 225, 262, 467, 545
family members, 173, 442, 459
family physician, 131
family studies, 137, 292, 481
fasting, 262, 278, 459
fat, 44, 76
fatigue, 464
fatty acids, 232
FDA, 15, 24, 134, 247, 282, 307, 311, 313, 316, 322, 335, 351, 394, 399, 412, 420, 425, 427, 494, 495, 496, 532
FDA approval, 532
fear, 320, 373
febrile seizure, 125, 289
feces, 354
feedback, 166, 189, 299
females, 124, 394, 455, 516, 547
fertilization, 468
fetal alcohol syndrome, 130
fever, 539
fibers, 42
fibrinogen, 42, 76, 522, 536, 560
fibroids, 441
fibrosis, 80, 255, 499
fidelity, 125
field trials, 316
filtration, 136
financing, 163
Finland, 209, 374
first generation, 148
fish, 571
fitness, 525
flexibility, 29, 32, 37, 145, 418
flexor, 86
flight, 388
flood, 6, 136
flora, 113, 318
fluid, 88, 244, 412, 467
fluorescence, 107, 158, 171, 210, 405, 416
fluoroquinolones, ix, 103, 105, 107, 111, 113, 120
fluoxetine, 159, 304, 363, 366, 414
fluvoxamine, 184, 294, 582
focus groups, 323
focusing, vii, 1, 5, 10, 11, 20, 189, 241, 246, 307, 322, 333, 349, 377, 440, 509, 517, 528, 529, 540, 546, 582
folate, 189, 356, 382, 418, 441, 473, 492, 498, 507, 508, 537
folic acid, 537
follicle, 468
food, 104, 365, 382, 531, 561, 564
food additives, 382
food production, 104
Ford, 207, 545
formal education, 225
Fourier analysis, 564
fractures, 371
France, 140, 155, 156, 158, 164, 204, 229, 230, 248, 299, 302, 316, 350, 355, 357, 363, 376, 421, 425, 430, 451, 478, 497, 513, 541, 568
freedom, 291
frequency distribution, 156, 374, 396
frontal lobe, 125, 143
fructose, 41
fruits, 544
fuel, 174, 435
functional analysis, 14, 174, 317, 333, 409, 461, 476, 547, 554
functional changes, 286
functional imaging, 94, 126, 133
funding, 241

G

gastrectomy, 194
gastrocnemius, 50
gastrointestinal tract, 200, 251
gel, 108, 135, 203, 354, 370, 583
gender, 128, 147, 168, 195, 213, 235, 236, 252, 304, 327, 375, 383, 384, 445, 452, 457, 459, 467, 477, 487, 497, 510, 553, 566
gene amplification, 146, 211, 356

gene arrays, viii, 39, 50, 286
gene expression, viii, 10, 17, 18, 24, 36, 39, 43, 44, 53, 62, 65, 68, 72, 74, 76, 79, 80, 81, 93, 126, 127, 133, 141, 142, 144, 145, 161, 169, 175, 178, 192, 205, 210, 211, 229, 238, 242, 246, 251, 254, 257, 260, 266, 267, 279, 280, 282, 286, 287, 288, 289, 294, 300, 303, 305, 307, 315, 317, 321, 325, 342, 351, 352, 353, 370, 372, 382, 384, 386, 392, 393, 407, 409, 413, 414, 416, 417, 438, 451, 453, 454, 471, 473, 485, 486, 488, 517, 518, 520, 529, 533, 540, 541, 550, 556, 557, 558, 560, 561, 563, 565, 567, 579
gene mapping, 440
gene promoter, 76, 162, 186, 339, 475
gene silencing, 372
gene targeting, 242
gene therapy, 136, 242, 437, 499, 535
gene transfer, ix, 103, 105, 115, 353
general anesthesia, 153
general practitioner, 457, 509
generalization, 99, 353
generation, 16, 17, 28, 49, 61, 62, 79, 80, 84, 86, 123, 294, 309, 370, 374, 387, 392, 407, 426, 441, 503, 556, 558, 575
generic drugs, 310, 497
genetic defect, 132, 194, 342, 403, 536, 582
genetic disease, 312, 493
genetic disorders, 4, 412
genetic diversity, 429
genetic factors, 3, 6, 14, 85, 88, 124, 126, 128, 157, 164, 166, 168, 202, 219, 241, 259, 269, 273, 301, 318, 322, 364, 371, 395, 414, 421, 423, 440, 448, 450, 458, 459, 463, 480, 481, 487, 488, 500, 508, 512, 513, 517, 521, 522, 526, 528, 531, 546, 547, 548
genetic information, 2, 6, 15, 25, 95, 123, 124, 136, 159, 219, 225, 242, 244, 250, 306, 323, 324, 353, 382, 445, 455, 456, 521, 523, 556
genetic linkage, 409, 526
genetic marker, 12, 21, 34, 35, 193, 347, 390, 396, 403, 508, 515, 534, 555
genetic mutations, 197
genetic screening, 124, 169, 339, 448, 581
genetic testing, 15, 35, 136, 155, 159, 173, 193, 209, 219, 225, 250, 254, 292, 314, 352, 373, 390, 395, 415, 421, 456, 500, 507
genetic traits, 202
genetics, 5, 6, 10, 20, 26, 28, 35, 99, 105, 114, 124, 125, 127, 130, 134, 137, 139, 141, 144, 150, 156, 158, 159, 161, 177, 202, 204, 209, 225, 226, 239, 242, 248, 250, 254, 260, 267, 274, 275, 277, 278, 283, 292, 293, 300, 302, 305, 309, 311, 312, 315, 318, 319, 321, 323, 325, 328, 333, 337, 340, 341, 342, 345, 346, 360, 361, 381, 387, 389, 403, 407, 409, 410, 414, 418, 422, 429, 430, 433, 456, 464, 489, 493, 494, 497, 498, 500, 517, 520, 521, 524, 527, 536, 546, 555, 573, 580, 581
genome, vii, 1, 2, 3, 6, 10, 12, 17, 20, 26, 28, 37, 72, 80, 81, 105, 125, 126, 139, 142, 160, 161, 175, 176, 178, 189, 192, 193, 194, 218, 222, 242, 244, 249, 263, 266, 276, 286, 302, 306, 311, 317, 348, 355, 364, 375, 388, 393, 394, 401, 408, 416, 417, 428, 430, 444, 483, 496, 502, 505, 514, 519, 521, 524, 525, 535, 537, 540, 549, 571, 574, 579
genomic regions, 406, 524, 560
genomics, 3, 4, 6, 10, 11, 16, 18, 20, 22, 26, 28, 29, 30, 32, 34, 128, 134, 136, 137, 147, 174, 175, 179, 193, 203, 225, 246, 257, 265, 284, 287, 302, 303, 322, 332, 335, 336, 347, 348, 350, 352, 353, 369, 373, 393, 407, 409, 413, 421, 425, 429, 430, 433, 435, 443, 444, 472, 479, 493, 511, 536, 537, 539, 541, 545, 547, 558, 559, 570, 571, 572, 574, 578, 580
genotype, 13, 37, 91, 92, 100, 116, 124, 129, 137, 145, 149, 151, 152, 153, 162, 164, 167, 178, 182, 184, 187, 197, 199, 203, 207, 208, 209, 211, 212, 213, 214, 217, 218, 223, 228, 231, 232, 235, 236, 253, 259, 260, 262, 270, 274, 275, 285, 291, 294, 295, 296, 297, 301, 302, 304, 305, 308, 316, 320, 325, 327, 329, 339, 341, 343, 348, 359, 360, 362, 363, 375, 377, 378, 379, 380, 383, 384, 391, 392, 394, 398, 405, 406, 409, 412, 415, 416, 427, 431, 432, 434, 437, 440, 442, 447, 450, 452, 455, 456, 458, 459, 460, 463, 464, 465, 467, 469, 470, 471, 473, 475, 476, 477, 478, 479, 481, 486, 487, 488, 492, 495, 502, 503, 504, 506, 512, 514, 516, 517, 519, 520, 521, 523, 525, 531, 535, 545, 548, 550, 551, 552, 553, 554, 566, 567, 569, 570, 574, 575, 578, 580, 583
Georgia, 208
germ cells, 345
germ line, 181
Germany, 145, 160, 165, 169, 173, 191, 202, 206, 214, 215, 216, 223, 226, 231, 232, 238, 245, 265, 268, 269, 271, 272, 287, 290, 294, 295, 301, 303, 312, 337, 339, 340, 342, 355, 358, 406, 426, 439, 446, 461, 462, 468, 473, 474, 475, 484, 494, 496, 504, 509, 511, 519, 526, 527, 528, 530, 532
gestation, 231
gestational diabetes, 263, 486

Gilbert's syndrome, 339
ginseng, 561
gizzard, 288
glaucoma, 447
glioblastoma, 444
glioma, 438
glucagon, 262, 454, 583
glucocorticoid receptor, 14, 44, 45, 79, 80, 440
gluconeogenesis, 41, 42, 43
glucose, 5, 40, 42, 43, 74, 78, 262, 278, 323, 473
glucose tolerance, 262
glucose tolerance test, 262
glutamate, 41, 42, 231
glutathione, 15, 38, 181, 199, 201, 227, 272, 315, 368, 402, 508, 550
glycerol, 41, 74
glycine, 196, 231, 447, 465, 548
glycogen, 40, 434
glycolysis, 41, 43, 445, 473
glycopeptides, ix, 104, 113
goals, 2, 128, 146, 147, 164, 201, 313, 316, 397, 428, 442, 487, 511
gold, 346
gonads, 243
government, 136, 146, 324
graph, 73, 81
Great Britain, 524
Greece, 1, 241, 459, 485, 498
grounding, 544
groundwater, 557
grouping, 52, 56
groups, 6, 17, 52, 58, 71, 85, 130, 145, 147, 150, 153, 154, 166, 183, 192, 199, 208, 218, 228, 229, 231, 245, 250, 266, 270, 271, 277, 297, 300, 301, 307, 316, 323, 327, 331, 343, 344, 346, 366, 370, 373, 375, 376, 392, 401, 403, 409, 415, 419, 420, 429, 450, 452, 454, 460, 468, 472, 479, 488, 495, 507, 515, 516, 517, 523, 545, 551, 553, 564, 574, 575
growth, 23, 42, 77, 78, 110, 132, 144, 177, 198, 211, 224, 225, 255, 256, 266, 272, 298, 300, 359, 364, 402, 421, 445, 454, 484, 498, 541, 542, 571
growth factor, 24, 42, 78, 132, 144, 145, 177, 211, 224, 256, 272, 364, 402, 454, 541, 542
growth hormone, 42, 77, 78, 298, 402, 421, 454
guanine, 156, 436
guidance, 114, 156, 247, 250, 260, 274, 311, 316, 335, 420, 427, 494
guidelines, 27, 123, 159, 217, 244, 253, 256, 290, 307, 316, 333, 426, 491, 511, 521, 532, 557, 570
gut, 113, 360, 361
gynecomastia, 359

H

HAART, 252
half-life, 196, 223, 415, 525
hallucinations, 88, 93, 372, 548
haplotypes, viii, 6, 12, 13, 16, 24, 27, 33, 83, 135, 138, 139, 151, 157, 167, 190, 214, 230, 231, 235, 248, 297, 332, 347, 384, 392, 396, 414, 418, 419, 462, 470, 474, 475, 476, 484, 506, 569
happiness, 548
harm, 173, 192, 245, 292, 453
hazards, 362, 453
HBV, 124, 582
HBV infection, 582
HDL, 41, 132, 168, 219, 378, 379
HE, 99, 162, 276, 378, 450, 576
headache, 450
health, 2, 5, 6, 17, 18, 19, 26, 27, 28, 30, 31, 34, 123, 130, 136, 149, 150, 159, 163, 178, 186, 204, 233, 239, 242, 249, 283, 284, 286, 292, 295, 308, 313, 321, 322, 323, 332, 348, 365, 373, 374, 375, 382, 387, 395, 400, 401, 402, 408, 418, 422, 427, 429, 430, 433, 440, 441, 454, 457, 466, 485, 492, 496, 510, 513, 520, 540, 544, 557, 561, 567, 571, 572, 575, 577
health care, 28, 31, 159, 163, 204, 323, 332, 348, 365, 373, 382, 387, 395, 401, 402, 408, 422, 433, 441, 457, 544, 577
health care professionals, 28, 323
health effects, 466
health insurance, 510
health services, 323
health status, 150, 567
heart attack, 422
heart disease, 11, 27, 239, 255, 547, 578
heart failure, 201, 202, 203, 206, 234, 239, 240, 322, 421, 460, 495, 578
heart rate, 484, 487, 547, 548
heat, 98, 393
height, 182, 359, 421, 549, 553
helicobacter pylori, 437
hematocrit, 233
hematology, 576
heme, 77, 260
hemoglobin, 359
hemolytic anemia, 5
hemostasis, 512, 562

hepatitis, 124, 139, 326, 394, 436, 481, 534, 535, 574, 582
hepatocytes, 79, 196, 287
hepatoma, 557, 563
hepatotoxicity, 217, 280, 282, 353, 399, 563
herbal medicine, 561
heredity, 149
heritability, 277, 491, 524, 535, 546
heroin, 149, 517
heterogeneity, 3, 7, 130, 142, 148, 198, 245, 278, 308, 319, 333, 392, 405, 456, 464, 519, 521, 580, 581
high density lipoprotein, 379
hip, 537, 547
hirsutism, 568
Hispanics, 129, 461
histamine, 530
histidine, 393
histology, 555
histone, 17, 18, 280, 472
HIV, 18, 19, 35, 128, 129, 130, 137, 142, 244, 251, 252, 265, 278, 279, 298, 299, 310, 321, 324, 327, 333, 337, 374, 378, 397, 464, 474, 479, 487, 500, 539, 555, 560
HIV infection, 142, 252, 299, 310
HIV/AIDS, 244
HIV-1, 19, 35, 128, 251, 479
HLA, 9, 19, 35, 90, 99, 139, 394, 418, 479, 560, 566, 582
homeostasis, 135, 219, 306, 312, 441, 513, 565
homocysteine, 492
homogeneity, 174, 357, 481
homovanillic acid, 88
homozygote, 447
Honda, 116, 364
Hong Kong, 209, 290, 478, 552
hormone, 78, 168, 243, 280, 298, 330, 356, 359, 410, 421, 432, 468, 523, 556
hospitalization, 234, 248, 288, 421
hospitals, 7, 105, 111, 265, 469
host, 87, 97, 124, 137, 144, 190, 210, 250, 251, 253, 279, 321, 324, 325, 337, 372, 440, 496, 500, 549, 571, 572
House, 76, 311, 328, 336
human behavior, 285
human brain, 436, 494
human development, 266
human exposure, 188, 284
human genome, 2, 29, 33, 126, 133, 153, 204, 209, 222, 246, 249, 256, 258, 259, 301, 313, 317, 322, 329, 348, 351, 375, 395, 400, 420, 430, 451, 484, 493, 508, 510, 515, 539, 544, 559, 578
human immunodeficiency virus, 222, 223, 452, 474, 479
human leukocyte antigen, 19, 582
human subjects, 142, 250, 384, 386, 458
Hungary, 432
hunting, 190
Huntington's disease, 8, 526
hybrid, 144
hybridization, ix, 51, 60, 61, 104, 105, 106, 107, 109, 111, 114, 116, 117, 178, 215, 224, 348, 409, 410, 416, 473
hydrocortisone, 79
hydrogen, 42
hydrolysis, 217
hydronephrosis, 314
hydroxyl, 411
hyperactivity, 99, 175, 277
hyperbilirubinemia, 483, 560
hypercholesterolemia, 241, 347, 391
hyperglycaemia, 79, 278
hyperglycemia, 40, 74, 84, 262, 263
hyperinsulinemia, 74
hyperlipemia, 233
hyperlipidemia, 7, 437
hyperparathyroidism, 465
hyperplasia, 144, 266, 398
hyperprolactinemia, 148
hyperpyrexia, 85, 89, 94, 96
hypersensitivity, 18, 19, 35, 129, 164, 222, 248, 360, 361, 418, 479, 500, 508, 516, 555, 560
hypertension, 7, 11, 30, 32, 40, 43, 44, 74, 77, 79, 86, 132, 135, 145, 183, 239, 244, 254, 255, 346, 376, 377, 378, 408, 410, 436, 437, 439, 467, 468, 515, 537, 545, 547, 568, 573, 577
hyperthermia, viii, 83, 85, 89, 98, 99, 548
hypertrophic cardiomyopathy, 11
hypertrophy, 44, 255, 276, 376, 562, 568
hypotension, 147
hypothalamus, 434, 513
hypothesis, 12, 90, 92, 125, 154, 162, 163, 168, 192, 202, 234, 265, 266, 279, 280, 290, 299, 309, 310, 314, 328, 331, 392, 394, 414, 434, 465, 469, 524, 525, 529, 539, 540, 542, 554, 556
hypothesis test, 524, 556
hypoxia, 445, 473
hypoxia-inducible factor, 445

I

iatrogenic, 546
IBD, 318, 321, 332, 372, 473
ideas, 5, 20, 543, 573, 579
identification, vii, x, 1, 10, 11, 12, 24, 25, 104, 105, 116, 118, 121, 123, 125, 139, 142, 161, 167, 169, 172, 173, 177, 178, 188, 190, 193, 197, 198, 199, 215, 242, 244, 245, 251, 254, 256, 264, 267, 279, 286, 288, 293, 294, 296, 303, 310, 311, 315, 316, 319, 320, 322, 335, 339, 342, 367, 369, 370, 371, 375, 382, 390, 391, 395, 403, 405, 406, 409, 410, 418, 426, 427, 428, 448, 451, 476, 482, 483, 489, 493, 496, 509, 515, 517, 518, 521, 527, 530, 533, 534, 536, 544, 546, 560, 567, 571, 576, 579
identity, 6, 332, 444, 454, 524
idiopathic, 80
idiosyncratic, 19, 24, 251, 261, 500
IFN, 327, 350, 394, 582
IL-6, 366, 392
imagination, 408
immune function, 312, 392
immune response, 164, 500
immune system, 40, 261, 274, 318, 382
immunity, 130, 150, 360, 361, 392
immunization, 139
immunodeficiency, 535
immunogenetics, 35, 248
immunohistochemistry, 158, 211
immunomodulation, 75
immunomodulatory, 337
immunosuppression, 136, 261, 326, 504, 505, 566, 567, 568
immunosuppressive agent, 156, 326, 550, 566
immunosuppressive drugs, 308, 504, 506, 566, 568, 569
implementation, 144, 146, 247, 252, 307, 309, 320, 322, 340, 405, 408, 426, 485, 491, 505, 519
imports, 72
impulsiveness, 277
in situ hybridization, 171
in vitro, 81, 89, 93, 125, 131, 154, 158, 171, 195, 196, 210, 211, 220, 237, 240, 242, 244, 246, 249, 268, 279, 287, 312, 318, 325, 331, 364, 380, 387, 392, 416, 417, 425, 441, 448, 451, 465, 468, 470, 525, 557, 558, 561, 563, 572, 583
inattention, 277
incentives, 423
incidence, 7, 13, 18, 19, 85, 88, 96, 99, 130, 153, 155, 206, 247, 248, 265, 296, 362, 395, 410, 415, 422, 455, 461, 487, 526, 539, 564, 570
inclusion, 265, 318, 351, 360, 377, 447, 492
incubation time, 357, 380
independence, 545, 557
independent variable, 452, 566
India, 156, 176, 252, 253, 257, 297, 320, 336, 505, 509, 538
Indians, 270, 296, 297, 374
indication, 149, 162, 477, 558
indicators, 15, 251, 386, 502
indices, 215, 453, 571
indirect effect, 48, 61
individual development, 165
individual differences, 129, 154, 168, 175, 226, 317, 342, 385, 420, 440, 455, 488, 528
individuality, 328, 572
individualization, 167, 220, 221, 258, 269, 313, 339, 372, 442, 464, 505, 524, 542, 555, 567
inducer, 279, 334, 344
induction, 33, 49, 66, 67, 68, 69, 78, 80, 164, 240, 243, 244, 290, 321, 325, 344, 345, 365, 413, 432, 445, 468, 520, 561, 563, 568
industrialized countries, 104, 193
industry, 104, 133, 136, 146, 150, 172, 188, 205, 238, 245, 260, 269, 311, 312, 316, 323, 324, 335, 416, 427, 429, 430, 505, 515, 556, 559, 574, 576, 580
inefficiency, 5, 7, 17
infancy, 253, 451, 502, 570
infants, 147, 366, 534, 570, 583
infarction, 163, 464, 552
infection, 124, 128, 139, 187, 222, 226, 288, 308, 310, 327, 346, 394, 438, 482, 537, 574, 582
infectious disease, 87, 278, 279
inferiority, 163
inflammation, 205, 226, 244, 251, 303, 334, 337, 360, 361, 392, 464, 555
inflammatory bowel disease, 40, 161, 169, 217, 221, 258, 265, 266, 318, 321, 332, 338, 372, 440, 448, 473
inflammatory disease, 440, 552
inflammatory responses, 42, 199, 226, 464
infliximab, 169, 440, 448, 494
information technology, 146, 163, 283, 406, 511
informed consent, 26, 173, 401, 415, 434, 510, 543
infrastructure, 25, 146, 150, 201, 283, 329, 406, 493
ingestion, 5, 221
inhaler, 237

inheritance, 11, 143, 292, 293, 338, 364, 371, 376, 403, 424, 442
inhibition, 33, 40, 47, 48, 63, 137, 154, 160, 181, 196, 228, 244, 256, 272, 280, 299, 365, 380, 401, 431, 432, 462, 498, 548, 561, 563, 565
inhibitor, 23, 35, 132, 149, 160, 163, 181, 185, 203, 210, 211, 220, 261, 273, 280, 299, 310, 337, 343, 344, 365, 366, 380, 439, 463, 474, 479, 500, 522, 547, 552, 560
initiation, 12, 15, 164, 199, 234, 239, 252, 262, 281, 321, 444, 504, 536, 552, 581
injections, 262, 264, 583
injury, 98, 251, 288, 386, 512, 555, 564
innate immunity, 150, 496
innovation, 163
inositol, 527
input, 46, 48, 165, 323, 333, 383, 559
insecticide, 466
insertion, 16, 135, 175, 185, 201, 203, 207, 236, 263, 276, 438, 522, 583
insight, 143, 161, 250, 284, 301, 305, 315, 329, 335, 337, 392, 394, 427, 442, 525
inspiration, 422
instability, 364, 503, 533
institutions, 147, 193, 267, 556
instruction, 504
instruments, 71
insulin, 42, 43, 70, 74, 75, 76, 78, 79, 225, 236, 261, 262, 263, 264, 278, 454, 486
insulin resistance, 43, 70, 74, 75, 76, 78, 79
insulin sensitivity, 43, 78, 263
insulin signaling, 74
insurance, 250, 351, 556
integration, 3, 11, 20, 25, 28, 166, 251, 260, 340, 387, 405, 407, 408, 425, 433, 446, 495, 496, 509, 522, 528, 562
integrin, 512, 543
integrity, 508
intellectual property, 26, 490, 504
intellectual property rights, 26, 490
intensity, 51, 54, 157, 164, 287, 372, 450, 476, 572
intent, viii, 39, 180, 353
interaction, 17, 43, 45, 74, 76, 97, 124, 126, 130, 166, 168, 171, 174, 193, 196, 197, 203, 240, 261, 269, 276, 278, 279, 285, 292, 293, 307, 317, 331, 345, 353, 360, 364, 409, 413, 422, 428, 431, 432, 459, 494, 496, 500, 509, 519, 531, 539, 545, 547, 578
interaction effect, 353, 364
interaction effects, 364
interactions, 3, 7, 11, 13, 14, 18, 20, 22, 23, 30, 45, 76, 130, 133, 135, 139, 140, 143, 150, 168, 172, 180, 194, 198, 199, 203, 205, 226, 243, 244, 245, 250, 251, 253, 268, 275, 284, 286, 307, 316, 328, 342, 345, 348, 360, 364, 365, 387, 424, 427, 428, 431, 475, 491, 496, 497, 498, 500, 506, 528, 543, 545, 559, 560, 561, 580, 583
interest, vii, 14, 15, 21, 22, 27, 51, 70, 71, 132, 148, 150, 176, 191, 209, 222, 226, 247, 265, 268, 284, 286, 290, 292, 293, 301, 303, 310, 311, 312, 324, 330, 336, 338, 343, 353, 360, 375, 377, 397, 403, 404, 410, 418, 429, 434, 456, 495, 499, 505, 511, 515, 538, 539, 545, 551, 569
interface, 71, 183, 188, 268, 298, 333, 334, 408, 450
interference, 17, 18, 34, 37, 175, 294, 308
interferon, 124, 326, 327, 365, 366, 381, 394, 574, 582
interferon (IFN), 327, 394, 582
interleukins, 244
interoperability, 511
interpersonal relations, 547
interpretation, 80, 130, 183, 184, 205, 293, 303, 309, 311, 338, 340, 365, 388, 448, 511, 513, 514, 519, 523, 535, 558, 572
interval, 184, 221, 229, 368, 546
intervention, 2, 12, 13, 28, 142, 150, 222, 272, 285, 315, 345, 387, 390, 496, 510
interview, 145, 319
intestine, 288, 404, 489
intramuscular injection, 87
intraocular, 447
intraocular pressure, 447
introns, 297
inversion, 177
investment, 515
ion channels, 2, 8, 38, 125, 134, 503, 556, 579
ionization, 217, 388
ions, 42
Iran, 242, 370
Ireland, 127, 186, 221, 299, 392, 440
iron, 315
irradiation, 87, 325
irritable bowel syndrome, 360, 361, 412
ischaemic heart disease, 459
Islam, 538
isolation, 11, 215, 317, 370, 409, 524
isoleucine, 519
isoniazid, 128, 403, 487
isotope, 410, 575
isozyme, 77, 91, 343, 442

isozymes, 343, 344, 383, 432, 442
Israel, 37, 151, 234, 322, 329, 330, 345, 427, 485, 511
Italy, 157, 182, 184, 187, 198, 210, 226, 261, 286, 321, 336, 354, 356, 357, 358, 371, 397, 413, 415, 420, 433, 434, 450, 463, 471, 480, 482, 489, 491, 499, 500, 507, 511, 514, 515, 516, 517, 528, 566, 567, 568, 581

J

Jamaica, 561
Japan, 83, 85, 97, 103, 107, 109, 114, 115, 131, 135, 152, 167, 169, 174, 194, 201, 218, 219, 230, 237, 256, 258, 270, 287, 289, 297, 338, 339, 344, 346, 364, 371, 385, 394, 396, 404, 405, 419, 430, 435, 436, 437, 443, 444, 458, 466, 477, 483, 490, 491, 529, 563, 582, 583
jaundice, 261
joint damage, 275
joint destruction, 275
Jordan, 174
judgment, 56
justice, 172, 283
justification, 281

K

K^+, 264
karyotype, 359
keratin, 279
kidney, 40, 42, 43, 44, 50, 53, 54, 74, 77, 136, 151, 200, 251, 280, 314, 385, 386, 404, 439, 489, 560, 564, 569
kidneys, 258, 543
kinase activity, 345, 534
kinetic parameters, 231, 268
kinetic studies, 351, 476
kinetics, 44, 62, 63, 171, 231, 286, 293, 380, 396, 453, 516, 539
knowledge, 3, 5, 6, 12, 13, 14, 20, 22, 23, 25, 29, 71, 126, 127, 141, 142, 151, 152, 156, 158, 159, 163, 164, 166, 175, 188, 193, 196, 200, 204, 209, 225, 232, 239, 243, 244, 245, 248, 250, 256, 278, 289, 293, 301, 302, 309, 311, 318, 323, 327, 338, 342, 346, 347, 348, 350, 358, 360, 361, 363, 375, 377, 381, 382, 387, 390, 396, 397, 402, 403, 404, 406, 408, 427, 428, 429, 430, 433, 441, 443, 451, 455, 483, 488, 494, 496, 503, 509, 514, 518, 524, 529, 539, 543, 544, 555, 559, 566, 568, 577, 580
Korea, 220, 491, 550
Kuwait, 401

L

labeling, 125, 314, 365, 497, 556
labor, 231, 252
labour, 179
lactate dehydrogenase, 445
land, 288
language, 358, 377
latency, 415, 556
later life, 340
laws, 408
lawyers, 283
LDL, 41, 43, 79, 132, 167, 168, 190, 191, 347, 371, 379, 459
lead, vii, 2, 7, 15, 16, 19, 24, 26, 28, 85, 86, 111, 139, 142, 155, 164, 170, 173, 178, 214, 217, 227, 237, 241, 242, 243, 245, 253, 261, 265, 278, 280, 286, 289, 290, 300, 303, 313, 316, 318, 319, 323, 325, 327, 335, 336, 342, 346, 358, 371, 408, 424, 425, 427, 428, 452, 464, 490, 505, 507, 517, 521, 536, 541, 542, 548, 558, 568, 581
learning, 26, 29, 256, 280, 559
Lebanon, 449
legality, 557
legislation, 26, 123, 146
leptin, 458, 530
lesions, 81, 291, 314, 347
leucine, 70, 347, 519
leucocyte, 139, 251
leukemia, 23, 35, 36, 40, 87, 126, 132, 160, 181, 248, 250, 325, 418, 436, 454, 498, 543
leukocytosis, 86
leukopenia, 217, 270
leukotriene antagonists, 254
leukotriene modifier, 241, 345, 514, 570
liability, 143, 324, 528
life cycle, 166, 252, 543
life expectancy, 368
life sciences, 400, 407, 511
lifestyle, 7, 85, 137, 284, 401, 434
lifestyle changes, 137
lifetime, 193, 368
ligand, 31, 125, 240, 268, 286, 411, 424, 565, 574
light transmittance, 180

likelihood, 25, 45, 168, 192, 212, 222, 254, 285, 299, 332, 368, 378, 392, 448, 484, 555
limitation, 160, 290, 483
linear function, 145
linear model, 352, 545
linkage, 21, 121, 127, 130, 133, 137, 141, 152, 157, 209, 227, 279, 289, 297, 304, 374, 381, 384, 409, 414, 422, 440, 466, 467, 474, 483, 506, 517, 519, 524, 560, 569
links, 174, 406, 434, 493
lipid metabolism, 183, 219, 312, 437, 459, 562, 578
lipids, 74, 79, 132, 184, 191, 219, 242
lipoproteins, 41, 42, 132, 219
liquid chromatography, 217, 295, 297, 298, 348, 349, 358, 411, 467, 471, 575
lithium, 293, 434, 463, 481, 512
liver, 13, 40, 41, 42, 43, 44, 48, 49, 50, 53, 54, 62, 64, 66, 67, 68, 69, 70, 74, 75, 76, 80, 81, 143, 153, 154, 167, 171, 195, 200, 229, 243, 251, 258, 261, 266, 280, 281, 301, 322, 364, 383, 384, 385, 386, 397, 404, 413, 419, 439, 470, 475, 476, 478, 487, 489, 518, 551, 559, 561, 563, 564, 567
liver disease, 551
liver metastases, 478
liver transplant, 397, 567
liver transplantation, 397, 567
localization, 333, 420, 439
location, 52, 72, 114, 466
locus, 33, 48, 100, 101, 117, 130, 139, 156, 157, 162, 167, 178, 219, 331, 391, 414, 524, 578
low risk, 216
low-density lipoprotein, 79, 131, 132, 347, 459
lower respiratory tract infection, 337
lumen, 347
lung cancer, 80, 132, 211, 224, 225, 252, 270, 398, 413, 445, 485, 533
lung function, 330
lupus, 40, 165
luteinizing hormone, 240
lymphedema, 398, 399
lymphocytes, 68, 69, 139, 465, 567
lymphoid, 325
lymphoma, 126, 206, 397, 449, 453
lysine, 416

M

machine learning, 480
machinery, 23, 514, 549
macromolecules, 22, 29
macrophages, 89, 239
magnesium, 201, 547
magnetic resonance, 581
magnetic resonance imaging, 581
major depression, 162, 414, 481
major depressive disorder, 149, 304, 530
major histocompatibility complex, 19, 500, 555
malaria, 5, 273, 296, 396, 420
Malaysia, 374
males, 124, 263, 394, 467, 516
malignancy, 308
malignant hyperthermia, 89, 90, 98, 155, 503
malignant tumors, 342, 385
malnutrition, 87, 244
management, 32, 75, 125, 126, 137, 146, 151, 155, 156, 163, 164, 167, 174, 182, 217, 220, 240, 241, 244, 247, 248, 251, 254, 255, 265, 283, 301, 307, 309, 310, 314, 317, 319, 321, 327, 337, 345, 346, 347, 348, 351, 358, 367, 373, 381, 387, 393, 399, 401, 402, 406, 419, 427, 428, 433, 441, 448, 497, 500, 502, 505, 508, 512, 522, 533, 535, 538, 544, 552, 570, 573
manganese, 90, 315
manic, 413, 527
manipulation, 353
manufacturing, 255
mapping, 10, 137, 161, 219, 264, 319, 329, 381, 400, 422, 428, 440, 453, 483, 533, 534, 561
marijuana, 171
market, 7, 10, 18, 25, 134, 146, 162, 166, 243, 269, 271, 324, 365, 395, 424, 497, 546
market segment, 162, 424
marketing, 134, 165, 274, 373, 374, 522
markets, 497, 544
marrow, 398, 402
mass, 11, 42, 176, 196, 216, 217, 237, 252, 255, 295, 323, 348, 349, 358, 366, 376, 388, 405, 458, 575
mass spectrometry, 216, 217, 295, 349, 358, 366, 388, 405, 575
mast cells, 205, 345
mathematics, 558, 559
matrix, 272, 319, 371, 388
matrix metalloproteinase, 272
maturation, 528
MCP, 392
meanings, 544
measurement, 27, 50, 156, 288, 304, 321, 325, 352, 372, 386, 417, 433, 533

measures, 124, 162, 179, 189, 191, 247, 249, 251, 263, 281, 288, 343, 344, 359, 368, 370, 372, 384, 396, 399, 401, 511, 538, 559
meat, 571
media, 441
median, 129, 151, 206, 212, 223, 232, 294, 321, 337, 384, 470, 537, 567
mediation, 205
medication, viii, 7, 30, 83, 87, 125, 127, 147, 149, 150, 169, 207, 241, 251, 265, 273, 275, 279, 290, 293, 294, 336, 345, 366, 373, 377, 390, 406, 420, 429, 453, 471, 477, 501, 510, 519, 531, 570, 578, 581, 582
Mediterranean, 517
melting, 478
membership, 221, 557
membranes, 200, 462, 583
men, 130, 132, 147, 168, 309, 359, 368, 378, 379, 459, 478, 489, 517, 534
meningitis, 105, 111, 119
mental disorder, 84, 332
mental health, 463
mental illness, 368
mental retardation, 98
mesothelioma, 157
messages, 127, 373
messenger ribonucleic acid, 78, 229, 366
messenger RNA, 123, 419
metabolic disorder, 204, 492
metabolic pathways, 513, 564
metabolic syndrome, 336, 497
metabolism, 12, 24, 43, 76, 89, 91, 98, 99, 100, 128, 129, 131, 134, 138, 141, 152, 153, 154, 156, 164, 166, 167, 171, 177, 178, 180, 183, 190, 195, 197, 200, 201, 204, 207, 208, 213, 215, 216, 218, 220, 232, 243, 245, 249, 266, 267, 268, 271, 275, 277, 285, 296, 297, 301, 307, 309, 314, 315, 318, 343, 349, 351, 354, 356, 364, 371, 372, 382, 383, 385, 387, 400, 403, 411, 419, 420, 422, 427, 435, 440, 441, 445, 446, 451, 455, 470, 471, 473, 477, 483, 485, 487, 491, 492, 500, 501, 503, 507, 510, 516, 518, 519, 520, 521, 523, 529, 532, 536, 539, 542, 543, 547, 548, 557, 558, 561, 563, 566, 569, 572, 575, 576, 581, 583
metabolites, 88, 164, 195, 196, 208, 217, 228, 237, 266, 295, 297, 298, 303, 321, 348, 362, 372, 404, 450, 477, 478, 560, 575
metabolizing, 8, 85, 90, 125, 126, 129, 130, 152, 159, 160, 161, 166, 168, 169, 170, 178, 188, 200, 202, 214, 216, 220, 226, 242, 243, 249, 251, 252, 258, 259, 260, 265, 269, 270, 271, 275, 276, 293, 298, 301, 305, 318, 327, 332, 338, 339, 342, 343, 362, 363, 365, 371, 372, 374, 375, 387, 390, 403, 411, 427, 445, 446, 448, 469, 473, 488, 491, 497, 500, 504, 505, 507, 508, 511, 514, 518, 519, 520, 521, 526, 537, 543, 548, 549, 550, 571, 580, 581, 582
metabolome, vii, 1, 410
metals, 399
metastasis, 126, 199, 334, 478
metastatic cancer, 142
metformin, 262
methanol, 358
methodology, 22, 94, 178, 222, 273, 279, 352, 353, 360, 373
methylation, 17, 18, 34, 156, 266, 359, 382, 397, 472, 525, 542, 548
methylphenidate, 176, 277
methylprednisolone, viii, 40, 44, 45, 50, 71, 77, 79, 80, 495
Mexico, 161, 180, 285, 536
MHC, 164
Miami, 153, 314, 383, 447
mice, 78, 206, 263, 281, 315, 379, 392, 411, 412, 428, 439, 471
microarray technology, 81, 192, 242, 257, 286, 294, 310, 399, 416, 557
microemulsion, 566
microorganism, 265
microscopy, 210
microsomes, 154, 171, 364, 383, 385, 470, 475
Middle East, 532
migraines, 450
milk, 221, 366, 453
milligrams, 234
mineralocorticoid, 42, 43, 77
mining, vii, viii, 2, 21, 40, 51, 53, 70, 71, 75, 251, 331, 333, 389, 556
minorities, 402
minority, 130
MIP, 392
mitochondria, 315
mitochondrial DNA, 363
mitogen, 393
MMA, 281
MMP, 217, 372
mode, 217, 256, 277, 288, 461, 521, 561
model specification, 545
model system, 170, 204, 211, 471, 527, 561

modeling, viii, 25, 36, 39, 45, 46, 48, 54, 60, 75, 76, 123, 145, 175, 204, 212, 302, 334, 352, 362, 382, 409, 461, 495, 503, 572
models, viii, 28, 39, 45, 48, 50, 62, 63, 70, 73, 74, 75, 76, 78, 80, 123, 127, 142, 146, 150, 160, 175, 189, 233, 246, 250, 257, 263, 280, 290, 294, 335, 349, 352, 367, 368, 383, 386, 387, 409, 426, 428, 451, 454, 477, 502, 530, 551, 558, 565, 572
moderate persistent asthma, 570
moderates, 87
modifier gene, 433
molar ratios, 383
mold, 172
molecular biology, vii, 1, 5, 6, 23, 26, 148, 154, 191, 259, 314, 353, 389, 401, 407, 435, 516, 533, 546, 559, 571, 573
molecular medicine, 3, 351, 497, 514, 541, 571
molecular pathology, 493
molecular targeting, 146
molecular weight, 10, 391
molecules, 14, 17, 22, 29, 42, 70, 85, 139, 142, 144, 147, 163, 179, 232, 246, 257, 286, 293, 303, 305, 312, 317, 337, 339, 394, 402, 408, 410, 440, 441, 443, 448, 454, 476, 525, 529, 554, 572
momentum, 514
money, 166, 401, 416
monitoring, 2, 3, 87, 94, 143, 173, 176, 188, 216, 217, 238, 251, 253, 265, 266, 273, 285, 308, 310, 314, 326, 338, 347, 372, 400, 436, 456, 490, 492, 537, 538, 548, 549, 551, 566, 567, 576
monoclonal antibody, 24, 169, 177, 494
monocyte chemoattractant protein, 392
monograph, 283
monolayer, 79
Montenegro, 359, 534
mood, 90, 99, 184, 277, 414, 434, 463, 464, 512, 527, 548
mood disorder, 90, 99, 184, 277, 414, 434, 463, 464, 512
morbidity, 88, 130, 139, 150, 198, 222, 248, 252, 273, 292, 321, 322, 340, 370, 399, 421, 456, 458, 463, 512, 515, 534
morphine, 194, 226, 379, 437, 450, 518, 519, 555
morphology, 579
mortality, 85, 87, 130, 139, 163, 198, 207, 222, 224, 225, 248, 252, 281, 292, 321, 399, 410, 421, 456, 515, 534, 537, 577, 578
mortality rate, 130, 410
mosaic, ix, 103, 105
mothers, 232, 366, 453
motion, viii, 39, 50, 54
motivation, 434
movement, 42, 69, 84, 89, 100, 309, 538, 542
movement disorders, 100
MRI, 581
mRNA, 44, 45, 48, 49, 50, 52, 53, 61, 62, 63, 64, 65, 66, 67, 68, 69, 78, 79, 80, 123, 251, 273, 276, 279, 288, 312, 356, 384, 385, 419, 444, 445, 475, 518, 555, 564
mtDNA, 363
mucosa, 33, 303, 494, 503
multidimensional, 158, 387, 453, 486, 572, 581
multiple factors, 488
multiple myeloma, 141, 169
multiple regression, 376, 477
multiple regression analysis, 376
multiple sclerosis, 40, 81, 381
multiplication, 69, 178
muscarinic receptor, 14
muscle atrophy, 74, 89
muscle relaxant, 87
muscles, 42, 79
muscular dystrophy, 8
Muslims, 156
mutant, 154, 181, 215, 218, 264, 297, 368, 379, 434, 524
mutation, 15, 88, 90, 92, 105, 125, 132, 139, 141, 152, 170, 177, 195, 214, 227, 239, 253, 262, 264, 265, 267, 277, 278, 297, 302, 312, 338, 339, 354, 355, 363, 398, 459, 460, 461, 474, 492, 499, 524, 538, 582
myelin, 414, 563
myelodysplastic syndromes, 326
myocardial infarction, 142, 163, 207, 209, 275, 391, 464, 552
myocardium, 255
myoclonus, 94
myocyte, 324
myosin, 11

N

NaCl, 50, 467
NAD, 206, 404
nanosystems, 242
nanotechnology, 6
nation states, 401
National Institutes of Health, 127, 130, 283, 284, 286, 345, 467, 483
National Research Council, 516

nausea, 153, 187, 212, 306, 546
necrosis, 159, 169, 239, 539, 560
needs, 12, 21, 36, 73, 94, 163, 165, 224, 246, 269, 363, 373, 388, 402, 403, 440, 481, 504, 564
negative mood, 531
neglect, 269
neonatal sepsis, 226
neonates, 226
neoplasm, 325
neoplastic tissue, 411
nephritis, 165
nephropathy, 40, 44, 431, 568
nephrotic syndrome, 40
nervous system, 90, 98, 129, 360, 361, 432, 450
nested PCR, 106, 111
Netherlands, 107, 172, 177, 200, 201, 210, 227, 230, 265, 275, 310, 343, 355, 360, 454, 455, 457, 485, 504, 542, 550, 552
network, 29, 73, 133, 184, 279, 317, 387, 407, 443, 483, 509, 549
neural network, 184, 527
neural networks, 185, 527
neurobiology, 390, 433, 491
neuroblastoma, 444
neurodegeneration, 315, 548
neurogenesis, 414
neuroimaging, 93, 433, 530, 581
neurokinin, 307
neuroleptic drugs, viii
neuroleptic malignant syndrome, viii, 83, 84, 85, 95, 96, 97, 98, 99, 100, 101, 102
neuroleptics, 84, 85, 86, 87, 88, 90, 91, 92, 93, 98
neurologic symptom, 84, 89
neurological disease, 381
neuronal circuits, 529, 540
neuronal systems, 175
neurons, 265, 304, 527
neuropathy, 201
neuropeptides, 513
neuroscience, 340, 381, 435
neurotransmission, 88, 90, 424, 548
neurotransmitter, 84, 134, 265, 342, 414, 455, 509, 548
neutropenia, 161, 187, 200, 212, 270
new market niches, 150
New Zealand, 221, 273, 372, 469, 491
next generation, 28, 142, 148, 397, 497
nicotinamide, 230, 473
nicotine, 149, 253, 363, 432, 435, 470, 501, 502, 575
nitric oxide, 11, 137, 138, 240, 276, 469
nitric oxide synthase, 138, 240, 276, 469
nitrogen, 41, 50
NMR, 410
nodes, 184
noise, 80, 123, 433
non-Hodgkin's lymphoma, 40
non-nucleoside reverse transcriptase inhibitors, 310
nonsense mutation, 201
nonsmokers, 132
non-steroidal anti-inflammatory drugs, 194, 196, 334, 423, 492
norepinephrine, 148, 450, 462, 463, 518, 547
normal distribution, 299
North Africa, 532
North America, 118, 120, 254
Norway, 153, 259, 262, 366, 450, 570
Nrf2, 565
NSAIDs, 194, 196, 197, 261, 323, 423
nuclear magnetic resonance, 348
nuclear receptors, 133, 243
nucleic acid, 17, 144, 178
nucleoside reverse transcriptase inhibitors, 555
nucleotide sequencing, ix, 104, 311
nucleotides, 6, 156, 216, 217, 239, 311, 320, 372, 574
nucleus, 45, 49, 62, 89
nurses, 225, 387
nursing, 147, 225, 387, 453
nutrients, 13, 382, 395
nutrition, 33, 130, 382

O

obesity, 78, 79, 244, 263, 303, 412, 462, 463, 513, 529
observations, viii, 83, 233, 250, 292, 299, 388, 389, 407, 421, 492, 525, 536, 546, 568
obstruction, 552
occupational health, 123
octopus, 390
oculomotor, 89
OECD, 202, 511
oedema, 555
ofloxacin, 113
OGSA, 405
oil, 395
olanzapine, 84, 95, 458, 538
oligonucleotide arrays, 233
omeprazole, 296, 297, 478
oncogenes, 144, 305

openness, 579
operator, 183
operon, 113
opiates, 194, 517
opioids, 194, 226, 517, 539, 546, 554, 555
optimism, 221
optimization, 158, 160, 178, 197, 215, 280, 339, 347
oral presentations, 131
orchestration, 29, 324
organ, 7, 33, 41, 244, 249, 252, 308, 326, 337, 339, 436, 448, 453, 505, 506, 507, 548, 566, 568
organic compounds, 147
organism, 4, 6, 17, 177, 178, 249, 288, 527, 548, 571
organization, viii, 40, 75, 147, 493, 562
organizations, 147, 238, 283, 351, 390, 497, 504
orientation, 299
osmolality, 244
osteoporosis, 272, 321, 371
otitis media, 111
outline, 22, 147, 251, 328, 493
outpatients, 367, 452
output, 334, 388, 533, 561
ovarian cancer, 142
overload, 562
overproduction, 266
oversight, 390
overweight, 513
ovulation, 314, 468
oxidation, 37, 92, 100, 171, 228, 260, 462, 548, 558
oxidation products, 558
oxidative stress, 81, 310, 315, 565
oxygen, 268, 570
ozone, 288

P

p53, 272, 402
Pacific, 418
paclitaxel, 212, 343, 358, 385, 394
pain, 193, 194, 226, 301, 349, 360, 361, 379, 414, 435, 450, 451, 539, 546
pain management, 301, 349
pairing, 424
pancreas, 210, 243, 567
pancreatic cancer, 210, 485
panic disorder, 340
paradigm shift, 348, 423, 529, 540
paralysis, 461
parameter, 184, 209, 295, 304, 310, 398, 486
parasite, 273, 571
parathyroid, 444, 465
parathyroid hormone, 465
parenting, 147
Parkinson's disease, 88
paroxetine, 162, 226, 294, 366
particles, 10
partition, 399
partnership, 159, 191, 359, 441
patents, 217
pathogenesis, 10, 11, 16, 24, 79, 87, 88, 90, 93, 127, 142, 143, 150, 157, 169, 204, 226, 240, 252, 290, 300, 332, 337, 342, 346, 377, 464, 493, 512, 534, 535, 544, 581
pathogens, ix, 103, 279
pathologist, 158, 559
pathology, 133, 191, 252, 314, 315, 382, 408, 493, 497, 536, 558, 559, 560, 562
pathophysiology, vii, viii, 1, 3, 7, 11, 22, 28, 83, 88, 90, 94, 161, 179, 189, 277, 303, 308, 337, 340, 347, 409, 411, 414, 433, 494, 498, 499, 509, 530, 541
pathways, vii, 1, 2, 11, 23, 28, 32, 72, 88, 89, 90, 127, 133, 134, 142, 145, 156, 172, 193, 197, 199, 200, 201, 239, 245, 246, 250, 257, 261, 265, 272, 274, 278, 286, 289, 294, 300, 303, 308, 315, 317, 326, 330, 331, 353, 357, 360, 361, 376, 397, 406, 408, 409, 410, 413, 414, 421, 427, 445, 453, 454, 472, 473, 485, 496, 507, 513, 526, 529, 533, 548, 549, 561, 564, 565, 575, 581
patient care, vii, 2, 3, 7, 8, 10, 11, 14, 15, 16, 17, 19, 20, 22, 24, 26, 27, 28, 29, 30, 34, 37, 163, 225, 242, 312, 316, 329, 390, 469
pattern recognition, 526, 559
PBMC, 233
PCP, 444
PCR, ix, 81, 104, 105, 106, 107, 109, 110, 111, 112, 113, 114, 116, 118, 119, 121, 152, 155, 156, 167, 171, 178, 191, 195, 199, 203, 210, 212, 213, 215, 217, 219, 224, 238, 266, 291, 295, 311, 312, 333, 339, 359, 381, 405, 411, 412, 413, 416, 446, 452, 473, 481, 482, 495, 516, 519, 551, 556, 563, 564, 566, 567, 574
pedigree, 174
penetrance, 302, 330, 456
penicillin, ix, 103, 104, 106, 111, 112, 115, 119, 121
peptides, 144, 255, 303, 496
percentile, 51
perceptions, 283
peripheral blood, 156, 220, 233, 464, 567
peripheral blood mononuclear cell, 233, 464, 567

peripheral neuropathy, 555
peripheral vascular disease, 110
peritonitis, 111
permeability, 105, 158, 239
permeation, 583
permit, ix, 22, 24, 28, 84, 88, 114, 138, 251, 316, 317, 353, 551, 555, 562
persistent asthma, 150
personality, 156
personality disorder, 156
perspective, 30, 35, 99, 126, 136, 147, 159, 184, 205, 237, 320, 323, 327, 346, 361, 368, 389, 407, 410, 425, 427, 484, 493, 496, 514, 559, 573, 577
Perth, 186, 500
pesticide, 282
PET, 436, 581
pH, 264, 461, 467
pharmaceuticals, 275, 282, 296, 547
pharmacogenomics, vii, 1, 2, 3, 5, 6, 8, 10, 12, 14, 15, 16, 17, 18, 19, 20, 21, 22, 24, 25, 26, 27, 28, 29, 30, 32, 33, 34, 36, 37, 38, 77, 80, 81, 126, 127, 134, 135, 136, 137, 140, 142, 146, 150, 151, 153, 155, 158, 161, 162, 166, 172, 175, 177, 179, 192, 194, 200, 201, 202, 204, 214, 220, 222, 239, 241, 242, 243, 244, 245, 246, 247, 250, 252, 253, 254, 256, 257, 258, 259, 260, 266, 267, 272, 275, 277, 282, 302, 305, 310, 314, 317, 321, 322, 323, 326, 328, 329, 332, 334, 335, 336, 338, 339, 351, 352, 354, 355, 364, 366, 372, 373, 377, 381, 395, 396, 397, 398, 399, 404, 406, 407, 408, 415, 420, 421, 423, 424, 425, 426, 427, 430, 439, 444, 445, 446, 448, 449, 450, 451, 453, 455, 456, 457, 481, 482, 483, 484, 485, 488, 489, 490, 491, 492, 493, 494, 495, 496, 499, 500, 502, 504, 508, 509, 510, 511, 513, 514, 515, 516, 525, 536, 537, 540, 541, 543, 544, 547, 549, 555, 570, 572, 580
pharmacokinetics, 5, 7, 22, 33, 49, 85, 128, 129, 131, 147, 148, 155, 165, 167, 198, 211, 212, 218, 221, 227, 228, 231, 232, 233, 235, 237, 242, 249, 258, 274, 301, 321, 326, 338, 339, 343, 357, 366, 378, 390, 394, 415, 420, 453, 464, 478, 487, 488, 497, 503, 505, 514, 515, 521, 547, 549, 550, 558, 567, 568, 572, 580, 583
pharmacological research, vii, 1
pharmacological treatment, 391, 431, 463, 482, 513, 517
pharmacology, vii, 1, 2, 3, 5, 6, 7, 8, 10, 13, 17, 20, 25, 32, 33, 36, 37, 133, 147, 153, 165, 190, 193, 220, 226, 240, 269, 272, 274, 276, 280, 292, 293, 322, 327, 328, 335, 341, 342, 358, 391, 403, 408, 409, 435, 485, 493, 494, 511, 527, 546, 547, 554, 572, 574, 578, 583
pharmacotherapy, 2, 3, 5, 7, 8, 11, 12, 13, 14, 15, 16, 17, 18, 19, 21, 23, 24, 26, 27, 28, 38, 85, 96, 149, 172, 195, 199, 200, 201, 202, 242, 258, 301, 310, 322, 342, 346, 358, 363, 365, 375, 412, 420, 432, 455, 463, 526, 539, 549, 581, 583
pharmacotyping, vii, 2, 3, 8, 16, 19, 21, 22, 23, 24, 25, 26, 27, 28, 242
pharyngitis, 357
pharynx, 118
phenol, 138
phenotype, 13, 16, 91, 92, 130, 152, 184, 194, 195, 202, 211, 213, 214, 230, 234, 235, 240, 254, 256, 264, 297, 300, 302, 303, 315, 318, 329, 332, 333, 350, 355, 358, 359, 366, 367, 371, 383, 384, 393, 394, 405, 409, 427, 433, 436, 440, 442, 444, 459, 469, 470, 473, 475, 476, 481, 483, 487, 499, 503, 515, 522, 527, 532, 534, 536, 537, 546, 548, 554, 562, 572, 580
phenylketonuria, 382
phenytoin, 171, 344, 470
phosphatidylcholine, 263
phosphatidylethanolamine, 263
phosphoenolpyruvate, 41, 76
phospholipids, 496, 563
phosphorylation, 109, 181, 210, 413
physical therapy, 399
physiology, 5, 6, 8, 26, 204, 278, 408, 527, 583
physiopathology, 198
pilot study, 92, 99, 273, 447
PK/PD models, viii, 39
placebo, 95, 185, 329, 331, 366, 432, 463, 494, 531, 545, 552
placenta, 444, 506
planning, 175, 290, 350, 351, 402, 564
plants, 288
plasma, 43, 47, 48, 49, 79, 91, 94, 128, 129, 141, 182, 188, 196, 203, 212, 218, 219, 223, 226, 228, 231, 234, 237, 253, 258, 262, 294, 295, 297, 301, 310, 313, 314, 347, 356, 358, 362, 378, 380, 383, 411, 415, 420, 435, 443, 452, 458, 459, 463, 464, 471, 474, 477, 479, 487, 492, 498, 521, 548, 555, 567
plasma cells, 141
plasma levels, 43, 380, 383, 555
plasmid, 107, 110, 113, 114, 118, 135
plasminogen, 522
plasticity, 35, 491, 528, 529, 540, 573
platelet aggregation, 180, 209, 334, 392, 535

platelet count, 327, 537
platelets, 512
platinum, 14, 201, 354, 446
plausibility, 289, 579
pleasure, 414
pleiotropy, 143
PM, 76, 91, 92, 145, 178, 195, 305, 329, 381, 421, 495, 512, 516, 517, 532
PMS, 274
pneumococcus, 119
pneumonia, 89, 337
point mutation, 107, 152, 265, 582
Poland, 131, 191, 391, 396, 403, 512
polarity, 444
policy makers, 174, 260, 441, 456, 496
policy making, 259
pollutants, 571
polycarbonates, 583
polycystic kidneys, 314
polymerase, ix, 104, 105, 106, 117, 135, 149, 152, 153, 161, 203, 213, 229, 265, 282, 291, 295, 297, 366, 367, 381, 392, 400, 406, 413, 447, 459, 465, 467, 519, 550, 566, 567
polymerase chain reaction, ix, 104, 105, 106, 117, 135, 149, 152, 153, 161, 203, 213, 229, 265, 282, 291, 295, 297, 366, 367, 381, 392, 400, 406, 413, 447, 459, 465, 467, 519, 550, 566, 567
polymerase chain reactions, ix, 104, 105
polymers, 10, 583
polymorphism, 13, 19, 31, 33, 34, 93, 99, 101, 125, 127, 135, 138, 142, 145, 148, 149, 152, 154, 156, 161, 162, 164, 168, 170, 175, 176, 178, 180, 182, 183, 184, 185, 186, 191, 193, 194, 195, 196, 197, 199, 201, 203, 206, 207, 208, 209, 210, 213, 214, 218, 220, 223, 226, 227, 230, 235, 236, 239, 240, 241, 250, 254, 258, 259, 260, 262, 270, 276, 277, 291, 296, 299, 304, 305, 311, 312, 322, 323, 329, 331, 333, 334, 340, 341, 344, 347, 351, 357, 359, 364, 368, 374, 375, 376, 378, 382, 383, 390, 396, 401, 402, 403, 405, 410, 412, 415, 416, 421, 432, 434, 435, 436, 437, 438, 442, 447, 450, 452, 455, 456, 458, 459, 461, 462, 463, 464, 465, 466, 467, 468, 469, 470, 474, 475, 476, 478, 479, 481, 486, 490, 498, 499, 501, 509, 512, 516, 517, 518, 519, 522, 523, 528, 531, 532, 534, 536, 549, 550, 551, 552, 555, 566, 569, 570, 577, 582
polyp, 196, 197
polypeptide, 31, 231, 237, 498
polyps, 196, 197
pools, 43
poor, 7, 91, 92, 142, 143, 153, 154, 160, 162, 178, 198, 215, 226, 234, 256, 267, 281, 293, 294, 295, 297, 329, 344, 352, 356, 364, 366, 367, 420, 433, 458, 469, 477, 479, 491, 501, 506, 508, 512, 516, 517, 534, 542, 548, 556
population, 11, 13, 15, 16, 44, 100, 119, 123, 129, 130, 135, 137, 140, 142, 150, 151, 156, 157, 159, 166, 167, 184, 188, 195, 198, 206, 208, 211, 213, 220, 222, 223, 232, 233, 236, 240, 243, 246, 248, 251, 255, 267, 270, 273, 274, 285, 289, 295, 296, 297, 299, 301, 303, 319, 327, 328, 331, 333, 334, 347, 351, 360, 363, 368, 371, 374, 378, 382, 387, 390, 394, 401, 410, 414, 415, 420, 422, 423, 427, 431, 440, 443, 451, 452, 453, 456, 458, 460, 462, 463, 466, 467, 470, 471, 477, 482, 487, 495, 503, 506, 514, 515, 516, 517, 521, 523, 524, 530, 536, 544, 547, 550, 552, 556, 564, 568, 572, 578
porphyria, 503
portfolio, 140, 490, 493
Portugal, 178, 296, 335, 537
positive correlation, 210, 302
positron, 307, 581
positron emission tomography, 307, 581
posttraumatic stress, 540
posture, 42
potassium, 9, 11, 274, 324, 557
power, 94, 140, 143, 145, 166, 199, 232, 294, 329, 369, 376, 424, 454, 513, 514, 519, 530, 545, 558, 579
PPAR agonists, 308
precipitation, 358
precursor cells, 248
predictability, 166, 205, 504
prediction, x, 18, 21, 25, 36, 38, 87, 88, 99, 104, 126, 133, 153, 158, 193, 195, 204, 205, 215, 221, 250, 253, 264, 280, 292, 309, 316, 317, 324, 347, 353, 362, 363, 364, 386, 393, 399, 412, 416, 426, 430, 453, 454, 478, 494, 498, 504, 509, 519, 542, 551, 560
predictors, 126, 131, 132, 138, 148, 183, 192, 202, 206, 226, 244, 249, 272, 278, 356, 386, 398, 452, 461, 463, 464, 475, 494, 495, 513, 529, 566, 569, 570, 577
prednisone, 79, 452
preference, 456
prefrontal cortex, 156
pregnancy, 85, 96, 130, 147, 231, 244
pressure, 104, 135, 137, 183, 245, 254, 334, 370, 376, 377, 431, 439, 510, 537
preterm delivery, 231

prevention, viii, 79, 83, 84, 87, 88, 124, 131, 146, 149, 150, 153, 159, 163, 164, 167, 179, 191, 204, 225, 241, 248, 272, 285, 292, 306, 316, 387, 402, 423, 430, 435, 441, 491, 504, 512, 520, 529, 535, 538, 554, 570, 582
pricing policies, 313
primary cells, 417
primary data, 406
primary tumor, 211
principle, 72, 138, 161, 178, 242, 262, 286, 299, 356, 386, 418, 476, 548, 564
prior knowledge, 214
privacy, 26, 27, 250, 320, 400, 406, 424, 488, 509, 540
probability, 53, 165, 198, 252, 348, 409, 414, 425, 506, 521
probe, 50, 51, 52, 53, 54, 55, 56, 57, 59, 60, 61, 64, 66, 67, 68, 69, 72, 73, 92, 116, 153, 233, 235, 280, 298, 408, 470, 495, 557
probiotic, 496
problem solving, 559
prodromal symptoms, 85, 88
prodrugs, 485
production, 10, 41, 42, 45, 46, 47, 65, 68, 69, 74, 78, 105, 107, 109, 112, 113, 121, 131, 182, 201, 260, 286, 353, 439
productivity, 162, 267
professions, 359
prognosis, 32, 85, 125, 198, 247, 255, 300, 305, 314, 342, 363, 364, 400, 478, 542, 579
program, 36, 45, 51, 76, 118, 120, 192, 284, 570
prolactin, 84, 93, 101
proliferation, 16, 20, 22, 181, 199, 248, 257, 272, 370, 472, 473, 533, 557, 562
prolyl oligopeptidase, 527
promoter, 13, 14, 33, 37, 93, 101, 117, 162, 197, 212, 230, 239, 262, 270, 304, 339, 344, 356, 434, 444, 458, 459, 466, 467, 474, 499, 512, 527, 528, 552
prophylactic, 139, 153, 481, 512
prophylaxis, 153, 306, 567
proposition, 57
propranolol, 9
propylene, 369
prostate, 81, 315, 359, 380, 410, 489
prostate cancer, 81, 315, 380, 489
prostate gland, 380
prosthesis, 537
protease inhibitors, 310
protective role, 486
protein family, 76
protein kinase C, 53, 402
protein misfolding, 525
protein sequence, 73, 239, 484
proteins, vii, ix, 1, 3, 10, 15, 16, 17, 23, 24, 29, 41, 42, 43, 72, 104, 112, 119, 124, 129, 133, 134, 138, 139, 144, 150, 159, 166, 183, 194, 200, 201, 211, 214, 219, 240, 251, 256, 260, 270, 277, 286, 289, 293, 303, 306, 312, 343, 348, 354, 357, 371, 394, 402, 403, 421, 430, 436, 443, 444, 448, 451, 454, 462, 473, 485, 487, 489, 503, 506, 507, 508, 511, 518, 519, 526, 527, 528, 558, 579
proteinuria, 136, 431
proteolytic enzyme, 74
proteome, vii, 1
proteomics, 10, 21, 126, 133, 142, 143, 179, 203, 204, 251, 252, 257, 302, 303, 328, 335, 341, 353, 372, 381, 397, 433, 444, 499, 536, 541, 562, 571, 572
prothrombin, 522
protocol, 181, 185, 188, 224, 299, 321, 327, 344, 390, 406, 408, 409, 541
proton pump inhibitors, 37, 269, 501
prototype, 290, 405, 413, 449
pruritus, 233
pseudocholinesterase, 299, 469
Pseudomonas aeruginosa, 288, 370
psoriasis, 189
psychiatric disorders, 143, 433, 482, 513, 527
psychiatric illness, 133, 143
psychiatric patients, 341
psychopathology, 340
psychopharmacology, 293, 367
psychoses, 96
psychosis, 99, 372, 455, 458, 538
psychosocial factors, 255
psychotic symptoms, 87
psychotropic drugs, 85, 87, 90, 94, 99, 168
PTSD, 530
public education, 147
public health, 124, 238, 283, 284, 285, 288, 310, 312, 323, 371, 395, 400, 433, 435, 456, 457, 489, 531, 546, 559, 564
public interest, 132, 284
public investment, 150
public policy, 147
pulse, 165, 354, 570
pumps, 200, 265, 306, 308
P-value, 330
pyrimidine, 161, 485

Pyszczynski, 80

Q

QT interval, 188, 324, 546
quality assurance, 146, 311
quality control, 54, 311, 358
quality of life, 325, 450, 541, 556, 578
quantum mechanics, 389
query, 70, 393
quetiapine, 84, 95
quinone, 230, 404

R

race, 150, 176, 223, 233, 267, 322, 373, 419, 430, 441, 467, 477, 510, 549, 551, 553, 580
racial differences, 394
radiation, 252, 541
Radiation, 156, 157, 317, 338
radiation therapy, 252
radiotherapy, 198, 363, 401
rain, 288
range, 42, 51, 55, 58, 127, 135, 138, 140, 146, 159, 173, 175, 176, 212, 214, 215, 223, 232, 234, 244, 252, 260, 272, 274, 277, 284, 290, 294, 298, 305, 313, 328, 330, 333, 335, 337, 346, 352, 358, 365, 372, 381, 382, 386, 405, 440, 461, 465, 482, 490, 528, 537, 556, 564, 567
rash, 224, 261, 539
ratings, 415
readership, 176
reading, 545
reagents, 249, 371, 413, 499
real time, 381, 473
reality, 2, 5, 20, 22, 28, 38, 185, 189, 214, 253, 267, 274, 275, 380, 489, 491, 520, 535
reasoning, 319
reception, 373
receptors, 2, 8, 9, 10, 11, 13, 31, 34, 41, 42, 43, 45, 68, 88, 90, 94, 98, 101, 125, 134, 143, 155, 167, 177, 201, 202, 207, 209, 214, 219, 226, 236, 239, 240, 242, 243, 257, 272, 273, 301, 308, 331, 332, 335, 342, 357, 368, 371, 379, 403, 412, 420, 421, 424, 436, 444, 454, 455, 462, 465, 474, 494, 501, 503, 504, 518, 526, 529, 530, 531, 535, 539, 543, 546, 549, 555, 556, 565, 574, 578, 582
reciprocal translocation, 23
recognition, 70, 85, 312, 337, 345, 407, 414, 424, 429, 572
recombinant DNA, 5, 10, 241, 252
recombination, ix, 103, 105, 152, 157
recovery, 44, 88, 196, 212, 402, 461, 481, 530
recurrence, 163, 196, 300, 363, 434, 534, 554
recycling, 240
redistribution, 402
reduction, 74, 132, 143, 149, 158, 167, 176, 183, 220, 227, 241, 290, 319, 322, 325, 372, 376, 405, 427, 431, 439, 455, 461, 463, 465, 487, 514, 553, 565, 578, 581
redundancy, 50, 333, 357, 495
refining, 192
reflection, 440
regeneration, 560, 564
Registry, 363
regression, 132, 137, 182, 187, 262, 291, 326, 329, 352, 353, 367, 368, 392, 419, 449, 452, 461, 466, 469, 509, 566
regression analysis, 132, 187, 262, 291, 327, 419, 452, 461, 466, 509, 566
regulation, 18, 32, 43, 49, 52, 54, 57, 76, 77, 93, 123, 140, 145, 147, 160, 167, 179, 180, 194, 224, 244, 259, 268, 272, 284, 333, 341, 352, 374, 376, 377, 395, 411, 418, 421, 442, 458, 473, 479, 497, 514, 518, 521, 528, 544, 556
regulations, 245, 375
regulators, 76, 179, 249, 328, 559
regulatory framework, 336, 395
regulatory oversight, 146
rejection, 151, 156, 308, 505, 551, 565, 566, 567, 568
relapses, 481, 582
relationship, 51, 53, 72, 73, 92, 93, 101, 117, 124, 141, 148, 151, 158, 160, 164, 172, 173, 174, 175, 181, 187, 195, 203, 209, 224, 251, 259, 269, 279, 280, 284, 292, 293, 294, 297, 305, 306, 314, 341, 344, 345, 362, 366, 375, 397, 401, 404, 429, 433, 436, 443, 447, 451, 466, 477, 488, 500, 503, 517, 521, 543, 553, 578, 582, 584
relationships, viii, 14, 39, 44, 72, 73, 101, 129, 167, 223, 270, 285, 310, 317, 318, 343, 349, 351, 355, 374, 404, 480, 500, 565
relatives, 526
relaxation, 331
relevance, 3, 5, 7, 10, 13, 17, 24, 25, 32, 99, 124, 125, 150, 159, 160, 166, 178, 205, 206, 211, 225, 235, 238, 244, 252, 256, 260, 268, 282, 305, 318, 325, 334, 338, 340, 353, 390, 404, 469, 471, 474,

484, 500, 506, 511, 519, 533, 561, 572, 573, 574, 578, 583, 584
reliability, 198, 199, 466
remission, 169, 400, 481, 482, 494, 581
remodelling, 199
renal failure, 185, 314, 465
renin, 136, 138, 202, 203, 207, 543
repair, 9, 15, 201, 382, 514, 533, 550, 565
replacement, 131, 136, 149, 150, 168, 298, 334, 341, 359, 363, 432, 477, 499, 502
replication, 125, 128, 148, 244, 253, 254, 434, 523, 549, 578
repression, 49, 63, 64, 67, 68
repressor, 444
reproduction, 571
resection, 194
residual disease, 325, 372, 400
residues, 472
resistance, ix, 9, 23, 33, 36, 43, 85, 90, 103, 104, 105, 106, 107, 108, 109, 110, 111, 112, 113, 114, 115, 116, 117, 118, 119, 120, 121, 125, 126, 128, 133, 135, 138, 146, 152, 157, 172, 181, 194, 206, 207, 210, 223, 224, 227, 252, 255, 256, 257, 264, 265, 272, 288, 290, 291, 292, 294, 305, 306, 307, 309, 317, 325, 332, 337, 338, 342, 344, 354, 355, 356, 357, 364, 369, 370, 373, 391, 392, 402, 411, 447, 448, 452, 473, 496, 498, 505, 506, 512, 524, 541, 542, 549, 551, 555, 566, 569, 570, 581, 583
resolution, viii, 40, 125, 138, 150, 253, 286, 582
resource allocation, 401
resources, 81, 193, 248, 260, 313, 370, 382, 387, 401, 405, 406, 407, 409, 418, 479, 480, 496
respiratory, 89, 111, 118, 139, 346, 436, 505, 513, 546, 570
respiratory acidosis, 89
respiratory problems, 513
respiratory rate, 570
response time, 528
responsiveness, 33, 93, 131, 292, 331, 372, 380, 421, 478, 506, 580, 582
resting potential, 461
restriction enzyme, 467, 551
restriction fragment length polymorphis, 217, 447, 519
retention, 42, 44, 135, 359
reticulum, 473, 562
retrieval, 406, 457
returns, 44, 48, 500
reverse transcriptase, 229, 265, 282, 479, 500, 560
rhabdomyolysis, 89, 94
rheumatic diseases, 159, 492
rheumatoid arthritis, 7, 38, 159, 170, 261, 275, 389, 437, 483, 498, 507
rhodopsin, 240
rhythm, 79
ribonucleic acid, 233, 348
ribozymes, 10, 144
rice, 12
rights, 271, 272, 275, 406, 441
rings, 107, 451
risk, viii, 2, 7, 9, 11, 15, 25, 28, 40, 83, 84, 86, 87, 88, 96, 97, 100, 123, 130, 134, 135, 136, 139, 142, 144, 150, 155, 156, 159, 160, 161, 163, 164, 165, 166, 167, 174, 180, 181, 188, 190, 192, 196, 197, 199, 202, 205, 207, 209, 216, 217, 222, 223, 225, 226, 227, 237, 241, 246, 248, 250, 252, 255, 258, 259, 261, 263, 266, 268, 270, 271, 273, 275, 277, 279, 282, 288, 292, 295, 296, 307, 309, 316, 317, 318, 319, 321, 322, 324, 325, 328, 329, 333, 336, 342, 344, 347, 348, 360, 362, 363, 368, 371, 375, 379, 381, 382, 387, 390, 394, 399, 411, 414, 418, 425, 427, 436, 442, 443, 449, 451, 453, 466, 467, 478, 479, 489, 500, 505, 512, 513, 517, 519, 522, 524, 525, 530, 531, 534, 537, 538, 539, 542, 543, 544, 546, 548, 551, 552, 553, 555, 557, 558, 564, 565, 566, 568, 569, 570, 572, 583
risk assessment, 123, 144, 159, 205, 237, 282, 325, 347, 362, 363, 489, 519, 544, 558, 564, 565
risk factors, viii, 7, 28, 83, 86, 87, 88, 96, 97, 130, 164, 188, 209, 248, 273, 278, 324, 427, 453, 534, 537, 538, 543, 546, 566, 570
risperidone, 84, 91, 95, 304, 366, 367, 435, 532
rituximab, 177, 453
RNA, vii, 1, 17, 18, 31, 34, 50, 106, 110, 133, 139, 152, 158, 175, 201, 242, 267, 294, 303, 308, 327, 336, 337, 344, 370, 382, 409, 454, 472, 535, 557, 560, 567, 575
RNAi, 17, 18
robustness, 238
rodents, 42, 150, 175, 298, 484
Romania, 354
rosiglitazone, 263
Royal Society, 186, 427
rubber, 401

S

sacrifice, 72, 74
safety, vii, viii, 2, 7, 8, 12, 14, 19, 22, 25, 26, 83, 133, 134, 140, 143, 144, 147, 155, 160, 162, 164,

166, 187, 188, 200, 205, 217, 221, 232, 233, 242, 246, 249, 255, 271, 274, 277, 282, 284, 293, 310, 314, 328, 337, 341, 365, 374, 376, 382, 395, 426, 428, 432, 445, 456, 463, 464, 488, 496, 504, 515, 521, 536, 549, 565, 581
salicylates, 476
salinity, 288
salts, 434, 463
sample, 68, 69, 99, 131, 139, 166, 173, 176, 179, 184, 209, 213, 214, 215, 229, 234, 241, 254, 279, 289, 299, 331, 350, 358, 368, 369, 375, 394, 399, 405, 414, 416, 422, 449, 457, 459, 464, 468, 474, 481, 520, 545, 556, 560
sampling, 49, 50, 211, 240, 349, 556
saturation, 210, 357, 570
Saudi Arabia, 482
scheduling, 440
schizophrenia, 7, 88, 91, 93, 100, 101, 124, 137, 143, 148, 272, 303, 304, 340, 341, 367, 374, 375, 420, 433, 435, 455, 458, 501, 509, 526, 538, 581
schizophrenic patients, 94, 99, 100, 101, 341, 420
school, 33, 37, 147, 277, 323, 485, 496, 504
scientific knowledge, 26, 299, 349
scientific understanding, 515
scores, 162, 216, 304, 435
SCP, 89, 257
search, 70, 127, 158, 168, 188, 193, 204, 320, 352, 377, 404, 406, 428, 455, 518, 526, 528, 537
searches, 54, 70, 71, 73, 185, 204, 235, 377, 413
searching, 185, 403, 409, 437, 556
secretion, 258, 262, 264, 278, 360, 361, 552
segregation, 52, 151, 370
seizure, 125, 290, 291, 292, 396
selecting, 14, 126, 128, 177, 204, 244, 324, 329, 344, 399, 418
selective serotonin reuptake inhibitor, 90, 99, 148, 162, 304, 340, 480, 482, 528, 582
selectivity, 144, 158, 160, 560
self, 135, 373, 441, 573
sensing, 240, 278, 465
sensitivity, 34, 50, 126, 134, 137, 142, 181, 210, 211, 214, 224, 234, 263, 264, 272, 277, 286, 291, 294, 300, 317, 325, 360, 361, 368, 379, 397, 409, 410, 413, 437, 438, 445, 465, 466, 468, 498, 502, 512, 515, 524, 527, 532, 560
sensitization, 360, 361, 570
sensors, 285
separation, 176, 251, 444
sepsis, 156, 226, 537
septic shock, 116
sequencing, ix, 2, 3, 10, 17, 28, 104, 105, 106, 107, 114, 166, 175, 229, 235, 246, 249, 258, 295, 297, 311, 339, 348, 401, 405, 417, 446, 452, 466, 475, 497, 506, 533, 565, 566, 574
series, viii, 40, 44, 48, 50, 51, 54, 55, 71, 73, 75, 127, 158, 190, 229, 291, 303, 340, 355, 363, 388, 398, 421, 447, 470, 495, 537, 561
serine, 447
serotonin, viii, 83, 88, 90, 94, 96, 98, 99, 102, 143, 148, 162, 193, 277, 304, 306, 342, 366, 384, 385, 390, 412, 414, 420, 435, 436, 458, 481, 482, 491, 512, 518, 526, 527, 528, 530, 531, 547, 582
serotonin syndrome, 94, 99, 102, 548
sertraline, 134, 294, 366, 532
serum, 42, 86, 125, 142, 165, 190, 191, 215, 255, 280, 327, 339, 357, 366, 392, 439, 450, 453, 459, 466, 486, 575
services, 183, 223, 324, 422, 504
set theory, 73
severe asthma, 523
severity, 7, 125, 136, 162, 208, 233, 252, 275, 294, 304, 331, 347, 456, 530, 537, 538, 542, 552, 560
sex, 124, 174, 196, 233, 262, 313, 325, 339, 371, 394, 431, 460, 488, 523, 536, 565
sex chromosome, 124
sex differences, 124, 395
sex hormones, 124, 371, 431
sex steroid, 565
shade, 13
shape, 208, 269, 435
shaping, 123, 518
shares, 173
sharing, 251, 413, 449, 460
shear, 512
sheep, 466
shock, 105, 393
siblings, 88, 93, 137, 400
sickle cell, 543
sickle cell anemia, 543
side effects, 30, 79, 90, 124, 129, 147, 154, 190, 194, 216, 245, 255, 265, 293, 294, 296, 299, 301, 303, 305, 308, 330, 336, 342, 397, 402, 403, 412, 429, 435, 446, 450, 451, 455, 473, 484, 491, 494, 499, 505, 506, 509, 526, 535, 539, 541, 555, 568, 578, 579, 582
signal transduction, 23, 28, 49, 81, 134, 145, 414, 421, 462, 526, 549
signaling pathway, 14, 22, 29, 142, 145, 224, 257, 393, 421, 441, 526
signalling, 193, 300, 357, 527, 565

signals, 50, 145, 152, 273, 412, 445, 571
signal-to-noise ratio, 329
significance level, 369
silk, 319
similarity, 51, 204
simulation, 123, 166, 283
Singapore, 193, 237, 238, 270, 491, 502
single-nucleotide polymorphism, 30, 191, 214, 220, 222, 319, 346, 405, 409, 414, 419, 422, 484, 525, 580
sinusitis, 111
siRNA, 17, 194, 370
sites, 12, 13, 72, 88, 104, 219, 285, 320, 333, 334, 346, 374, 388, 443, 449, 474, 506, 512, 519, 544
skeletal muscle, 40, 42, 43, 44, 48, 50, 51, 52, 54, 55, 56, 57, 58, 60, 61, 74, 77, 78, 89, 251, 495
skills, 26, 36, 159, 183, 225
skin, 105, 281, 489, 570
skin cancer, 489
small intestine, 13, 33
smallpox, 396
smoke, 363
smokers, 132, 294, 363, 432, 455, 531
smoking, 147, 149, 253, 435, 460, 498, 502, 523, 531, 548, 575
SNP, 125, 126, 145, 152, 170, 183, 194, 201, 222, 230, 258, 259, 333, 344, 346, 375, 376, 388, 403, 405, 406, 409, 414, 416, 417, 434, 437, 462, 474, 476, 484, 506, 519, 556, 569, 584
sociability, 548
social cognition, 358
social injustices, 422
socialization, 193
sodium, 11, 42, 50, 97, 281, 351, 461, 469
soft tissue sarcomas, 508
software, 51, 52, 71, 174, 188, 196, 204, 280, 334, 387, 405, 406, 409, 449, 497
soil, 288
solid tumors, 212, 343, 542
solubility, 158
somatic mutations, 224, 326, 363, 364, 485
South Asia, 422, 569
South Korea, 228, 393
Southeast Asia, 544
Spain, 128, 180, 186, 245, 255, 298, 305, 443, 445, 459, 487, 489, 508, 534, 547, 573
species, ix, 4, 28, 72, 103, 105, 111, 121, 196, 205, 282, 333, 334, 357, 380, 383, 416, 428, 472, 492, 555
specificity, 50, 77, 142, 175, 176, 191, 214, 234, 280, 368, 404, 415, 442
spectrophotometry, 237
spectroscopy, 348, 525
spectrum, 85, 94, 130, 135, 181, 236, 240, 274, 291, 314, 340, 354, 455, 498, 502, 521, 537
speculation, 307
speed, 144, 175, 193, 404, 416, 513, 519
sperm, 468
spindle, 519
spleen, 392
spontaneity, 89
Sprague-Dawley rats, 560
squamous cell, 542
squamous cell carcinoma, 542
stability, 65, 66, 117, 475
stabilization, 544
stages, 7, 24, 142, 147, 165, 191, 199, 205, 274, 279, 311, 341, 407, 426, 430, 564
stakeholders, 146, 282, 441, 564
standard deviation, 54, 556, 567
standardization, 189, 198, 282
standards, 176, 204, 312, 359, 360, 422, 423, 504, 511, 544, 573
staphylococci, ix, 103, 105, 116, 117, 135
statin, 131, 137, 167, 168, 219, 241, 336, 347, 421, 459, 460, 464, 578
statistics, 319, 388, 449
stem cells, 278
stenosis, 560
steroids, 42, 48, 75, 76, 268, 337, 440, 443, 523, 568
stigmatized, 395
stimulant, 414
stimulus, 189
stochastic model, 123
stock, 283
stomach, 423, 500
storage, 41, 250, 404, 406, 548, 556, 563
strain, 280, 284, 354, 370, 439
strategies, 28, 36, 104, 127, 131, 132, 133, 136, 139, 141, 142, 146, 147, 148, 160, 165, 167, 175, 178, 185, 197, 198, 204, 223, 225, 240, 247, 248, 249, 255, 292, 299, 306, 307, 317, 322, 326, 329, 339, 342, 345, 346, 347, 353, 357, 369, 380, 381, 398, 401, 404, 422, 423, 433, 435, 436, 446, 456, 481, 491, 495, 496, 500, 511, 522, 544, 558, 567, 568, 574
stratification, 17, 27, 141, 172, 250, 267, 289, 351, 414, 493, 514, 573
strength, 159, 318, 388

streptococci, 119
streptokinase, 522
stress, 25, 40, 87, 133, 272, 315, 347, 360, 361, 390, 417, 428, 473, 491, 512, 557
stressors, 5, 284, 287, 288
striatum, 93, 101
stroke, 27, 163, 207, 245, 272, 275, 545, 546, 554
structure formation, 22
structuring, 319
students, 25
stupor, 86
subacute, 222
substance abuse, 130, 277, 340, 363
substance use, 147
substitution, 231, 239, 270, 298, 331, 359, 394, 481, 486
substrates, 13, 37, 41, 44, 91, 134, 148, 154, 194, 210, 219, 226, 235, 250, 258, 290, 296, 298, 306, 311, 382, 384, 385, 442, 459, 479, 581
success rate, 166, 167, 320, 502, 520
sugar, 74
suicidal behavior, 538
suicide, 538
suicide attempts, 538
sulfonylurea, 261, 262, 264
sulfur, 492
Sun, 32, 78, 79, 80, 81, 247, 303, 465
suppliers, 179
suppression, 77, 222, 244, 256, 263, 359, 392, 398, 413, 550
suprachiasmatic nucleus, 434
surface area, 233, 390, 477
surveillance, 111, 118, 274, 292, 374
survival, 135, 140, 141, 142, 165, 169, 186, 187, 202, 211, 233, 250, 315, 362, 363, 382, 397, 398, 411, 445, 446, 449, 478, 486, 541, 542, 551, 566, 568
survival rate, 364
survivors, 391
susceptibility, viii, x, 6, 11, 27, 30, 83, 91, 104, 105, 111, 115, 116, 119, 120, 124, 128, 129, 133, 137, 143, 145, 148, 156, 161, 184, 202, 226, 249, 250, 252, 259, 264, 266, 273, 279, 289, 310, 318, 323, 324, 329, 332, 340, 363, 371, 376, 388, 401, 403, 405, 437, 438, 455, 464, 467, 470, 494, 500, 506, 509, 517, 521, 526, 538, 547, 570, 582
Sweden, 130, 166, 183, 188, 199, 212, 271, 279, 301, 321, 376, 517, 520, 554, 556, 571, 573
Switzerland, 115, 185, 205, 231, 278, 280, 307, 341, 381, 402, 408, 411, 416, 429, 433, 454, 464, 474, 490, 546, 548, 564
symbols, 62, 65, 206
sympathetic nervous system, 203
symptom, 89, 143, 176, 303, 304, 341, 360, 361, 527
symptoms, viii, 83, 84, 85, 87, 88, 89, 93, 94, 129, 143, 153, 159, 275, 277, 304, 358, 366, 373, 433, 450, 455, 509, 530, 539, 548, 581
synaptic plasticity, 527
synchronization, 189
syndrome, viii, 9, 11, 83, 84, 85, 92, 94, 96, 97, 98, 102, 105, 179, 195, 208, 248, 324, 339, 358, 361, 373, 457, 508, 542, 546
synergistic effect, 464
synthesis, 10, 42, 43, 51, 62, 63, 65, 66, 67, 74, 75, 76, 106, 114, 147, 196, 197, 201, 210, 268, 311, 371, 382, 414, 439, 542, 549, 565, 567
synthetic polymers, 369
systems, 10, 13, 20, 23, 84, 88, 105, 114, 126, 131, 137, 143, 146, 163, 166, 167, 170, 188, 200, 202, 204, 240, 242, 249, 252, 256, 265, 266, 267, 277, 284, 285, 293, 313, 351, 357, 369, 371, 374, 387, 406, 409, 416, 417, 428, 433, 451, 456, 457, 490, 493, 495, 499, 509, 514, 517, 527, 528, 530, 548, 555, 558, 565, 572, 573, 577, 583
systolic blood pressure, 183

T

T cell, 139
T lymphocytes, 164
tachycardia, 86, 89
Taiwan, 112, 120, 195, 204, 304, 352, 491, 570
tamoxifen, 343, 362, 443
tandem repeats, 350, 582
tardive dyskinesia, 84, 90, 92, 99, 100, 148, 309, 342, 368, 455, 481, 527, 538
target identification, 142, 204
target organs, 251
targets, 10, 20, 23, 35, 76, 81, 104, 120, 128, 135, 141, 142, 144, 166, 169, 172, 174, 177, 193, 196, 240, 241, 245, 257, 272, 280, 294, 301, 303, 305, 309, 354, 355, 372, 391, 392, 413, 416, 423, 444, 448, 494, 496, 500, 521, 525, 526, 529, 530, 533, 540, 567, 571, 572, 573, 576
tau, 322, 427, 461, 485
taxonomy, 348
teachers, 496
teaching, 13, 25, 225

technical change, 104
technological advancement, 133, 176
technology, 3, 5, 6, 10, 16, 31, 32, 126, 136, 141, 142, 144, 146, 158, 163, 166, 169, 172, 173, 175, 205, 222, 223, 238, 241, 242, 246, 247, 248, 249, 252, 254, 268, 271, 284, 286, 311, 312, 313, 314, 323, 324, 336, 352, 369, 376, 381, 387, 389, 393, 395, 396, 399, 405, 412, 415, 416, 490, 496, 497, 505, 514, 520, 533, 534, 539, 558, 559, 576
technology gap, 249
teicoplanin, ix, 104, 110, 113
telephone, 189, 509
temperature, 50, 86, 288
tenure, 268
teratogen, 279
test data, 556
testosterone, 133, 358, 380, 410
text mining, 54
Thailand, 396
thalassemia, 543
theory, 26, 81, 88, 145, 389, 478, 573
therapeutic agents, 127, 133, 134, 146, 160, 235, 240, 293, 300, 352, 408, 443, 445, 516, 549
therapeutic approaches, 23, 303
therapeutic goal, 136
therapeutic targets, 35, 136, 141, 158, 169, 305, 337, 440, 513, 569, 572
therapeutics, 3, 8, 10, 15, 17, 20, 23, 27, 29, 31, 34, 37, 127, 132, 143, 144, 146, 150, 156, 177, 190, 194, 221, 241, 242, 254, 274, 294, 300, 305, 307, 335, 342, 348, 351, 356, 369, 371, 378, 418, 498, 522, 540, 541, 555, 578
thiazolidinediones, 263
thinking, 172
threat, 118, 264, 288
three-dimensional model, 554
threshold, 210, 449
thresholds, 289
thrombocytopenia, 233
thrombolytic therapy, 163
thrombosis, 163, 164, 180, 492, 512, 522
thrombus, 209
thyroid, 133, 243, 280, 432
thyrotropin, 240
tics, 416
time, vii, viii, x, 2, 5, 12, 13, 18, 22, 39, 42, 44, 45, 46, 47, 48, 49, 50, 51, 52, 53, 54, 55, 57, 59, 61, 62, 63, 64, 65, 66, 67, 68, 69, 71, 72, 73, 74, 80, 81, 85, 104, 105, 106, 111, 114, 116, 119, 121, 123, 127, 128, 129, 141, 151, 155, 158, 159, 166, 175, 179, 190, 193, 195, 199, 203, 210, 211, 215, 219, 223, 224, 228, 229, 231, 237, 238, 247, 249, 255, 265, 266, 295, 296, 298, 302, 308, 311, 312, 334, 336, 345, 349, 362, 368, 371, 375, 380, 386, 388, 392, 397, 402, 404, 405, 406, 408, 411, 415, 416, 417, 429, 435, 436, 441, 449, 450, 451, 452, 456, 457, 461, 462, 472, 477, 479, 488, 495, 497, 515, 520, 523, 530, 536, 542, 553, 560, 562, 563, 567
time series, viii, 39, 44, 50, 51, 53, 55, 57, 71, 73, 74, 80, 495
timing, 562
tissue, 24, 40, 41, 42, 49, 50, 54, 70, 71, 72, 74, 77, 78, 80, 105, 133, 140, 157, 243, 244, 255, 290, 291, 294, 306, 348, 363, 371, 401, 409, 410, 420, 424, 439, 442, 445, 446, 471, 476, 483, 503, 514, 519, 522, 556, 563, 567
tissue plasminogen activator, 522
TLR4, 464
TNF, 239, 494, 511
TNF-alpha, 239, 494
tobacco, 149, 303, 363, 432, 435, 470
tobacco smoke, 149, 470
tonic, 42
total cholesterol, 348, 459
total costs, 301
Tourette's syndrome, 412
toxic effect, 130, 177, 259, 281, 284, 396, 401, 548, 567
toxic products, 286
toxic side effect, 252, 356, 498
toxicity, 2, 5, 7, 8, 14, 15, 17, 19, 29, 34, 35, 126, 128, 133, 141, 144, 155, 156, 158, 160, 161, 163, 165, 169, 177, 186, 187, 188, 190, 192, 196, 197, 198, 201, 205, 208, 212, 216, 217, 220, 227, 229, 238, 242, 243, 246, 249, 251, 252, 253, 258, 260, 261, 266, 280, 282, 286, 287, 293, 298, 305, 309, 310, 316, 317, 319, 321, 325, 328, 331, 335, 338, 339, 342, 349, 355, 356, 364, 372, 386, 393, 394, 397, 416, 417, 423, 425, 426, 428, 441, 445, 446, 448, 451, 455, 456, 464, 466, 467, 472, 473, 476, 485, 487, 498, 499, 500, 507, 508, 519, 523, 525, 534, 536, 539, 541, 542, 548, 549, 557, 559, 560, 562, 567, 568, 569, 572
toxicology, 81, 126, 131, 147, 165, 205, 238, 246, 251, 252, 268, 271, 284, 285, 286, 287, 289, 328, 338, 341, 349, 386, 387, 393, 401, 412, 416, 417, 428, 493, 499, 533, 544, 555, 558, 559, 562, 572
toxicology studies, 205, 341, 558, 559
toxin, 393

TPA, 281
trade, 490
tradition, 133, 577
traffic, 104
training, 3, 25, 28, 97, 147, 281, 413, 559
traits, x, 27, 104, 105, 114, 128, 157, 190, 221, 254, 269, 329, 340, 359, 389, 395, 403, 430, 451, 487, 524, 549
transaminases, 41, 74, 125, 261
transcription, 41, 42, 43, 45, 53, 63, 65, 66, 67, 70, 74, 77, 145, 201, 239, 243, 245, 262, 289, 308, 333, 334, 348, 351, 365, 366, 381, 393, 401, 444, 473, 475, 479, 518, 565
transcription factors, 41, 42, 43, 45, 65, 70, 74, 145, 262, 308, 518, 565
transcriptomics, 21, 251, 328, 562
transcriptone, vii, 1
transcripts, vii, 1, 193, 233, 251, 473, 556
transducer, 365, 366
transduction, 66, 105, 421
transfection, 194, 350, 370, 421, 472
transformation, 5, 20, 105, 134, 246, 445
transfusion, 327
transgene, 369
transition, 6, 24, 144, 165, 211, 328, 442, 444
transitions, 147
translation, 15, 65, 163, 253, 262, 275, 313, 318, 365, 376, 401, 423, 425, 442, 469, 486, 577
translocation, 23, 62, 169
transmission, 104, 121, 128, 143, 277, 293, 396
transplant recipients, 151, 326, 398, 505, 566, 567, 568, 569
transplantation, 40, 75, 151, 185, 257, 308, 325, 326, 452, 505, 506, 507, 543, 566, 568, 569
transport, 2, 13, 24, 78, 155, 200, 207, 208, 237, 244, 258, 291, 309, 333, 343, 346, 356, 402, 414, 422, 440, 445, 448, 451, 467, 473, 474, 489, 500, 507, 543, 555, 557, 563, 572
transportation, 201
trastuzumab therapy, 146
trees, 51, 53, 54, 55, 56, 57, 58
tremor, 84, 94
trend, 146, 165, 187, 197, 211, 236, 252, 278, 322, 343, 359, 375, 378, 384, 501, 538, 567
trial, 132, 140, 145, 163, 166, 187, 188, 189, 207, 211, 212, 233, 244, 247, 269, 290, 316, 326, 327, 329, 330, 335, 337, 342, 360, 362, 402, 403, 414, 418, 432, 433, 447, 483, 523, 538, 541, 545, 552, 568, 577, 579
tricyclic antidepressant, 501, 532
tricyclic antidepressants, 501, 532
triggers, 272
triglycerides, 41, 43, 132
trihybrid, 572
troubleshooting, 311
trust, 434
tryptophan, 481, 482, 528
tuberculosis, 264, 276
tumor, 24, 126, 144, 146, 178, 192, 208, 212, 224, 246, 247, 252, 254, 256, 258, 272, 305, 317, 334, 362, 363, 364, 397, 411, 443, 445, 446, 454, 490, 492, 503, 514, 519, 530, 533, 541, 542, 549, 564, 572
tumor cells, 212, 246, 256, 272, 397, 514, 549
tumor growth, 334
tumor necrosis factor, 454, 530
tumors, 23, 31, 198, 247, 254, 256, 273, 301, 317, 342, 364, 411, 446, 448, 503, 507, 534, 546, 564
tumour growth, 401
tumours, 199, 227, 300, 306, 355, 443, 478
Turkey, 574
turnover, 45, 62, 77, 88, 224, 518
twins, 526, 575
type 2 diabetes, 73, 78, 79, 261, 262, 263, 547
tyrosine, 23, 24, 43, 44, 79, 80, 144, 145, 181, 224, 345, 393, 444, 534, 550

U

UK, 141, 151, 155, 161, 172, 175, 188, 189, 192, 198, 205, 241, 250, 251, 253, 259, 260, 261, 267, 271, 288, 293, 303, 308, 309, 311, 312, 313, 318, 328, 332, 335, 336, 341, 355, 356, 370, 373, 379, 381, 382, 391, 396, 397, 417, 419, 422, 429, 430, 434, 440, 457, 458, 463, 464, 466, 473, 479, 483, 490, 493, 497, 501, 502, 505, 520, 521, 526, 533, 537, 543, 544, 545, 565, 569, 571, 578
ulcer, 110
ulcerative colitis, 318, 321, 332, 473
ultrasonography, 314
ultrasound, 142
uncertainty, 163, 184, 332, 373, 395, 409, 572
underlying mechanisms, 36, 534
uniform, 50
United Kingdom, 182, 271, 274, 292, 313, 318, 338, 400, 429, 522, 527, 555, 561
United States, 76, 78, 80, 85, 96, 115, 118, 132, 134, 149, 150, 202, 237, 260, 314, 315, 328, 346, 363, 375, 378, 420, 488
universe, 281

universities, 469, 556
unstable angina, 391
untranslated regions, 229, 344
updating, 307, 513
urea, 41, 74
urinary tract, 113, 314
urinary tract infection, 113
urine, 110, 196, 228, 231, 233, 295, 471, 477, 478, 560, 575
usual dose, 194, 578
uterus, 444
UV, 203, 288, 365
UV light, 203

V

vaccine, 139
Valencia, 459
validation, 20, 21, 27, 81, 142, 144, 148, 155, 163, 165, 177, 189, 204, 255, 267, 272, 285, 309, 312, 316, 331, 335, 351, 426, 451, 472, 493, 509, 514, 523, 571
validity, 15, 21, 27, 182, 313, 522
values, 51, 52, 54, 62, 157, 184, 218, 231, 268, 298, 345, 351, 369, 379, 385, 394, 431, 459, 472, 474, 475, 524, 525, 563
vancomycin, ix, 103, 104, 110, 113, 114, 115, 118, 120, 121
variability, vii, 1, 4, 5, 6, 7, 8, 13, 17, 18, 20, 33, 85, 96, 128, 134, 137, 149, 154, 155, 159, 160, 163, 165, 167, 169, 175, 191, 192, 197, 198, 200, 208, 213, 218, 220, 221, 226, 227, 229, 230, 231, 235, 243, 245, 250, 251, 254, 256, 265, 270, 275, 287, 293, 301, 302, 305, 314, 316, 322, 324, 327, 328, 338, 339, 342, 345, 348, 355, 364, 375, 377, 382, 384, 385, 390, 392, 397, 417, 419, 420, 422, 431, 432, 433, 443, 445, 449, 450, 451, 456, 460, 464, 465, 470, 471, 475, 477, 481, 482, 484, 487, 489, 497, 500, 502, 505, 509, 510, 512, 514, 515, 516, 518, 523, 528, 529, 535, 536, 539, 542, 543, 548, 549, 554, 558, 567, 569, 571, 572, 580
variable, 46, 47, 48, 120, 135, 136, 141, 156, 161, 166, 170, 174, 193, 202, 212, 219, 252, 263, 276, 305, 317, 332, 335, 349, 350, 395, 403, 407, 414, 459, 465, 484, 486, 487, 488, 505, 506, 514, 520, 577
variables, 132, 145, 182, 184, 187, 212, 287, 325, 366, 367, 368, 411, 414, 415, 445, 449, 475, 481, 515, 553, 581
variance, 188, 319, 419, 471, 516
variation, vii, 6, 17, 18, 28, 31, 57, 79, 91, 127, 128, 130, 131, 134, 135, 138, 140, 142, 145, 148, 152, 155, 164, 166, 167, 170, 173, 175, 190, 197, 199, 200, 207, 209, 219, 227, 229, 236, 239, 240, 241, 243, 244, 248, 249, 250, 251, 253, 258, 259, 261, 263, 265, 273, 289, 292, 293, 299, 301, 309, 326, 329, 330, 331, 332, 337, 340, 341, 343, 348, 351, 359, 363, 372, 376, 380, 381, 382, 385, 390, 392, 395, 406, 408, 419, 421, 422, 424, 425, 428, 429, 430, 433, 439, 440, 443, 446, 450, 453, 455, 458, 462, 463, 464, 466, 467, 468, 470, 471, 472, 473, 474, 476, 484, 485, 486, 487, 488, 489, 490, 491, 500, 502, 504, 517, 523, 535, 539, 540, 550, 553, 554, 559, 563, 573, 574, 575, 582
vasoconstriction, 465
vasopressin, 240
vector, 280, 339, 560
vegetation, 287
vein, 50, 164, 236, 465, 492, 522
velocity, 359
venlafaxine, 294, 366, 532
Vietnam, 550
viral infection, 492
viral vectors, 242, 370
virology, 252
virus infection, 139, 574, 582
viruses, 139
vision, 29, 285, 580
visualization, 51, 55, 436, 453, 572
vitamin D, 42, 182, 321
vitamin K, 419
VLDL, 41
vocabulary, 72
vomiting, 153, 261, 306, 546
vulnerability, 85, 90, 99, 277, 491

W

Wales, 175, 290
war, 322
warrants, 92, 143, 145, 373
water, 44, 135, 243, 281, 350, 441, 557
wealth, 50, 70, 126, 200, 402, 541
web, 5, 173, 182, 183, 188, 272, 406, 409, 519
web service, 406
web sites, 409
weight gain, 99, 147, 342, 458, 513, 526, 529, 531
weight loss, 445, 462, 463
welfare, 456
well-being, 548

West Indies, 561
Western Europe, 237
white blood cell count, 537
white matter, 89
wild type, 170, 171, 196, 215, 217, 229, 232, 239, 268, 296, 302, 349, 351, 357, 368, 386, 523, 553, 575
withdrawal, 88, 150, 156, 390, 491, 530
women, 132, 136, 142, 147, 168, 179, 231, 236, 252, 263, 309, 362, 363, 366, 368, 431, 459, 468, 478, 517, 532, 534
wood, 353
workers, 190
workflow, 182, 183, 418
workplace, 124, 225
wound infection, 113

X

xenografts, 411
XML, 334

Y

yeast, 174, 289, 526
yield, 55, 57, 65, 152, 171, 192, 201, 332, 430, 571
young adults, 325

Z

zinc, 444
ziprasidone, 367